Biomechanics-Based Motion Analysis

Biomechanics-Based Motion Analysis

Editors

Christina Zong-Hao Ma
Zhengrong Li
Chen He

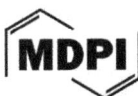

Basel • Beijing • Wuhan • Barcelona • Belgrade • Novi Sad • Cluj • Manchester

Editors
Christina Zong-Hao Ma
The Hong Kong Polytechnic University
Hong Kong
China

Zhengrong Li
Tongji University
Shanghai
China

Chen He
University of Shanghai for
Science and Technology
Shanghai
China

Editorial Office
MDPI
St. Alban-Anlage 66
4052 Basel, Switzerland

This is a reprint of articles from the Special Issue published online in the open access journal *Bioengineering* (ISSN 2306-5354) (available at: www.mdpi.com/journal/bioengineering/special_issues/biomechanics_motion_analysis).

For citation purposes, cite each article independently as indicated on the article page online and as indicated below:

Lastname, A.A.; Lastname, B.B. Article Title. *Journal Name* **Year**, *Volume Number*, Page Range.

ISBN 978-3-0365-8027-2 (Hbk)
ISBN 978-3-0365-8026-5 (PDF)
doi.org/10.3390/books978-3-0365-8026-5

© 2023 by the authors. Articles in this book are Open Access and distributed under the Creative Commons Attribution (CC BY) license. The book as a whole is distributed by MDPI under the terms and conditions of the Creative Commons Attribution-NonCommercial-NoDerivs (CC BY-NC-ND) license.

Contents

About the Editors ix

Christina Zong-Hao Ma, Zhengrong Li and Chen He
Advances in Biomechanics-Based Motion Analysis
Reprinted from: *Bioengineering* **2023**, *10*, 677, doi:10.3390/bioengineering10060677 1

Jialing Cao, Hangyu Li, Hongyan Tang, Xuenan Gu, Yan Wang, Dongshi Guan, et al.
Stiff Extracellular Matrix Promotes Invasive Behaviors of Trophoblast Cells
Reprinted from: *Bioengineering* **2023**, *10*, 384, doi:10.3390/bioengineering10030384 5

Dai-Soon Kwak, Yong Deok Kim, Nicole Cho, Yong In, Man Soo Kim, Dohyung Lim and In Jun Koh
Restoration of the Joint Line Configuration Reproduces Native Mid-Flexion Biomechanics after Total Knee Arthroplasty: A Matched-Pair Cadaveric Study
Reprinted from: *Bioengineering* **2022**, *10*, 564, doi:10.3390/bioengineering9100564 19

Tanja Lerchl, Kati Nispel, Thomas Baum, Jannis Bodden, Veit Senner and Jan S. Kirschke
Multibody Models of the Thoracolumbar Spine: A Review on Applications, Limitations, and Challenges
Reprinted from: *Bioengineering* **2023**, *10*, 202, doi:10.3390/bioengineering10020202 31

Janine Huthwelker, Jürgen Konradi, Claudia Wolf, Ruben Westphal, Irene Schmidtmann, Philipp Drees and Ulrich Betz
Reference Values for 3D Spinal Posture Based on Videorasterstereographic Analyses of Healthy Adults
Reprinted from: *Bioengineering* **2022**, *9*, 809, doi:10.3390/bioengineering9120809 49

Chiara Palmisano, Laura Beccaria, Stefan Haufe, Jens Volkmann, Gianni Pezzoli and Ioannis U. Isaias
Gait Initiation Impairment in Patients with Parkinson's Disease and Freezing of Gait
Reprinted from: *Bioengineering* **2022**, *9*, 639, doi:10.3390/bioengineering9110639 71

Xin Li, Zhenghui Lu, Dong Sun, Rongrong Xuan, Zhiyi Zheng and Yaodong Gu
The Influence of a Shoe's Heel-Toe Drop on Gait Parameters during the Third Trimester of Pregnancy
Reprinted from: *Bioengineering* **2022**, *9*, 241, doi:10.3390/bioengineering9060241 87

Cagla Fadillioglu, Felix Möhler, Marcel Reuter and Thorsten Stein
Changes in Key Biomechanical Parameters According to the Expertise Level in Runners at Different Running Speeds
Reprinted from: *Bioengineering* **2022**, *9*, 616, doi:10.3390/bioengineering9110616 99

Aléxia Fernandes, José Afonso, Francisco Noronha, Bruno Mezêncio, João Paulo Vilas-Boas and Ricardo J. Fernandes
Intracycle Velocity Variation in Swimming: A Systematic Scoping Review
Reprinted from: *Bioengineering* **2023**, *10*, 308, doi:10.3390/bioengineering10030308 109

Michiel Herteleer, Armin Runer, Magdalena Remppis, Jonas Brouwers, Friedemann Schneider, Vasiliki C. Panagiotopoulou, et al.
Continuous Shoulder Activity Tracking after Open Reduction and Internal Fixation of Proximal Humerus Fractures
Reprinted from: *Bioengineering* **2023**, *10*, 128, doi:10.3390/bioengineering10020128 133

Vincenzo Giordano, Anderson Freitas, Robinson Esteves Pires,
Leonardo Rigobello Battaglion, Mariana de Oliveira Lobo and William Dias Belangero
Evaluation of a Locking Autocompression Screw Model in Pauwels Type-3 Femoral Neck Fracture: In Vitro Analysis
Reprinted from: *Bioengineering* 2022, 9, 464, doi:10.3390/bioengineering9090464 147

Chia-En Wong, Hsuan-Teh Hu, Yu-Heng Huang and Kuo-Yuan Huang
Optimization of Spinal Reconstructions for Thoracolumbar Burst Fractures to Prevent Proximal Junctional Complications: A Finite Element Study
Reprinted from: *Bioengineering* 2022, 9, 491, doi:10.3390/bioengineering9100491 159

Kati Nispel, Tanja Lerchl, Veit Senner and Jan S. Kirschke
Recent Advances in Coupled MBS and FEM Models of the Spine—A Review
Reprinted from: *Bioengineering* 2023, 10, 315, doi:10.3390/bioengineering10030315 173

Chen He, Jian-Tao Yang, Qian Zheng, Zhao Mei and Christina Zong-Hao Ma
How do Paraspinal Muscles Contract during the Schroth Exercise Treatment in Patients with Adolescent Idiopathic Scoliosis (AIS)?
Reprinted from: *Bioengineering* 2022, 9, 234, doi:/10.3390/bioengineering9060234 189

KeunBaDa Son, Ji-Min Lee, Young-Tak Son, Jin-Wook Kim, Myoung-Uk Jin
and Kyu-Bok Lee
How Does the Use of an Intraoral Scanner Affect Muscle Fatigue? A Preliminary In Vivo Study
Reprinted from: *Bioengineering* 2022, 9, 358, doi:10.3390/bioengineering9080358 199

Le Li, Huijing Hu, Bo Yao, Chengjun Huang, Zhiyuan Lu, Cliff S. Klein and Ping Zhou
Electromyography–Force Relation and Muscle Fiber Conduction Velocity Affected by Spinal Cord Injury
Reprinted from: *Bioengineering* 2023, 10, 217, doi:10.3390/bioengineering10020217 211

Haoran Li, Hongshi Huang, Shuang Ren and Qiguo Rong
Leveraging Multivariable Linear Regression Analysis to Identify Patients with Anterior Cruciate Ligament Deficiency Using a Composite Index of the Knee Flexion and Muscle Force
Reprinted from: *Bioengineering* 2023, 10, 284, doi:10.3390/bioengineering10030284 223

Huan Zhao, Junyi Cao and Wei-Hsin Liao
Simultaneous Estimation of the Vertical Stiffness in the Knee and Hip for Healthy Human Subjects during Walking
Reprinted from: *Bioengineering* 2023, 10, 187, doi:10.3390/bioengineering10020187 235

Óscar Agudelo-Varela, Julio Vargas-Riaño and Ángel Valera
Turmell-Meter: A Device for Estimating the Subtalar and Talocrural Axes of the Human Ankle Joint by Applying the Product of Exponentials Formula
Reprinted from: *Bioengineering* 2022, 9, 199, doi:10.3390/bioengineering9050199 251

Stefan Haufe, Ioannis U. Isaias, Franziska Pellegrini and Chiara Palmisano
Gait Event Prediction Using Surface Electromyography in Parkinsonian Patients
Reprinted from: *Bioengineering* 2023, 10, 212, doi:10.3390/bioengineering10020212 287

Tasriva Sikandar, Sam Matiur Rahman, Dilshad Islam, Md. Asraf Ali,
Md. Abdullah Al Mamun, Mohammad Fazle Rabbi, et al.
Walking Speed Classification from Marker-Free Video Images in Two-Dimension Using Optimum Data and a Deep Learning Method
Reprinted from: *Bioengineering* 2022, 9, 715, doi:10.3390/bioengineering9110715 303

Hui Tang, Jiahao Pan, Barry Munkasy, Kim Duffy and Li Li
Comparison of Lower Extremity Joint Moment and Power Estimated by Markerless and Marker-Based Systems during Treadmill Running
Reprinted from: *Bioengineering* **2022**, *9*, 574, doi:10.3390/bioengineering9100574 317

Hongmin Wang, Chi Gao, Hong Fu, Christina Zong-Hao Ma, Quan Wang, Ziyu He and Maojun Li
Automated Student Classroom Behaviors' Perception and Identification Using Motion Sensors
Reprinted from: *Bioengineering* **2023**, *10*, 127, doi:10.3390/bioengineering10020127 333

Kang Xia, Xianglei Chen, Xuedong Chang, Chongshuai Liu, Liwei Guo, Xiaobin Xu, et al.
Hand Exoskeleton Design and Human–Machine Interaction Strategies for Rehabilitation
Reprinted from: *Bioengineering* **2022**, *9*, 682, doi:10.3390/bioengineering9110682 351

About the Editors

Christina Zong-Hao Ma

Dr. Christina Zong-Hao Ma is an Assistant Professor, a Certified Prosthetist and Orthotist (CPO, ISPO Category I), and a Certified Rehabilitation Therapist (CRT) at the Department of Biomedical Engineering, The Hong Kong Polytechnic University (PolyU). Before her appointment at PolyU, she served as a Lecturer, later promoted to Assistant Professor (permanent position), in Prosthetics and orthotics at the Department of Rehabilitation, Jönköping University, Sweden, from 2018 to 2020. She received her PhD from the Faculty of Engineering, The Hong Kong Polytechnic University (2018) and her BSc from the West China School of Medicine, Sichuan University (2012). She also used to work as a Certified Prosthetist and Orthotist and a Clinical Instructor at the China Rehabilitation Research Center (permanent employment, 2012–2013) and as a Visiting Research Scholar in Mechanical Engineering at the University of Michigan, Ann Arbor (2017). Dr. Ma's research focuses on (1) investigating the mechanisms of human posture and motion control; (2) promoting physical activity and active health; and (3) developing solutions for improving balance and preventing falls in older/disabled people. As a CPO and CRT who used to work in hospitals and rehabilitation centers, Dr. Ma is well aware of how physical disability could significantly affect the quality of life of older adults, patients, and their families. She has a genuine interest in promoting these people's quality of life through research and development. Dr. Ma's multidisciplinary academic background in healthcare and engineering and her clinical experience enabled her to employ various interdisciplinary approaches such as biomechanics, electronics, rehabilitation, assistive technology, biomedical ultrasound imaging, and smart wearable technology to achieve her research goals. Her research outcomes can benefit older adults, stroke survivors, trainers/trainees of muscular fitness training, lower-limb amputees, patients with low back pain, etc.

Zhengrong Li

Prof. Dr. Zhengrong Li is currently a Full Professor at Tongji University and was awarded her PhD degree by Tongji University, China. Over the past twenty years, she has been active in the interdisciplinary area, mainly focusing on: (1) occupant human behavior and its mechanisms in the built environment; and (2) passive technology for a healthy indoor thermal-illuminance environment. She currently holds more than 150 web-of-science-listed articles, has authored about 10 chapters in scientific books, edited five scientific books, and published 10 national and Shanghai standards. Besides, she is an editorial board member of several distinguished journals.

Chen He

Dr. Chen He is an Assistant Professor at the Institute of Rehabilitation Engineering and Technology, University of Shanghai for Science and Technology (USST), Shanghai, China. She obtained her PhD degree from the Hong Kong Polytechnic University in 2018. Her research interests include spinal deformity, spinal orthosis, spine exoskeleton, intelligent orthosis, and scoliosis. She was funded by the Shanghai Sailing Plan (2020) and the National Key Research and Development Program of China (2020). She also participated in two national research projects as a main investigator, including the National Natural Science Foundation of China (2019) and the National Key Research and Development Program of China (2021).

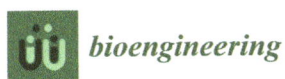

Editorial

Advances in Biomechanics-Based Motion Analysis

Christina Zong-Hao Ma [1,2,*], Zhengrong Li [3] and Chen He [4]

1. Department of Biomedical Engineering, The Hong Kong Polytechnic University, Hong Kong SAR 999077, China
2. Research Institute for Smart Ageing, The Hong Kong Polytechnic University, Hong Kong SAR 999077, China
3. School of Mechanical Engineering, Tongji University, Shanghai 200082, China; lizhengrong@tongji.edu.cn
4. Institute of Rehabilitation Engineering and Technology, University of Shanghai for Science and Technology, Shanghai 200093, China; hechen@usst.edu.cn
* Correspondence: czh.ma@polyu.edu.hk; Tel.: +852-2766-7671; Fax: +852-2334-2429

Motion patterns in humans have been closely associated with neurological/musculoskeletal/behavioral/psychological health issues and competitive sports performance. Recent decades have witnessed the development of a number of motion capture and analysis techniques to assist professionals in quantitatively evaluating motion patterns. However, current assessments still mainly rely on the professionals' experience, questionnaires or scales, and functional tests. As a result, some pathological or elite athletes' motion patterns remained unclear. Moreover, the in-depth biomechanical/neuromuscular mechanisms of motion patterns are poorly understood. Therefore, in this Special Issue, we have assembled 23 research articles and review papers on the state-of-the-art advances in motion analysis from fundamental in vitro cell [1] and cadaveric studies [2] to in vivo experiments on human subjects. These studies have either applied validated biomechanical models and neuromuscular analyses to answer unresolved clinical/sports-related questions or focused on the development of novel motion analysis methods. We expect this Special Issue to shed light on future research and developments in biomechanics and motion analysis.

1. Evaluation of Motion Patterns Using Validated Biomechanical Analysis

Biomechanical motion analysis is generally based on two types of models: multibody models and finite element models (FEMs) [3]. A multibody model refers to a set of rigid bodies connected by joints; inverse dynamics are normally incorporated to calculate joint kinetics from the measurable kinematics of body segments [4]. In contrast, FEMs reconstruct internal strain, stress, or deformation in flexible bodies based on continuum mechanics theories [3,5]. These validated models have been instrumental in exploring the motion patterns in specific patients/athletes and examining the effects of specific interventions/treatments on motion patterns. The analyzed body parts range from global posture, balance, gait, or sports performance to localized trunk, upper-limb, or lower-limb joint motions.

Regarding global motion analyses, validated multibody models have been used to quantify postures in healthy adults, gait initiation in patients with Parkinson's disease, walking patterns in pregnant women, running performance, and swimming performance. Huthwelker et al. [6] quantitatively measured the spine postures in healthy adults of different age and gender groups, serving as reference data for studies of abnormal spine postures. The freezing of gait is common in patients with Parkinson's disease and may lead to falls; thus, Palmisano et al. [7] investigated underlying balance control in gait initiation and identified that the center of pressure parameters, rather than the center of mass parameters, could be related to the freezing of gait. Li et al. [8] investigated the effects of different shoe-heel heights on pregnant women's walking balance, providing new insights on reducing fall risks in this population. Fadillioglu et al. [9] compared running patterns in novice runners vs. expert runners, and identified the key spatiotemporal and kinematic parameters indicating better running performance. In addition, Fernandes et al. [10] con-

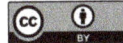

Citation: Ma, C.Z.-H.; Li, Z.; He, C. Advances in Biomechanics-Based Motion Analysis. *Bioengineering* **2023**, *10*, 677. https://doi.org/10.3390/bioengineering10060677

Received: 14 May 2023
Revised: 24 May 2023
Accepted: 31 May 2023
Published: 2 June 2023

Copyright: © 2023 by the authors. Licensee MDPI, Basel, Switzerland. This article is an open access article distributed under the terms and conditions of the Creative Commons Attribution (CC BY) license (https://creativecommons.org/licenses/by/4.0/).

ducted a comprehensive review on whether swimming performance is related to kinematic parameters, i.e., intracycle velocity variations.

Regarding the motion analyses of localized body components, both validated multibody models and FEMs have been used. Using multibody models, Herteleer et al. [11] continuously monitored shoulder joint angles in patients after surgeries of humerus fractures, and examined the effects of different rehabilitation protocols, i.e., early postoperative mobilization vs. immobilization, on the shoulder joint motions. Similarly, Kwak et al. [2] compared knee joint kinematics following two different protocols of total knee arthroplasty to evaluate the effectiveness of the treatments. However, when some newly proposed interventions cannot be conducted directly on human subjects due to ethical reasons, FEMs can help simulate how interventions may cause changes in specific biomechanical indicators in vitro and simulate the possible clinical outcomes. Giordano et al. [12] used FEMs to examine mechanical properties within the femur (such as stress distribution) by simulating different constructions of implants for treating femur head fractures, and evaluated the treatment effects of different implant construction methods. Similarly, Wong et al. [13] used FEMs to evaluate the stress of different thoracolumbar reconstruction constructs on proximal junctional levels, providing insights on the optimal selection of reconstruction constructs to treat thoracolumbar burst fractures and minimize postoperative complications. In addition, Nispel et al. [14] reviewed the contemporary use of coupled multibody models and FEM simulations to analyze both the holistic biomechanics of the spine and the stress distribution within flexible components (e.g., intervertebral discs), providing a more comprehensive view of facilitating the evaluations and diagnoses of spine-related health issues.

2. Evaluation of Motion Patterns Using Validated Neuromuscular Analysis

The in-depth analysis of surface electromyography (sEMG) signals can also be used to explain abnormal motion patterns. He et al. [15] investigated how Schroth exercises, one of the commonly used training methods for patients with adolescent idiopathic scoliosis in clinical settings, activate the paraspinal muscles in concave and convex sides; the findings provide evidence for the effectiveness of this treatment. Son et al. [16] analyzed the sEMG signals of neck, shoulder, and arm muscles during dentists' daily occupational tasks, and found that the repetition of one task causes muscle fatigue, a finding which supports the importance of rest for reducing occupation-related musculoskeletal disorders. By examining elbow flexor sEMG signals in patients after spinal cord injuries (SCIs) vs. healthy controls, Li et al. [17] found that both the muscle fiber conduction velocity (indicating muscle properties) and the sEMG–force relationship (indicating central neural drive) had been altered after SCI. These applications of validated neuromuscular analyses have complemented biomechanical analyses in advancing the assessment and management of motor function impairments.

3. Methodological Optimization and Development in Motion Analysis

To meet the huge demands for wearable motion capture and remote motion analysis in healthcare sectors [18–21], new trends are emerging to optimize existing motion analysis models or combine them with the novel statistical, machine learning, or deep learning algorithms. Li et al. [22] proposed the use of multivariable linear regression models and a composite index, which was derived from the most significant differences in patients with anterior cruciate ligament deficiency (ACLD) vs. healthy controls, to facilitate the clinical diagnosis of ACLD. Zhao et al. [23] proposed a new model of using only the easily available anthropometric data (i.e., leg length, body weight, and walking cadence) to estimate vertical stiffness in hip and knee joints, providing alternative insights for gait analysis. Human ankle subtalar and talocrural joint motions are difficult to quantitatively measure in outdoor environments; therefore, Agudelo-Varela et al. [24] proposed a wearable device using a new statistical method of angle calculation. Machine/deep learning algorithms have further facilitated marker-free motion capture and analysis. Using machine learning algorithms, Haufe et al. [25] found that the gait events could accurately be determined by as few as two lower-limb muscles' sEMG signals in patients with Parkinson's disease. Sikandar et al. [26] used deep learning algorithms to classify walking speeds based on two-dimensional marker-free video images. Similarly, Tang et al. [27] attempted to estimate joint moments and power using video data and deep learning algorithms; however, differences existed when comparing marker-free and marker-based estimates, which indicated that their marker-free approach could be further improved to identify the joint centers/center of segment mass more accurately. In addition to video images, Wang et al. [28] utilized motion data collected by two inertial measuring units (IMUs) to identify students' classroom behaviors using deep learning algorithms. Similarly, Xia et al. [29] used IMUs and thin-film force sensors in hand exoskeletons designed for stroke survivors, enabling intention recognition based on the biomechanical data collected using the deep learning algorithms.

4. Conclusions

Collectively, the studies presented in this Special Issue have used various validated biomechanical models or proposed novel methods of motion analysis to gain new insights into health-related problems and sports performance. As the editors of this Special Issue, we look forward to the continuous efforts of applying novel biomechanics-based motion analysis to support clinical practice and overcome any unsolved challenges. We expect that further steps are needed to translate the methodological developments of motion analysis methods into broader applications.

Author Contributions: Conceptualization, C.Z.-H.M., C.H. and Z.L.; writing—original draft preparation, C.Z.-H.M.; writing—review and editing, C.H. and Z.L. All authors have read and agreed to the published version of the manuscript.

Funding: This editorial received no external funding.

Acknowledgments: We would like to express our sincere gratitude to all contributors for their submissions to this Special Issue of *Bioengineering*.

Conflicts of Interest: The authors declare no conflict of interest.

References

1. Cao, J.; Li, H.; Tang, H.; Gu, X.; Wang, Y.; Guan, D.; Du, J.; Fan, Y. Stiff Extracellular Matrix Promotes Invasive Behaviors of Trophoblast Cells. *Bioengineering* **2023**, *10*, 384. [CrossRef] [PubMed]
2. Kwak, D.-S.; Kim, Y.D.; Cho, N.; In, Y.; Kim, M.S.; Lim, D.; Koh, I.J. Restoration of the Joint Line Configuration Reproduces Native Mid-Flexion Biomechanics after Total Knee Arthroplasty: A Matched-Pair Cadaveric Study. *Bioengineering* **2022**, *9*, 564. [CrossRef] [PubMed]
3. Lerchl, T.; Nispel, K.; Baum, T.; Bodden, J.; Senner, V.; Kirschke, J.S. Multibody Models of the Thoracolumbar Spine: A Review on Applications, Limitations, and Challenges. *Bioengineering* **2023**, *10*, 202. [CrossRef] [PubMed]
4. Xin, H.; Diao, H. Computational biomechanical modelling of the spine. In *Computational Modelling of Biomechanics and Biotribology in the Musculoskeletal System*; Elsevier: Amsterdam, The Netherlands, 2021; pp. 577–597.
5. Parashar, S.K.; Sharma, J.K. A review on application of finite element modelling in bone biomechanics. *Perspect. Sci.* **2016**, *8*, 696–698. [CrossRef]
6. Huthwelker, J.; Konradi, J.; Wolf, C.; Westphal, R.; Schmidtmann, I.; Drees, P.; Betz, U. Reference Values for 3D Spinal Posture Based on Videorasterstereographic Analyses of Healthy Adults. *Bioengineering* **2022**, *9*, 809. [CrossRef]
7. Palmisano, C.; Beccaria, L.; Haufe, S.; Volkmann, J.; Pezzoli, G.; Isaias, I.U. Gait Initiation Impairment in Patients with Parkinson's Disease and Freezing of Gait. *Bioengineering* **2022**, *9*, 639.
8. Li, X.; Lu, Z.; Sun, D.; Xuan, R.; Zheng, Z.; Gu, Y. The Influence of a Shoe's Heel-Toe Drop on Gait Parameters during the Third Trimester of Pregnancy. *Bioengineering* **2022**, *9*, 241.
9. Fadillioglu, C.; Möhler, F.; Reuter, M.; Stein, T. Changes in Key Biomechanical Parameters According to the Expertise Level in Runners at Different Running Speeds. *Bioengineering* **2022**, *9*, 616. [CrossRef]
10. Fernandes, A.; Afonso, J.; Noronha, F.; Mezêncio, B.; Vilas-Boas, J.P.; Fernandes, R.J. Intracycle Velocity Variation in Swimming: A Systematic Scoping Review. *Bioengineering* **2023**, *10*, 308. [CrossRef]
11. Herteleer, M.; Runer, A.; Remppis, M.; Brouwers, J.; Schneider, F.; Panagiotopoulou, V.C.; Grimm, B.; Hengg, C.; Arora, R.; Nijs, S.; et al. Continuous Shoulder Activity Tracking after Open Reduction and Internal Fixation of Proximal Humerus Fractures. *Bioengineering* **2023**, *10*, 128. [CrossRef]

12. Giordano, V.; Freitas, A.; Pires, R.E.; Battaglion, L.R.; Lobo, M.d.O.; Belangero, W.D. Evaluation of a Locking Autocompression Screw Model in Pauwels Type-3 Femoral Neck Fracture: In Vitro Analysis. *Bioengineering* **2022**, *9*, 464. [CrossRef]
13. Wong, C.-E.; Hu, H.-T.; Huang, Y.-H.; Huang, K.-Y. Optimization of Spinal Reconstructions for Thoracolumbar Burst Fractures to Prevent Proximal Junctional Complications: A Finite Element Study. *Bioengineering* **2022**, *9*, 491. [CrossRef]
14. Nispel, K.; Lerchl, T.; Senner, V.; Kirschke, J.S. Recent Advances in Coupled MBS and FEM Models of the Spine—A Review. *Bioengineering* **2023**, *10*, 315.
15. He, C.; Yang, J.-T.; Zheng, Q.; Mei, Z.; Ma, C.Z.-H. How do Paraspinal Muscles Contract during the Schroth Exercise Treatment in Patients with Adolescent Idiopathic Scoliosis (AIS)? *Bioengineering* **2022**, *9*, 234. [CrossRef]
16. Son, K.; Lee, J.-M.; Son, Y.-T.; Kim, J.-W.; Jin, M.-U.; Lee, K.-B. How Does the Use of an Intraoral Scanner Affect Muscle Fatigue? A Preliminary In Vivo Study. *Bioengineering* **2022**, *9*, 358. [CrossRef]
17. Li, L.; Hu, H.; Yao, B.; Huang, C.; Lu, Z.; Klein, C.S.; Zhou, P. Electromyography—Force Relation and Muscle Fiber Conduction Velocity Affected by Spinal Cord Injury. *Bioengineering* **2023**, *10*, 217.
18. Ma, C.Z.-H.; Bao, T.; DiCesare, C.A.; Harris, I.; Chambers, A.; Shull, P.B.; Zheng, Y.-P.; Cham, R.; Sienko, K.H. Reducing Slip Risk: A Feasibility Study of Gait Training with Semi-Real-Time Feedback of Foot–Floor Contact Angle. *Sensors* **2022**, *22*, 3641. [CrossRef]
19. Ma, C.Z.-H.; Ling, Y.T.; Shea, Q.T.K.; Wang, L.-K.; Wang, X.-Y.; Zheng, Y.-P. Towards Wearable Comprehensive Capture and Analysis of Skeletal Muscle Activity during Human Locomotion. *Sensors* **2019**, *19*, 195. [CrossRef]
20. Lyu, P.-Z.; Zhu, R.T.-L.; Ling, Y.T.; Wang, L.-K.; Zheng, Y.-P.; Ma, C.Z.-H. How paretic and non-paretic ankle muscles contract during walking in stroke survivors: New insight using novel wearable ultrasound imaging and sensing technology. *Biosensors* **2022**, *12*, 349. [CrossRef]
21. Ma, C.Z.-H.; Zheng, Y.-P.; Lee, W.C.-C. Changes in gait and plantar foot loading upon using vibrotactile wearable biofeedback system in patients with stroke. *Top. Stroke Rehabil.* **2018**, *25*, 20–27. [CrossRef]
22. Li, H.; Huang, H.; Ren, S.; Rong, Q. Leveraging Multivariable Linear Regression Analysis to Identify Patients with Anterior Cruciate Ligament Deficiency Using a Composite Index of the Knee Flexion and Muscle Force. *Bioengineering* **2023**, *10*, 284. [CrossRef] [PubMed]
23. Zhao, H.; Cao, J.; Liao, W.-H. Simultaneous Estimation of the Vertical Stiffness in the Knee and Hip for Healthy Human Subjects during Walking. *Bioengineering* **2023**, *10*, 187. [CrossRef] [PubMed]
24. Agudelo-Varela, Ó.; Vargas-Riaño, J.; Valera, Á. Turmell-Meter: A Device for Estimating the Subtalar and Talocrural Axes of the Human Ankle Joint by Applying the Product of Exponentials Formula. *Bioengineering* **2022**, *9*, 199. [CrossRef] [PubMed]
25. Haufe, S.; Isaias, I.U.; Pellegrini, F.; Palmisano, C. Gait Event Prediction Using Surface Electromyography in Parkinsonian Patients. *Bioengineering* **2023**, *10*, 212. [CrossRef] [PubMed]
26. Sikandar, T.; Rahman, S.M.; Islam, D.; Ali, M.A.; Mamun, M.A.A.; Rabbi, M.F.; Ghazali, K.H.; Altwijri, O.; Almijalli, M.; Ahamed, N.U. Walking Speed Classification from Marker-Free Video Images in Two-Dimension Using Optimum Data and a Deep Learning Method. *Bioengineering* **2022**, *9*, 715. [CrossRef]
27. Tang, H.; Pan, J.; Munkasy, B.; Duffy, K.; Li, L. Comparison of Lower Extremity Joint Moment and Power Estimated by Markerless and Marker-Based Systems during Treadmill Running. *Bioengineering* **2022**, *9*, 574. [CrossRef]
28. Wang, H.; Gao, C.; Fu, H.; Ma, C.Z.-H.; Wang, Q.; He, Z.; Li, M. Automated Student Classroom Behaviors' Perception and Identification Using Motion Sensors. *Bioengineering* **2023**, *10*, 127. [CrossRef]
29. Xia, K.; Chen, X.; Chang, X.; Liu, C.; Guo, L.; Xu, X.; Lv, F.; Wang, Y.; Sun, H.; Zhou, J. Hand Exoskeleton Design and Human-Machine Interaction Strategies for Rehabilitation. *Bioengineering* **2022**, *9*, 682. [CrossRef]

Disclaimer/Publisher's Note: The statements, opinions and data contained in all publications are solely those of the individual author(s) and contributor(s) and not of MDPI and/or the editor(s). MDPI and/or the editor(s) disclaim responsibility for any injury to people or property resulting from any ideas, methods, instructions or products referred to in the content.

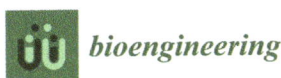

Article

Stiff Extracellular Matrix Promotes Invasive Behaviors of Trophoblast Cells

Jialing Cao [1,2], Hangyu Li [3,4], Hongyan Tang [1], Xuenan Gu [1], Yan Wang [5,*], Dongshi Guan [3,4,*], Jing Du [1,*] and Yubo Fan [1,*]

[1] Key Laboratory for Biomechanics and Mechanobiology of the Ministry of Education, Institute of Nanotechnology for Single Cell Analysis, Beijing Advanced Innovation Center for Biomedical Engineering, School of Biological Science and Medical Engineering, Beihang University, Beijing 100083, China
[2] Sino-French Engineer School, Beihang University, Beijing 100083, China
[3] State Key Laboratory of Nonlinear Mechanics, Institute of Mechanics, Chinese Academy of Sciences, Beijing 100190, China
[4] School of Engineering Science, University of Chinese Academy of Sciences, Beijing 100049, China
[5] Department of Obstetrics and Gynecology, Peking University Third Hospital, Beijing 100191, China
* Correspondence: wjgqhn@263.net (Y.W.); dsguan@imech.ac.cn (D.G.); dujing@buaa.edu.cn (J.D.); yubofan@buaa.edu.cn (Y.F.)

Abstract: The effect of extracellular matrix (ECM) stiffness on embryonic trophoblast cells invasion during mammalian embryo implantation remains largely unknown. In this study, we investigated the effects of ECM stiffness on various aspects of human trophoblast cell behaviors during cell–ECM interactions. The mechanical microenvironment of the uterus was simulated by fabricating polyacrylamide (PA) hydrogels with different levels of stiffness. The human choriocarcinoma (JAR) cell lineage was used as the trophoblast model. We found that the spreading area of JAR cells, the formation of focal adhesions, and the polymerization of the F-actin cytoskeleton were all facilitated with increased ECM stiffness. Significantly, JAR cells also exhibited durotactic behavior on ECM with a gradient stiffness. Meanwhile, stiffness of the ECM affects the invasion of multicellular JAR spheroids. These results demonstrated that human trophoblast cells are mechanically sensitive, while the mechanical properties of the uterine microenvironment could play an important role in the implantation process.

Keywords: embryo implantation; human choriocarcinoma cell; extracellular matrix; stiffness; durotaxis

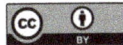

1. Introduction

Embryo implantation is a critical feature of mammalian pregnancy and requires a series of interactions between the embryo and the uterus, which can be divided into three different steps: apposition, attachment, and invasion [1]. In brief, after hatching from the zona pellucida, the spheroid of cells floats freely and finds the proper implantation site (apposition), and the trophoblasts firmly attach to the uterine wall (adhesion). The trophoblasts then differentiate into cytotrophoblasts and syncytiotrophoblasts under tight regulation, thereby invading the endometrium (invasion) and leading to compromised placental development and pregnancy complications [2].

Recent research on embryo implantation primarily focused on biochemical aspects, including some molecular mechanisms and related signaling pathways. During the early stages of implantation, there are many molecular mediators coordinated by ovarian steroid hormones involved in the initial maternal-fetal communication and interaction. These mediators include adhesion molecules, cytokines, growth factors, and lipids [3,4]. Meanwhile, using human endometrium Ishikawa and PL95-2 cells, Ming Yu et al. found that N-glycosylation of the endometrium is necessary to maintain the receptive functions of the uterus [5].

Several studies recently uncovered the role of mechanical forces before and during human embryo implantation [6–8]. The mechanical properties of the human endometrium are complex, and spatiotemporal changes exist during embryo implantation [8,9]. Mechanical indentation was used to demonstrate that mechanical properties significantly differ between anatomical locations in both nonpregnant and pregnant uterine tissue [10]. For instance, in pregnant tissue, Young's modulus of fundus tissue is higher than that of the posterior and anterior tissue. The stiffness of decidual basalis (implantation site) is much higher than the decidua parietalis, nonpregnant endometrium, and placenta (~10^3 Pa vs. ~10^2 Pa) [11]. When the uterus is in a pathological state or there is a scar in the endometrium, the stiffness will increase [12,13]. For example, the shear modulus in a pathological state is about 7 kPa (calculated elastic modulus: 18.2 kPa), and the shear modulus in an extreme pathological state is about 17.4 kPa (calculated elastic modulus: 45.2 kPa) [6,13]. Endometrium extracellular matrix (ECM) stiffness is lower during the secretory phase than during the proliferative phase (shear modulus: 3.34 kPa vs. 1.97 kPa; calculate elastic modulus: 8.68 kPa vs. 5.12 kPa) [14].

Recent work demonstrated that the implantation process may be regulated by mechanical factors. Firm adhesion between trophoblast-type cells and endometrium epithelial cells was only observed when the trophoblast-functionalized tip indented the apical surface of the epithelial cell [15], indicating the role of mechanical forces during the maternal-fetal interaction [7]. Meanwhile, recent work studied the mechanobiological regulation of placental trophoblast fusion through ECM stiffness [6]. Using a stiffness-tunable hydrogel culture system, Ma et al. suggested that stiffer ECM promotes the spreading and fusion of trophoblast cells [6]. Wong et al. demonstrated that thicker ECM promotes the self-assembly of 3D trophoblast cells spheroids [16]. These might suggest an effect of ECM stiffness on the invasion of trophoblast cells, but they do not directly demonstrate how substrate stiffness regulates the invasion behaviors of trophoblast cells. Therefore, it is important to reveal the effect of ECM stiffness on trophoblast cell adhesion, migration, and invasion of multicellular spheroids.

Polyacrylamide hydrogels are widely used as a biocompatible material with easy fabrication and adjustable stiffness to study the effect of substrate stiffness on cell behaviors [17–19]. In this study, we generated collagen-coated polyacrylamide (PA) hydrogels with different stiffness gradients to mimic the microenvironment of the uterus and investigate the role of ECM stiffness in trophoblast cell morphology, migration, and invasion. We chose the human choriocarcinoma (JAR) cell lineage, which is derived from human choriocarcinoma and is the most widely-used cytotrophoblast-like cell model [20–27]. Our results showed that as the simulated ECM stiffness increased, the spreading area of JAR cells gradually promoted, and the number of focal adhesions increased, while the cytoskeleton became more robust and filamentous. We also found that individual trophoblast cells exhibited durotaxis behavior, and simulated ECM stiffness enhanced the invasion capacity of trophoblast spheroids. This study complements the effect of mechanical forces on the invasion behaviors of trophoblast cells, revealing the important role of ECM stiffness in embryonic implantation, while being able to provide some references for the study of diseases related to implantation.

2. Materials and Methods

2.1. General Cell Culture

The JAR human choriocarcinoma cell line (TCHu156 ATCC) was maintained in RPMI 1640 medium (Hyclone) at 37 °C under 5% CO_2 in incubator. The culture media was supplemented with 10% (v/v) fetal bovine serum (FBS, SERANA), 100 units/mL penicillin, and 100 units/mL streptomycin.

2.2. JAR Spheroid Formation

For the spheroid formation assay, we seeded 100 μL of JAR cells at a density of 1×10^5 cells/mL in each well of an ultra-low attachment 96-well round bottom plate (Corning, NY, USA).

Cells were incubated overnight at 37 °C in a 5% CO_2 incubator. During this incubation, JAR cells formed spheroids of 50–200 µm in diameter via natural aggregation. The aggregate diameter of the spheroids was measured by CellSens standard software (Olympus, Tokyo, Japan).

2.3. Fabrication of Polyacrylamide Hydrogels with Stiffness Gradients

A polymer solution containing 20% (v/v) acrylamide monomer (Bio-Rad) and 0.4% (v/v) N,N′-methylenebisacrylamide cross-linker (Bio-Rad) was prepared in 1× Dulbecco's phosphate-buffered saline (PBS, Life Technologies, Gaithersburg, MD, USA) without Mg^{2+} and Ca^{2+}. An amount of 1 mL aliquots were degassed for 5 min, and 4 µL of 10% (w/v) ammonium persulfate (APS) (Sigma-Aldrich) was added and mixed for 0.5 s; then, 1.2 µL of N,N,N′,N′-tetramethylethylenediamine (TEMED) (Bio-Rad) was quickly added and mixed for 1 s. An amount of 120 µL of this solution was transferred into a glass mold, and a functionalized glass coverslip was placed over the solution at an angle so that no air remained under the coverslip. The solution was allowed to polymerize for 30 min at room temperature, after which the coverslip was removed from the mold. The gels were rinsed and stored in 1× PBS without Mg^{2+} and Ca^{2+} for subsequent use. For cell adhesion, Sulfosuccinimidyl 6-(4′-azido-2′-nitrophenylamino) hexanoate (sulfo-SANPAH, Thermo Fisher Scientific, Waltham, MA, USA) was applied to the PA gel surface for 15 min under 365 nm UV light (2 times). Then, the gel was coated with collagen I (100 µg/mL) overnight at 4 °C. Before the cell seeding, PA gels were washed 3 times with PBS. PA hydrogels with this structure have thickness gradient and apparent stiffness gradient [28].

To measure the thickness of the gel, PA gel was stained with Coomassie brilliant blue G-250 for about 10 min. Using confocal microscope (Leica TCS SP8 X, Germany, Wetzlar, Germany), we obtained a series of Z-stack images and reconstructed to measure the thickness of the PA gel.

An atomic force microscope (AFM, MFP-3D, Asylum Research Inc., Santa Barbara, CA, USA) with the colloidal probe cantilever was used for the apparent Young's modulus measurement. The cantilever used in the experiments was a non-tip cantilever (NSC36, MikroMasch, Watsonville, CA, USA) with a spring constant of 2 N/m. The colloidal probe was assembled, as described previously, by adhering a glass sphere of diameter d = 26.3 µm to the front end of the cantilever [29]. To effectively reduce the adhesion between the probe and the PA gel, the surface of the colloidal probe was coated with a thin layer of PLL-g-PEG (SuSoS AG.) [30]. The AFM measurements were carried out in contact mode with 1~8 µm indentation depths. The measured force–distance curves were recorded and fitted with Hertz model $F = \frac{4}{3(1-v^2)} E R^{0.5} \delta^{1.5}$ to calculate the reduced Young's modulus E [31], where F is the measured force, R is the probe radius, δ is the indentation distance, and $v = 0.33$ is the Poisson ratio. Prior to each force measurement, the spring constant of the colloidal probe is calibrated in situ using the thermal power spectral density method [29].

The topography of PA gel surface was visualized using scanning electron microscopy (SEM, Quanta 200 FEG). PA gels were flash frozen and were then lyophilized overnight. A layer of platinum (Pt) was deposited on the gel surface using a turbomolecular pump coater (Q150T, Quorum Technologies, Lewis, UK) prior to observation to enhance the electrical conductivity of the gel.

In each independent experiment, the PA gel was fabricated under the same condition. The size, thickness, and partitioning of the PA were controlled consistently. The reproducibility of the gel fabrication was verified.

2.4. Cell Immunofluorescence

JAR cells in hydrogel substrates were fixed in 4% (w/v) paraformaldehyde in PBS for 15 min at room temperature. The hydrogel was washed twice with PBS, permeabilized in 0.1% (v/v) triton X-100 in PBS for 15 min, and washed twice more with PBS. JAR cells were blocked in 2.5% (v/v) goat serum in PBS for 2 h at room temperature to prevent non-specific binding. Then, cells were incubated with anti-vinculin antibody (1:200, Abcam,

GR3270283-14, overnight, 4 °C) in goat serum. For secondary staining, cells were washed twice with PBS and incubated with goat anti-rabbit IgH H&L (488 nm) antibody (Abcam, 1:500, GR320844-3, 3 h, room temperature). Directly stained cells were incubated with 1:200 DAPI and phalloidin (546 nm) in goat serum solution (2 h, room temperature) and thoroughly washed with PBS. Confocal microscope (Leica TCS SP8 X, Germany, Wetzlar, Germany) was used for acquiring images.

2.5. Image Analysis and Figure Preparation

Unless otherwise stated, images were adjusted and analyzed using the Fiji distribution of ImageJ. R was used to generate all graphs and perform all statistical analyses. Figures were made using Photoshop Creative Cloud and PowerPoint.

2.6. Live Cell Imaging, Cell Tracking, and Migration Analyses

Cells plated on PA hydrogels were incubated overnight in RPMI 1640 with 10% FBS. For cell tracking, 1×10^6 cells were seeded in the confocal dishes (BioFroxx, BDD-12-35) and incubated overnight. Cells were monitored using an automated live-cell imager (Leica, Germany) with a 10× dry objective and maintained at 37 °C in a 5% CO_2 environment during imaging. Phase-contrast images were captured every 15 min for 14 h. Imaris' cell tracking module was used to track individual cells and obtain (x, y) coordinates to calculate displacement, track length, and cell velocity (track_length/time). Migrating cells were identified as those that migrated beyond a circular area 2 times the diameter of the cell over 14 h of imaging. The maximum displacement was calculated as the maximum change in the Euclidean distance of a particular cell throughout the imaging process.

2.7. F-Actin Skeletonization

F-actin skeletonization was performed using a steerable filter with MATLAB and ImageJ [32]. In brief, multiple-scale steerable filtering was used to enhance the curvilinear features, and centerlines of curvilinear features were extracted. Next, the filament fragments were clustered into high and low confidence and the fragments were connected with a graph matching. A network of F-actin was obtained after the reconstruction and each filament was represented by an ordered chain of pixels and a local filament orientation. ImageJ was used to determine the length of detected filaments (Plugins > NeuronJ) and enhance filament thickness for visualization.

2.8. Focal Adhesion Area Measurement

Focal adhesion area was measured using ImageJ software [33]. Briefly, the original image of immunofluorescence was firstly subtracted the local background by applying SUBSTRACT BACKGROUND. Then, the local contrast of the image was enhanced by adjusting Contrast Limit Histogram Equalization. Mathematical exponential and BRIGHT-NESS & CONTRAST tool were used for further minimizing the background. Next, we used the LOD3D plugin to filter the image and ran the THRESHOLD command to convert the image to a binary image. Finally, ANALYSE PARTICLES command was executed to scan the binary image and find the edge of focal adhesions.

2.9. Particle Image Velocimetry (PIV) Measurement

PIV analysis was performed using a custom algorithm based on MATLAB's PIVlab software package (Matlab2020a, PIVlab2.36). We used live cell image sequences of JAR cells to analyze the direction and magnitude of cell movement. To avoid the influence of the background movement on the calculated results, the calculated velocity field was subtracted from the average velocity. For the velocity vectors arrows, each pixel of length represents 0.05 µm/min.

2.10. Durotaxis Assays

Cells were seeded on PA hydrogels with stiffness gradients. The cells were mounted and maintained on the microscope as described above. After live cell imaging and cell tracking, the direction of cell movement was calculated based on the results of the PIV analysis (fractional velocities in the x and y directions).

2.11. Spheroid Spreading Assay

Multicellular spheroids were generated as described above. Diameters of JAR spheroids were similar to those of human embryos at the periods of implantation (5–6 days after fertilization), with an average of 150 ± 15 µm [34,35]. By observation under a stereomicroscope (Olympus, Japan), each spheroid at the bottom of the well was carefully aspirated with a disposable pipette tip and transferred into a small dish (LABSELECT 12111). Spheroids with proper size were gently collected and evenly dispersed into six-well plates containing hydrogel-coated coverslips. Spheroids were then incubated for 24 h for attachment and spreading before imaging with 10× or 20× objectives. To quantify the degree of dispersion, images were firstly converted into 8-bit image and then thresholded using ImageJ (Image > Adjust > Threshold) to outline the periphery of the aggregate, and the spreading area (total area–spheroid area) of the 24 h image was divided by the area of the spheroid, which was considered the spreading ratio.

2.12. Statistical Analysis

All statistical analyses were performed using R software (version 4.1.1). Results were expressed as the mean ± standard deviation (SD). Every experiment was repeated three times (n = 3). After confirming that the data were normally distributed and homogeneous in variance using the Shapiro–Wilk significance test as well as the Bartlett test, Student's t-test was used for analysis. For all comparisons, $p < 0.05$ was considered statistically significant.

3. Results

3.1. Simulated ECM Stiffness Regulates Trophoblast Cell Morphology and Spreading Area

Numerous studies demonstrated that cell spreading and focal adhesion maturation are positively correlated with ECM rigidity in various cells [36–42]. However, this correlation was not investigated in cytotrophoblasts. Therefore, we fabricated PA hydrogels (Figure S1), examined the surface morphology of the gels by SEM (Figure S2), and measured the apparent elastic modulus by AFM (Figure S3), which represent varying ECM stiffnesses independently of topographical and compositional cues [28]. We cultured JAR cells on simulated ECM with stiffness gradients ranging from 10 kPa to 100 kPa (Figure 1A,B). We then divided the hydrogel into three regions according to their stiffness: a stiff region (46.7 ± 25 kPa), an intermediate region (14.6 ± 8.0 kPa), and a soft region (6.9 ± 0.5 kPa).

After 24 h incubation, the cells were observed by phase-contrast microscope (Figure 1C). Cells growing on simulated ECM with different stiffness showed significant changes in cell morphology and spreading area. On the stiffer simulated ECM, JAR cells were polygonal with a larger cell spreading area, while the spreading area of the cells tended to decrease as stiffness decreased, and the cell morphology gradually became round (Figure 1D). These results demonstrate that JAR cell morphology and spreading area are regulated by simulated ECM stiffness.

3.2. F-Actin Organization and Focal Adhesion Formation Are Affected by Simulated ECM Stiffness in JAR Cells

Since cell spreading is regulated by the cytoskeleton and focal adhesion complex [43], we measured the assembly of F-actin and the focal adhesion in JAR cells on simulated ECM with different stiffnesses (Figure 2A). The images revealed significant differences in actin organization and focal adhesion formation between three simulated ECM regions with different stiffnesses. The focal adhesion area indicated by the staining of vinculin, which was measured by ImageJ software, increased as simulated ECM stiffness increased (Figure 2B). To quantify the F-actin cytoskeleton structure differences, we applied a steerable filter to extract F-actin bundles [32] (Figure 2C). The results demonstrated that JAR cells in the stiff simulated ECM region had longer and more robust stress fibers compared to other simulated ECM regions (Figure 2D). This demonstrates that stiff simulated ECM enhanced the F-actin organization and focal adhesion assembly of JAR cells.

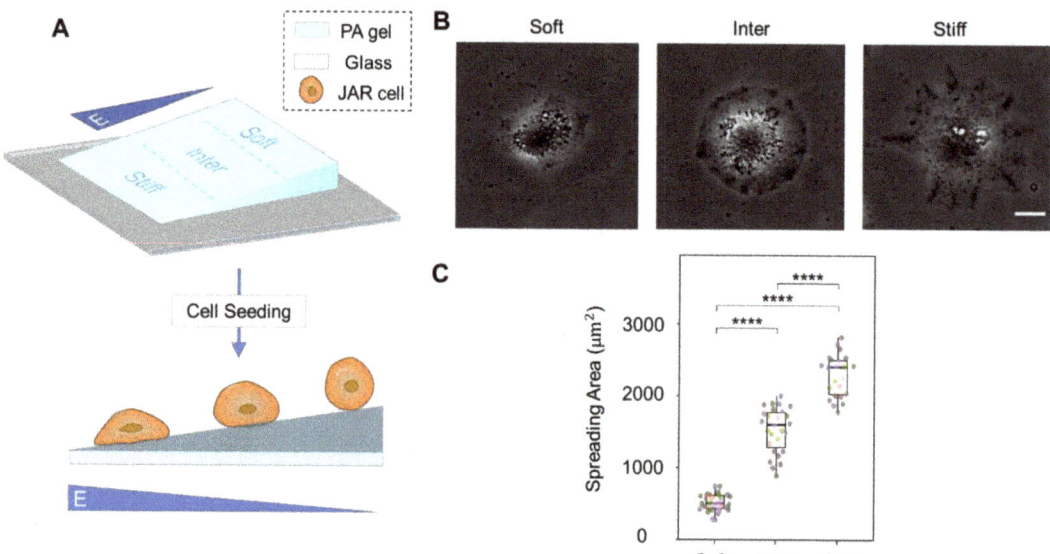

Figure 1. Simulated ECM stiffness regulates trophoblast cell morphology and spreading area. (**A**) (**Top**): schematic diagram of PA gel with stiffness gradient. The Young's modulus of the PA gel is 1 kPa, and its apparent Young's modulus gradually increases with the decrease in the gel thickness. According to the change of the apparent Young's modulus, the surface of the PA gel is evenly divided into three regions, namely Stiff, Intermediate, and Soft. (**Bottom**): schematic representation of JAR cells cultured on different regions. E indicates the apparent Young's modulus. (**B**) Phase contrast images of JAR cells cultures on different regions scale bar: 20 µm. The yellow dashed line indicates the boundary of cells. (**C**) Measured average cell spreading area of JAR cells cultured on different regions. **** $p < 1 \times 10^{-6}$, n = 31, 27, 23 for Soft, Inter and Stiff, respectively. Data reported as mean ± standard deviation for N = 3 independent experiments. Each scatter indicates each cell being measured, and each color indicates an independent experiment.

3.3. Stiff Simulated ECM Enhances JAR Cell Motility

Several studies demonstrated that cell migration is regulated by ECM stiffness [44–48]. To investigate cell migration behavior on ECM with different stiffness, we used a time-lapse microscope to visualize the motility of JAR cells. To examine the relationship between ECM stiffness and JAR cell migration, we used particle image velocity (PIV) to analyze the movement of JAR cells on simulated ECM with different stiffnesses (Figure 3A). Meanwhile, we selected JAR cells in different simulated ECM regions (stiff, intermediate, and soft) and tracked their migration for 5 h (Figure 3B). The migration distance (track length) as well as the migration velocity (track_length/time) of JAR cells on the inter and stiff regions were significantly increased compared to JAR cells on the soft region (Figure 3C,D). The displacement of JAR cells significantly increased as simulated ECM stiffness increased (Figure 3E). These results indicate that stiff simulated ECM increases cell motility in JAR cells.

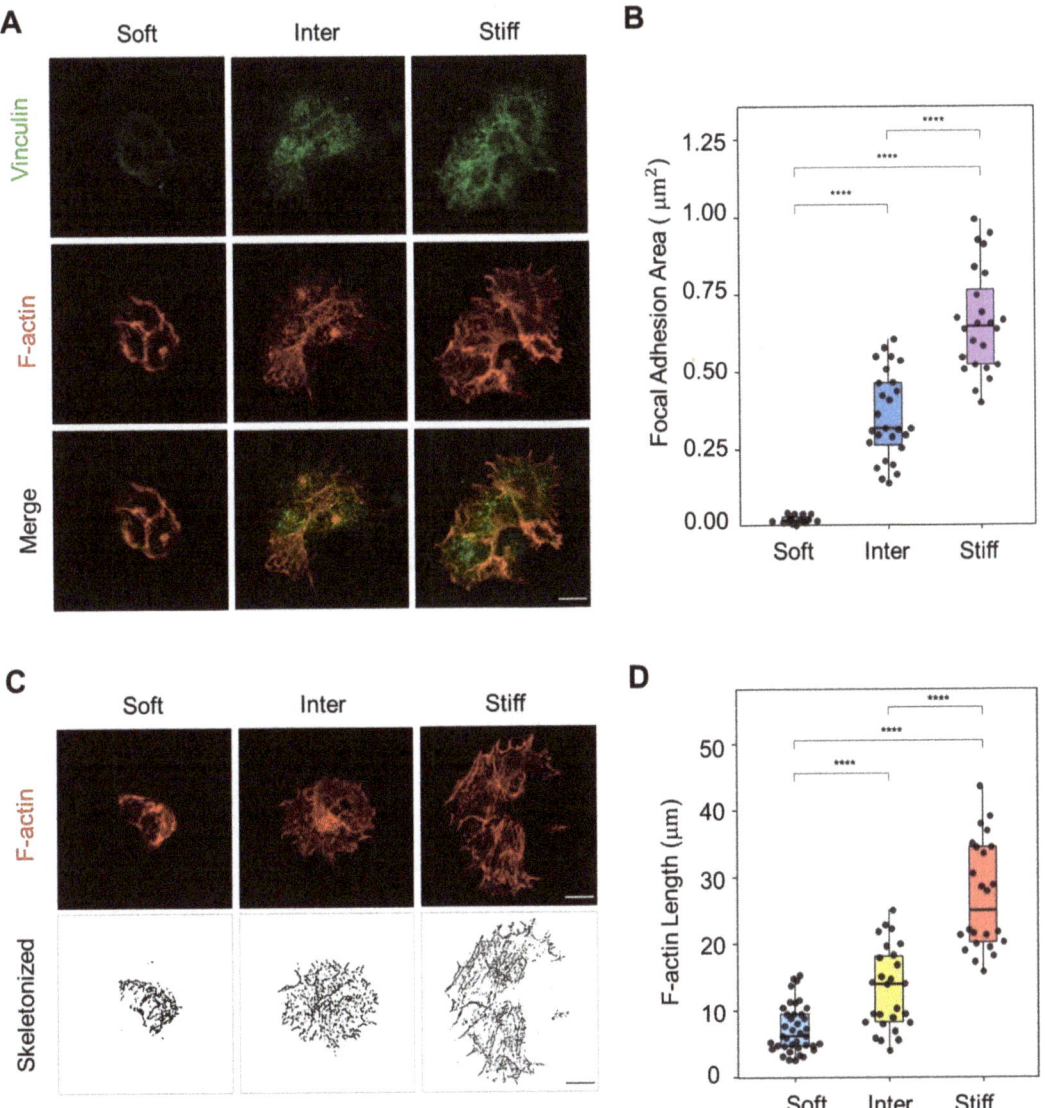

Figure 2. F-actin organization and focal adhesion formation are affected by simulated ECM stiffness in JAR cells. (**A**) Immunofluorescence staining of JAR cells cultured on different regions (red: F-actin; green: vinculin, scale bar: 20 µm). (**B**) Measured focal adhesion area of JAR cells cultured on different regions. **** 1×10^{-6}, n = 18, 27, 24 for Soft, Inter, and Stiff, respectively. Data reported as mean ± standard deviation for N = 3 independent experiments. Each scatter indicates each focal adhesion being measured. (**C**) Skeletonization of F-actin in JAR cells cultured on different regions (scale bar: 20 µm). (**D**) Measured cytoskeleton length of JAR cells cultured on different regions. **** 1×10^{-6}, n = 35, 27, 24 for Soft, Inter, and Stiff, respectively. Data reported as mean ± standard deviation for N = 3 independent experiments. Each scatter indicated each F-actin filament being measured.

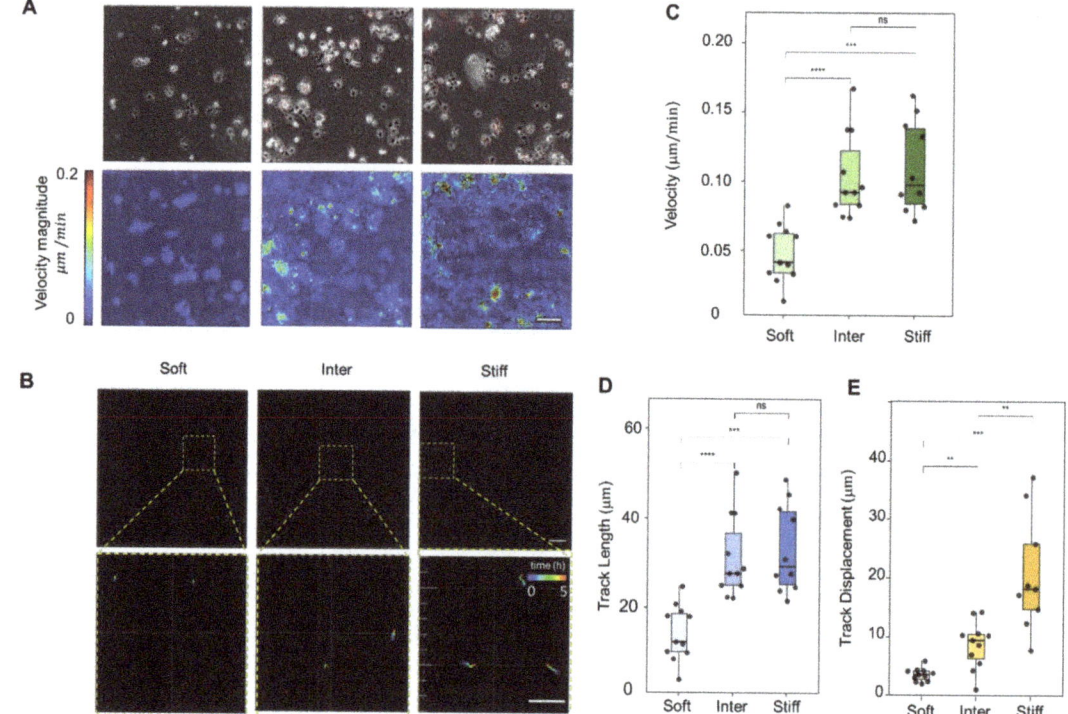

Figure 3. Stiff simulated ECM enhances JAR cell motility (**A**) (**Top**): Vectors of JAR cell migration. (**Bottom**): heatmap of velocity magnitude on different regions of simulated ECM (scale bar: 50 μm, color bar: 0~0.2 μm/min). (**B**) Tracking of JAR cells cultured on different regions (scale bar: 100 μm, time bar: 5 h). Each scatter indicated each cell being analyzed. (**C,D**) Velocity and track length of JAR cell migration. **** $p < 1 \times 10^{-6}$, *** $p < 0.001$, $n = 11, 11, 9$ for Soft, Inter, and Stiff, respectively. Data reported as mean ± standard deviation for $N = 3$ independent experiments. Each scatter indicated each cell being analyzed. (**E**) Track displacement of JAR cells cultured on different regions. *** $p < 0.001$, ** $p < 0.01$, $n = 11, 11, 9$ for Soft, Inter, and Stiff, respectively. Data reported as mean ± standard deviation for $N = 3$ independent experiments.

3.4. JAR Cells Exhibit Durotaxis

Spatial changes in ECM stiffness were shown to induce migration toward increased stiffness in numerous cell types both in vitro and in vivo [49]. This process, which is a key regulator of cell migration and invasion, is called durotaxis [50–52]. Although durotaxis was observed in many cell types [53–56], few studies described durotaxis in the context of human trophoblast cells. Therefore, we performed tracing for JAR cells grown on simulated ECM with a large stiffness gradient for 9.5 h (Figure 4A). By analyzing these trajectories, we found that most cells tended to migrate toward the stiffer simulated ECM region (Figure 4B,D). PIV analysis that was performed on two adjacent frames also demonstrated that the migratory direction of most cells coincided with the positive direction of the stiffness gradient (Figure 4C). These results demonstrate that JAR cells exhibit durotaxis.

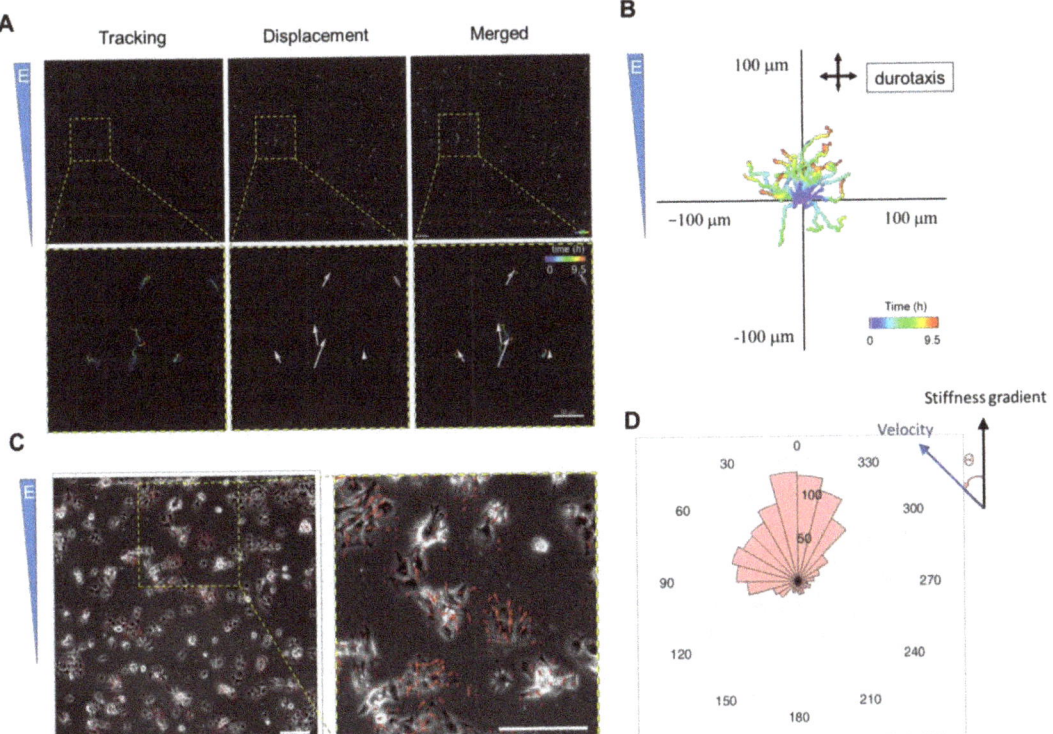

Figure 4. JAR cells exhibit durotaxis. (**A**) Tracking of JAR cells cultured on stiff region (scale bar: 50 μm, time bar: 9.5 h). E indicates the apparent Young's modulus. Arrows indicated the displacement of each cell, (**B**) Representative JAR cell migration plots on stiff region over 9.5 h. The total cell number $n = 56$, number of independent experiments $N = 3$. (**C**) Vector map of JAR cell migration on stiff region (scale bar: 150 μm). Arrows indicated the vector of velocity. (**D**) Rose diagram of cell migration direction, which displays the angular between migration and stiffness gradient and the frequency of each class. The total cell number $n = 56$, number of independent experiments $N = 3$.

3.5. Stiff Simulated ECM Enhances the Adhesion and Invasion of Multicellular JAR Spheroids

During the complex biophysical process of embryo implantation, trophoblasts contribute to successful implantation via attachment and invasion. Numerous studies demonstrated many similarities between embryo implantation and tumor progression [57–60]. Components that are crucial to tumor cell migration and invasion are shared by the human trophoblast, including the involvement of the extracellular matrix (ECM), proteases (including serine proteases, cathepsins, and matrix-metalloproteinases), and cell-surface receptors (integrins) [59]. F-actin remodeling regulated by fascin plays a critical role in both cancer metastasis and trophoblast migration and invasion [60,61].

As such, we inferred that if the migration of individual JAR cells is affected by the mechanical forces of their microenvironment, the invasion behaviors of multicellular JAR spheroids could also be regulated by ECM stiffness. During the first step of the embryo implantation process, the blastocyst, a spheroid, establishes adhesion to the endometrium. Wong et al. demonstrated that ECM stiffness regulates the self-assembling of 3D placental trophoblast spheroids [16], but few studies directly demonstrated how ECM stiffness affects adhesion or spreading of 3D human trophoblast spheroids.

Based on this, we referred to tumor research methods to study the effect of ECM stiffness on invasion of multicellular JAR spheroid [62]. Multicellular JAR spheroids were formed in ultra-low attachment 96-well plates, as described in Methods, and were then seeded onto PA hydrogels with different stiffness and allowed to attach for 24 h (Figure 5A). JAR spheroids on stiff and intermediate-stiff simulated ECM had larger adhesion areas and showed a higher degree of invasion compared to spheroids on soft simulated ECM (Figure 5B–D). No significant difference was found in the degree of spheroid invasion on the stiff and intermediate-stiff simulated ECM. This demonstrated that the invasion of multicellular JAR cell spheroids is regulated by simulated ECM stiffness.

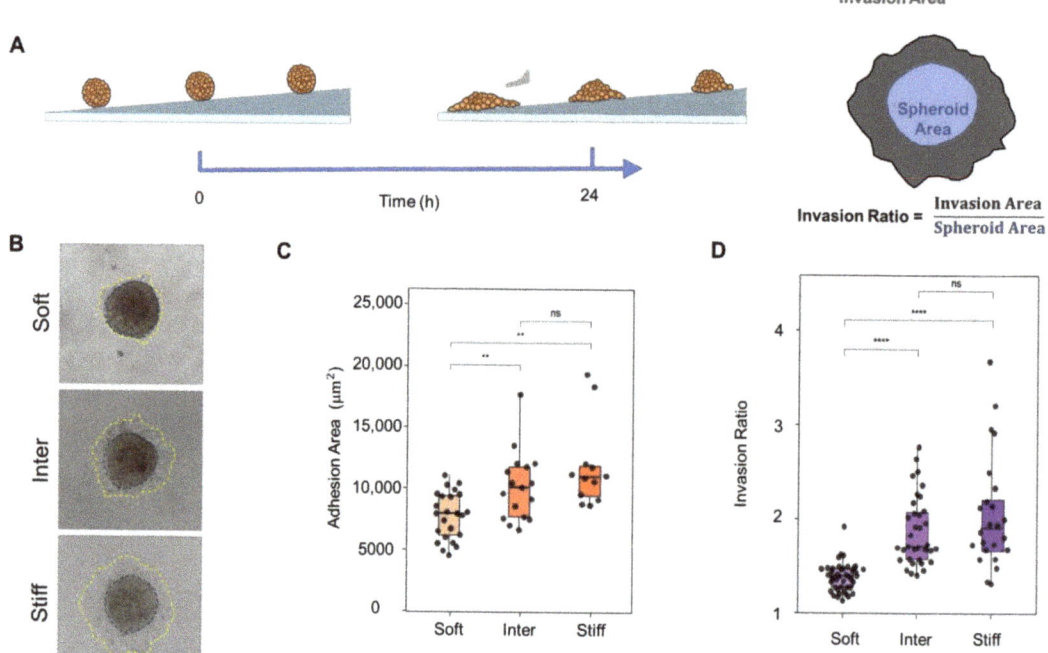

Figure 5. Stiff simulated ECM enhances the adhesion and invasion of multicellular JAR spheroids. (**A**) (**Left**): schematic diagram of JAR spheroid invasion assay. (**Right**): schematic diagram of the calculation of the invasion ratio. (**B**) Image of JAR spheroid invasion taken by an inverted microscope (scale bar: 200 μm). (**C**) Calculated adhesion area of JAR spheroids on different regions. ** $p < 0.01$, $n = 24, 17, 12$ for Soft, Inter, and Stiff, respectively. Data reported as mean ± standard deviation for $N = 3$ independent experiments. Each scatter indicated each spheroid being measured. (**D**) Calculated invasion ratio of JAR spheroids on different regions. **** $p < 1 \times 10^{-6}$, $n = 43, 35, 25$ for Soft, Inter, and Stiff, respectively. Data reported as mean ± standard deviation for $N = 3$ independent experiments. Each scatter indicated each spheroid being analyzed.

4. Discussion

Although ECM stiffness was demonstrated to be a key regulator of several developmental processes, the importance of extracellular mechanics for embryo implantation, especially for embryo attachment, was not established. This work identified trophoblasts as mechano-responding malignant tumor-like cells. Using PA hydrogels that mimic Young's modulus values of the human endometrium, we demonstrated that stiffer substrate enhances various cellular processes closely related to trophoblast adhesion and invasion, including JAR cell morphology, migration, contractility, and multicellular spheroid disaggregation. Our results demonstrate that adhesion and invasion of trophoblasts could be regulated by the mechanical properties (e.g., stiffness) of the endometrium. Altogether, these results suggest that mechanobiological properties may regulate the adhesion and invasion of human embryo during the process of implantation, and that the stiffness of the endometrium may affect the selection of embryo implantation sites and the subsequent invasion process.

Scar pregnancy (CSP) occurs when an embryo implants on a scar in the uterus, and the incidence of CSP increases with the number of previous cesarean deliveries [63]. The exact pathogenesis of CSP is not known, but the mechanical properties of the uterine scar significantly differ from other sites. The stiffness of the uterine scar appears to be significantly increased compared to the intact myometrium, as measured by ultrasound elastography [12], which could also affect embryo implantation. In addition, the stiffness of the endometrium in the pathological state is significantly higher than that of the normal state [6,13]. Our experiments demonstrated that in the context of normal and diseased human endometrium tissue characteristics (difference in stiffness), the mechanobiological regulation of trophoblast migration and attachment likely plays a critical role in implantation.

More broadly, this work demonstrated that trophoblast migration and adhesion are mechanically sensitive, which highlights the importance of strategies using extracellular tissue engineering to better understand and develop treatments for diseases related to implantation. This knowledge of mechanically mediated mechanisms for migration and adhesion can be further leveraged to create better technologies to increase the success rate of in vitro fertilization (IVF). In addition, the identification of this process will help to identify new regulatory mechanisms of embryonic adhesion and provide new ideas for the development of therapeutic strategies related to pregnancy.

Considering the difficulty in obtaining pure, primary, first-trimester human trophoblast cells, we used human choriocarcinoma (JAR) cell lineage instead of primary trophoblast cell line in this study. However, compared with primary trophoblast cells, choriocarcinoma cell lines have different transcriptomic profiles, are malignant and contain an abnormal number of chromosomes, which is unfavorable for studying the uniquely invasive extravillous trophoblast (EVT) cell behavior [64]. Therefore, in the subsequent study of embryo invasion, we will choose human embryonic stem cell (hESCs) or adult progenitor cells to derive trophoblast organoids. Endometrial epithelial cells are also involved in the embryo implantation process [65,66]. Under normal conditions, the trophoblast cells interact with endometrial epithelial cells to achieve maternal–fetal adhesion. The stiffness of the ECM could also affect the function of endometrial epithelial cells and the expression of related proteins. Therefore, to better simulate the in vivo environment, it is necessary to consider the mechanism of interaction between these two cells under the regulation of mechanical properties. Furthermore, since mechanical stiffness affects the invasion behaviors of trophoblast cells, the mechanobiological regulation of trophoblast migration and adhesion is most likely to be related to integrin-related signaling pathways. The integrin protein mediates the adhesion between cells and ECM. After being affected by mechanical forces, integrin binds to its ligands and mediates FAK, PI3K, AKT/PKB, and other signaling pathways that regulate cell proliferation, migration, and epithelial-mesenchymal transition [67,68]. By upregulating integrin-β1, the invasion of human trophoblasts can be promoted [69]. We also examined the expression of integrin-β1 of JAR cells on different regions and found no significant differences either between soft and inter or between inter and stiff, with stiff being slightly higher than soft (Figure S4), and the expression of other subunits of integrin did not change significantly with substrate stiffness [16]. In addition, several studies demonstrated the significant role of Rho protein in the process of implantation [26,70,71]. For example, Rho GTPase, most likely RhoA, regulates the adhesion of human trophoblasts to uterine epithelial RL95-2 cells [26].RhoA can also regulate trophoblast migration through cytoskeleton reorganization [70]. By interfering with related proteins such as integrin and Rho, we can further study the precise molecular mechanism of this phenomenon, which is also the content of our follow-up research.

Supplementary Materials: The following supporting information can be downloaded at: https://www.mdpi.com/article/10.3390/bioengineering10030384/s1, Figure S1: Fabricated sample of polyacrylamide hydrogel with stiffness gradient. Scale bar = 10 mm. Figure S2: SEM analysis of PA gel surface. Scale bar = 30 μm. Figure S3: Elastic modulus measured by AFM. Data reported as mean ± standard deviation for N = 3 independent experiments. Figure S4: Left: Immunofluorescence staining of JAR cells cultured on different regions (green: integrin-β1; blue: DAPI, scale bar: 20 μm). Right: mean fluorescence intensity of integrin-β1 in JAR cells cultured on different regions. n = 12, 13, 13 for Soft, Inter and Stiff, respectively. Data reported as mean ± standard deviation.

Author Contributions: J.C., Y.W., X.G., D.G., J.D. and Y.F. designed the study; J.C., H.L. and H.T. performed experiments and data analysis; Y.W., J.D. and Y.F. conceived and supervised this project and prepared the paper. All authors have read and agreed to the published version of the manuscript.

Funding: This work was supported by the National Natural Science Foundation of China (12222201, 82273500, U20A20390, 11827803 and 11972351), Fundamental Research Funds for the Central Universities (ZG140S1971), National Key R&D Program of China (2021YFA0719302), Peking University Health Science Center-X Cross Seed Fund (BMU2020MX014), and Incubation fund for reserve candidates of Peking University Third Hospital (BYSYFY2021007).

Institutional Review Board Statement: Not applicable.

Informed Consent Statement: Not applicable.

Data Availability Statement: The data presented in this study are available on request from the corresponding author. The data are not publicly available due to privacy.

Conflicts of Interest: The authors declare no conflict of interest.

References

1. Norwitz, E.R.; Schust, D.J.; Fisher, S.J. Implantation and the Survival of Early Pregnancy. *N. Engl. J. Med.* **2001**, *345*, 1400–1408. [CrossRef] [PubMed]
2. Foulk, R.A. *Implantation of the Human Embryo*; IntechOpen: London, UK, 2012.
3. Fitzgerald, H.C.; Salamonsen, L.A.; Rombauts, L.J.; Vollenhoven, B.J.; Edgell, T.A. The proliferative phase underpins endometrial development: Altered cytokine profiles in uterine lavage fluid of women with idiopathic infertility. *Cytokine* **2016**, *88*, 12–19.f. [CrossRef] [PubMed]
4. Zhao, Y.; Garcia, J.; Kolp, L.; Cheadle, C.; Rodriguez, A.; Vlahos, N.F. The impact of luteal phase support on gene expression of extracellular matrix protein and adhesion molecules in the human endometrium during the window of implantation following controlled ovarian stimulation with a GnRH antagonist protocol. *Fertil. Steril.* **2010**, *94*, 2264–2271. [CrossRef] [PubMed]
5. Yu, M.; Qin, H.; Wang, H.; Liu, J.; Liu, S.; Yan, Q. N-glycosylation of uterine endometrium determines its receptivity. *J. Cell. Physiol.* **2020**, *235*, 1076–1089. [CrossRef]
6. Ma, Z.; Sagrillo-Fagundes, L.; Mok, S.; Vaillancourt, C.; Moraes, C. Mechanobiological regulation of placental trophoblast fusion and function through extracellular matrix rigidity. *Sci. Rep.* **2020**, *10*, 5837. [CrossRef]
7. Sternberg, A.K.; Buck, V.U.; Classen-Linke, I.; Leube, R.E. How Mechanical Forces Change the Human Endometrium during the Menstrual Cycle in Preparation for Embryo Implantation. *Cells* **2021**, *10*, 2008. [CrossRef]
8. Matsuzaki, S. Mechanobiology of the female reproductive system. *Reprod. Med. Biol.* **2021**, *20*, 371–401. [CrossRef]
9. Kurek, A.; Kłosowicz, E.; Sofińska, K.; Jach, R.; Barbasz, J. Methods for Studying Endometrial Pathology and the Potential of Atomic Force Microscopy in the Research of Endometrium. *Cells* **2021**, *10*, 219. [CrossRef]
10. Fang, S.; McLean, J.; Shi, L.; Vink, J.Y.; Hendon, C.P.; Myers, K.M. Anisotropic Mechanical Properties of the Human Uterus Measured by Spherical Indentation. *Ann. Biomed. Eng.* **2021**, *49*, 1923–1942. [CrossRef]
11. Abbas, Y.; Carnicer-Lombarte, A.; Gardner, L.; Thomas, J.; Brosens, J.J.; Moffett, A.; Sharkey, A.M.; Franze, K.; Burton, G.J.; Oyen, M.L. Tissue stiffness at the human maternal-fetal interface. *Hum. Reprod.* **2019**, *34*, 1999–2008. [CrossRef]
12. Di Pasquo, E.; Kiener, A.J.O.; DallAsta, A.; Commare, A.; Angeli, L.; Frusca, T.; Ghi, T. Evaluation of the uterine scar stiffness in women with previous Cesarean section by ultrasound elastography: A cohort study. *Clin. Imaging* **2020**, *64*, 53–56. [CrossRef]
13. Kılıç, F.; Kayadibi, Y.; Yüksel, M.A.; Adaletli, İ.; Ustabaşıoğlu, F.E.; Öncül, M.; Madazlı, R.; Yılmaz, M.H.; Mihmanlı, İ.; Kantarcı, F. Shear wave elastography of placenta: In vivo quantitation of placental elasticity in preeclampsia. *Diagn. Interv. Radiol.* **2015**, *21*, 202–207. [CrossRef]
14. Jiang, X.; Asbach, P.; Streitberger, K.J.; Thomas, A.; Hamm, B.; Braun, J.; Sack, I.; Guo, J. In vivo high-resolution magnetic resonance elastography of the uterine corpus and cervix. *Eur. Radiol.* **2014**, *24*, 3025–3033. [CrossRef]
15. Thie, M.; Röspel, R.; Dettmann, W.; Benoit, M.; Ludwig, M.; Gaub, H.E.; Denker, H.W. Interactions between trophoblast and uterine epithelium: Monitoring of adhesive forces. *Hum. Reprod.* **1998**, *13*, 3211–3219. [CrossRef]

16. Wong, M.K.; Shawky, S.A.; Aryasomayajula, A.; Green, M.A.; Ewart, T.; Selvaganapathy, P.R.; Raha, S. Extracellular matrix surface regulates self-assembly of three-dimensional placental trophoblast spheroids. *PLoS ONE* **2018**, *13*, e0199632. [CrossRef]
17. Kandow, C.E.; Georges, P.C.; Janmey, P.A.; Beningo, K.A. Polyacrylamide hydrogels for cell mechanics: Steps toward optimization and alternative uses. *Methods Cell Biol.* **2007**, *83*, 29–46.
18. Dupont, S.; Morsut, L.; Aragona, M.; Enzo, E.; Giulitti, S.; Cordenonsi, M.; Zanconato, F.; Le Digabel, J.; Forcato, M.; Bicciato, S.; et al. Role of YAP/TAZ in mechanotransduction. *Nature* **2011**, *474*, 179–183. [CrossRef]
19. Wen, J.H.; Vincent, L.G.; Fuhrmann, A.; Choi, Y.S.; Hribar, K.C.; Taylor-Weiner, H.; Chen, S.; Engler, A.J. Interplay of matrix stiffness and protein tethering in stem cell differentiation. *Nat. Mater.* **2014**, *13*, 979–987. [CrossRef]
20. Grümmer, R.; Hohn, H.P.; Mareel, M.M.; Denker, H.W. Adhesion and invasion of three human choriocarcinoma cell lines into human endometrium in a three-dimensional organ culture system. *Placenta* **1994**, *15*, 411–429. [CrossRef]
21. Wang, H.; Pilla, F.; Anderson, S.; Martínez-Escribano, S.; Herrer, I.; Moreno-Moya, J.M.; Musti, S.; Bocca, S.; Oehninger, S.; Horcajadas, J.A. A novel model of human implantation: 3D endometrium-like culture system to study attachment of human trophoblast (Jar) cell spheroids. *Mol. Hum. Reprod.* **2012**, *18*, 33–43. [CrossRef]
22. Schmitz, C.; Yu, L.; Bocca, S.; Anderson, S.; Cunha-Filho, J.S.; Rhavi, B.S.; Oehninger, S. Role for the endometrial epithelial protein MFG-E8 and its receptor integrin $\alpha v \beta 3$ in human implantation: Results of an in vitro trophoblast attachment study using established human cell lines. *Fertil. Steril.* **2014**, *101*, 874–882. [CrossRef] [PubMed]
23. Evron, A.; Goldman, S.; Shalev, E. Effect of primary human endometrial stromal cells on epithelial cell receptivity and protein expression is dependent on menstrual cycle stage. *Hum. Reprod.* **2011**, *26*, 176–190. [CrossRef] [PubMed]
24. Harduf, H.; Goldman, S.; Shalev, E. Human uterine epithelial RL95-2 and HEC-1A cell-line adhesiveness: The role of plexin B1. *Fertil. Steril.* **2007**, *87*, 1419–1427. [CrossRef] [PubMed]
25. Kodithuwakku, S.P.; Ng, P.Y.; Liu, Y.; Ng, E.H.; Yeung, W.S.; Ho, P.C.; Lee, K.F. Hormonal regulation of endometrial olfactomedin expression and its suppressive effect on spheroid attachment onto endometrial epithelial cells. *Hum. Reprod.* **2011**, *26*, 167–175. [CrossRef]
26. Heneweer, C.; Kruse, L.H.; Kindhäuser, F.; Schmidt, M.; Jakobs, K.H.; Denker, H.W.; Thie, M. Adhesiveness of human uterine epithelial RL95-2 cells to trophoblast: Rho protein regulation. *Mol. Hum. Reprod.* **2002**, *8*, 1014–1022. [CrossRef]
27. Heneweer, C.; Schmidt, M.; Denker, H.W.; Thie, M. Molecular mechanisms in uterine epithelium during trophoblast binding: The role of small GTPase RhoA in human uterine Ishikawa cells. *J. Exp. Clin. Assist. Reprod.* **2005**, *2*, 4. [CrossRef]
28. Cai, P.; Layani, M.; Leow, W.R.; Amini, S.; Liu, Z.; Qi, D.; Hu, B.; Wu, Y.L.; Miserez, A.; Magdassi, S.; et al. Bio-Inspired Mechanotactic Hybrids for Orchestrating Traction-Mediated Epithelial Migration. *Adv. Mater.* **2016**, *28*, 3102–3110. [CrossRef]
29. Guan, D.; Hang, Z.H.; Marcet, Z.; Liu, H.; Kravchenko, I.I.; Chan, C.T.; Chan, H.B.; Tong, P. Direct Measurement of Optical Force Induced by Near-Field Plasmonic Cavity Using Dynamic Mode AFM. *Sci. Rep.* **2015**, *5*, 16216. [CrossRef]
30. Guan, D.; Shen, Y.; Zhang, R.; Huang, P.; Lai, P.-Y.; Tong, P. Unified description of compressive modulus revealing multiscale mechanics of living cells. *Phys. Rev. Res.* **2021**, *3*, 043166. [CrossRef]
31. Hertz, H. On the contact of elastic solids. *J. Reine Angew. Math.* **1881**, *92*, 156–171.
32. Gan, Z.; Ding, L.; Burckhardt, C.J.; Lowery, J.; Zaritsky, A.; Sitterley, K.; Mota, A.; Costigliola, N.; Starker, C.G.; Voytas, D.F.; et al. Vimentin Intermediate Filaments Template Microtubule Networks to Enhance Persistence in Cell Polarity and Directed Migration. *Cell Syst.* **2016**, *3*, 252–263.e8. [CrossRef]
33. Sigaut, L.; von Bilderling, C.; Bianchi, M.; Burdisso, J.E.; Gastaldi, L.; Pietrasanta, L.I. Live cell imaging reveals focal adhesions mechanoresponses in mammary epithelial cells under sustained equibiaxial stress. *Sci. Rep.* **2018**, *8*, 9788. [CrossRef]
34. Shigehito, Y.; Mark, H.; Tetsuya, T. Human Embryology. In *New Discoveries in Embryology*; Bin, W., Ed.; IntechOpen: Rijeka, Croatia, 2015; Chapter 5.
35. Kim, S.E.; Lee, J.E.; Han, Y.H.; Lee, S.I.; Kim, D.K.; Park, S.R.; Yu, S.L.; Kang, J. Decursinol from Angelica gigas Nakai enhances endometrial receptivity during implantation. *BMC Complement. Med. Ther.* **2020**, *20*, 36. [CrossRef]
36. Tee, S.Y.; Fu, J.; Chen, C.S.; Janmey, P. Cell shape and substrate rigidity both regulate cell stiffness. *Biophys. J.* **2011**, *100*, L25–L27. [CrossRef]
37. Yeung, T.; Georges, P.C.; Flanagan, L.A.; Marg, B.; Ortiz, M.; Funaki, M.; Zahir, N.; Ming, W.; Weaver, V.; Janmey, P.A. Effects of substrate stiffness on cell morphology, cytoskeletal structure, and adhesion. *Cell Motil. Cytoskelet.* **2005**, *60*, 24–34. [CrossRef]
38. Nicolas, A.; Besser, A.; Safran, S.A. Dynamics of cellular focal adhesions on deformable substrates: Consequences for cell force microscopy. *Biophys. J.* **2008**, *95*, 527–539. [CrossRef]
39. Prager-Khoutorsky, M.; Lichtenstein, A.; Krishnan, R.; Rajendran, K.; Mayo, A.; Kam, Z.; Geiger, B.; Bershadsky, A.D. Fibroblast polarization is a matrix-rigidity-dependent process controlled by focal adhesion mechanosensing. *Nat. Cell Biol.* **2011**, *13*, 1457–1465. [CrossRef]
40. Wormer, D.B.; Davis, K.A.; Henderson, J.H.; Turner, C.E. The focal adhesion-localized CdGAP regulates matrix rigidity sensing and durotaxis. *PLoS ONE* **2014**, *9*, e91815. [CrossRef]
41. Califano, J.P.; Reinhart-King, C.A. Substrate Stiffness and Cell Area Predict Cellular Traction Stresses in Single Cells and Cells in Contact. *Cell. Mol. Bioeng.* **2010**, *3*, 68–75. [CrossRef]
42. McKenzie, A.J.; Hicks, S.R.; Svec, K.V.; Naughton, H.; Edmunds, Z.L.; Howe, A.K. The mechanical microenvironment regulates ovarian cancer cell morphology, migration, and spheroid disaggregation. *Sci. Rep.* **2018**, *8*, 7228. [CrossRef]

43. Pelham, R.J., Jr.; Wang, Y. Cell locomotion and focal adhesions are regulated by substrate flexibility. *Proc. Natl. Acad. Sci. USA* **1997**, *94*, 13661–13665. [CrossRef] [PubMed]
44. Pandya, P.; Orgaz, J.L.; Sanz-Moreno, V. Actomyosin contractility and collective migration: May the force be with you. *Curr. Opin. Cell Biol.* **2017**, *48*, 87–96. [CrossRef] [PubMed]
45. Lintz, M.; Muñoz, A.; Reinhart-King, C.A. The Mechanics of Single Cell and Collective Migration of Tumor Cells. *J. Biomech. Eng.* **2017**, *139*, 0210051–02100519. [CrossRef] [PubMed]
46. Schiffhauer, E.S.; Robinson, D.N. Mechanochemical Signaling Directs Cell-Shape Change. *Biophys. J.* **2017**, *112*, 207–214. [CrossRef]
47. Stroka, K.M.; Konstantopoulos, K. Physical biology in cancer. 4. Physical cues guide tumor cell adhesion and migration. *Am. J. Physiol. Cell Physiol.* **2014**, *306*, C98–C109. [CrossRef]
48. Wang, Y.; Wang, G.; Luo, X.; Qiu, J.; Tang, C. Substrate stiffness regulates the proliferation, migration, and differentiation of epidermal cells. *Burns* **2012**, *38*, 414–420. [CrossRef]
49. Lo, C.M.; Wang, H.B.; Dembo, M.; Wang, Y.L. Cell movement is guided by the rigidity of the substrate. *Biophys. J.* **2000**, *79*, 144–152. [CrossRef]
50. Plotnikov, S.V.; Waterman, C.M. Guiding cell migration by tugging. *Curr. Opin. Cell Biol.* **2013**, *25*, 619–626. [CrossRef]
51. Aubry, D.; Gupta, M.; Ladoux, B.; Allena, R. Mechanical link between durotaxis, cell polarity and anisotropy during cell migration. *Phys. Biol.* **2015**, *12*, 026008. [CrossRef]
52. Roca-Cusachs, P.; Sunyer, R.; Trepat, X. Mechanical guidance of cell migration: Lessons from chemotaxis. *Curr. Opin. Cell Biol.* **2013**, *25*, 543–549. [CrossRef]
53. DuChez, B.J. Durotaxis by Human Cancer Cells. *Biophys. J.* **2019**, *116*, 670–683. [CrossRef]
54. Evans, E.B.; Brady, S.W.; Tripathi, A.; Hoffman-Kim, D. Schwann cell durotaxis can be guided by physiologically relevant stiffness gradients. *Biomater. Res.* **2018**, *22*, 14. [CrossRef]
55. Martinez, J.S.; Schlenoff, J.B.; Keller, T.C., 3rd. Collective epithelial cell sheet adhesion and migration on polyelectrolyte multilayers with uniform and gradients of compliance. *Exp. Cell Res.* **2016**, *346*, 17–29.
56. Shellard, A.; Mayor, R. Collective durotaxis along a self-generated stiffness gradient in vivo. *Nature* **2021**, *600*, 690–694. [CrossRef]
57. Murray, M.J.; Lessey, B.A. Embryo implantation and tumor metastasis: Common pathways of invasion and angiogenesis. *Semin. Reprod. Endocrinol.* **1999**, *17*, 275–290. [CrossRef]
58. Pilka, R.; Kudela, M.; Procházka, M. Matrix metalloproteinases, embryo implantation and tumor invasion. *Ceska Gynekol.* **2003**, *68*, 179–185.
59. Soundararajan, R.; Rao, A.J. Trophoblast 'pseudo-tumorigenesis': Significance and contributory factors. *Reprod. Biol. Endocrinol.* **2004**, *2*, 15. [CrossRef]
60. Lamptey, J.; Czika, A.; Aremu, J.O.; Pervaz, S.; Adu-Gyamfi, E.A.; Otoo, A.; Li, F.; Wang, Y.X.; Ding, Y.B. The role of fascin in carcinogenesis and embryo implantation. *Exp. Cell Res.* **2021**, *409*, 112885. [CrossRef]
61. Grasset, E.M.; Bertero, T.; Bozec, A.; Friard, J.; Bourget, I.; Pisano, S.; Lecacheur, M.; Maiel, M.; Bailleux, C.; Emelyanov, A.; et al. Matrix Stiffening and EGFR Cooperate to Promote the Collective Invasion of Cancer Cells. *Cancer Res.* **2018**, *78*, 5229–5242. [CrossRef]
62. Vinci, M.; Box, C.; Eccles, S.A. Three-dimensional (3D) tumor spheroid invasion assay. *J. Vis. Exp.* **2015**, e52686.
63. Timor-Tritsch, I.E.; Monteagudo, A.; Calì, G.; D'Antonio, F.; Kaelin Agten, A. Cesarean Scar Pregnancy: Diagnosis and Pathogenesis. *Obstet. Gynecol. Clin. N. Am.* **2019**, *46*, 797–811. [CrossRef] [PubMed]
64. Abbas, Y.; Turco, M.Y.; Burton, G.J.; Moffett, A. Investigation of human trophoblast invasion in vitro. *Hum. Reprod. Update* **2020**, *26*, 501–513. [CrossRef] [PubMed]
65. Bortolotti, D.; Soffritti, I.; D'Accolti, M.; Gentili, V.; Di Luca, D.; Rizzo, R.; Caselli, E. HHV-6A Infection of Endometrial Epithelial Cells Affects miRNA Expression and Trophoblast Cell Attachment. *Reprod. Sci.* **2020**, *27*, 779–786. [CrossRef] [PubMed]
66. Soni, U.K.; Chadchan, S.B.; Gupta, R.K.; Kumar, V.; Kumar Jha, R. miRNA-149 targets PARP-2 in endometrial epithelial and stromal cells to regulate the trophoblast attachment process. *Mol. Hum. Reprod.* **2021**, *27*, gaab039. [CrossRef]
67. Ma, H.; Wang, J.; Zhao, X.; Wu, T.; Huang, Z.; Chen, D.; Liu, Y.; Ouyang, G. Periostin Promotes Colorectal Tumorigenesis through Integrin-FAK-Src Pathway-Mediated YAP/TAZ Activation. *Cell Rep.* **2020**, *30*, 793–806.e6. [CrossRef]
68. Li, N.; Zhang, X.; Zhou, J.; Li, W.; Shu, X.; Wu, Y.; Long, M. Multiscale biomechanics and mechanotransduction from liver fibrosis to cancer. *Adv. Drug Deliv. Rev.* **2022**, *188*, 114448. [CrossRef]
69. Zhu, S.; Li, Z.; Cui, L.; Ban, Y.; Leung, P.C.K.; Li, Y.; Ma, J. Activin A increases human trophoblast invasion by upregulating integrin β1 through ALK4. *FASEB J.* **2021**, *35*, e21220. [CrossRef]
70. Han, J.; Li, L.; Hu, J.; Yu, L.; Zheng, Y.; Guo, J.; Zheng, X.; Yi, P.; Zhou, Y. Epidermal growth factor stimulates human trophoblast cell migration through Rho A and Rho C activation. *Endocrinology* **2010**, *151*, 1732–1742. [CrossRef]
71. Shiokawa, S.; Iwashita, M.; Akimoto, Y.; Nagamatsu, S.; Sakai, K.; Hanashi, H.; Kabir-Salmani, M.; Nakamura, Y.; Uehata, M.; Yoshimura, Y. Small guanosine triphospatase RhoA and Rho-associated kinase as regulators of trophoblast migration. *J. Clin. Endocrinol. Metab.* **2002**, *87*, 5808–5816. [CrossRef]

Disclaimer/Publisher's Note: The statements, opinions and data contained in all publications are solely those of the individual author(s) and contributor(s) and not of MDPI and/or the editor(s). MDPI and/or the editor(s) disclaim responsibility for any injury to people or property resulting from any ideas, methods, instructions or products referred to in the content.

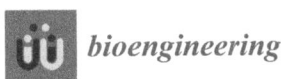

Article

Restoration of the Joint Line Configuration Reproduces Native Mid-Flexion Biomechanics after Total Knee Arthroplasty: A Matched-Pair Cadaveric Study

Dai-Soon Kwak [1], Yong Deok Kim [2,3], Nicole Cho [4], Yong In [3,5], Man Soo Kim [3,5], Dohyung Lim [6] and In Jun Koh [2,3,*]

1. Catholic Institute for Applied Anatomy, Department of Anatomy, College of Medicine, The Catholic University of Korea, Seoul 06591, Korea
2. Joint Replacement Center, Eunpyeong St. Mary's Hospital, Seoul 03312, Korea
3. Department of Orthopaedic Surgery, College of Medicine, The Catholic University of Korea, Seoul 06591, Korea
4. Boston College, Morrissey College of Arts and Sciences, Chestnut Hill, MA 02467, USA
5. Department of Orthopaedic Surgery, Seoul St. Mary's Hospital, Seoul 06591, Korea
6. Department of Mechanical Engineering, Sejong University, Seoul 05006, Korea
* Correspondence: esmh.jrcenter@gmail.com; Tel.: +82-2-2030-2655; Fax: +82-2-2030-4629

Abstract: Background: Recent evidence supports that restoration of the pre-arthritic condition via total knee arthroplasty (TKA) is associated with improved post-TKA performance and patient satisfaction. However, whether the restored pre-arthritic joint line simulates the native mid-flexion biomechanics remains unclear. Objective: We performed a matched-pair cadaveric study to explore whether restoration of the joint line via kinematically aligned (KA) TKA reproduced native knee biomechanics more accurately than the altered joint line associated with mechanically aligned (MA) TKA. Methods: Sixteen fresh-frozen cadaveric knees (eight pairs) were affixed onto a customized knee-squatting simulator for measurement of femoral rollback and medial collateral ligament (MCL) strain during mid-flexion. One knee from each cadaver was randomly designated to the KA TKA group (with the joint line restored to the pre-arthritic condition) and the other to the MA TKA group (with the joint line perpendicular to the mechanical axis). Optical markers were attached to all knees and rollback was analyzed using motion capture cameras. A video extensometer measured real-time variations in MCL strain. The kinematics and MCL strain prior to and following TKA were measured for all specimens. Results: KA TKA was better for restoring the knee kinematics to the native condition than MA TKA. The mid-flexion femoral rollback and axial rotation after KA TKA were consistently comparable to those of the native knee. Meanwhile, those of MA TKA were similar only at ≤40° of flexion. Furthermore, KA TKA better restored the mid-flexion MCL strain to that of the native knee than MA TKA. Over the entire mid-flexion range, the MCL strain of KA TKA and native knees were similar, while the strains of MA TKA knees were more than twice those of native knees at >20° of flexion. Conclusions: The restored joint line after KA TKA effectively reproduced the native mid-flexion rollback and MCL strain, whereas the altered joint line after MA TKA did not. Our findings may explain why patients who undergo KA TKA experience superior outcomes and more natural knee sensations during daily activities than those treated via MA TKA.

Keywords: rollback; ligament strain; kinematic alignment; mechanical alignment; total knee arthroplasty

Citation: Kwak, D.-S.; Kim, Y.D.; Cho, N.; In, Y.; Kim, M.S.; Lim, D.; Koh, I.J. Restoration of the Joint Line Configuration Reproduces Native Mid-Flexion Biomechanics after Total Knee Arthroplasty: A Matched-Pair Cadaveric Study. *Bioengineering* 2022, 9, 564. https://doi.org/10.3390/bioengineering9100564

Academic Editors: Christina Zong-Hao Ma, Zhengrong Li and Chen He

Received: 26 September 2022
Accepted: 14 October 2022
Published: 17 October 2022

Publisher's Note: MDPI stays neutral with regard to jurisdictional claims in published maps and institutional affiliations.

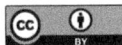

Copyright: © 2022 by the authors. Licensee MDPI, Basel, Switzerland. This article is an open access article distributed under the terms and conditions of the Creative Commons Attribution (CC BY) license (https://creativecommons.org/licenses/by/4.0/).

1. Introduction

Despite advances in technology and surgical technique, recent evidence indicates that mechanically aligned (MA) total knee arthroplasty (TKA) does not improve residual symptoms, natural knee sensations, or patient satisfaction [1–5]. In addition, neutrally aligned TKA fails to reproduce patient-specific knee kinematics [6–8]. Thus, kinematic alignment that restores patient-specific pre-arthritic alignment, joint line obliquity, and soft tissue laxity has attracted increasing interest [9,10]. Many studies have shown that kinematically aligned (KA) TKA better restores the pre-arthritic knee kinematics and functional performance than MA TKA, thereby increasing patient satisfaction [11–18]. However, biomechanical data explaining these improvements are lacking.

Many daily activities, including walking and rising from a chair, are performed in the mid-flexion range [19]; restoration of preoperative knee performance within that range is essential for TKA to be successful. It has been suggested that mid-flexion instability is inevitable after well-balanced MA TKA [20]; joint line elevation after MA TKA was a risk factor for instability [21–23]. Theoretically, KA TKA that restores both the joint line height and obliquity of the pre-arthritic knee should provide more natural mid-flexion kinematics and laxity than MA TKA. However, reports on the relationship between restoration of the joint line configuration (height and obliquity) and mid-flexion biomechanics/laxity have been inconsistent [12,15,21,24–26].

The objective of this matched-pair study was to determine whether the restored pre-arthritic joint line configuration after KA TKA provided femoral rollback closer to that of the native knee than the altered joint line perpendicular to the mechanical axis created after MA TKA, and whether KA TKA more effectively restored MCL strain in comparison to MA TKA. We hypothesized that KA TKA reproduced the natural mid-flexion knee kinematics (rollback and tibiofemoral axial rotation) better than MA TKA. In addition, we proposed that KA TKA would more naturally reproduce MCL strain in the mid-flexion range than MA TKA.

2. Materials and Methods

2.1. Participants

Eight freshly frozen full-body specimens (human cadavers, donated to the College of Medicine, The Catholic university of Korea, 16 knees; five male pairs and three female pairs; mean age, 76 years; range: 58–86 years) were used (Table 1). The two knees of each cadaver were randomly assigned to either the KA TKA or the MA TKA group. All specimens were macroscopically intact, and none exhibited any gross pathology. This cadaveric study was approved by Institutional Cadaver Research Committee (College of Medicine, The Catholic University of Korea) (R19-A018).

Table 1. Demographic variables of the specimens.

Specimen Number	Age (y)	Hight (cm)	Weight (kg)	Sex	Left Knee HKA (°)	Right Knee Alignment	OA Severity	HKA (°)	Alignment	OA Severity
1	85	163	74	Male	3.6	MA	Mild	5.2	KA	Mild
2	71	175	64	Male	2.9	KA	Mild	2.9	MA	Mild
3	84	163	50	Male	7.1	MA	Mild	8.0	KA	Mild
4	58	166	78	Male	5.1	MA	Mild	2.1	KA	Mild
5	86	167	48	Female	4.0	MA	Mild	0	KA	Mild
6	79	164	58	Female	3.3	KA	Moderate	4.4	MA	Moderate
7	63	170	56	Male	7.6	MA	Mild	4.6	KA	Mild
8	81	160	48	Female	3.5	KA	Mild	1.0	MA	Mild

2.2. Preparation of Specimens

The specimens were frozen at 20 °C until they were thawed to room temperature on the evening prior to dissection. All skin and subcutaneous tissues were dissected away, leaving only the extensor mechanism, knee capsule, and periarticular soft tissues intact. We took high-resolution anterior-to-posterior photographs of each leg and measured the anatomical and mechanical axes of both the femur and tibia and the hip–knee–ankle axis.

The severity of osteoarthritis (OA) in each cadaveric specimen was graded as mild (no articular cartilage lesions), moderate (focal lesion present), or severe (extensive lesion present) (Table 1). Separation of the quadriceps femoris revealed the vastus medialis, rectus femoris/vastus intermedius, and vastus lateralis. Additionally, separation of the hamstring muscles revealed the biceps femoris and semimembranosus/semitendinosus. Then, suturing the parted muscle branches with wire ensured the connection between the muscles. The femur and the tibia were cut 30 cm proximal and 25 cm distal to the joint line, respectively.

2.3. Surgical Procedure

A senior surgeon (one of the authors) performed all arthroplasties following a standard posterior-substituting (PS) prosthetic system (Legion Total Knee System; Smith & Nephew, Memphis, TN, USA). Furthermore, a subvastus approach ensured exposure of the knee joint; the patella was not resurfaced in any case. We sought to ensure that all medial (distal and posterior femoral) resections were 9.5 mm in thickness, because the thicknesses of the distal and posterior femoral implants were 9.5 mm. KA TKA was performed using the previously described calipered technique [27,28]. The femur and tibia resection thicknesses were equivalent to those of the implants placed in the native joint lines; there was no manipulation of soft tissue. Calipers were used to measure the thickness of each resected osteochondral fragment, followed by adjustment of each resection until it matched the thickness of the implant (Figure 1). The angle of the tibial resection guide was altered until the saw slot and angle were parallel to the coronal and sagittal proximal articular surfaces (after compensating for wear). In the MA TKA group, TKA was performed with the conventional measured resection technique. Resection of the distal femur proceeded using intramedullary instrumentation that considered the difference between the mechanical and anatomical axes of each individual specimen; the trans-epicondylar axis was used as the reference for determining the femoral component external rotation. Extramedullary instrumentation was then used to perform resections of the coronal and sagittal proximal tibias at a cutting angle of 90° relative to the tibial axis (Figure 1). Lastly, a tensor device (B Braun-Aesculap, Tuttlingen, Germany) under a 200-N distraction force was used to measure the 0° and 90° flexion gaps. The resected osteochondral fragment thickness and gap after bone resection with KA TKA contrasted with those after MA TKA (Table 2).

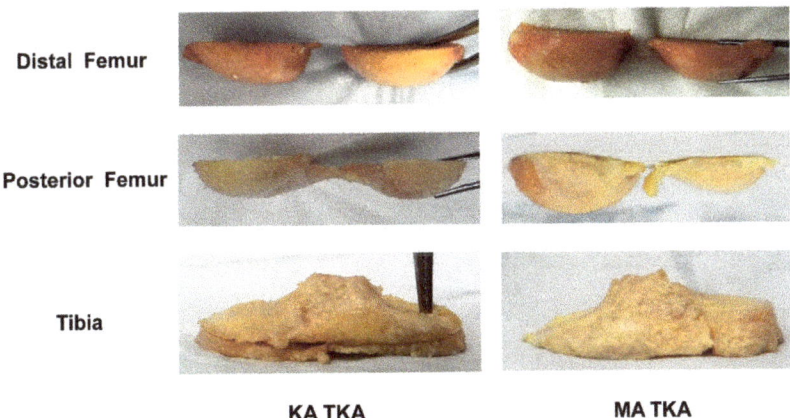

Figure 1. The resected osteochondral fragments. During KA TKA, the femur and tibia resection thicknesses were the same as those of the implants placed in the native joint lines. In the MA TKA group, distal femoral resection was performed perpendicular to the mechanical axis of the femur; the trans-epicondylar axis served as the reference when determining the external rotation of the femoral component. Tibial resection was then performed perpendicular to the mechanical axis of the tibia.

Table 2. Resected osteochondral fragment thickness and gaps after KA and MA TKA.

	KA TKA (n = 8)	MA TKA (n = 8)	Significance
Resected bone thickness (mm)			
Distal femur			
Medial	9.6 (0.7)	10.1 (0.8)	0.227
Lateral	9.8 (0.7)	7.0 (1.1)	<0.001
Posterior femur			
Medial	10.4 (1.5)	11.5 (1.5)	0.158
Lateral	10.5 (1.6)	8.3 (1.0)	<0.001
Tibia			
Medial	6.3 (1.5)	2.1 (0.3)	<0.001
Lateral	6.9 (0.8)	9.6 (1.7)	<0.001
Gap (mm)			
Full extension			
Medial	11.1 (2.2)	12.8 (1.0)	0.076
Lateral	11.8 (2.4)	12.8 (1.0)	0.293
90° flexion			
Medial	12.8 (2.4)	13.4 (1.2)	0.525
Lateral	16.0 (2.3)	13.9 (1.3)	0.078

All data are the mean (standard deviation). KA, kinematic alignment; MA, mechanical alignment; TKA, total knee arthroplasty.

2.4. Test Procedure

Following preparation, each knee was affixed in its original axial position onto a customized knee-squatting simulator system (RNX and Corentec, Seoul, Korea) [18]; this induces continuous flexion–extension knee motion under physiological muscle loading and allows both the femur and the tibia to be positioned with six degrees of freedom (Figure 2A). The ratio between the physiological cross-sectional multiplane loading of the quadriceps and hamstring muscles simulated physiological knee joint loading [29].

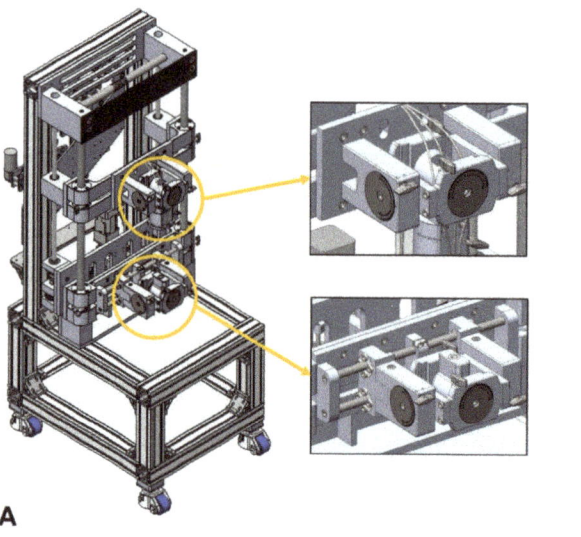
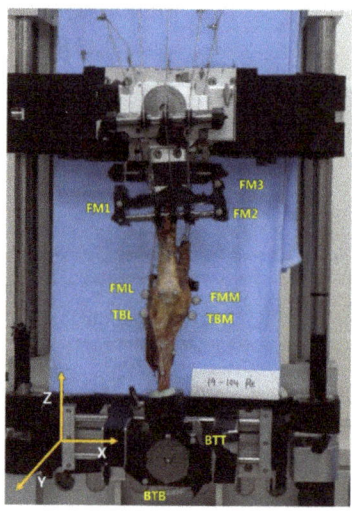

Figure 2. Schematic of the knee-squatting simulator with six degrees-of-freedom (**A**) and locations of the optical markers (**B**) on the femur (FML and FMM); tibia (TBL and TBM); and RIG system (FM1, FM2, and FM3 BTT and BTB).

2.4.1. Knee Kinematics

A motion capture system combined with optical markers (Cortex 8.1; Motion Analysis, Rohnert Park, CA, USA) was used to measure knee kinematics. Five motion capture cameras (Kestrel 1300; Motion Analysis) were employed. Optical markers were attached to the medial and lateral epicondyles of the femur (the FML and FMM); medial and lateral ends of the longest medial-lateral axis of the tibia (the TBL and TBM); and RIG system (FM1, FM2, and FM3 BTT and BTB) to analyze the medial and lateral femoral rollback (Figure 2B). We used an L-frame and 200-mm wand to calibrate the system. After calibration, the wand length was typically 199.99~200.02 mm. We checked the accuracy during continuous movement by measuring the distance between two markers on the rotational disk. Over 60 s at 60 Hz, the root mean square error was 0.012 mm. Samples fixed to the knee rig system were tested from 20° to 80° of flexion. The marker positions were measured at 60 Hz by the motion capture cameras, and the positional coordinates were calculated (Figure 3A).

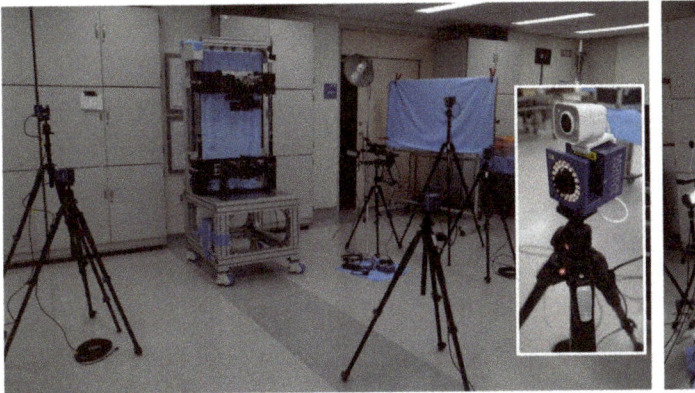
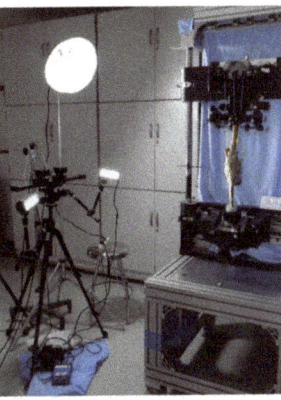

Figure 3. Biomechanical test setup. The motion capture system included five cameras; optical markers were placed when measuring knee kinematics (**A**). Real-time changes in MCL strain during flexion were analyzed using a noncontact video extensometer with a high-resolution digital camera and real-time image-processing software. A camera was placed 1 m from each specimen mounted in a customized knee-squatting simulator (**B**).

2.4.2. MCL Strain

Real-time variations in the mid-flexion MCL strain were examined with a noncontact video extensometer featuring a high-resolution digital camera (ISG Monet 3D; Sobriety s.r.o., Kuřim, Czech Republic) and real-time image processing software (ISG; Mercury RT × 64 2.7; Sobriety). The camera was placed 1 m from each knee (field of view, 485 × 383 mm; resolution, 1.87 μm). In order to minimize the effects of illumination, each test was completed under two 36-W light-emitting diodes. The MCL strain was assessed at knee flexion angles from 20 to 80° at intervals of 10°. The strain was measured over the entire MCL area; measurements were performed on each specimen prior to and following TKA (Figure 3B).

2.5. Statistical Analysis

All data were displayed as means with their corresponding standard deviations. We used the paired t-test to determine whether the medial and lateral rollback, axial rotation, and MCL strain differed between the preoperative and post-TKA specimens. All analyses were completed using SPSS for Windows software (ver. 26.0; IBM Corp., Armonk, NY, USA), and a p-value < 0.05 indicated statistical significance. Additionally, an a priori power analysis based on a pilot test of changes in the femoral rollback and MCL strain of native knees was performed to determine the required sample size. We found that, for two-sided hypothesis testing at an alpha value of 0.05 and power of 90%, seven pairs of knees (14 knees) were needed to detect a 1-mm difference in the rollback and 5% difference in the MCL strain.

3. Results

3.1. Femoral Rollback

KA TKA restored the mid-flexion medial and lateral rollback and tibiofemoral axial rotation to levels closer to those of the native knee than MA TKA. The medial and lateral rollback of KA TKA and native knees was similar over the entire mid-flexion range (Figures 4A and 5A). The medial and lateral rollback after MA TKA were significantly lower compared with native knees at both > 40° (Figure 4B) and >20° (Figure 5B) of flexion. In addition, tibiofemoral axial rotation during flexion after KA TKA was similar to that of the native knee (Figure 6A), while that of MA TKA differed from the native knee in the mid-flexion range (Figure 6B). Remarkably, the femur moved forward during flexion after MA TKA over the entire mid-flexion range, except at 20° of flexion (Figures 4B, 5B and 6B).

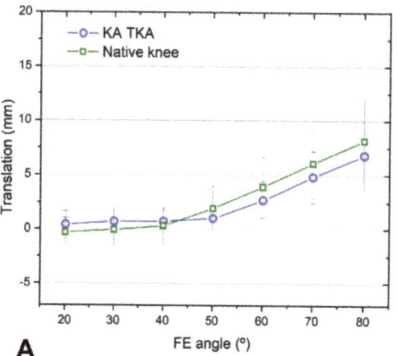 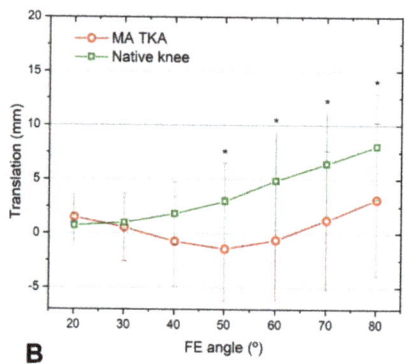

Figure 4. Medial femoral rollback after KA TKA (**A**) and MA TKA (**B**). Rollback following KA TKA and of the native knees were similar at all flexion angles. Meanwhile, rollback following MA TKA was reduced at flexion angles > 40°. Error bars denote standard deviations. Significant differences ($p < 0.05$) are marked with asterisks.

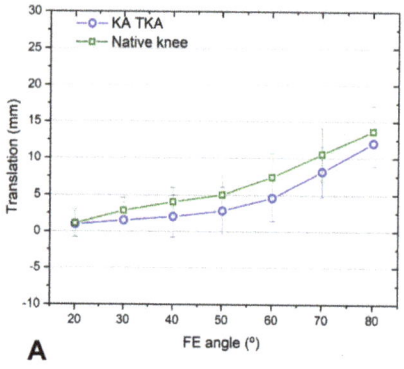 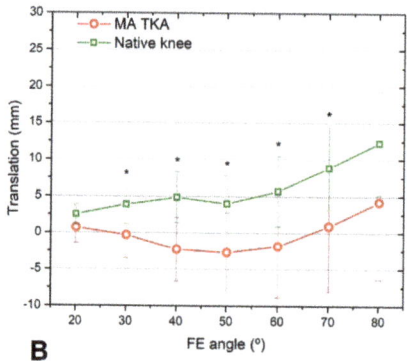

Figure 5. Lateral femoral rollback after KA TKA (**A**) and MA TKA (**B**). Rollback after KA TKA compared to native knee rollback over the entire mid-flexion range, but in the case of MA TKA, the rollback was significantly smaller, except at a flexion angle of 20°. A paradoxical forward movement was observed after MA TKA. Error bars denote standard deviations. Significant differences ($p < 0.05$) are marked with asterisks.

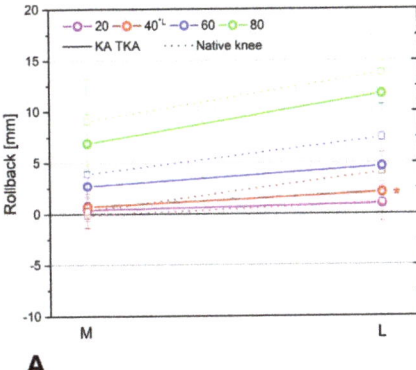
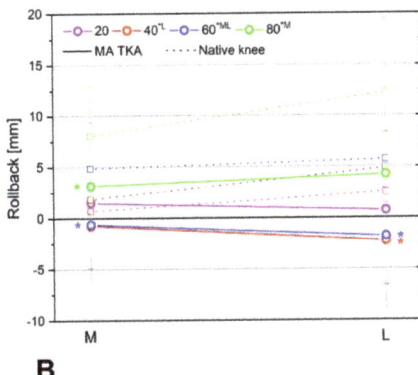

Figure 6. Tibiofemoral axial rotations after KA TKA (**A**) and MA TKA (**B**). During flexion, KA TKA and native knee rotations were similar, while rotation following MA TKA was quite different from that of the native knee. A paradoxical forward movement was observed after MA TKA. Significant differences ($p < 0.05$) are marked with asterisks.

3.2. MCL Strain

KA TKA was better for restoring the MCL strain to that of the native knee over the entire mid-flexion range than MA TKA. The mean strain measurements following KA TKA and those of the native knee were alike over all ranges (Figure 7A). The MCL strain after MA TKA was two-fold greater than that of the native knee at flexion angles > 20° (Figure 7B).

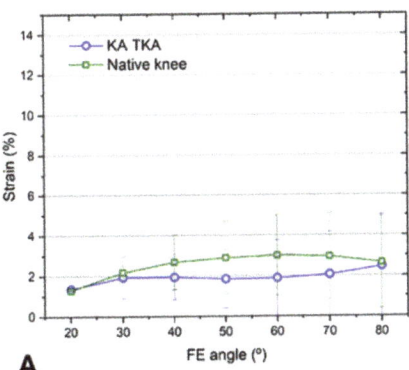
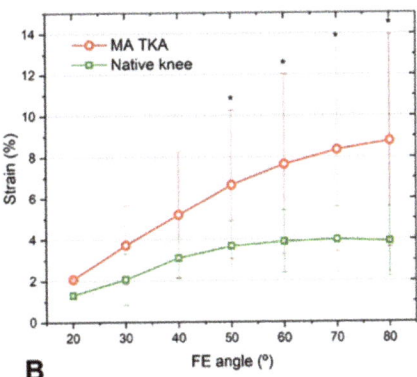

Figure 7. MCL strain after KA TKA (**A**) and MA TKA (**B**). The mean strains following KA TKA and that of the native knee were consistently similar, while the mean strain after MA TKA was about two-fold higher at >30° of flexion. Error bars denote standard deviations. Significant differences ($p < 0.05$) are marked with asterisks.

4. Discussion

Despite advancements in both technology and surgical techniques of MA TKA, patient dissatisfaction with post-TKA pain relief and overall outcomes remains high; a substantial proportion of patients report knee abnormalities [1,2,5,30,31]. KA TKA seeks to restore the anatomy of each individual patient; the kinematic and clinical outcomes are better than those of MA TKA [14–16,18]. Joint line elevation after MA TKA is associated with a risk of mid-flexion instability; theoretically, KA TKA restoration of native joint line height and obliquity makes mid-flexion biomechanics more natural than MA TKA [20,21,25,32].

However, it remains unclear whether restoration of the joint line configuration affects post-TKA mid-flexion kinematics and laxity [12,18,21,24–26]. Therefore, this matched pair cadaveric study tested which TKA alignment concept, KA or MA, would reproduce more native mid-flexion rollback and MCL strain.

The present study's results endorse that KA TKA provides better physiological kinematics over the mid-flexion range than MA TKA, as hypothesized. We found that after KA TKA, medial and lateral femoral rollback, and axial rotation, were consistently similar to those of the native knee, whereas for MA TKA this was the case only at $\leq 40°$ of flexion. In addition, a paradoxical femoral forward movement during flexion was observed after MA TKA. Our findings agree with those of recent cadaveric studies, which suggest that compared to MA TKA, knee kinematics after KA TKA were more alike to those of native knees [14,15,26]. Our results, and those of previous studies, reveal why patients who undergo KA TKA often report superior mid-flexion functional performance compared with those who undergo MA TKA.

Our findings also support the hypothesis that the joint line following KA TKA is better for restoring natural MCL strain during mid-flexion than the perpendicular joint line after MA TKA. KA TKA resulted in MCL strain that was consistently comparable to that of native knees, whereas, in the case of MA TKA, it was twice as high. Our findings agree with those of a recent cadaveric study: KA TKA was better for restoring the magnitude and distribution of MCL strain to natural levels than MA TKA [18]. Although it is challenging to directly liken our results with those of prior studies that assessed MCL strain via linear, two-dimensional measurements of length changes under valgus stress, our findings support previous studies that report that restoration of the pre-arthritic joint line provided a more physiological MCL strain than traditional MA TKA [12,14,15,26,33]. Furthermore, our results, when taken into consideration with the widely acknowledged existence of a nociceptor in the MCL [34], indicate that patients may experience less pain and more native knee sensations during mid-flexion after KA TKA, as opposed to MA TKA.

The results of the present study propose that restoration of natural MCL strain via KA TKA may explain the more physiological knee kinematics evident after KA TKA compared to MA TKA. In this study, KA TKA reproduces more physiological medial pivot motion, while MA TKA results in paradoxical anterior motion during mid-flexion. Given that the MCL serves as the fundamental restraint in ACL-deficient, prosthetic knees, our findings suggest that MCL strain may be strongly associated with restoration of knee kinematics. Interestingly, a recent cadaveric study reported that restoration of joint line obliquity was not associated with mid-flexion coronal plane laxity, if the medial joint line height was restored [21]. However, although we restored the medial joint line height in all knees, our study found a significant difference between KA and MA TKA knees in the MCL strain. Still, the correlation between these findings is limited, since the previous study assessed soft tissue laxity by the length changes of MCL after the valgus load, and information on knee kinematics was not presented. Although the cause of the inconsistencies is unclear, one plausible explanation is that, although valgus stress increases the MCL strain, the MCL length may not change if the stress is lower than the threshold required for such change.

Due to the use of a cadaveric model, this study has some limitations. First, specimen preparation and the squatting loads used may not have been entirely natural. Second, as the tissue quality around the knee joint is associated with the severity of knee OA, the experimental results could be affected by the OA status of the cadaver. However, most knees in this study lacked advanced osteoarthritis necessitating TKA, so caution is required when extrapolating our findings to clinical practice. Third, this study featured PS prosthesis, which requires consideration of the implant feature prior to any broad generalizations, as implant design has been shown to be strongly correlated with knee kinematics [26,35]. Generally, when performing KA TKA, a cruciate-retaining (CR) prosthesis is recommended. However, a recent study found that native knees, and knees in which CR and PS prostheses were placed during KA TKA, had similar kinematics and soft tissue laxity [14]. Fourth, because the thresholds for pain and mechanical failure in the human knee are unknown, assessing the clinical significance of MCL strain was difficult. Fifth, it is possible that the study was underpowered and subject type-II error with respect to detecting all relevant outcomes. Sixth, the group assignment for the knees were not kept blinded to all investigators, which could have raised ascertainment bias. Finally, biofeedback, which is natural in knee function and enhanced by the innovative TKA surgical technique, could have introduced nonlinearity in the feedback and improved the signal-to-noise ratio in the loop [36]. Thus, the video extensometer that we used does not process data with 100% accuracy; changes in illumination may affect image processing, because illumination affects the properties of biomaterials. Nevertheless, we used a matched-pair design to minimize confounders, and this is the first study to simultaneously measure femoral rollback and MCL strain. These results provide valuable insight on the differences regarding mid-flexion kinematics and patterns of MCL strain between KA TKA and MA TKA.

5. Conclusions

We investigated whether restoration of the pre-arthritic joint line following TKA would affect post-TKA biomechanics. Restoration of the height and obliquity of the pre-arthritic joint line following KA TKA reproduces more natural rollback and MCL strain than alteration of the joint line following MA TKA over the entire mid-flexion range. Future studies focused on the development of both the motion analysis system that assesses the knee kinematics of patients in real clinical practice and the algorithm that recommends the optimal implant position restoring native knee kinematics are required.

Author Contributions: Conceptualization, I.J.K., D.-S.K. and D.L.; methodology, D.-S.K. and M.S.K.; software, D.-S.K. and M.S.K.; validation, D.-S.K. and D.L.; formal analysis, D.-S.K.; investigation, I.J.K. and Y.I.; resources, D.-S.K., D.L. and I.J.K.; data curation, D.-S.K., N.C. and M.S.K.; writing—original draft preparation, Y.D.K. and D.-S.K.; writing—review and editing, I.J.K. and N.C.; visualization, D.-S.K. and I.J.K.; supervision, I.J.K. and Y.I.; project administration, I.J.K., D.-S.K. and D.L.; funding acquisition, I.J.K., D.-S.K. and D.L. All authors have read and agreed to the published version of the manuscript.

Funding: This work was supported by the National Research Foundation of Korea (NRF) grant funded by the Korea government (MSIT) (No. 2019 R1F1A 1057842 and No. 2017M3A9E9073545) and the Industry-Academy Cooperation Program through the Industry Academic Cooperation Foundation of the Catholic University of Korea (5-2020-D0721-00001). The funding source did not play any scientific role in performing this study.

Institutional Review Board Statement: This cadaveric study was conducted in compliance with the Act on Dissection and Preservation of Corpses of the Republic of Korea (act number: 14885) and approved by the Institutional Cadaver Research Committee of College of Medicine, The Catholic University of Korea (code number: R19-A018).

Informed Consent Statement: Written informed consent for use of the cadavers and consent for use of future research on the related materials were provided by all donors or authorized representatives.

Data Availability Statement: All data are presented in the article. Instrumental readings are available upon request from the corresponding author.

Acknowledgments: We thank Smith & Nephew (Seoul, Korea) for providing all surgical instruments. In particular, we thank Su Gu Chai B.S. and Seung Jun Lee P.R.S. of Smith & Nephew and Ki Joon Yoo B.A., Jae Young Sung B.S. and Hyunggu Han B.A. of Daon HealthCare (Seoul, Korea) for their assistance. We also thank the cadaver donors and their families.

Conflicts of Interest: The authors declare that they have no conflict of interest.

References

1. Bourne, R.B.; Chesworth, B.M.; Davis, A.M.; Mahomed, N.N.; Charron, K.D. Patient satisfaction after total knee arthroplasty: Who is satisfied and who is not? *Clin. Orthop. Relat. Res.* **2010**, *468*, 57–63. [CrossRef] [PubMed]
2. Nam, D.; Nunley, R.M.; Barrack, R.L. Patient dissatisfaction following total knee replacement: A growing concern? *Bone Joint J.* **2014**, *96-B*, 96–100. [CrossRef] [PubMed]

3. Pawar, P.; Naik, L.; Sahu, D.; Bagaria, V. Comparative Study of Pinless Navigation System versus Conventional Instrumentation in Total Knee Arthroplasty. *Clin. Orthop. Surg.* **2021**, *13*, 358–365. [CrossRef] [PubMed]
4. Park, C.H.; Song, S.J. Sensor-Assisted Total Knee Arthroplasty: A Narrative Review. *Clin. Orthop. Surg.* **2021**, *13*, 1–9. [CrossRef]
5. Halawi, M.J.; Jongbloed, W.; Baron, S.; Savoy, L.; Williams, V.J.; Cote, M.P. Patient Dissatisfaction after Primary Total Joint Arthroplasty: The Patient Perspective. *J. Arthroplasty* **2019**, *34*, 1093–1096. [CrossRef]
6. Bellemans, J.; Colyn, W.; Vandenneucker, H.; Victor, J. The Chitranjan Ranawat award: Is neutral mechanical alignment normal for all patients? The concept of constitutional varus. *Clin. Orthop. Relat. Res.* **2012**, *470*, 45–53. [CrossRef]
7. Hirschmann, M.T.; Moser, L.B.; Amsler, F.; Behrend, H.; Leclercq, V.; Hess, S. Phenotyping the knee in young non-osteoarthritic knees shows a wide distribution of femoral and tibial coronal alignment. *Knee Surg. Sports Traumatol. Arthrosc.* **2019**, *27*, 1385–1393. [CrossRef]
8. Thienpont, E.; Schwab, P.E.; Cornu, O.; Bellemans, J.; Victor, J. Bone morphotypes of the varus and valgus knee. *Arch. Orthop. Trauma. Surg.* **2017**, *137*, 393–400. [CrossRef]
9. Abdel, M.P.; Oussedik, S.; Parratte, S.; Lustig, S.; Haddad, F.S. Coronal alignment in total knee replacement: Historical review, contemporary analysis, and future direction. *Bone Joint J.* **2014**, *96-b*, 857–862. [CrossRef]
10. Riviere, C.; Iranpour, F.; Auvinet, E.; Howell, S.; Vendittoli, P.A.; Cobb, J.; Parratte, S. Alignment options for total knee arthroplasty: A systematic review. *Orthop. Traumatol. Surg. Res.* **2017**, *103*, 1047–1056. [CrossRef]
11. Courtney, P.M.; Lee, G.C. Early Outcomes of Kinematic Alignment in Primary Total Knee Arthroplasty: A Meta-Analysis of the Literature. *J. Arthroplasty* **2017**, *32*, 2028–2032.e2021. [CrossRef]
12. Delport, H.; Labey, L.; Innocenti, B.; De Corte, R.; Vander Sloten, J.; Bellemans, J. Restoration of constitutional alignment in TKA leads to more physiological strains in the collateral ligaments. *Knee Surg. Sports Traumatol. Arthrosc.* **2015**, *23*, 2159–2169. [CrossRef]
13. Dossett, H.G.; Estrada, N.A.; Swartz, G.J.; LeFevre, G.W.; Kwasman, B.G. A randomised controlled trial of kinematically and mechanically aligned total knee replacements: Two-year clinical results. *Bone Joint J.* **2014**, *96-b*, 907–913. [CrossRef]
14. Koh, I.J.; Chalmers, C.E.; Lin, C.C.; Park, S.B.; McGarry, M.H.; Lee, T.Q. Posterior stabilized total knee arthroplasty reproduces natural joint laxity compared to normal in kinematically aligned total knee arthroplasty: A matched pair cadaveric study. *Arch. Orthop. Trauma. Surg.* **2021**, *141*, 119–127. [CrossRef]
15. Koh, I.J.; Lin, C.C.; Patel, N.A.; Chalmers, C.E.; Maniglio, M.; Han, S.B.; McGarry, M.H.; Lee, T.Q. Kinematically aligned total knee arthroplasty reproduces more native rollback and laxity than mechanically aligned total knee arthroplasty: A matched pair cadaveric study. *Orthop. Traumatol. Surg. Res.* **2019**, *105*, 605–611. [CrossRef]
16. Koh, I.J.; Park, I.J.; Lin, C.C.; Patel, N.A.; Chalmers, C.E.; Maniglio, M.; McGarry, M.H.; Lee, T.Q. Kinematically aligned total knee arthroplasty reproduces native patellofemoral biomechanics during deep knee flexion. *Knee Surg. Sports Traumatol. Arthrosc.* **2019**, *27*, 1520–1528. [CrossRef]
17. Lee, Y.S.; Howell, S.M.; Won, Y.Y.; Lee, O.S.; Lee, S.H.; Vahedi, H.; Teo, S.H. Kinematic alignment is a possible alternative to mechanical alignment in total knee arthroplasty. *Knee Surg. Sports Traumatol. Arthrosc.* **2017**, *25*, 3467–3479. [CrossRef]
18. Lim, D.; Kwak, D.S.; Kim, M.; Kim, S.; Cho, H.J.; Choi, J.H.; Koh, I.J. Kinematically aligned total knee arthroplasty restores more native medial collateral ligament strain than mechanically aligned total knee arthroplasty. *Knee Surg. Sports Traumatol. Arthrosc.* **2022**, *30*, 2815–2823. [CrossRef]
19. Rowe, P.J.; Myles, C.M.; Walker, C.; Nutton, R. Knee joint kinematics in gait and other functional activities measured using flexible electrogoniometry: How much knee motion is sufficient for normal daily life? *Gait Posture* **2000**, *12*, 143–155. [CrossRef]
20. Shalhoub, S.; Moschetti, W.E.; Dabuzhsky, L.; Jevsevar, D.S.; Keggi, J.M.; Plaskos, C. Laxity Profiles in the Native and Replaced Knee-Application to Robotic-Assisted Gap-Balancing Total Knee Arthroplasty. *J. Arthroplasty* **2018**, *33*, 3043–3048. [CrossRef]
21. Luyckx, T.; Vandenneucker, H.; Ing, L.S.; Vereecke, E.; Ing, A.V.; Victor, J. Raising the Joint Line in TKA is Associated with Mid-flexion Laxity: A Study in Cadaver Knees. *Clin. Orthop. Relat. Res.* **2018**, *476*, 601–611. [CrossRef]
22. Van Lieshout, W.A.M.; Valkering, K.P.; Koenraadt, K.L.M.; van Etten-Jamaludin, F.S.; Kerkhoffs, G.; van Geenen, R.C.I. The negative effect of joint line elevation after total knee arthroplasty on outcome. *Knee Surg. Sports Traumatol. Arthrosc.* **2019**, *27*, 1477–1486. [CrossRef]
23. Abdel, M.P.; Ollivier, M.; Parratte, S.; Trousdale, R.T.; Berry, D.J.; Pagnano, M.W. Effect of Postoperative Mechanical Axis Alignment on Survival and Functional Outcomes of Modern Total Knee Arthroplasties with Cement: A Concise Follow-up at 20 Years. *J. Bone Joint. Surg. Am.* **2018**, *100*, 472–478. [CrossRef]
24. Minoda, Y.; Sugama, R.; Ohta, Y.; Ueyama, H.; Takemura, S.; Nakamura, H. Joint line elevation is not associated with mid-flexion laxity in patients with varus osteoarthritis after total knee arthroplasty. *Knee Surg. Sports Traumatol. Arthrosc.* **2020**, *28*, 3226–3231. [CrossRef]
25. Vajapey, S.P.; Pettit, R.J.; Li, M.; Chen, A.F.; Spitzer, A.I.; Glassman, A.H. Risk Factors for Mid-Flexion Instability after Total Knee Arthroplasty: A Systematic Review. *J. Arthroplasty* **2020**, *35*, 3046–3054. [CrossRef]
26. Maderbacher, G.; Keshmiri, A.; Krieg, B.; Greimel, F.; Grifka, J.; Baier, C. Kinematic component alignment in total knee arthroplasty leads to better restoration of natural tibiofemoral kinematics compared to mechanic alignment. *Knee Surg. Sports Traumatol. Arthrosc.* **2019**, *27*, 1427–1433. [CrossRef]
27. Howell, S.M.; Papadopoulos, S.; Kuznik, K.T.; Hull, M.L. Accurate alignment and high function after kinematically aligned TKA performed with generic instruments. *Knee Surg. Sports Traumatol. Arthrosc.* **2013**, *21*, 2271–2280. [CrossRef] [PubMed]

28. Nedopil, A.J.; Singh, A.K.; Howell, S.M.; Hull, M.L. Does Calipered Kinematically Aligned TKA Restore Native Left to Right Symmetry of the Lower Limb and Improve Function? *J. Arthroplasty* **2018**, *33*, 398–406. [CrossRef] [PubMed]
29. Wickiewicz, T.L.; Roy, R.R.; Powell, P.L.; Edgerton, V.R. Muscle architecture of the human lower limb. *Clin. Orthop. Relat. Res.* **1983**, *179*, 275–283. [CrossRef]
30. Simcox, T.; Singh, V.; Oakley, C.T.; Barzideh, O.S.; Schwarzkopf, R.; Rozell, J.C. A comparison of utilization and short-term complications of technology-assisted versus conventional total knee arthroplasty. *Knee Surg. Relat. Res.* **2022**, *34*, 14. [CrossRef] [PubMed]
31. Tanifuji, O.; Mochizuki, T.; Yamagiwa, H.; Sato, T.; Watanabe, S.; Hijikata, H.; Kawashima, H. Comparison of post-operative three-dimensional and two-dimensional evaluation of component position for total knee arthroplasty. *Knee Surg. Relat. Res.* **2021**, *33*, 21. [CrossRef]
32. Cross, M.B.; Nam, D.; Plaskos, C.; Sherman, S.L.; Lyman, S.; Pearle, A.D.; Mayman, D.J. Recutting the distal femur to increase maximal knee extension during TKA causes coronal plane laxity in mid-flexion. *Knee* **2012**, *19*, 875–879. [CrossRef]
33. Watanabe, M.; Kuriyama, S.; Nakamura, S.; Nishitani, K.; Tanaka, Y.; Sekiguchi, K.; Ito, H.; Matsuda, S. Abnormal knee kinematics caused by mechanical alignment in symmetric bicruciate-retaining total knee arthroplasty are alleviated by kinematic alignment. *Knee* **2020**, *27*, 1385–1395. [CrossRef]
34. Cabuk, H.; Kusku Cabuk, F. Mechanoreceptors of the ligaments and tendons around the knee. *Clin. Anat.* **2016**, *29*, 789–795. [CrossRef]
35. Chang, M.J.; Kang, S.B.; Chang, C.B.; Han, D.H.; Park, H.J.; Hwang, K.; Park, J.; Hwang, I.U.; Lee, S.A.; Oh, S. Posterior condylar offset changes and its effect on clinical outcomes after posterior-substituting, fixed-bearing total knee arthroplasty: Anterior versus posterior referencing. *Knee Surg. Relat. Res.* **2020**, *32*, 10. [CrossRef]
36. Bucolo, M.; Buscarino, A.; Fortuna, L.; Gagliano, S. Can Noise in the Feedback Improve the Performance of a Control System? *J. Phys. Soc. Jpn.* **2021**, *90*, 075002. [CrossRef]

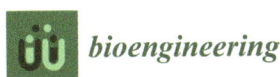

Review

Multibody Models of the Thoracolumbar Spine: A Review on Applications, Limitations, and Challenges

Tanja Lerchl [1,2,*], Kati Nispel [1,2], Thomas Baum [2], Jannis Bodden [2], Veit Senner [1] and Jan S. Kirschke [2]

[1] Sport Equipment and Sport Materials, School of Engineering and Design, Technical University of Munich, 85748 Garching, Germany
[2] Department of Diagnostic and Interventional Neuroradiology, School of Medicine, Klinikum Rechts der Isar, Technical University of Munich, 81675 Munich, Germany
* Correspondence: tanja.lerchl@tum.de; Tel.: +49-89-289-15365

Abstract: Numerical models of the musculoskeletal system as investigative tools are an integral part of biomechanical and clinical research. While finite element modeling is primarily suitable for the examination of deformation states and internal stresses in flexible bodies, multibody modeling is based on the assumption of rigid bodies, that are connected via joints and flexible elements. This simplification allows the consideration of biomechanical systems from a holistic perspective and thus takes into account multiple influencing factors of mechanical loads. Being the source of major health issues worldwide, the human spine is subject to a variety of studies using these models to investigate and understand healthy and pathological biomechanics of the upper body. In this review, we summarize the current state-of-the-art literature on multibody models of the thoracolumbar spine and identify limitations and challenges related to current modeling approaches.

Keywords: musculoskeletal multibody dynamics; spinal biomechanics; spinal alignment; spinal loading; muscle force computation; thoracolumbar spine; biomechanical model

Citation: Lerchl, T.; Nispel, K.; Baum, T.; Bodden, J.; Senner, V.; Kirschke, J.S. Multibody Models of the Thoracolumbar Spine: A Review on Applications, Limitations, and Challenges. *Bioengineering* **2023**, *10*, 202. https://doi.org/10.3390/bioengineering10020202

Academic Editors: Christina Zong-Hao Ma, Zhengrong Li and Chen He

Received: 29 December 2022
Revised: 30 January 2023
Accepted: 31 January 2023
Published: 3 February 2023

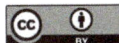

Copyright: © 2023 by the authors. Licensee MDPI, Basel, Switzerland. This article is an open access article distributed under the terms and conditions of the Creative Commons Attribution (CC BY) license (https://creativecommons.org/licenses/by/4.0/).

1. Introduction

Chronic back pain is one of the major health issues worldwide. Though general risk factors such as occupation, obesity or anthropometric parameters could be identified in the past years [1], the specification of individual biomechanical indicators for the prediction of symptoms and chronicity is challenging, as it requires an in-depth knowledge of spinal kinematics and resulting loads. Even though experimental methods are essential to help build this knowledge, they come with limitations. In vitro studies can help understand segment mechanics but are not applicable when it comes to the investigation of complex in vivo biomechanics of the whole torso [2]. The invasive character of the in vivo measurement of these parameters via intradiscal pressure sensors [3,4] or instrumented vertebral implants [5,6] makes these methods unsuitable for clinical analysis. Computational, biomechanical models can provide a valuable alternative when it comes to the estimation of spinal loads. There are two approaches for the numerical analysis of spinal loading. While finite element models (FEM) hold the potential to investigate internal stress states in flexible bodies and their underlying or resulting deformation, multibody models (multibody system, MBS) can help analyze mechanical loads on the musculoskeletal system at a holistic level. Breaking the system down to its essential mechanical components, classic MBS models incorporate rigid bodies connected by joints and, depending on the respective research question, force elements representing flexible structures such as intervertebral discs (IVD), ligaments, cartilage, and other connective tissue. This way, MBS models represent a valuable tool to increase a profound understanding of healthy and pathological biomechanics. Gould et al. published a review on FEM and MBS models of the healthy and scoliotic spine in 2021 [7]. Focusing on the latter one, the authors state that their review provides solely a brief overview on MBS models of the healthy spine and refer the reader to the review on MBS modeling of the cervical spine by Alizadeh et al. [8] and the review by Dreischarf et al. on in vivo studies and computational models, published in 2016 [9].

The wide range of applications, improved technical capabilities, and increasing knowledge of spinal biomechanics, which answer old questions and raise new ones, mean that the demand for high-quality MBS models is not abating. As a consequence, the number of published models is increasing every year providing new opportunities and insight.

In recent years, models have been introduced that extend the classic notion of a multibody or musculoskeletal models. These models incorporate flexible bodies such as beam elements into rigid body models and thus soften the boundary between FEM and MBS models [10,11]. However, within the scope of this work, we want to review the developments in the field of multibody models of the healthy thoracolumbar spine, focusing on classical rigid body models. Hereby, we shed light on common modeling methods and applications, as well as identify and discuss related limitations and challenges in state-of-the-art spine modeling.

2. Methods

To generate a list of potentially relevant publications, a systematic search was carried out in PubMed and Scopus in November and December 2022. The search included the keywords "spine AND model AND ((multi AND body) OR musculoskeletal)". Excluding results prior to 2013 left 1288 publications on PubMed and 1304 on Scopus. However, relevant citations in the articles were also included, if they were published before 2013. Subsequently, duplicates were removed by identical PubMedIDs and titles. Remaining articles were then filtered by title and abstract and the full text eventually analyzed. Publications were excluded if they featured at least one of the following topics:

- Finite element modeling;
- Models of the cervical spine;
- Models without muscle incorporation;
- Models of the scoliotic spine;
- Models of the nonhuman spine;
- Studies with a medical scope other than biomechanics.

Inclusion criteria were set to

- Musculoskeletal models;
- Multibody models;
- Models of the thoracolumbar spine;
- Models of the healthy spine.

We analyzed the remaining studies systematically according to the represented modeling methods and applications and identified existing limitations and challenges.

3. Multibody Modeling of the Healthy Spine

After filtering a total of 2592 articles, 81 articles remained, which were included in this review. Focusing on extensive musculoskeletal models of the thoracolumbar spine, we discuss models with reduced complexity, such as abstracted models [12–16], skeletal models neglecting muscular effects [17,18] or models of the lumbar spine [19–29] only in passing.

Overall, our literature review revealed that a large proportion of published studies was based on a few original models [30–33]. Due to the accessibility of these models via the commercially available software AnyBody (AnyBody Technology A/S, Aalborg, Denmark) [30,33] or the open-source software OpenSim [31,32,34], numerous studies can be found that used, modified, and extended these models, beyond the boundaries of the respective research groups as well [35–58]. Apart from these widely reused models, further original models can be found in the literature using alternative software [59–64]. Table 1 provides an overview of the original models found and subsequent studies associated with them.

Table 1. Overview of original models of the musculoskeletal thoracolumbar spine and related modeling methods. Semi-individualized models are those that contain both individualized and generic musculoskeletal components. Joint definitions include potentially assigned constraints.

Reference	Included Segments	Joint Definition	Generic/Indiv.	Passive Force Elements	Muscle Model and Force Estimation	Software	Related Studies
de Zee et al. [30]	Pelvis, sacrum, L1-L5, thorax	3 rot. DOFs (IV)	Generic	-	Act., ID, SO	AnyBody	[33,35,36,39,44,45,47,65]
Christophy et al. [31]	Pelvis, sacrum, L1-L5, thorax	3 rot. DOFs (IV)	Generic	-	Hill type	OpenSim	[37,40,41,46,48–53]
Bruno et al. [32]	Pelvis, sacrum, T1-L5, ribs, sternum, upper limbs, head–neck	3 rot. DOFs (IV) 1 rot. DOFs (CV)	Generic	-	Hill type, ID, SO	OpenSim	[38,42,43,54–58]
Ignasiak et al. [33]	Pelvis, sacrum, T1-L5, ribs, sternum head–neck	6 rot. DOFs (IV) 1 rot. DOFs (CV/CT) 3 rot. DOFs (CS I) 6 rot. DOFs (CS II-X)	Generic	CS, CT, CV, IV joint (lin.)	Act., ID, FSK [66], SO	AnyBody	[39,67,68]
Lerchl et al. [59]	Pelvis, sacrum, L1-L5, thorax, upper limbs, head–neck	3 rot. DOFs (IV)	Semi-indiv.	Lig. (nonlin.) IVD (nonlin.)	Actuators, ID, SO	Simpack	-
Favier et al. [69]	Lower limbs pelvis, sacrum, L1-L5, thorax (3 segments), upper limbs, head–neck	3 rot. DOFs (IV)	Semi-indiv.	Joint (lin.)	Hill type, IK, ID, SO	OpenSim	-
Malakoutian et al. [60]	Pelvis, sacrum, L1-L5, thorax, humeri	6 DOFs (IV)	generic	Joint, IAP	Hill type, FD-assisted SO	AriSynth	[70]
Rupp et al. [61]	Pelvis, sacrum, L1-L5, thorax	6 DOFs (IV)	Generic	Lig. (nonlin.) IVD (nonlin.)	Hill type, FD	In-house	-
Fasser et al. [62]	Pelvis, sacrum, L1-L5, thorax	3 rot. DOFs (IV)	Semi-indiv.	-	Hill type, IK, ID, SO	Matlab	[71]
Bayoglu et al. [72]	Pelvis, sacrum, C1-L5, ribs, sternum, skull (3 segments), shoulder (3 Segments)	3 rot. DOFs (IV) 6 DOFs (CS) 1 DOF (CV/CT)	Individ.	Joint (lin.)	Act., ID, SO	AnyBody	[73–75]
Huynh et al. [63]	Full-body, C1-L5	3 rot. DOFs (IV)	Generic	Lig. (lin.) IVD (lin.), IAP	IK, ID, SO	LifeMOD	[76]
Khurelbaatar et al. [64]	Pelvis, sacrum, C1-L5, ribs, sternum, upper limbs, head	6 DOFs (IV/CS) 3 rot. DOFs (CV)	Semi-indiv. (bones)	Lig. (nonlin.), IVD (nonlin.), CS cartilage (lin.), facet joints	Act., ID, SO	RECURDYN	-
Guo et al. [77]	Pelvis, sacrum, C1-L5, ribs, sternum, upper limbs, head	6 DOFs (IV)	Generic	Lig. (nonlin.), IVD (lin.), facet joints, IAP	Hill type, ALE, FD	OpenSim	-

The definition of the abbreviations can be found at the end of this article.

3.1. General Model Setup and Kinematics

In the past two decades, simplified models of the whole torso with a detailed lumbar spine were developed to investigate lumbar loads [30,31,59,61,69]. One of the first generic models for lumbar load estimation was introduced by de Zee et al. in 2007 [30], which comprised seven rigid bodies for the pelvis including the sacrum, five lumbar vertebrae, and one lumped segment representing the thoracic spine including the rib cage and cervical spine. The model anatomy was based on publications by Hansen et al. [78] and Bodguk et al. [79]. De Zee defined intervertebral joints as spherical joints with their respective center of rotation (COR) located in the intersection of the instantaneous axis of rotation and the midsagittal plane according to Pearcy and Bodguk [80]. A total of 154 actuators representing muscle fascicles for the erector spinae (ES), rectus abdominis (RA), internal obliques (IO), external obliques (EO), psoas major (PM), quadratus lumborum (QL), and multifidus (MF) were implemented in the model either as a straight line between insertion and origin or, in order to mimic more realistic lines of action, redirected using so-called via points or wrapping surfaces [30].

Inspired by de Zee's model, Christophy et al. published a generic multibody model of the lumbar spine in 2012 [31], incorporating a more detailed muscle architecture regarding the latissimus dorsi (LD) and the MF muscle. Using the open-source software OpenSim [34], the model has been widely used and extended in the past years [31,37,40,41,48–52,81,82]. In recent years, other models with simplified thorax have been published [59,61,69].

Favier et al. published a full-body model with a detailed lumbar spine in 2021 [69]. The model was created in OpenSim and included in total 20 rigid bodies including the head–neck, three-segment thoracic and cervical spine (spherical joints in T7-T8 and C7-T1), five lumbar vertebrae, pelvis with sacrum, as well as upper and lower extremities. The model incorporated a total of 538 muscle actuators for the lower limbs and lumbar spine [69].

Lerchl et al. introduced a pipeline for the semiautomated generation of individualized MBS models with a detailed lumbar spine created in the commercial multibody modeling software Simpack (Dassault Systèmes, France) in 2022 [59]. Based on CT data, the models included individual vertebrae T1-L5 with a fused thoracic part and rib cage and spherical lumbar intervertebral joints, and generic segments for the head–neck, pelvis, sacrum, and simplified arms. A total number of 103 actuators representing the muscles of the lower back were incorporated [59].

Research devoted to the loading of the thoracic spine is less common and therefore, only few models incorporating a detailed thoracic spine and rib cage can be found in the literature [32,33,72]. As opposed to musculoskeletal models with a rigid thorax, these models allow a comprehensive analysis of spinal loading for load cases involving thoracic movement. Based on the generic model of the lumbar spine by de Zee et al. [30], Ignasiak et al. introduced a musculoskeletal model of the thoracolumbar spine with a detailed articulated rib cage [33]. Ignasiak et al. extended the model by individual rigid bodies of 12 vertebrae, 10 pairs of ribs, and a sternum. Intervertebral thoracic joints were defined as six-DOF joints and lumbar joints, originally modeled as spherical joints [30], were also modified, respectively. Costovertebral (CV) and costotransverse (CT) joints were defined as revolute joints with the rotation axis in the frontal direction and all joints between the ribs and the sternum were modeled with six DOFs, except the first pair, which were modeled as spherical joints. The model was validated against in vivo data and used in follow-up studies [33,39,67,68].

A comprehensive model of the upper body including 60 segments (vertebrae, ribs, skull, sternum, hyoid, thyrohyoid, clavicles, scapulas, humeri, sacrum, and pelvis) created in AnyBody was published by Bayoglu et al. in 2019 [72].

Based on the lumbar spine model of Christophy et al. [31], Bruno et al. developed and validated a fully articulated model of the thoracolumbar spine in OPENSIM including individual vertebrae, ribs, and sternum [32]. Like Christophy's model, the thoracolumbar model of Bruno et al. has been widely used and adapted since its publication [32,43,54,56–58,83,84].

In biomechanical MBS modeling, intersegmental connections are usually implemented as joints with defined DOFs, which can either be defined directly in the joint or are implemented as constraints, limiting the joint's effective degrees of freedom to its relevant components. It is common practice to model intervertebral joints as spherical joints allowing rotation around three spatial axes [31,62]. Few models exist, that defined intervertebral joints with six DOFs, additionally accounting for translational motion [33,37,41,61]. The centers of rotation are located either in the geometrical center of the IVD [33,59,62] or in the instantaneous axis of rotation according to Pearcy and Bodguk [30,31,69,80]. CV joints are modeled as pin joints rotating around the vector between the costovertebral and costotransverse joints [32,33,72] or spherical joints [64] and CS joints as six DOFs [33,64,72]. Depending on the simulation approach (Section 3.4), kinematic data have been most commonly assigned to the respective DOFs according to findings from our own experimental studies or the literature (Section 3.3). This way, model kinematics are usually described using relative minimum coordinates. However, for inverse kinematic approaches, absolute coordinates are assigned to the end link of the kinematic chain. Providing stable boundary conditions for the mechanical analyses, the models are usually connected to the inertial frame of reference and therefore leaving the head–neck complex as the end link of the open kinematic chain. Upper-body weight is either combined and included in the center of mass of the lumped thoracic body [61], distributed according to the literature [85,86] or derived from patient-specific CT or MRI data and distributed levelwise along the thoracolumbar spine [59,62].

3.2. Passive (Visco)elastic Components

Various approaches have been taken regarding the modeling of viscoelastic structures that passively stabilize the spine, such as IVD, spinal ligaments, or the (cartilage) tissue of the thorax. The modeling approach can vary both in the level of detail and in the mechanical characteristics considered. Thus, some models neglect the effects of these components entirely [30–32,62], whereas others combine them partially or completely into one single stabilizing element per joint [60,69,72], or even integrate individual components explicitly [59,61,64,77]. The majority of approaches simplify the mechanical properties of connective tissue to linear elastic force elements, which produce corresponding forces and moments exclusively depending on their deformation. In multibody models, such material behavior is described via spring elements with constant stiffness for the corresponding DOFs. Only a few models incorporate the nonlinear mechanical behavior of biological passive structures [87]. However, modeling these components as purely elastic does not account for viscous effects that influence the mechanical response as a function of the deformation rate, also known as damping behavior. A detailed nonlinear viscoelastic modeling of IVDs and spinal ligaments, such as the anterior and posterior longitudinal ligament, the flavum ligament, as well as the interspinal and supraspinal ligament, can be found in only a few models [59,61]. The respective parameters are usually taken from in vitro studies available in the literature [88–92].

To examine thoracic loads, models require an appropriate force transmission from the rib cage to the thoracic spine in addition to intervertebral passive structures. In this context, costosternal (CS), costotransverse (CT) and costovertebral (CV) articulations are a central issue. Commonly, these connections are constrained and modeled as linear elastic elements according to the resulting DOFs. Stiffness parameters are usually taken from in vitro studies or adapted from previously published in silico studies. Bruno et al. included point-to-point actuators, which were placed between the ends of the ribs and the sternum (ribs 1–7) or between the ends of adjacent ribs (ribs 8–10) to represent forces transmitted by costal cartilage. As a result of a sensitivity analysis, forces generated by the actuators were set to 1000 N allowing the costal cartilage to provide a high supporting force to the end of the ribs [32].

Mechanical properties are usually incorporated either directly from mechanical testing, such as ligament tensile tests [88,93] or by simulating in vitro protocols, such as stepwise reduction studies, where individual connective structures are gradually removed from functional biological units, such as the FSU or the rib cage, while measuring the mechanical properties of the units after every resection [89,94,95]. However, due to the high level of intra- and interindividual variability regarding the mechanical characteristics of biological materials, the resulting parameters usually come with high standard deviations [96].

3.3. Scaling and Individualization

Spinal loading is highly dependent on a variety of subject-specific characteristics, such as spinal alignment, anthropometry, body weight distribution, or kinematics. While finite element models exist that account for individual characteristics [97–104], multibody models are predominantly generic in nature. In the past years, an increasing number of studies have been published, putting an emphasis on the individualization of the models [54,55,58,59,62].

A wide range of MBS models are based on measurements available in respective databases, e.g., in the OpenSim database (https://simtk.org/projects/osimdatabase, accessed on 27 December 2022). To gain reliable insights for the examined load cases, it is important to match the subject characteristics to the investigated kinematics as congruently as possible. It is common scientific practice to use available data based on measurements of bone geometries derived from imaging data or cadaver studies of individuals and scale and adapt the relevant parameters to the desired anthropometry depending on the characteristics of the studied target group. The need to make use of various sources in this regard makes it essential to be clear about the underlying data sets, in order to draw meaningful conclusions from simulation results. Thus, segment masses and body weight distribution and simplified kinematics are usually taken from the literature [85,86,105]. Some studies include experimental data collection of kinematics to scale the existing model appropriately [45,51,83] and include muscle activity from electromyography (EMG) measurement to drive the model [52]. This usually does not incorporate individual bone geometries, muscle morphology, or the mechanical properties of viscoelastic components.

However, the neglect or only limited consideration of interindividual variation makes these models poorly suitable for a detailed subject-specific analysis. Models based on coherent datasets regarding bone geometry, anthropometry, and muscle architecture, and kinematics are rare in the literature. Bayoglu et al. built a model based on extensive measurements of one cadaver, incorporating general kinematic data from the literature [72–74]. Dao et al. published a patient-specific model based on CT and MRI data [20] of the lumbar spine. Bruno et al. used their generic model [32] for the investigation of the impact of the integration of subject-specific properties [42]. Therefore, they incorporated CT-based measurements of trunk anatomy, such as spinal alignment and muscle morphology, indicating the relevance of considering these factors [42]. Based on this publication, Banks et al. investigated lumbar load in a patient-specific MBS model using CT data and marker-based motion capturing to combine individual musculoskeletal geometry and coherent kinematics [58]. However, the individualization of those models usually involves a time-consuming, manual, or semiautomated process which requires expert knowledge. To the best of our knowledge, only two publications can be found that deal with the topic of automating the individualization of MBS models [59,62].

Fasser at al. used annotated bi-planar radiography images (EOS imaging, Paris, France) for the automated generation of semi-subject-specific MBS models of the torso. The models included individual size and the alignment of bony structures as well as an individual body mass distribution. In the process, 112 and 109 points were marked in the frontal and sagittal plane, respectively, and converted into 3D coordinates. The body mass distribution was determined using the individual body contour of the imaging data. Individual bone geometries, muscle morphology, and passive elements were not included in the model. [62]

Based on the use of artificial neural networks (ANN), Lerchl et al. introduced a pipeline for the automated segmentation of vertebrae [106] and soft tissue of the torso, as well as the generation of the points of interest defining muscles and ligaments' attachment points and the location and orientation of intervertebral joints. All data were derived from CT imaging and the model generation required minimal manual interaction, making it suitable for the analysis of large patient cohorts. However, the individual characteristics of the muscles and connective tissue could not yet be integrated in the process [59].

3.4. Muscle Force Estimation

A mechanical analysis with multibody systems can follow two approaches, which define the necessary input data. Forward dynamic simulations (FD) require kinetic data to drive the model to generate specific kinematics. This usually means that muscle forces are applied directly or indirectly to the model to produce a desired motion. This is contrasted with the idea of inverse dynamic simulations(ID), which use kinematic data as input to calculate the required kinetic data. Thus, joint kinematics during as specific movement is imposed to the model and necessary joint moments and therefore, associated muscle forces are calculated. However, having more control variables, namely, muscle fascicles, than DOFs, the human musculoskeletal system is redundant. This leads to an infinite number of solutions for each load case. In order to determine the most suitable solutions, a mathematical optimization is a commonly used method. Numerous algorithms are available to find the optimal solution. Hereby, depending on the chosen algorithm, control variables, namely, muscle activation, excitation, or forces are varied in a deterministic or stochastic way until some given optimality criteria and constraints are met. Most commonly, a combination of inverse dynamics and static optimization (SO) is used [30,32,45], sometimes including inverse kinematics (IK) to determine individual joint kinematics [62,63,69]. The inverse dynamic simulation provides joint moments necessary to generate the simulated movement. Subsequently, the static optimization solves the redundancy problem for each time frame sequentially under the consideration of meeting equilibrium conditions.

In MBS models of the spine, muscles of interest are usually modeled as multiple fascicles, which comprehensively consider the respective lines of action (Section 3.1). Individual fascicles are modeled either as simple force actuators or, more complex, as Hill type muscles [107]. The classic muscle model according to Hill comprises serial and parallel elastic elements, representing passive elastic properties of the muscle–tendon complex as well as a contractile element representing the active component, namely, the function of myofilaments. This element can include muscle-specific characteristics, such as the force–length and force–velocity relationship as well as activation dynamics. Depending on how far these dynamics are taken into account, the muscle excitation, activation, or force can drive the model and therefore represent control variables for optimization routines. Detailed definitions of muscle-specific dynamics can be found in the literature [108,109].

4. Applications of MBS Models

MBS models can be used to address a wide range of questions. There are numerous publications devoted to the evaluation of methods in numerical modeling, including sensitivity analys or validation studies. Furthermore, validated models can help to gain valuable insights into biomechanically or clinically relevant load cases. However, depending on the investigated load case and subject collective, model extensions, and modifications are usually necessary. Table 2 provides an overview of the most relevant studies using existing models to address specific research questions.

Table 2. Overview of representative studies using available original models to address methodological or biomechanical research questions.

Study	Focus	Modifications	Original Model
Actis et al. [48]	Methodological Validation for flexion, extension, lateral bending, axial rotation for participants with and without transtibial amputation	model extension by lower body [110], muscle strength [32], and body mass distribution [86] inclusion of experimental protocol for EMG and kinematic data collection	[31]
Arshad et al. [38]	Biomechanical Influence of spinal rhythm and IAP on lumbar loads during trunk inclination	Adapted spinal rhythm, inclusion of ligaments, IVD, and IAP	[30]
Arx et al. [83]	Biomechanical Lumbar loading during different lifting styles	Integration of measured kinematic data	[32]

Table 2. Cont.

Study	Focus	Modifications	Original Model
Banks et al. [58]	Biomechanical Comparison of static and dynamic vertebral loading during lifting patient-specific models in an older study population	CT-based individualization and integration of patient-specific kinematic data	[32]
Bassani et al. [45]	Methodological Model validation for various loading tasks via spinopelvic rhythm and IDP according to [4]	Integration of kinematic data	[30]
Bassani et al. [47]	Biomechanical Effect of spinopelvic sagittal alignment on lumbar loads	Variation of spinal alignment based on four parameters	[30].
Bayoglu et al. [75]	Methodological Sensitivity of muscle and IV disc force computations to variations in muscle attachment sites	Variation of the location of muscle insertion	[72]
Raabe et al. [40]	Biomechanical Jogging biomechanics	Combination with full-body model by [111]	[31]
Beaucage-Gauvreau et al. [49–51]	Biomechanical Effects of lifting techniques on lumbar loads	Adjust all spinal joints with 3 DOFs and inclusion of kinematic data from motion capturing during lifting	[31,40]
Burkhart et al. [54]	Methodological Reliability of optoelectronic motion capturing for subject-specific spine model generation	Combination with model of lower limbs [110]	[32]
Malakoutian et al. [70]	Methodological Effect of muscle parameters on spinal loading	Variation of biomechanical parameters of paraspinal muscles	[60]
Senteler et al. [41]	Methodological Joint reaction forces for flexion and lifting	Combination with models of upper limbs and neck, IV joints set to 6 DOFs, added passive lin. joint stiffness	[31]
Meng et al. [37]	Methodological Force-motion coupling in 6-DOF joint	6 DOFs (IV), added 6-DOF stiffness	[31]
Molinaro et al. [52]	Biomechanical Effects of throwing technique solid waste collection occupation on lumbar loads	Incorporation of collected kinematics and EMG data, EMG-assisted muscle force estimation and SO	[49]
Schmid et al. [56]	Methodological Validation of a thoracolumbar model for children and adolescents	Combination with model of the lower limbs [112], scaling to anthropometry of children and adolescents	[32]
Schmid et al. [57]	Methodological Feasibility of a skin-marker based method for spinal alignment modeling	Reduction of muscle architecture, implementation of skin-marker derived alignment	[56]
Wang et al. [84]	Methodological Implementation of a physiological FSU	Adaption of IV joints to represent passive properties of a physiological FSU	[32]
Overbergh et al. [55]	Methodological Workflow for generation of an image-based (CT), subject-specific thoracolumbar model of spinal deformity	Addition of kinematic coupling constraints, personalization of bone geometries, alignment, IV joint definitions and kinematics	[32]
Han et al. [36]	Methodological Effect of centers of rotation on spinal loads and muscle forces in total disc replacement of lumbar spine	Ligaments and facet joints added, altering location of CoR	[30]
Zhu et al. [46]	Biomechanical Effects of lifting techniques on lumbar loads	Combining with models of upper and lower limbs, 6-DOF IV joint, integration of a customized marker set	[31]
Kuai et al. [44]	Biomechanical Influence of disc herniation on kinematics of the spine and lower limbs	Integration of kinematic data from patients with lumbar disc herniation	[30]
Senteler et al. [113]	Methodological Sensitivity of intervertebral joint forces to CoR location	Altering location of CoR	[41]

4.1. Studies with Methodological Focus

Various publications can be found in the literature evaluating and validating new approaches in MBS modeling [19,30–32,45,63,64,69]. For the purpose of validating these approaches, it is common scientific practice to compare simulation results with existing results from in vivo or in vitro measurements. Of note, those comparisons are mainly relative, as few in vivo measurements are available and exact boundary conditions are hard to control. Frequently used in vivo studies to validate results on spinal loading from simulation are intradiscal pressure measurements [4,114]. Estimated muscle forces are usually compared to EMG measurements from one's own experimental studies [48] or the literature [59].

Apart from evaluating the validity of the modeling approach, the simulation results of generated MBS models can be used to validate novel methods in data processing regarding the derivation of both relevant modeling data from imaging [19–21] and kinematic data motion capture [54]. Due to the usually extensive effort connected to the processing of individual data, recent publications have focused on the automation of the process [59,62].

Simplifications are an integral part of any model and have to be taken into consideration when it comes to the interpretation of the results. To understand and evaluate their influence, MBS models have been used to systematically investigate common assumptions, such as the reduction of complex mechanics of the functional spine unit (FSU) [37,115]. Further, the sensitivity of the model accuracy to assumed positions of intervertebral centers of rotation [23,36] or muscle insertions [75] have been analyzed. Rockenfeller et al. investigated the effect of muscle- or torque-driven centrodes using an MBS model of the lumbar spine.

Furthermore, a systematic model-based analysis can help standardize clinical procedures, such as the classification of spinal shapes [116] or to define boundary conditions for experimental protocols [24].

4.2. Studies with Biomechanical or Clinical Focus

Validated models are used to comprehensively investigate biomechanical and clinical aspects of a wide range from routine scenarios to nonphysiological, or even traumatic events.

The relevance of low-dynamic everyday or work-related activities for the general population, as well as their experimental accessibility, make these scenarios among the most studied in biomechanical simulations. Therefore, numerous models exist that deal with the mechanical effects of lifting [12,13,25,46,76,77,82], everyday activities such as walking, flexion, extension, or lateral bending [15,43,69] or work-related situations such as high-frequency axial loading [17,18]. In this context, different lifting techniques were evaluated [50,51,83,117]. Accident situations were investigated by Wei et al. [16] for snowboarding and for frontal impact by Valdano et al. [14]. Incorporating noncritical higher dynamics, Raabe et al. combined a generic model of the lumbar spine [31] with a model of the lower limbs [111] to analyze the biomechanics of jogging [40]. Studies investigating specific kinematic boundary conditions usually involve an experimental setup to collect kinematic data in a healthy adult population [46,47,52,58,83]. Comparably few studies target more vulnerable populations, such as amputees [48,53] or children [27,56], who used validated models of adults and scales them according to the literature to match the average anthropometric data of children.

Regarding the influence of healthy anatomical and anthropometric and anatomical characteristics, biomechanical modeling have been used to determine the effect of spinal alignment [28,43,47], to gain insight into load sharing of passive structures of the FSU [22], the effect of ligament stiffness [65] or muscle strengthening [118].

Furthermore, MBS models can help to understand and treat pathological developing or surgically induced pathological biomechanics. Kuai et al. analyzed the impact of disc herniation on the kinetics of the spine and lower extremities during everyday activities [44].

Surgical interventions always represent a major intervention in the natural biomechanics of the musculoskeletal system. Thus, several studies on the effects of spinal fusion can be found in the literature [29,71,119]. The resulting kinematic effects of spinal fusion were investigated by Ignasiak et al., who proposed a method for the prediction of a full-body sagittal alignment including reciprocal changes as a reaction to spinal fusion [68].

5. Limitations and Challenges

It is in the nature of numerical models that they come with limitations. One of the great challenges is to keep the balance between necessary accuracy and reasonable complexity. This requires not only in-depth knowledge of the object to be modeled but also the corresponding data from experimental studies and the appropriate technical solutions for implementation. During our literature research, we were able to identify several core limitations that could be found in a wide range of MBS models of the spine and the related challenges when it came to addressing these limitations.

5.1. Database

Any model can only be as good as its input data. In the context of biomechanical models, this comprises bony geometry, anthropometry, muscle architecture, the mechanical parameters of viscoelastic components and kinematic data. Due to the necessary measurements to determine these parameters, it is currently not possible to build models based on fully consistent datasets. While anthropometric and kinematic data can be determined via noninvasive measures in biomechanics labs, such as marker-based motion capturing, the derivation of bony geometries, muscle architecture, and a detailed distribution of soft tissue usually need medical imaging or are performed in cadaver studies. However, the mechanical properties of viscoelastic components such as ligaments or the IVD can currently only be determined with the help of in vitro studies, which require the isolation of the structure of interest to mount them in respective testing machines. Consequently, these measurements are also usually performed with specimens from cadaver studies and highly dependent on the experimental conditions.

In the past years, more studies including widely individualized models were published [55,59,62]. However, even these models can only offer a limited customization.

In order to obtain consistent data sets for biomechanical models, alternative, noninvasive methods must be developed to determine these parameters in large subject cohorts. Here, the combination of experimental studies, multimodal imaging, and ANNs could be a possible solution to increase the level of model individualization beyond its anthropometric and skeletal characteristics. Thus, the individual mechanical condition of functional components can be evaluated partly on the basis of imaging data. For instance, according to the Pfirrmann scale, a potential degradation of the IVD can be determined via the height and signal intensity from MRI data [120]. Correlating this degradation with the mechanical alteration of IVD [121], this can be used to consider the individual mechanical state of connective tissue, when it is implemented in respective models. Training ANNs with these data will provide large, more diverse datasets for individualized multibody models.

Furthermore, invasive experimental studies on spinal loading for model validation are rare and are not widely feasible due to ethical reasons. Accordingly, even consistently constructed models cannot ultimately be validated against data pertaining to the individual in question. Additionally, the high level of variability in mechanical properties of biological materials as mentioned in Section 3.2, and therefore, the integration of parameters with high standard deviations inevitably leads to models containing inaccuracies. Depending on the complexity of the model, these inaccuracies can accumulate and further blur the generated results. It is necessary to be aware of existing inconsistencies and imprecision when interpreting simulation results in order not to draw incorrect conclusions.

5.2. Joint Definition

Intervertebral connections are a complex combination of the IVD, ligaments, facet joints, and articulated capsules. Depending on the applied load, this leads to complicated kinematics in which the instantaneous center of rotation migrates in the course of the motion [122]. However, in the vast majority of spine models, intervertebral joints are simplified to spherical joints allowing three rotational DOFs around a fixed center of rotation. The sensitivity of this assumption has been subject to several in silico studies [23,113,123], indicating that the effect of this assumption on the calculated muscle forces and spinal loading should not be neglected. Detailed modeling requires six degrees of freedom and the consideration of appropriate stabilizing structures, the validity of which depends primarily on the definition of their mechanical parameters (Section 5.1). There are some models to be found in the literature incorporating such detailed representation of intervertebral connection [22], mainly focusing on load sharing in passive structures.

Larger data sets could also help to better understand intervertebral dynamics in order to develop corresponding valid modeling approaches. As already mentioned in Section 5.1, the combination of imaging, machine learning for process automation, and in vitro studies can contribute to progress.

5.3. Intra-Abdominal Pressure

The stabilizing influence of intra-abdominal pressure (IAP) on the spine has been widely studied [124,125]. However, only a few MBS models consider its effects [38,60,63,70,77]. In consequence, spinal loads in lifting tasks or the inclination of the upper body are assumed to be overestimated in the MBS modeling of the spine. Arshad et al. observed a decrease of up to 514 N in lumbar compression force and 279 N in global muscle force due to the inclusion of intra-abdominal pressure [38]. These results indicated that it was necessary to consider the effects of IAP to obtain reliable quantitative results on spinal loads.

5.4. Muscle Modeling and Muscle Force Estimation

A valid representation of relevant muscles is crucial to gain meaningful findings on the biomechanics of the spine. Most of the models contain a detailed muscle architecture consisting of multiple fascicles spanning between origin and insertion according to the literature. Deploying modeling components, that are usually defined as point-to-point force elements, can lead to nonphysiological lever arms depending on the imposed movement. De Zee's model used so-called via points to redirect the lines of action of the modeled long muscle fascicles along the rib cage and thus create more realistic lines of action compared to simple straight lines [30]. However, this approach came with an increased computational cost, making it only conditionally suited for a systematic analysis of large participant cohorts.

Another aspect that has to be critically discussed is the applied muscle model. While simple force actuators are considered sufficient for a static investigation, high-dynamic load situations require the consideration of activation and contraction dynamics. This requires an in-depth knowledge of the characteristics of individual muscle morphology such as optimal fiber length, physiological cross-sectional area (PCSA), or pennation angle. Again, the need for subject-specific solutions is evident, as muscle morphology is highly dependent on the individual.

The vast majority of currently published models use a combination of inverse dynamics and static optimization for muscle force calculation. This approach provides a sufficient accuracy in static and quasi-static simulations but is dependent on the defined cost function, constraints, and used algorithm. Most commonly used are criteria for minimum fatigue [126], or the sum of squared muscle strength [127] or activation [34], and the maximum muscle stress is defined as the upper-bound constraint, which is usually set to 100 MPa [32,49,59] to guarantee that equilibrium conditions are met reliably. However, this value does not correspond to a physiological value [49]. Furthermore, SO neglects cocontraction, which incorporates the activation of the antagonist in addition to the agonist stabilizing the respective joint and therefore increasing muscle activation. This is in contradiction to the idea of static optimization, which aims at minimizing the defined cost function (e.g., muscle activation) [128]. In high-dynamic load cases, where the role of cocontraction is more evident, this leads to an underestimation of spinal loading.

One way to address this problem is to use dynamic optimization (DO). In contrast to static optimization, the entire time history of the motion under investigation is taken into account [128]. Integrating the respective criteria in the optimization objective, stabilizing effects such as cocontraction can come into play [25]. However, this method comes with a massive increase of computational cost [129]. Another possibility would be to train models with the help of artificial intelligence. However, such training requires large quantities of data, which is not possible due to the still widely manual and therefore time-consuming process of modeling [128]. Anderson et al. compared both approaches for the simulation of normal gait in 2001, stating that both provided equivalent results for low-dynamic simulations [129]. A similar comparison was made by Morrow et al. for wheelchair propulsion, noticing significant differences in estimated muscle activations [130]. Keeping in mind that wheelchair propulsion comprises higher dynamics than normal gait, these findings indicate that the validity of the chosen approach was largely dependent on the investigated load case.

6. Conclusions

Multibody models are a powerful tool to gain insight into the healthy and pathological musculoskeletal system. They can promote a general understanding of the pathobiomechanics of a large set of medical impairments and might even be able to support diagnostics and therapy planning in the future. Although simplifications and assumptions are an integral part of any model, it is essential to look closely at the implications of these assumptions, potential interactions, and possible solutions. Modern technology holds the potential to provide some of these solutions. Thus, artificial intelligence and state-of-the-art medical imaging can provide the necessary extensive data basis to systematically investigate critical parameters to derive appropriate solutions. These technical approaches coupled with a distinct awareness of existing limitations will lead us towards a growing, more profound understanding of musculoskeletal mechanics.

Author Contributions: Conceptualization, T.L. and J.S.K.; writing—original draft preparation, T.L.; writing—review and editing, K.N., T.B., J.B., V.S. and J.S.K.; supervision, J.S.K.; project administration, J.S.K.; funding acquisition, J.S.K. All authors have read and agreed to the published version of the manuscript.

Funding: This research was funded by the European Research Council (ERC) under the European Union's Horizon 2020 research and innovation program. Grant no.: 101045128—iBack-epic—ERC-2021-COG.

Institutional Review Board Statement: Not applicable.

Informed Consent Statement: Not applicable.

Data Availability Statement: Not applicable.

Conflicts of Interest: J.S.K. is a co-founder of Bonescreen GmbH. All other authors declare that the research was conducted in the absence of any commercial or financial relationships that could be construed as a potential conflict of interest.

Abbreviations

The following abbreviations are used in this manuscript:

MBS	Multibody system
FEM	Finite element method
DOF	Degree of freedom
FSU	Functional spine unit
IAP	Intra-abdominal pressure
EMG	Electromyography
COR	Center of rotation
IVD	Intervertebral disc
IV	Intervertebral
CS	Costosternal
CV	Costovertebral
CT	Costotransversal
FD	Forward dynamic
ID	Inverse dynamic
IK	Inverse kinematic
SO	Static optimization
DO	Dynamic optimization
ANN	Artificial neural network
ALE	Arbitrary Langrangian–Eulerian

References

1. Murtezani, A.; Ibraimi, Z.; Sllamniku, S.; Osmani, T.; Sherifi, S. Prevalence and risk factors for low back pain in industrial workers. *Folia Med.* **2011**, *53*, 68–74. [CrossRef]
2. Fu, L.; Ma, J.; Lu, B.; Jia, H.; Zhao, J.; Kuang, M.; Feng, R.; Xu, L.; Bai, H.; Sun, L.; et al. Biomechanical effect of interspinous process distraction height after lumbar fixation surgery: An in vitro model. *Proc. Inst. Mech. Eng. Part H J. Eng. Med.* **2017**, *231*, 663–672. [CrossRef]
3. Sato, K.; Kikuchi, S.; Yonezawa, T. In vivo intradiscal pressure measurement in healthy individuals and in patients with ongoing back problems. *Spine* **1999**, *24*, 2468. [CrossRef]
4. Wilke, H.J.; Neef, P.; Hinz, B.; Seidel, H.; Claes, L. Intradiscal pressure together with anthropometric data—A data set for the validation of models. *Clin. Biomech.* **2001**, *16*, S111–S126. [CrossRef] [PubMed]
5. Dreischarf, M.; Rohlmann, A.; Graichen, F.; Bergmann, G.; Schmidt, H. In vivo loads on a vertebral body replacement during different lifting techniques. *J. Biomech.* **2016**, *49*, 890–895. [CrossRef] [PubMed]
6. Rohlmann, A.; Graichen, F.; Kayser, R.; Bender, A.; Bergmann, G. Loads on a Telemeterized Vertebral Body Replacement Measured in Two Patients. *Spine* **2008**, *33*, 1170–1179. [CrossRef]
7. Gould, S.L.; Cristofolini, L.; Davico, G.; Viceconti, M. Computational Modelling of the Scoliotic Spine: A Literature Review. *Int. J. Numer. Methods Biomed. Eng.* **2021**, *37*, e3503. [CrossRef] [PubMed]
8. Alizadeh, M.; Knapik, G.G.; Mageswaran, P.; Mendel, E.; Bourekas, E.; Marras, W.S. Biomechanical musculoskeletal models of the cervical spine: A systematic literature review. *Clin. Biomech.* **2020**, *71*, 115–124. [CrossRef]
9. Dreischarf, M.; Shirazi-Adl, A.; Arjmand, N.; Rohlmann, A.; Schmidt, H. Estimation of loads on human lumbar spine: A review of in vivo and computational model studies. *J. Biomech.* **2016**, *49*, 833–845. [CrossRef]
10. Heidari, E.; Arjmand, N.; Kahrizi, S. Comparisons of lumbar spine loads and kinematics in healthy and non-specific low back pain individuals during unstable lifting activities. *J. Biomech.* **2022**, *144*, 111344. [CrossRef] [PubMed]
11. Khoddam-Khorasani, P.; Arjmand, N.; Shirazi-Adl, A. Effect of changes in the lumbar posture in lifting on trunk muscle and spinal loads: A combined in vivo, musculoskeletal, and finite element model study. *J. Biomech.* **2020**, *104*, 109728. [CrossRef] [PubMed]
12. Breloff, S.P.; Chou, L.S. Three-dimensional multi-segmented spine joint reaction forces during common workplace physical demands/activities of daily living. *Biomed. Eng.-Appl. Basis Commun.* **2017**, *29*, 1750025. [CrossRef]
13. Zaman, R.; Xiang, Y.; Cruz, J.; Yang, J. Three-dimensional asymmetric maximum weight lifting prediction considering dynamic joint strength. *Proc. Inst. Mech. Eng. Part H J. Eng. Med.* **2021**, *235*, 437–446. [CrossRef] [PubMed]
14. Valdano, M.; Asensio-Gil, J.M.; Jiménez-Octavio, J.R.; Cabello-Reyes, M.; Vasserot-Tolmos, R.; López-Valdés, F.J. Parametric Analysis of The Effect of CRS Seatback Angle in Dummy Measurements in Frontal Impacts. In Proceedings of the IRCOBI Conference 2022, Porto, Portugal, 14–16 September 2022; Volume 2022, pp. 519–531.
15. Panero, E.; Digo, E.; Ferrarese, V.; Dimanico, U.; Gastaldi, L. Multi-segments kinematic model of the human spine during gait. In Proceedings of the 2021 IEEE International Symposium on Medical Measurements and Applications (MeMeA), Lausanne, Switzerland, 23–25 June 2021. [CrossRef]
16. Wei, W.; Evin, M.; Bailly, N.; Arnoux, P.J. Biomechanical evaluation of Back injuries during typical snowboarding backward falls. *Scand. J. Med. Sci. Sport.* **2022**, 1–11. [CrossRef]

17. Valentini, P.P.; Pennestrì, E. An improved three-dimensional multibody model of the human spine for vibrational investigations. *Multibody Syst. Dyn.* **2016**, *36*, 363–375. [CrossRef]
18. Low, L.; Newell, N.; Masouros, S. A Multibody Model of the Spine for Injury Prediction in High-Rate Vertical Loading. In Proceedings of the IRCOBI Conference 2022, , Porto, Portugal, 14–16 September 2022.
19. Dao, T.T.; Pouletaut, P.; Charleux, F.; Lazáry, Á.; Eltes, P.; Varga, P.P.; Tho, M.C.H.B. Estimation of patient specific lumbar spine muscle forces using multi-physical musculoskeletal model and dynamic MRI. In *Knowledge and Systems Engineering*; Springer International, Basel, Switzerland, 2014; pp. 411–422.
20. Dao, T.T.; Pouletaut, P.; Charleux, F.; Lazáry, Á.; Eltes, P.; Varga, P.P.; Tho, M.C.H.B. Multimodal medical imaging (CT and dynamic MRI) data and computer-graphics multi-physical model for the estimation of patient specific lumbar spine muscle forces. *Data Knowl. Eng.* **2015**, *96*, 3–18. [CrossRef]
21. Dao, T.T.; Pouletaut, P.; Lazáry, Á.; Tho, M.C.H.B. Multimodal Medical Imaging Fusion for Patient Specific Musculoskeletal Modeling of the Lumbar Spine System in Functional Posture. *J. Med. Biol. Eng.* **2017**, *37*, 739–749. [CrossRef]
22. Abouhossein, A.; Weisse, B.; Ferguson, S.J. A multibody modelling approach to determine load sharing between passive elements of the lumbar spine. *Comput. Methods Biomech. Biomed. Eng.* **2011**, *14*, 527–537. [CrossRef]
23. Abouhossein, A.; Weisse, B.; Ferguson, S.J. Quantifying the centre of rotation pattern in a multi-body model of the lumbar spine. *Comput. Methods Biomech. Biomed. Eng.* **2013**, *16*, 1362–1373. [CrossRef] [PubMed]
24. Borrelli, S.; Putame, G.; Pascoletti, G.; Terzini, M.; Zanetti, E.M. In Silico Meta-Analysis of Boundary Conditions for Experimental Tests on the Lumbar Spine. *Ann. Biomed. Eng.* **2022**, *50*, 1243–1254. [CrossRef]
25. Ghiasi, M.S.; Arjmand, N.; Boroushaki, M.; Farahmand, F. Investigation of trunk muscle activities during lifting using a multi-objective optimization-based model and intelligent optimization algorithms. *Med Biol. Eng. Comput.* **2016**, *54*, 431–440. [CrossRef] [PubMed]
26. Bauer, S.; Hausen, U.; Gruber, K. Effects of individual spine curvatures—A comparative study with the help of computer modelling. *Biomed. Tech. Biomed. Eng.* **2012**, *57* (Suppl. 1), 132–135. [CrossRef] [PubMed]
27. Bauer, S.; Wasserhess, C.; Paulus, D. Quantification of loads on the lumbar spine of children with different body weight—A comparative study with the help of computer modelling. *Biomed. Tech.* **2014**, *59*, S913–S916.
28. Müller, A.; Rockenfeller, R.; Damm, N.; Kosterhon, M.; Kantelhardt, S.R.; Aiyangar, A.K.; Gruber, K. Load Distribution in the Lumbar Spine During Modeled Compression Depends on Lordosis. *Front. Bioeng. Biotechnol.* **2021**, *9*, 661258. [CrossRef] [PubMed]
29. Kantelhardt, S.; Hausen, U.; Kosterhon, M.; Amr, A.; Gruber, K.; Giese, A. Computer simulation and image guidance for individualised dynamic spinal stabilization. *Int. J. Comput. Assist. Radiol. Surg.* **2015**, *10*, 1325–1332. [CrossRef]
30. de Zee, M.; Hansen, L.; Wong, C.; Rasmussen, J.; Simonsen, E.B. A generic detailed rigid-body lumbar spine model. *J. Biomech.* **2007**, *40*, 1219–1227. [CrossRef]
31. Christophy, M.; Faruk Senan, N.A.; Lotz, J.C.; O'Reilly, O.M. A musculoskeletal model for the lumbar spine. *Biomech. Model. Mechanobiol.* **2012**, *11*, 19–34. [CrossRef]
32. Bruno, A.G.; Bouxsein, M.L.; Anderson, D.E. Development and Validation of a Musculoskeletal Model of the Fully Articulated Thoracolumbar Spine and Rib Cage. *J. Biomech. Eng.* **2015**, *137*, 081003. [CrossRef]
33. Ignasiak, D.; Dendorfer, S.; Ferguson, S.J. Thoracolumbar spine model with articulated ribcage for the prediction of dynamic spinal loading. *J. Biomech.* **2016**, *49*, 959–966. [CrossRef]
34. Delp, S.L.; Anderson, F.C.; Arnold, A.S.; Loan, P.; Habib, A.; John, C.T.; Guendelman, E.; Thelen, D.G. OpenSim: Open-source software to create and analyze dynamic simulations of movement. *IEEE Trans. Bio-Med. Eng.* **2007**, *54*, 1940–1950. [CrossRef]
35. Han, K.S.; Zander, T.; Taylor, W.R.; Rohlmann, A. An enhanced and validated generic thoraco-lumbar spine model for prediction of muscle forces. *Med. Eng. Phys.* **2012**, *34*, 709–716. [CrossRef] [PubMed]
36. Han, K.S.; Kim, K.; Park, W.M.; Lim, D.S.; Kim, Y.H. Effect of centers of rotation on spinal loads and muscle forces in total disk replacement of lumbar spine. *Proc. Inst. Mech. Eng. Part H J. Eng. Med.* **2013**, *227*, 543–550. [CrossRef]
37. Meng, X.; Bruno, A.G.; Cheng, B.; Wang, W.; Bouxsein, M.L.; Anderson, D.E. Incorporating Six Degree-of-Freedom Intervertebral Joint Stiffness in a Lumbar Spine Musculoskeletal Model-Method and Performance in Flexed Postures. *J. Biomech. Eng.* **2015**, *137*, 101008. [CrossRef] [PubMed]
38. Arshad, R.; Zander, T.; Dreischarf, M.; Schmidt, H. Influence of lumbar spine rhythms and intra-abdominal pressure on spinal loads and trunk muscle forces during upper body inclination. *Med. Eng. Phys.* **2016**, *38*, 333–338. [CrossRef] [PubMed]
39. Ignasiak, D.; Ferguson, S.J.; Arjmand, N. A rigid thorax assumption affects model loading predictions at the upper but not lower lumbar levels. *J. Biomech.* **2016**, *49*, 3074–3078. [CrossRef]
40. Raabe, M.E.; Chaudhari, A.M. An investigation of jogging biomechanics using the full-body lumbar spine model: Model development and validation. *J. Biomech.* **2016**, *49*, 1238–1243. [CrossRef]
41. Senteler, M.; Weisse, B.; Rothenfluh, D.A.; Snedeker, J.G. Intervertebral reaction force prediction using an enhanced assembly of OpenSim models. *Comput. Methods Biomech. Biomed. Eng.* **2016**, *19*, 538–548. [CrossRef]
42. Bruno, A.G.; Mokhtarzadeh, H.; Allaire, B.T.; Velie, K.R.; De Paolis Kaluza, M.C.; Anderson, D.E.; Bouxsein, M.L. Incorporation of CT-based measurements of trunk anatomy into subject-specific musculoskeletal models of the spine influences vertebral loading predictions. *J. Orthop. Res.: Off. Publ. Orthop. Res. Soc.* **2017**, *35*, 2164–2173. [CrossRef]

43. Bruno, A.G.; Burkhart, K.; Allaire, B.; Anderson, D.E.; Bouxsein, M.L. Spinal loading patterns from biomechanical modeling explain the high incidence of vertebral fractures in the thoracolumbar region. *J. Bone Miner. Res.* **2017**, *32*, 1282–1290. [CrossRef]
44. Kuai, S.; Zhou, W.; Liao, Z.; Ji, R.; Guo, D.; Zhang, R.; Liu, W. Influences of lumbar disc herniation on the kinematics in multi-segmental spine, pelvis, and lower extremities during five activities of daily living. *BMC Musculoskelet. Disord.* **2017**, *18*, 1–13. [CrossRef]
45. Bassani, T.; Stucovitz, E.; Qian, Z.; Briguglio, M.; Galbusera, F. Validation of the AnyBody full body musculoskeletal model in computing lumbar spine loads at L4L5 level. *J. Biomech.* **2017**, *58*, 89–96. [CrossRef] [PubMed]
46. Zhu, X.Y.; Kim, H.K.; Zhang, Y. Development of an enhanced musculoskeletal model for simulating lumbar spine loading during manual lifting tasks. *Lect. Notes Comput. Sci. (Incl. Subser. Lect. Notes Artif. Intell. Lect. Notes Bioinform.)* **2017**, *10286*, 229–237. [CrossRef]
47. Bassani, T.; Casaroli, G.; Galbusera, F. Dependence of lumbar loads on spinopelvic sagittal alignment: An evaluation based on musculoskeletal modeling. *PLoS ONE* **2019**, *14*, e0207997. [CrossRef] [PubMed]
48. Actis, J.A.; Honegger, J.D.; Gates, D.H.; Petrella, A.J.; Nolasco, L.A.; Silverman, A.K. Validation of lumbar spine loading from a musculoskeletal model including the lower limbs and lumbar spine. *J. Biomech.* **2018**, *68*, 107–114. [CrossRef] [PubMed]
49. Beaucage-Gauvreau, E.; Robertson, W.S.P.; Brandon, S.C.E.; Fraser, R.; Freeman, B.J.C.; Graham, R.B.; Thewlis, D.; Jones, C.F. Validation of an OpenSim full-body model with detailed lumbar spine for estimating lower lumbar spine loads during symmetric and asymmetric lifting tasks. *Comput. Methods Biomech. Biomed. Eng.* **2019**, *22*, 451–464. [CrossRef]
50. Beaucage-Gauvreau, E.; Brandon, S.C.; Robertson, W.S.; Fraser, R.; Freeman, B.J.; Graham, R.B.; Thewlis, D.; Jones, C.F. A braced arm-to-thigh (BATT) lifting technique reduces lumbar spine loads in healthy and low back pain participants. *J. Biomech.* **2020**, *100*, 109584. [CrossRef]
51. Beaucage-Gauvreau, E.; Brandon, S.C.; Robertson, W.S.; Fraser, R.; Freeman, B.J.; Graham, R.B.; Thewlis, D.; Jones, C.F. Lumbar spine loads are reduced for activities of daily living when using a braced arm-to-thigh technique. *Eur. Spine J.* **2021**, *30*, 1035–1042. [CrossRef]
52. Molinaro, D.D.; King, A.S.; Young, A.J. Biomechanical analysis of common solid waste collection throwing techniques using OpenSim and an EMG-assisted solver. *J. Biomech.* **2020**, *104*, 109704. [CrossRef]
53. Honegger, J.D.; Actis, J.A.; Gates, D.H.; Silverman, A.K.; Munson, A.H.; Petrella, A.J. Development of a multiscale model of the human lumbar spine for investigation of tissue loads in people with and without a transtibial amputation during sit-to-stand. *Biomech. Model. Mechanobiol.* **2021**, *20*, 339–358. [CrossRef]
54. Burkhart, K.; Grindle, D.; Bouxsein, M.L.; Anderson, D.E. Between-session reliability of subject-specific musculoskeletal models of the spine derived from optoelectronic motion capture data. *J. Biomech.* **2020**, *112*, 110044. [CrossRef]
55. Overbergh, T.; Severijns, P.; Beaucage-Gauvreau, E.; Jonkers, I.; Moke, L.; Scheys, L. Development and validation of a modeling workflow for the generation of image-based, subject-specific thoracolumbar models of spinal deformity. *J. Biomech.* **2020**, *110*, 109946. [CrossRef] [PubMed]
56. Schmid, S.; Burkhart, K.A.; Allaire, B.T.; Grindle, D.; Anderson, D.E. Musculoskeletal full-body models including a detailed thoracolumbar spine for children and adolescents aged 6–18 years. *J. Biomech.* **2020**, *102*, 109305. [CrossRef]
57. Schmid, S.; Connolly, L.; Moschini, G.; Meier, M.L.; Senteler, M. Skin marker-based subject-specific spinal alignment modeling: A feasibility study. *J. Biomech.* **2022**, *137*, 111102. [CrossRef]
58. Banks, J.J.; Alemi, M.M.; Allaire, B.T.; Lynch, A.C.; Bouxsein, M.L.; Anderson, D.E. Using static postures to estimate spinal loading during dynamic lifts with participant-specific thoracolumbar musculoskeletal models. *Appl. Ergon.* **2023**, *106*, 103869. [CrossRef] [PubMed]
59. Lerchl, T.; El Husseini, M.; Bayat, A.; Sekuboyina, A.; Hermann, L.; Nispel, K.; Baum, T.; Löffler, M.T.; Senner, V.; Kirschke, J.S. Validation of a Patient-Specific Musculoskeletal Model for Lumbar Load Estimation Generated by an Automated Pipeline From Whole Body CT. *Front. Bioeng. Biotechnol.* **2022**, *10*, 862804. [CrossRef]
60. Malakoutian, M.; Street, J.; Wilke, H.J.; Stavness, I.; Fels, S.; Oxland, T. A musculoskeletal model of the lumbar spine using ArtiSynth–development and validation. *Comput. Methods Biomech. Biomed. Eng. Imaging Vis.* **2018**, *6*, 483–490. [CrossRef]
61. Rupp, T.K.; Ehlers, W.; Karajan, N.; Günther, M.; Schmitt, S. A forward dynamics simulation of human lumbar spine flexion predicting the load sharing of intervertebral discs, ligaments, and muscles. *Biomech. Model. Mechanobiol.* **2015**, *14*, 1081–1105. [CrossRef]
62. Fasser, M.R.; Jokeit, M.; Kalthoff, M.; Gomez Romero, D.A.; Trache, T.; Snedeker, J.G.; Farshad, M.; Widmer, J. Subject-Specific Alignment and Mass Distribution in Musculoskeletal Models of the Lumbar Spine. *Front. Bioeng. Biotechnol.* **2021**, *9*, 745. [CrossRef]
63. Huynh, K.; Gibson, I.; Jagdish, B.; Lu, W. Development and validation of a discretised multi-body spine model in LifeMOD for biodynamic behaviour simulation. *Comput. Methods Biomech. Biomed. Eng.* **2015**, *18*, 175–184. [CrossRef]
64. Khurelbaatar, T.; Kim, K.; Kim, Y.H. A cervico-thoraco-lumbar multibody dynamic model for the estimation of joint loads and muscle forces. *J. Biomech. Eng.* **2015**, *137*, 111001. [CrossRef]
65. Putzer, M.; Auer, S.; Malpica, W.; Suess, F.; Dendorfer, S. A numerical study to determine the effect of ligament stiffness on kinematics of the lumbar spine during flexion. *BMC Musculoskelet. Disord.* **2016**, *17*, 1–7. [CrossRef] [PubMed]

66. Andersen, M.S.; Damsgaard, M.; Rasmussen, J. Force-dependent kinematics: A new analysis method for non-conforming joints. In Proceedings of the XIII International Symposium on Computer Simulation in Biomechanics, Leuven, Belgium, 30 June–2 July 2011.
67. Ignasiak, D.; Valenzuela, W.; Reyes, M.; Ferguson, S.J. The effect of muscle ageing and sarcopenia on spinal segmental loads. *Eur. Spine J.* **2018**, *27*, 2650–2659. [CrossRef]
68. Ignasiak, D. A novel method for prediction of postoperative global sagittal alignment based on full-body musculoskeletal modeling and posture optimization. *J. Biomech.* **2020**, *102*, 109324. [CrossRef]
69. Favier, C.D.; Finnegan, M.E.; Quest, R.A.; Honeyfield, L.; McGregor, A.H.; Phillips, A.T.M. An open-source musculoskeletal model of the lumbar spine and lower limbs: A validation for movements of the lumbar spine. *Comput. Methods Biomech. Biomed. Eng.* **2021**, *24*, 1310–1325. [CrossRef] [PubMed]
70. Malakoutian, M.; Sanchez, C.A.; Brown, S.H.; Street, J.; Fels, S.; Oxland, T.R. Biomechanical properties of paraspinal muscles influence spinal loading—A musculoskeletal simulation study. *Front. Bioeng. Biotechnol.* **2022**, *10*, 852201. [CrossRef] [PubMed]
71. Fasser, M.R.; Gerber, G.; Passaplan, C.; Cornaz, F.; Snedeker, J.G.; Farshad, M.; Widmer, J. Computational model predicts risk of spinal screw loosening in patients. *Eur. Spine J.* **2022**, *31*, 2639–2649. [CrossRef]
72. Bayoglu, R.; Galibarov, P.E.; Verdonschot, N.; Koopman, B.; Homminga, J. Twente Spine Model: A thorough investigation of the spinal loads in a complete and coherent musculoskeletal model of the human spine. *Med. Eng. Phys.* **2019**, *68*, 35–45. [CrossRef]
73. Bayoglu, R.; Geeraedts, L.; Groenen, K.H.J.; Verdonschot, N.; Koopman, B.; Homminga, J. Twente spine model: A complete and coherent dataset for musculo-skeletal modeling of the lumbar region of the human spine. *J. Biomech.* **2017**, *53*, 111–119. [CrossRef]
74. Bayoglu, R.; Geeraedts, L.; Groenen, K.H.J.; Verdonschot, N.; Koopman, B.; Homminga, J. Twente spine model: A complete and coherent dataset for musculo-skeletal modeling of the thoracic and cervical regions of the human spine. *J. Biomech.* **2017**, *58*, 52–63. [CrossRef]
75. Bayoglu, R.; Guldeniz, O.; Verdonschot, N.; Koopman, B.; Homminga, J. Sensitivity of muscle and intervertebral disc force computations to variations in muscle attachment sites. *Comput. Methods Biomech. Biomed. Eng.* **2019**, *22*, 1135–1143. [CrossRef]
76. Huang, M.; Hajizadeh, K.; Gibson, I.; Lee, T. Analysis of compressive load on intervertebral joint in standing and sitting postures. *Technol. Health Care* **2016**, *24*, 215–223. [CrossRef] [PubMed]
77. Guo, J.; Guo, W.; Ren, G. Embodiment of intra-abdominal pressure in a flexible multibody model of the trunk and the spinal unloading effects during static lifting tasks. *Biomech. Model. Mechanobiol.* **2021**, *20*, 1599–1626. [CrossRef] [PubMed]
78. Hansen, L.; de Zee, M.; Rasmussen, J.; Andersen, T.B.; Wong, C.; Simonsen, E.B. Anatomy and biomechanics of the back muscles in the lumbar spine with reference to biomechanical modeling. *Spine* **2006**, *31*, 1888–1899. [CrossRef] [PubMed]
79. Bogduk, N. *Clinical Anatomy of the Lumbar Spine and Sacrum*; Elsevier Health Sciences: Amsterdam, The Netherlands, 1997.
80. Pearcy, M.J.; Bogduk, N. Instantaneous axes of rotation of the lumbar intervertebral joints. *Spine* **1988**, *13*, 1033–1041. [CrossRef]
81. Byrne, R.M.; Aiyangar, A.K.; Zhang, X. Sensitivity of musculoskeletal model-based lumbar spinal loading estimates to type of kinematic input and passive stiffness properties. *J. Biomech.* **2020**, *102*, 109659. [CrossRef]
82. Kim, H.K.; Zhang, Y. Estimation of lumbar spinal loading and trunk muscle forces during asymmetric lifting tasks: Application of whole-body musculoskeletal modelling in OpenSim. *Ergonomics* **2017**, *60*, 563–576. [CrossRef]
83. von Arx, M.; Liechti, M.; Connolly, L.; Bangerter, C.; Meier, M.L.; Schmid, S. From Stoop to Squat: A comprehensive analysis of lumbar loading among different lifting styles. *Front. Bioeng. Biotechnol.* **2021**, *9*, 769117. [CrossRef]
84. Wang, W.; Wang, D.; De Groote, F.; Scheys, L.; Jonkers, I. Implementation of physiological functional spinal units in a rigid-body model of the thoracolumbar spine. *J. Biomech.* **2020**, *98*, 109437. [CrossRef]
85. Pearsall, D.J.; Reid, J.G.; Livingston, L.A. Segmental inertial parameters of the human trunk as determined from computed tomography. *Ann. Biomed. Eng.* **1996**, *24*, 198–210. [CrossRef]
86. Winter, D.A. *Biomechanics and Motor Control of Human Movement*; Wiley, Weilheim, Germany, 2009.
87. Fung, Y.C. *Biomechanics: Mechanical Properties of Living Tissues*; Springer Science & Business Media: Luxemburg, 2013.
88. Pintar, F.A.; Yoganandan, N.; Myers, T.; Elhagediab, A.; Sances, A., Jr. Biomechanical properties of human lumbar spine ligaments. *J. Biomech.* **1992**, *25*, 1351–1356. [CrossRef]
89. Heuer, F.; Schmidt, H.; Klezl, Z.; Claes, L.; Wilke, H.J. Stepwise reduction of functional spinal structures increase range of motion and change lordosis angle. *J. Biomech.* **2007**, *40*, 271–280. [CrossRef] [PubMed]
90. Ashton-Miller, J.A.; Schultz, A.B. Biomechanics of the human spine. *Basic Orthop. Biomech.* **1997**, *2*, 353–385.
91. Panjabi, M.M.; Brand, R., Jr.; White, A., 3rd. Mechanical properties of the human thoracic spine as shown by three-dimensional load-displacement curves. *JBJS* **1976**, *58*, 642–652. [CrossRef]
92. White, A.A. *Clinical Biomechanics of the Spine*; Lippincott Williams & Wilkins: Philadelphia, PA, USA, 2022.
93. Myklebust, J.B.; Pintar, F.; Yoganandan, N.; Cusick, J.F.; Maiman, D.; Myers, T.J.; Sances, A., Jr. Tensile strength of spinal ligaments. *Spine* **1988**, *13*, 526–531. [CrossRef]
94. Liebsch, C.; Graf, N.; Appelt, K.; Wilke, H.J. The rib cage stabilizes the human thoracic spine: An in vitro study using stepwise reduction of rib cage structures. *PLoS ONE* **2017**, *12*, e0178573. [CrossRef]
95. Wilke, H.J.; Grundler, S.; Ottardi, C.; Mathew, C.E.; Schlager, B.; Liebsch, C. In vitro analysis of thoracic spinal motion segment flexibility during stepwise reduction of all functional structures. *Eur. Spine J.* **2020**, *29*, 179–185. [CrossRef]
96. Cook, D.; Julias, M.; Nauman, E. Biological variability in biomechanical engineering research: Significance and meta-analysis of current modeling practices. *J. Biomech.* **2014**, *47*, 1241–1250. [CrossRef]

97. Akhavanfar, M.H.; Kazemi, H.; Eskandari, A.H.; Arjmand, N. Obesity and spinal loads; a combined MR imaging and subject-specific modeling investigation. *J. Biomech.* **2018**, *70*, 102–112. [CrossRef]
98. El Ouaaid, Z.; Shirazi-Adl, A.; Plamondon, A. Effects of variation in external pulling force magnitude, elevation, and orientation on trunk muscle forces, spinal loads and stability. *J. Biomech.* **2016**, *49*, 946–952. [CrossRef]
99. Eskandari, A.H.; Arjmand, N.; Shirazi-Adl, A.; Farahmand, F. Hypersensitivity of trunk biomechanical model predictions to errors in image-based kinematics when using fully displacement-control techniques. *J. Biomech.* **2019**, *84*, 161–171. [CrossRef]
100. Ghezelbash, F.; Shirazi-Adl, A.; Arjmand, N.; El-Ouaaid, Z.; Plamondon, A. Subject-specific biomechanics of trunk: Musculoskeletal scaling, internal loads and intradiscal pressure estimation. *Biomech. Model. Mechanobiol.* **2016**, *15*, 1699–1712. [CrossRef] [PubMed]
101. Little, J.P.; Adam, C.J. Geometric sensitivity of patient-specific finite element models of the spine to variability in user-selected anatomical landmarks. *Comput. Methods Biomech. Biomed. Eng.* **2015**, *18*, 676–688. [CrossRef] [PubMed]
102. Naserkhaki, S.; Jaremko, J.L.; El-Rich, M. Effects of inter-individual lumbar spine geometry variation on load-sharing: Geometrically personalized Finite Element study. *J. Biomech.* **2016**, *49*, 2909–2917. [CrossRef] [PubMed]
103. Périé, D.; Sales De Gauzy, J.; Hobatho, M.C. Biomechanical evaluation of Cheneau-Toulouse-Munster brace in the treatment of scoliosis using optimisation approach and finite element method. *Med. Biol. Eng. Comput.* **2002**, *40*, 296–301. [CrossRef] [PubMed]
104. Vergari, C.; Courtois, I.; Ebermeyer, E.; Bouloussa, H.; Vialle, R.; Skalli, W. Experimental validation of a patient-specific model of orthotic action in adolescent idiopathic scoliosis. *Eur. Spine J.* **2016**, *25*, 3049–3055. [CrossRef]
105. Wong, K.W.N.; Luk, K.D.K.; Leong, J.C.Y.; Wong, S.F.; Wong, K.K.Y. Continuous Dynamic Spinal Motion Analysis. *Spine* **2006**, *31*, 414–419. [CrossRef]
106. Sekuboyina, A.; Husseini, M.E.; Bayat, A.; Löffler, M.; Liebl, H.; Li, H.; Tetteh, G.; Kukačka, J.; Payer, C.; Štern, D. VerSe: A vertebrae labelling and segmentation benchmark for multi-detector CT images. *arXiv* **2020**, arXiv:2001.09193.
107. Hill, A.V. The heat of shortening and the dynamic constants of muscle. *Proc. R. Soc. London. Ser. B-Biol. Sci.* **1938**, *126*, 136–195.
108. Thelen, D.G. Adjustment of muscle mechanics model parameters to simulate dynamic contractions in older adults. *J. Biomech. Eng.* **2003**, *125*, 70–77. [CrossRef]
109. Millard, M.; Uchida, T.; Seth, A.; Delp, S.L. Flexing computational muscle: Modeling and simulation of musculotendon dynamics. *J. Biomech. Eng.* **2013**, *135*, 021005. [CrossRef]
110. Delp, S.L.; Loan, J.P.; Hoy, M.G.; Zajac, F.E.; Topp, E.L.; Rosen, J.M. An interactive graphics-based model of the lower extremity to study orthopaedic surgical procedures. *IEEE Trans. Biomed. Eng.* **1990**, *37*, 757–767. [CrossRef]
111. Hamner, S.R.; Seth, A.; Delp, S.L. Muscle contributions to propulsion and support during running. *J. Biomech.* **2010**, *43*, 2709–2716. [CrossRef]
112. Anderson, F.C.; Pandy, M.G. A dynamic optimization solution for vertical jumping in three dimensions. *Comput. Methods Biomech. Biomed. Eng.* **1999**, *2*, 201–231. [CrossRef] [PubMed]
113. Senteler, M.; Aiyangar, A.; Weisse, B.; Farshad, M.; Snedeker, J.G. Sensitivity of intervertebral joint forces to center of rotation location and trends along its migration path. *J. Biomech.* **2018**, *70*, 140–148. [CrossRef] [PubMed]
114. Takahashi, I.; Kikuchi, S.i.; Sato, K.; Sato, N. Mechanical load of the lumbar spine during forward bending motion of the trunk-a biomechanical study. *Spine* **2006**, *31*, 18–23. [CrossRef] [PubMed]
115. Wang, Q.D.; Guo, L.X. Biomechanical role of osteoporosis in the vibration characteristics of human spine after lumbar interbody fusion. *Int. J. Numer. Methods Biomed. Eng.* **2020**, *36*, e3402. [CrossRef]
116. Rockenfeller, R.; Müller, A. Augmenting the Cobb angle: Three-dimensional analysis of whole spine shapes using Bézier curves. *Comput. Methods Programs Biomed.* **2022**, *225*, 107075. [CrossRef]
117. Kim, J.W.; Eom, G.M.; Kwon, Y.R. Analysis of maximum joint moment during infant lifting-up motion. *Technol. Health Care* **2022**, *30*, S441–S450. [CrossRef]
118. Nowakowska-Lipiec, K.; Michnik, R.; Linek, P.; Myśliwiec, A.; Jochymczyk-Woźniak, K.; Gzik, M. A numerical study to determine the effect of strengthening and weakening of the transversus abdominis muscle on lumbar spine loads. *Comput. Methods Biomech. Biomed. Eng.* **2020**, *23*, 1287–1296. [CrossRef]
119. Bauer, S.; Paulus, D. Analysis of the biomechanical effects of spinal fusion to adjacent vertebral segments of the lumbar spine using multi body simulation. *Int. J. Simulation: Syst. Sci. Technol.* **2014**, *15*, 1–7. [CrossRef]
120. Pfirrmann, C.W.; Metzdorf, A.; Zanetti, M.; Hodler, J.; Boos, N. Magnetic resonance classification of lumbar intervertebral disc degeneration. *Spine* **2001**, *26*, 1873–1878. [CrossRef]
121. Foltz, M.H.; Kage, C.C.; Johnson, C.P.; Ellingson, A.M. Noninvasive assessment of biochemical and mechanical properties of lumbar discs through quantitative magnetic resonance imaging in asymptomatic volunteers. *J. Biomech. Eng.* **2017**, *139*, 111002. [CrossRef]
122. Bogduk, N.; Macintosh, J.E.; Pearcy, M.J. A universal model of the lumbar back muscles in the upright position. *Spine* **1992**, *17*, 897–913. [CrossRef] [PubMed]
123. Aiyangar, A.; Zheng, L.; Anderst, W.; Zhang, X. Instantaneous centers of rotation for lumbar segmental extension in vivo. *J. Biomech.* **2017**, *52*, 113–121. [CrossRef]
124. Daggfeldt, K.; Thorstensson, A. The mechanics of back-extensor torque production about the lumbar spine. *J. Biomech.* **2003**, *36*, 815–825. [CrossRef] [PubMed]

125. Hodges, P.W.; Cresswell, A.G.; Daggfeldt, K.; Thorstensson, A. In vivo measurement of the effect of intra-abdominal pressure on the human spine. *J. Biomech.* **2001**, *34*, 347–353. [CrossRef] [PubMed]
126. Rasmussen, J.; Damsgaard, M.; Voigt, M. Muscle recruitment by the min/max criterion—A comparative numerical study. *J. Biomech.* **2001**, *34*, 409–415. [CrossRef]
127. Crowninshield, R.D.; Brand, R.A. A physiologically based criterion of muscle force prediction in locomotion. *J. Biomech.* **1981**, *14*, 793–801. [CrossRef]
128. Ezati, M.; Ghannadi, B.; McPhee, J. A review of simulation methods for human movement dynamics with emphasis on gait. *Multibody Syst. Dyn.* **2019**, *47*, 265–292. [CrossRef]
129. Anderson, F.C.; Pandy, M.G. Static and dynamic optimization solutions for gait are practically equivalent. *J. Biomech.* **2001**, *34*, 153–161. [CrossRef]
130. Morrow, M.M.; Rankin, J.W.; Neptune, R.R.; Kaufman, K.R. A comparison of static and dynamic optimization muscle force predictions during wheelchair propulsion. *J. Biomech.* **2014**, *47*, 3459–3465. [CrossRef] [PubMed]

Disclaimer/Publisher's Note: The statements, opinions and data contained in all publications are solely those of the individual author(s) and contributor(s) and not of MDPI and/or the editor(s). MDPI and/or the editor(s) disclaim responsibility for any injury to people or property resulting from any ideas, methods, instructions or products referred to in the content.

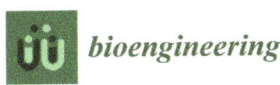

Article

Reference Values for 3D Spinal Posture Based on Videorasterstereographic Analyses of Healthy Adults

Janine Huthwelker [1,*], Jürgen Konradi [1], Claudia Wolf [1], Ruben Westphal [2], Irene Schmidtmann [2], Philipp Drees [3] and Ulrich Betz [1]

1. Institute of Physical Therapy, Prevention and Rehabilitation, University Medical Center of the Johannes Gutenberg University Mainz, Langenbeckstraße 1, D-55131 Mainz, Germany
2. Institute of Medical Biostatistics, Epidemiology and Informatics, University Medical Center of the Johannes Gutenberg University Mainz, Obere Zahlbacher Straße 69, D-55131 Mainz, Germany
3. Department of Orthopedics and Trauma Surgery, University Medical Center of the Johannes Gutenberg University Mainz, Langenbeckstraße 1, D-55131 Mainz, Germany
* Correspondence: janine.huthwelker@unimedizin-mainz.de

Abstract: Visual examinations are commonly used to analyze spinal posture. Even though they are simple and fast, their interrater reliability is poor. Suitable alternatives should be objective, non-invasive, valid and reliable. Videorasterstereography (VRS) is a corresponding method that is increasingly becoming established. However, there is a lack of reference data based on adequate numbers of participants and structured subgroup analyses according to sex and age. We used VRS to capture the spinal posture of 201 healthy participants (aged 18–70 years) divided into three age cohorts. Three-dimensional reference data are presented for the global spine parameters and for every vertebral body individually (C7-L4) (here called the specific spine parameters). The vertebral column was found to be systematically asymmetric in the transverse and the coronal planes. Graphical presentations of the vertebral body posture revealed systematic differences between the subgroups; however, large standard deviations meant that these differences were not significant. In contrast, several global parameters (e.g., thoracic kyphosis and lumbar lordosis) indicated differences between the analyzed subgroups. The findings confirm the importance of presenting reference data not only according to sex but also according to age in order to map physiological posture changes over the life span. The question also arises as to whether therapeutic approximations to an almost symmetrical spine are biomechanically desirable.

Keywords: surface topography; rasterstereographic back shape analysis; normative data; healthy adults; posture analysis; spine

1. Introduction

The spine connects the pelvis and the head with 24 vertebral bodies that can move against each other in three directions of movement. It stabilizes the torso and enables verticalization. The posture and movements of the spine are individually varied and highly characteristic of each person [1]. Visual inspection and posture analyses are important aspects of the basic examination of patients affected by spinal disorders [2]. Many musculoskeletal examiners have reported that visual estimations are one of their most commonly used assessment tools when analyzing spinal posture in clinical practice [3]. Although these visual assessments are simple and quick to perform, their results are relatively subjective, and their interrater reliability is statistically poor [3,4]. This becomes problematic when the results contribute to the clinical decision making process or are used in follow-up examinations to assess the progress and outcomes of the initiated therapies [5]. In order to address this problem, the collection of data regarding spinal posture should be objective and standardized using valid, reliable and reproducible measurement approaches. It is crucial for the assessments to be non-invasive for the patient and quick and easy to conduct in daily clinical routines. Videorasterstereography (VRS) seems to be a corresponding method that is increasingly becoming established in clinical practice [6–8].

The VRS system is based on a horizontal light line pattern projected onto the patient's unclothed back and creates a virtual plaster cast of the individual back surface within only a few seconds [7]. In addition to information about the surface topographic curvature picture, the system is able to precisely estimate the position of every vertebral body (from C7 to L4) and the pelvis in a virtually constructed three-dimensional model of the human vertebral column [7,9–12]. VRS has evolved since its initial development in the 1980s and has been described in various publications [6,7,13]. The system has been proven to be valid and highly reliable compared to the clinical gold standard (X-ray imaging) [8,14–17].

In order to implement VRS for spinal posture analysis as a routine assessment in clinical practice, it is essential to have systematic reference data available for comparison with the potential pathological findings. Unfortunately, the current datasets are only conditionally able to fulfill these requirements, as they have several limitations.

Thus far, there are reference data for the global spine parameters of children [18], young adults [19–21] and young and middle-aged adults [22,23]. Either relatively heterogeneous study cohorts with very small numbers of participants have been analyzed without any further subgroup specifications [22,23], or subgroup-analyses have focused only on the potential differences between female and male participants in young, relatively homogenous study cohorts [19–21]. Possible changes in physiologic spinal posture according to sex and/or age over the adult life span have not yet been investigated. This knowledge, however, is essential for the consultation of reference data in clinical practice, in which not only young but also older patients are examined using VRS measurement devices.

In order to close this gap in our knowledge, the first aim of the current study was to provide practitioners and researchers with an additional set of VRS reference data that, firstly, included a preferably high number of healthy participants. Secondly, structured subgroup analyses were used depict possible physiologic changes in the spinal posture parameters according to sex and age over an adult life span of 18 to 70 years.

The second aim of this study was to provide the respective reference data for specific spine parameters: the isolated position of each vertebral body from C7 to L4 in all three dimensions of movement. These data are currently missing from the literature. As of up to a few years ago, only global spine parameters such as the thoracic kyphosis and lumbar lordosis angles were exportable from the DICAM 3 software. Meanwhile, the three-dimensional position of each vertebral body can be analyzed using an additional export interface.

In contrast to the work previously published by our own research group, describing a subgroup analysis of 100 asymptomatic females based on the dataset included here [24], this project involved a more differentiated analysis providing reference data for three different age cohorts (18–30 years, 31–50 years and 51–70 years) and for both sexes, respectively.

2. Materials and Methods

The data analyzed in this work were part of a prospective, explorative, cross-sectional and monocentric study assessing the three-dimensional spinal posture and movement behavior of healthy participants in the upright standing position and at four different walking speeds (2 km/h, 3 km/h, 4 km/h and 5 km/h). Ethical approval was obtained from the responsible ethics committee of the Rhineland-Palatinate Medical Association, and the study is registered with the World Health Organization (WHO) (INT: DRKS00010834). Based on a statistical sample size calculation, 201 healthy participants (sex ratio of 2/3 females to 1/3 males, aged 18–70 years) who gave their informed consent prior to participation were included in three different age cohorts (young (18–30 years), middle (31–50 years) and old (51–70 years)).

2.1. Participants

In order to participate, the volunteers had to be free of pain, and due to data capture requirements, their body mass index (BMI) had to be ≤ 30.0 kg/m^2. All the participants had to demonstrate adequate gait stability (timed up-and-go test [25]), an age- and sex-accorded walking speed (two-minute walk test [26]) and spinal function (back performance scale [27]), as well as an appropriate joint mobility in order, theoretically, to be able to perform a physiological gait pattern [28]. Interested volunteers were excluded from participation in cases where they reported a history of surgery or fracture between the spinal segments of C7 and the pelvis. Further exclusion criteria were medical or therapeutic treatments due to spinal or pelvic girdle complaints (C7-pelvis) within the last 12 months or medical or therapeutic treatments due to musculoskeletal problems (musculoskeletal system except for C7-pelvis) within the last six months prior to the investigation.

2.2. Experimental Setup and Data Capture

In the study, "4D average" posture analyses were performed on all the participants using the DIERS Formetric III 4D measuring device (software versions DICAM v3.7.1.7 (DIERS International GmbH, Schlangenbad, Germany) for the data collection and DICAM v3.5.0Beta11 (DIERS International GmbH, Schlangenbad, Germany) for the data export), a VRS system based on the principle of triangulation [13]. A slide projector, used as the optical equivalent to an inverse camera, projects horizontal and parallel light lines onto the unclothed back of the participant, who is standing upright on a treadmill (height: ~18 cm) at a predefined distance from the measuring device (~2 m), with the eyes looking towards a standardized point ~2 m away and 20 cm below the individual's body height (measured from the ground). Twelve series recordings of the transformed line pattern (due to back surface curvatures) were captured for a period of 6 s with an associated camera system. The three-dimensional scatter plot derived (consisting of up to 150,000 individual data points, depending on the body size) was used to create a virtual plaster cast of the surface of the participant's back. The three-dimensional position of the underlying spine and the pelvis was estimated based on this information in combination with a clinically validated correlational model [11–13].

Even though it is technically not required for static VRS posture analyses, all the participants were marked with seven reflective markers prior to the data capture (on the spinal process of C7, the spinous processes between the medial parts of the spinae scapulae (~T3) and the thoracolumbar transitions (~T12), the left and right posterior superior iliac spine (PSIS) and on both acromia). This was necessary because the superior study protocol meant that the data for the dynamic gait analyses were also captured on the same measurement appointment. In order to best control for potential palpation or measurement bias, however, the same investigator (physical therapist) always performed the complete procedure themselves, including the entrance examinations (checking for inclusion and exclusion criteria), palpation, marker attachments and the VRS measurements, following a strict and standardized protocol. A static control scan was also performed to check for the correct placement of the markers. Where there were clinically inconclusive measurement results or any uncertainty on the part of the investigator, the placement of the markers was checked, palpated again, and corrected, if necessary, until the final marker position was defined. The measurements were repeated if the first graphical data output revealed clinically incomprehensible, inconsistent measuring artefacts or apparent software misinterpretations. For reasons of quality assurance, the investigator and an additional technician, who were both highly familiar with the software and the measuring device, further inspected all the pictures and the graphical data output visually after completion of the data collection phase for further abnormal spinal representations or other measuring artefacts and corrected them if necessary. In total, 46 specific and 14 global spine parameters were exported using the export interface of the DICAM v3.5.0Beta11 software. The Statistical Analysis System (SAS version 9.4) was used to combine all the exported files into one editable sheet of raw data. Figure 1 provides a schematic flow chart of the experimental process.

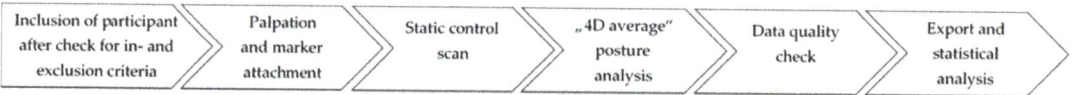

Figure 1. Schematic flow chart of the experimental process.

2.3. Data Analysis

The "4D average" measurement approach used meant that 12 individual values per participant were exported for every spine parameter. Several clinically inconclusive extreme values and, for one participant, isolated missing data points were identified in a preliminary visual data review. The Statistical Package of the Social Sciences (IBM SPSS Statistics for Windows, Version 23.0. Armonk, NY, USA: IBM Corp.) was used to systematically identify these values for every analyzed parameter, and all the extreme outliers revealed by the stem-and-leaf plot were removed from the raw dataset. The missing values were treated as extreme outliers, and the respective cells were removed from the raw dataset as well. The remaining values for every parameter were aggregated to finally create one mean value for every participant and for every parameter of interest.

Descriptive statistics were used to describe the reference values for all the specific (C7–L4 and the pelvis) and global spine parameters according to the mean of means (MoM) and the standard deviation (SD) in all three dimensions for the entire group, for all the female and all the male participants, and for the female and male participants within the three different age cohorts, respectively. An explorative two-way analysis of variance (two-way ANOVA) was used to check for possible differences between the groups according to sex, age cohort or a combination of both (level of significance $p < 0.05$). Possible deviations from the symmetrical zero positions of the different spine parameters were checked by one-sample Wilcoxon signed rank tests (level of significance $p < 0.05$). Graphical figures were created using Microsoft Excel (Microsoft Corporation, Version 2016. Redmond, WA, USA).

The authors do not include a detailed definition or description of the analyzed global and specific spine parameters. Instead, the reader is referred to the respective previous publications [19,24].

3. Results

3.1. Participants

A total of 201 healthy participants (132 females and 69 males) were included in the data analyses and were subdivided into three different age cohorts (67 participants per group). Their detailed characteristics, according to age and BMI, are presented in Table 1.

3.2. Data Analysis

The spinal posture data were analyzed using descriptive and explorative statistics. Reference values for the specific and global spine parameters are presented in Table 2 for the transversal plane, in Table 3 for the coronal plane and in Table 4 for the sagittal plane. Figure 2 (transversal), Figure 3 (coronal) and Figure 4 (sagittal) are the respective graphical representations of the specific spine parameters for those three investigated planes. The results of the explorative statistical analyses are presented in Table 5.

Table 1. Participant characteristics.

		All Participants	Sex		Age Cohort "Young"			Age Cohort "Middle"			Age Cohort "Old"		
			All Females	All Males	All Young Participants	Young Females	Young Males	All Middle Participants	Middle Females	Middle Males	All Old Participants	Old Females	Old Males
N		201	132	69	67	44	23	67	44	23	67	44	23
Age (years)	Mean	41.3	41.3	41.3	25.9	26.0	25.6	41.4	42.2	39.8	56.6	55.7	58.3
	SD	13.4	13.0	14.3	2.9	2.7	3.3	6.4	6.5	6.2	4.3	3.9	4.5
BMI (kg/m²)	Mean	23.5	22.9	24.6	22.7	22.0	23.9	23.7	23.0	25.0	24.1	23.6	25.0
	SD	2.8	2.8	2.4	2.9	2.9	2.6	2.8	2.8	2.3	2.5	2.5	2.2

Table 2. Results of the descriptive statistical analyses (MoM ± SD) of the spinal parameters in the transversal plane.

		Specific Parameters																			Global Parameters			
		Sh (°)	C7 (°)	T1 (°)	T2 (°)	T3 (°)	T4 (°)	T5 (°)	T6 (°)	T7 (°)	T8 (°)	T9 (°)	T10 (°)	T11 (°)	T12 (°)	L1 (°)	L2 (°)	L3 (°)	L4 (°)	Pel (°)	Surface Rotation RMS (°)	Surface Rotation MAX (°)	(Right Side) Surface Rotation +Max (°)	(Left Side) Surface Rotation −Max (°)
All Participants	N	198	199	201	200	200	197	197	198	198	198	200	201	201	201	201	200	200	200	200	200	201	198	201
	MoM	−0.3	0.2	0.0	0.1	0.0	−0.2	−0.5	−1.0	−1.6	−1.9	−2.3	−2.2	−2.4	−2.2	−1.9	−1.4	−0.7	−0.2	0.0	2.3	−1.9	1.5	−3.3
	SD	2.0	0.2	0.4	0.8	1.4	2.2	3.2	3.9	4.0	3.9	3.8	3.6	3.3	3.3	3.3	3.0	2.4	1.4	0.5	0.9	4.0	1.5	2.3
All Females	N	130	131	132	131	131	129	129	130	130	130	131	132	132	132	132	131	131	131	132	131	132	130	132
	MoM	−0.3	0.0	0.1	0.1	1.3	−0.1	−0.4	−0.8	−1.4	−1.9	−2.2	−2.2	−2.1	−2.0	−1.7	−1.2	−0.6	−0.1	0.0	2.2	−1.8	1.5	−3.2
	SD	2.0	0.4	0.1	0.1	1.3	2.0	3.0	3.6	3.8	3.6	3.3	3.3	3.5	3.6	3.6	3.3	2.6	1.4	0.5	0.9	4.0	1.4	2.3
All Males	N	68	68	69	69	69	68	68	68	68	68	69	69	69	69	69	69	69	69	68	69	69	68	69
	MoM	−0.3	0.2	0.0	0.9	−0.1	2.5	3.6	4.3	−2.1	−2.6	−2.7	−2.6	−2.8	−2.7	−2.3	−1.6	−0.9	−0.2	0.1	2.3	−2.1	1.7	−3.6
	SD	2.0	0.2	0.5	0.9	1.6	2.5	3.6	4.3	4.4	4.2	4.1	3.6	3.2	2.8	2.7	2.5	2.1	1.3	0.4	1.0	4.0	1.4	2.3
All Young Participants	N	67	67	67	67	67	67	67	67	67	66	66	67	67	67	67	66	66	66	66	66	67	66	67
	MoM	−0.1	0.0	0.0	−0.1	−0.2	−0.5	−1.0	−1.5	−2.1	−2.7	−2.9	−2.7	−2.7	−2.5	−2.1	−1.5	−0.6	0.0	0.1	2.3	−2.3	1.2	−3.5
	SD	2.1	0.2	0.4	0.7	1.3	2.1	3.1	3.7	3.9	3.4	3.4	3.4	3.1	3.1	3.2	2.9	2.3	1.3	0.5	0.9	3.6	1.4	2.2
Young Females	N	44	44	44	44	44	44	44	44	44	43	43	44	44	44	44	43	43	43	44	43	44	43	44
	MoM	0.1	0.2	0.0	−0.2	−0.2	−0.4	−0.9	−1.5	−2.0	−2.8	−2.8	−2.5	−2.4	−2.3	−1.9	−1.4	−0.5	0.0	0.0	2.4	−2.4	1.3	−3.5
	SD	2.0	0.2	0.4	0.7	1.3	2.1	3.1	3.7	3.9	3.4	3.3	3.4	3.3	3.3	3.3	3.2	2.3	1.4	0.5	0.9	3.8	1.3	2.3
Young Males	N	23	23	23	23	23	23	23	23	23	23	23	23	23	23	23	23	23	23	22	23	23	23	23
	MoM	−0.4	0.0	−0.1	−0.1	−0.3	−0.6	−1.1	−1.7	−2.3	−2.8	−3.0	−3.0	−3.2	−3.0	−2.6	−1.9	−0.9	−0.1	0.3	2.2	−2.3	1.2	−3.6
	SD	2.2	0.2	0.4	0.7	1.3	2.0	3.2	3.8	4.1	4.0	3.7	3.7	3.5	3.0	2.4	2.2	1.8	1.1	0.4	0.8	3.4	1.2	2.2
All Middle Participants	N	66	67	67	67	67	67	67	67	67	67	67	67	67	67	67	67	67	67	66	67	67	66	67
	MoM	−0.4	0.2	0.1	0.1	0.1	0.0	−0.2	−0.6	−1.2	−1.5	−2.1	−2.3	−2.3	−2.3	−2.0	−1.5	−0.8	−0.3	−0.1	2.1	−2.3	1.4	−3.4
	SD	2.1	0.2	0.4	0.7	1.3	2.2	3.2	3.7	3.8	3.8	3.6	3.5	3.5	3.4	3.3	3.3	2.7	1.6	0.4	1.0	3.6	1.4	2.2
Middle Females	N	43	44	44	44	44	43	44	44	44	44	44	44	44	44	44	44	44	44	44	44	44	43	44
	MoM	−0.6	0.0	0.1	0.2	0.1	0.2	0.0	−0.4	−0.9	−1.4	−1.9	−2.1	−2.3	−2.3	−2.0	−1.5	−0.9	−0.3	−0.1	2.0	−2.2	1.3	−3.3
	SD	2.0	0.2	0.4	0.6	1.2	1.9	2.8	3.2	3.4	3.4	3.4	3.4	3.5	3.4	3.5	3.5	2.8	1.6	0.4	0.8	3.4	1.4	2.0
Middle Males	N	23	23	23	23	23	23	23	23	23	23	23	23	23	23	23	23	23	23	22	23	23	23	23
	MoM	−0.6	0.2	0.3	0.3	0.2	−0.3	−0.6	−1.1	−1.7	−2.3	−2.6	−2.6	−2.5	−2.3	−2.0	−1.3	−0.5	−0.5	−0.2	2.3	−2.4	1.5	−3.6
	SD	2.1	0.2	0.4	0.9	1.5	2.6	3.8	4.5	4.7	4.5	4.3	3.9	3.5	3.2	3.0	2.9	2.6	1.7	0.4	1.1	3.8	1.5	2.6
All Old Participants	N	65	65	67	66	66	63	63	64	64	65	66	67	67	67	67	67	67	67	66	67	67	65	67
	MoM	−0.3	0.0	0.0	0.2	0.2	−0.1	−0.4	−0.8	−1.5	−2.0	−2.1	−2.2	−2.1	−1.9	−1.6	−1.1	−0.6	−0.1	0.1	2.3	−1.1	1.8	−3.1
	SD	2.0	0.5	0.5	0.6	1.6	2.4	3.4	4.2	4.3	4.0	3.9	3.9	3.6	3.4	3.2	2.9	2.2	1.3	0.4	0.9	4.6	1.7	2.4
Old Females	N	43	43	44	43	43	41	41	42	42	42	43	44	44	44	44	44	44	44	44	44	44	43	44
	MoM	−0.6	0.2	0.1	0.3	0.3	0.0	−0.3	−0.5	−1.3	−1.7	−1.8	−1.9	−1.7	−1.5	−1.2	−0.8	−0.3	0.0	0.1	2.3	−0.9	1.8	−2.9
	SD	2.0	0.2	0.4	0.8	1.4	2.2	3.2	3.9	4.1	4.0	4.3	4.0	3.8	3.5	3.5	3.1	2.4	1.4	0.4	0.9	4.6	1.8	2.4
Old Males	N	22	22	23	23	23	22	22	22	22	23	23	23	23	23	23	23	23	23	22	23	23	22	23
	MoM	0.3	0.3	0.0	0.1	0.1	−0.4	−1.4	−1.4	−2.1	−2.5	−2.5	−2.6	−2.8	−2.6	−2.2	−1.7	−1.2	−0.5	−0.2	2.5	−1.4	1.8	−3.5
	SD	1.8	0.2	0.6	1.1	1.9	2.9	4.3	4.6	4.3	4.3	4.4	3.8	3.1	2.8	2.4	2.4	1.8	1.0	0.4	0.9	4.8	1.7	2.3

Abbreviations: MoM = mean of means; SD = standard deviation; Sh = shoulder; Pel = pelvis; N = number.

Table 3. Results of the descriptive statistical analyses (MoM ± SD) of the spinal parameters in the coronal plane.

			Specific Parameters																Global Parameters			
			Sh (°)	C7 (°)	T1 (°)	T2 (°)	T3 (°)	T4 (°)	T5 (°)	T6 (°)	T7 (°)	T8 (°)	T9 (°)	T10 (°)	T11 (°)	T12 (°)	L1 (°)	L2 (°)	L3 (°)	L4 (°)	Pel (°)	Trunk Imbalance VP-DM (°)	Trunk Imbalance VP-DM (mm)	Apical Deviation RMS (mm)	Apical Deviation MAX (mm)	(Right Side) Apical Deviation VP-DM +Max (mm)	(Left Side) Apical Deviation VP-DM −Max (mm)
Sex	All Participants	N	200	197	195	194	199	198	198	198	201	201	200	200	200	199	198	198	198	200	194	194	195	196	201	198	198
		MoM	−1.1	−1.1	−1.5	−1.7	−1.3	−0.5	0.3	1.0	1.2	1.1	0.8	0.5	0.3	0.3	0.0	−0.2	0.1	0.2	−0.1	−0.2	−1.7	3.6	−1.8	3.2	−4.9
		SD	1.3	2.1	2.3	2.6	3.1	3.0	2.6	2.1	2.0	2.2	2.1	1.9	1.9	1.9	1.6	1.7	2.4	3.1	0.8	0.8	7.3	1.7	7.1	3.0	3.3
	All Females	N	131	129	128	127	132	131	131	131	132	132	131	131	131	130	129	129	129	131	127	126	128	130	132	131	130
		MoM	−1.3	−1.2	−1.6	−1.8	−1.4	−0.7	0.1	0.8	1.1	1.1	0.8	0.5	0.3	0.3	0.1	−0.1	0.3	1.0	−0.1	−0.2	−1.6	3.5	−2.3	2.9	−4.9
		SD	1.4	2.2	2.3	2.5	3.1	3.0	2.5	1.9	1.7	2.1	2.0	2.0	2.0	2.0	1.7	1.8	2.5	3.2	0.8	0.9	7.7	1.7	6.7	2.8	3.3
	All Males	N	69	68	67	67	67	67	67	67	69	69	69	69	69	69	69	69	69	69	67	68	67	66	69	67	68
		MoM	−0.9	−1.0	−1.3	−1.3	−1.1	−0.3	0.6	1.2	1.4	1.1	0.8	0.5	0.4	0.2	−0.1	−0.4	−0.3	0.2	−0.3	−0.2	−2.0	3.8	−0.8	3.8	−4.7
		SD	1.3	2.1	2.3	2.8	3.1	3.2	2.8	2.3	2.3	2.4	2.3	2.0	1.8	1.8	1.5	1.5	2.2	2.8	0.8	0.8	6.6	1.6	7.7	3.4	3.2
Age Cohort "Young"	All Young Participants	N	67	66	66	66	66	66	67	66	67	67	67	67	67	67	67	67	66	66	64	66	66	65	67	66	66
		MoM	−1.0	−0.9	−1.2	−1.3	−0.6	0.2	0.9	1.2	1.0	0.7	0.5	0.4	0.4	0.4	0.0	−0.3	−0.3	0.8	−0.1	−0.3	−2.5	3.5	−0.9	3.3	−4.4
		SD	1.2	1.7	2.0	2.4	2.8	2.7	2.4	1.9	1.8	1.9	1.9	2.0	2.0	1.9	1.6	1.8	2.6	3.0	0.9	0.8	6.5	1.6	7.0	2.9	3.2
	Young Females	N	44	43	43	43	44	43	43	43	44	44	44	44	44	44	44	44	43	43	42	43	43	42	44	43	43
		MoM	−1.1	−1.1	−1.4	−1.4	−0.6	0.4	0.9	1.1	0.9	0.7	0.5	0.4	0.5	0.4	0.1	−0.1	0.6	1.5	−0.1	−0.3	−2.6	3.4	−1.1	3.1	−4.4
		SD	1.3	1.7	2.0	2.5	3.0	2.7	2.2	1.7	1.7	1.8	1.7	2.3	2.1	2.0	1.9	1.9	2.7	3.2	0.9	0.8	6.7	1.6	7.2	2.7	3.1
	Young Males	N	23	23	23	23	23	23	23	23	23	23	23	23	23	23	23	23	23	23	22	23	23	23	23	23	23
		MoM	−0.7	−0.6	−0.9	−1.1	−0.7	0.0	0.7	1.3	1.3	0.7	0.4	0.2	0.3	0.3	−0.2	−0.5	−0.2	0.6	−0.1	−0.2	−2.3	3.6	−0.4	3.8	−4.4
		SD	1.1	1.8	2.0	2.3	2.4	2.8	2.7	2.2	1.9	2.1	2.3	2.1	1.9	2.0	1.7	1.6	2.2	2.6	0.8	0.7	6.3	1.6	6.7	3.1	3.1
Age Cohort "Middle"	All Middle Participants	N	67	65	63	63	67	67	67	67	67	67	66	66	66	65	66	66	66	67	64	66	66	66	67	66	66
		MoM	−1.2	−1.1	−1.6	−1.9	−1.5	−0.8	0.0	0.7	1.1	1.1	1.0	0.8	0.4	0.4	0.1	−0.2	0.4	0.8	−0.2	−0.2	−1.9	3.8	−2.9	2.9	−5.3
		SD	1.3	2.4	2.2	2.7	3.3	3.2	2.7	2.2	2.1	2.1	2.0	1.9	2.1	2.2	1.9	1.9	2.2	2.6	0.8	0.8	7.0	1.8	7.0	3.2	3.3
	Middle Females	N	44	42	41	41	44	44	44	44	44	44	44	43	43	42	43	42	43	44	41	43	43	44	44	44	43
		MoM	−1.2	−1.0	−1.7	−2.2	−1.7	−0.8	−0.3	0.5	1.0	1.1	1.1	0.9	0.5	0.4	0.2	−0.1	0.6	1.5	−0.1	−0.2	−1.8	3.6	−3.3	2.8	−5.3
		SD	1.3	2.4	2.4	2.7	3.3	2.9	2.4	1.9	2.0	2.0	1.9	1.9	2.0	2.2	1.9	1.4	2.3	3.3	0.7	0.9	7.4	1.9	6.4	2.9	3.1
	Middle Males	N	23	23	22	22	23	23	23	23	23	23	23	23	23	23	23	23	23	23	23	23	23	23	23	23	23
		MoM	−1.0	−1.3	−1.3	−1.3	−1.1	−0.4	0.4	1.1	1.3	1.2	0.9	0.6	0.3	0.3	−0.3	−0.3	0.0	0.2	−0.4	−0.4	−2.2	4.1	−2.2	3.2	−5.4
		SD	1.1	2.3	2.3	2.7	3.5	3.7	3.2	2.8	2.5	2.2	2.3	2.0	2.3	2.0	1.4	2.0	2.0	2.8	0.9	0.7	6.2	1.7	8.0	3.7	3.4
Age Cohort "Old"	All Old Participants	N	66	66	66	65	65	65	65	65	67	67	67	67	67	67	65	66	66	67	66	62	63	65	67	66	66
		MoM	−1.2	−1.3	−1.7	−1.8	−1.7	−1.0	0.0	1.0	1.6	1.5	1.0	0.7	0.1	0.0	0.0	−0.2	−0.2	0.2	−0.1	−0.1	−0.8	3.6	−1.5	3.3	−4.8
		SD	1.4	2.2	2.4	2.7	3.0	3.1	2.8	2.3	2.3	2.4	2.2	1.9	1.7	1.7	0.0	1.8	2.5	3.0	0.8	0.9	8.3	1.6	7.3	3.1	3.3
	Old Females	N	43	44	44	43	44	44	44	44	44	44	44	44	44	44	42	43	43	44	44	40	42	44	44	44	44
		MoM	−1.3	−1.3	−1.6	−1.9	−1.9	−1.2	−0.2	0.8	1.5	1.4	0.9	0.3	0.0	0.0	0.0	−0.1	−0.1	0.6	0.0	−0.2	−0.4	3.5	−2.4	2.8	−5.1
		SD	1.3	2.3	2.4	2.4	2.9	3.1	2.9	2.1	1.9	2.2	2.2	1.9	1.6	1.8	2.5	2.0	2.5	3.0	0.8	1.0	8.8	1.7	6.5	2.7	3.5
	Old Males	N	23	22	22	22	21	21	21	21	23	23	23	23	23	23	23	23	23	23	22	22	21	21	23	22	22
		MoM	−1.0	−1.2	−1.3	−1.6	−1.3	−0.4	0.6	1.4	1.7	1.6	1.2	0.7	0.3	0.0	−0.3	−0.5	−0.7	−0.6	−0.2	−0.1	−1.4	3.7	0.3	4.4	−4.3
		SD	1.6	2.0	2.5	3.4	3.3	3.3	2.5	2.6	2.8	2.8	2.3	2.0	1.9	1.6	1.3	1.5	2.3	2.8	0.7	0.9	7.4	1.6	8.5	3.6	3.0

Abbreviations: MoM = mean of means; SD = standard deviation; Sh = shoulder; Pel = pelvis; N = number.

Table 4. Results of the descriptive statistical analyses (MoM ± SD) of the spinal parameters in the sagittal plane.

			Sh (°)	C7 (°)	T1 (°)	T2 (°)	T3 (°)	T4 (°)	T5 (°)	T6 (°)	T7 (°)	T8 (°)	T9 (°)	T10 (°)	T11 (°)	T12 (°)	L1 (°)	L2 (°)	L3 (°)	L4 (°)	Pel (°)	Trunk Inclination (VP-DM) (°)	Trunk Inclination (VP-DM) (mm)	Thoracic Kyphosis (ICT-ITL) (°)	Lumbar Lordosis (ITL-ILS) (°)
											Specific Parameters													Global Parameters		
Sex	All Participants	N	-	201	201	200	200	199	200	199	200	201	201	201	200	200	200	199	201	201	201	198	198	200	201
		MoM		25.5	25.5	23.6	18.6	13.7	10.0	7.2	4.4	0.2	−5.4	−11.0	−15.3	−17.6	−17.4	−13.7	−2.7	10.7	18.4	3.1	26.0	49.9	40.9
		SD		7.5	6.3	6.4	6.5	5.3	4.6	3.9	3.7	3.8	3.9	4.2	4.5	4.9	5.1	5.7	7.4	7.7	8.9	2.1	17.5	8.3	9.2
	All Females	N		132	132	131	131	132	132	131	132	132	132	132	131	131	131	130	132	132	132	130	130	131	132
		MoM		26.2	25.6	22.5	16.9	12.1	8.8	6.3	3.6	−0.6	−6.3	−11.9	−16.3	−18.5	−17.7	−13.0	−0.6	13.9	19.1	3.1	25.6	50.1	44.0
		SD		7.6	6.4	6.4	6.3	5.1	4.4	3.8	3.7	3.6	3.7	4.2	4.5	5.1	5.8	6.3	7.5	6.6	8.9	2.1	17.6	8.2	8.5
	All Males	N		69	69	69	69	67	68	68	68	69	69	69	69	69	69	69	67	69	69	68	68	69	69
		MoM		24.1	25.4	25.7	21.9	16.7	12.4	9.0	6.0	1.9	−3.7	−9.1	−13.5	−16.0	−16.9	−15.1	−6.7	4.5	17.0	3.0	26.7	49.6	34.9
		SD		7.1	6.0	5.7	5.4	4.3	4.0	3.4	3.3	3.7	3.6	3.7	4.0	4.1	4.3	5.2	5.5	5.5	8.7	2.0	17.4	8.6	7.3
Age Cohort "Young"	All Young Participants	N		67	67	66	66	67	67	67	67	67	67	67	66	67	66	66	67	67	67	66	66	66	67
		MoM		23.4	23.7	22.2	17.1	12.5	9.2	6.8	4.4	0.5	−5.0	−10.5	−14.7	−16.9	−16.8	−13.4	−2.7	10.9	21.6	2.9	24.8	46.5	40.1
		SD		6.9	6.0	5.9	6.2	5.3	4.7	4.0	3.8	3.9	3.8	4.2	4.5	5.0	5.8	6.2	7.0	7.7	8.3	2.2	18.4	7.1	8.9
	Young Females	N		44	44	44	44	44	44	44	44	44	44	44	44	44	44	43	44	44	44	43	43	43	44
		MoM		23.9	23.4	20.7	15.0	10.7	7.9	5.7	3.3	−0.4	−5.8	−11.1	−15.3	−17.6	−17.0	−12.9	−1.3	13.2	22.1	2.8	22.6	46.9	43.0
		SD		7.4	6.5	5.5	5.5	4.9	4.6	4.0	3.9	4.1	4.0	4.6	5.1	5.5	5.4	5.9	7.3	7.7	8.9	2.1	17.5	6.9	8.7
	Young Males	N		23	23	23	23	23	23	23	23	23	23	23	23	23	23	23	23	23	23	23	23	23	23
		MoM		22.6	24.3	25.0	21.2	16.1	11.8	9.0	6.4	2.2	−3.5	−9.1	−13.4	−15.6	−16.5	−14.6	−5.4	6.5	20.7	3.3	28.9	45.8	34.5
		SD		5.8	5.1	5.7	5.4	4.3	3.8	3.2	2.7	2.9	2.8	3.1	3.5	3.7	4.7	5.8	5.6	5.6	6.9	2.2	19.7	7.7	6.5
Age Cohort "Middle"	All Middle Participants	N		67	67	67	67	66	66	66	66	67	67	67	67	67	67	66	67	67	67	67	67	67	67
		MoM		27.7	26.7	23.1	17.9	13.3	10.1	7.7	4.9	0.6	−5.1	−10.6	−15.3	−18.1	−17.9	−14.5	−3.8	9.9	17.8	3.2	27.0	49.7	41.0
		SD		6.8	5.9	6.5	6.4	4.7	3.7	3.2	3.3	3.6	3.9	4.2	4.9	4.9	5.2	5.6	5.6	7.4	8.8	2.0	17.0	7.7	9.0
	Middle Females	N		44	44	44	44	44	44	44	44	44	44	44	43	44	44	43	44	44	44	44	44	44	44
		MoM		28.5	26.7	21.7	16.0	11.9	9.4	6.9	4.1	−0.4	−6.3	−11.9	−16.8	−19.5	−18.2	−13.5	−1.0	13.5	18.4	3.2	26.3	49.3	43.7
		SD		6.0	5.5	6.5	6.0	4.4	3.4	3.0	3.3	3.3	3.6	4.0	4.2	4.9	5.4	5.6	7.1	5.6	8.6	2.1	17.3	7.6	9.0
	Middle Males	N		23	23	23	23	22	22	22	22	23	23	23	23	23	23	23	23	23	23	23	23	23	23
		MoM		26.1	26.8	25.7	21.4	16.1	12.3	9.4	6.3	2.6	−2.8	−8.2	−12.4	−15.4	−17.2	−16.3	−9.2	3.0	16.7	3.2	28.3	50.5	35.7
		SD		8.1	6.6	5.7	5.8	3.9	3.5	2.9	2.7	3.4	3.5	3.4	3.7	3.8	3.6	4.9	4.9	5.2	9.1	1.9	16.7	7.9	6.2
Age Cohort "Old"	All Old Participants	N		67	67	67	67	66	67	66	67	67	67	67	67	66	67	67	66	67	67	65	65	67	67
		MoM		25.4	26.1	25.5	20.8	15.2	10.7	7.2	3.9	−0.4	−6.2	−11.8	−16.0	−17.9	−17.6	−13.2	−1.7	11.3	15.7	3.1	26.1	53.4	41.6
		SD		8.2	6.5	6.3	6.3	5.1	4.2	4.0	3.3	3.9	3.8	4.4	4.8	4.9	5.4	6.1	7.7	7.9	8.6	2.1	17.4	8.7	9.7
	Old Females	N		44	44	43	43	44	44	43	44	44	44	44	44	43	44	44	43	44	44	43	43	44	44
		MoM		26.3	26.7	25.0	19.6	13.8	9.5	6.5	3.3	−1.1	−6.9	−12.7	−16.8	−18.3	−17.8	−12.6	0.4	15.0	16.8	3.4	27.8	54.0	45.3
		SD		8.7	6.7	6.5	6.7	5.5	4.9	4.1	3.4	3.4	3.4	4.0	4.1	4.8	5.6	6.0	8.0	6.4	8.4	2.2	18.2	8.7	7.7
	Old Males	N		23	23	23	23	22	23	23	23	23	23	23	23	23	23	23	23	23	23	22	22	23	23
		MoM		23.5	25.0	26.4	23.2	18.1	13.0	8.7	5.2	0.8	−4.7	−10.1	−14.6	−17.0	−17.1	−14.3	−5.7	4.1	13.7	2.6	22.8	52.4	34.4
		SD		6.9	6.1	6.0	4.9	4.5	4.7	4.1	4.1	4.5	4.2	4.2	4.8	4.7	5.1	6.0	5.3	5.2	8.9	1.8	15.5	9.0	9.1

Abbreviations: MoM = mean of means; SD = standard deviation; Sh = shoulder; Pel = pelvis; N = number.

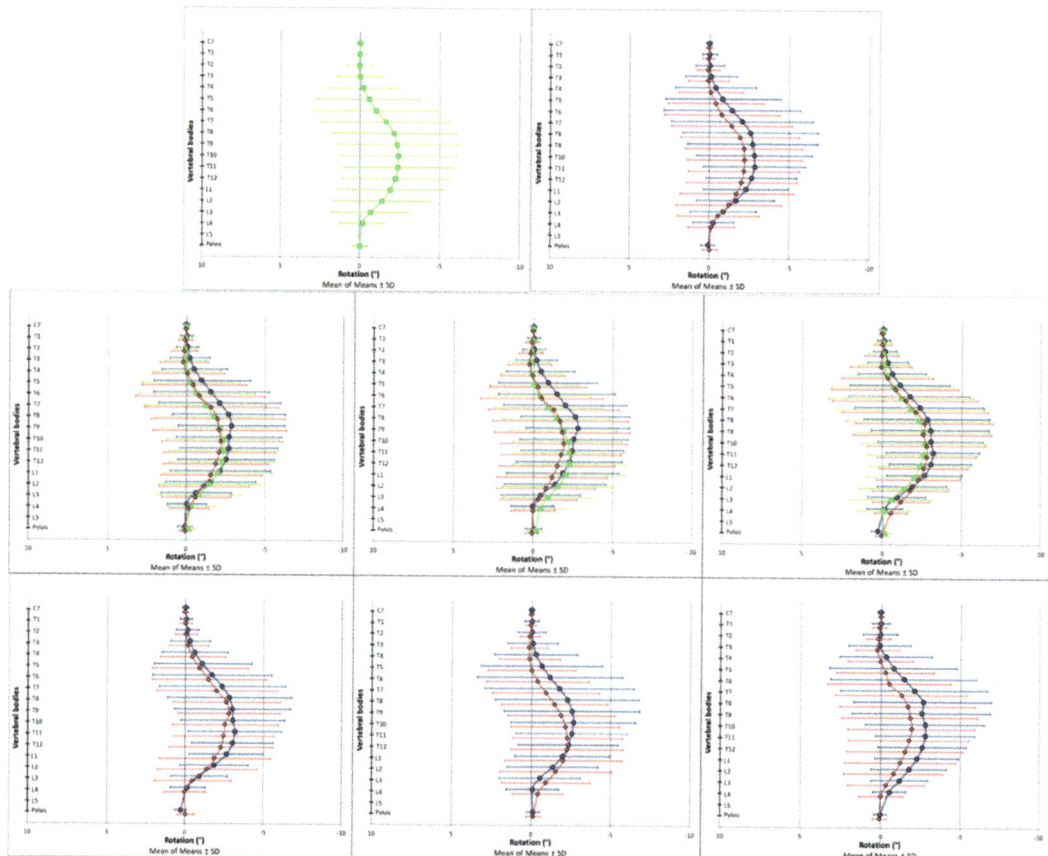

Figure 2. Vertebral body positions in the transversal plane. Positive values represent a rotation of the vertebral bodies to the left (counterclockwise), and negative values represent a rotation of the vertebral bodies to the right (clockwise). The scale of the x-axis is turned to enhance the intuitive visual interpretability of the results: (**Upper row**) (left picture: all participants (■, green); right picture: all female (◆, red) and all male (●, blue) participants). (**Middle row**) (left picture: all participants of the respective age cohorts: young (●, blue), middle (■, green) and old (◆, red); middle picture: all female participants of the respective age cohorts: young (●, blue), middle (■, green) and old (◆, red); right picture: all male participants of the respective age cohorts: young (●, blue), middle (■, green) and old (◆, red)). (**Lower row**) (left picture: all young female (◆, red) and all young male (●, blue) participants; middle picture: all middle-aged female (◆, red) and all middle-aged male (●, blue) participants; right picture: all old female (◆, red) and all old male (●, blue) participants).

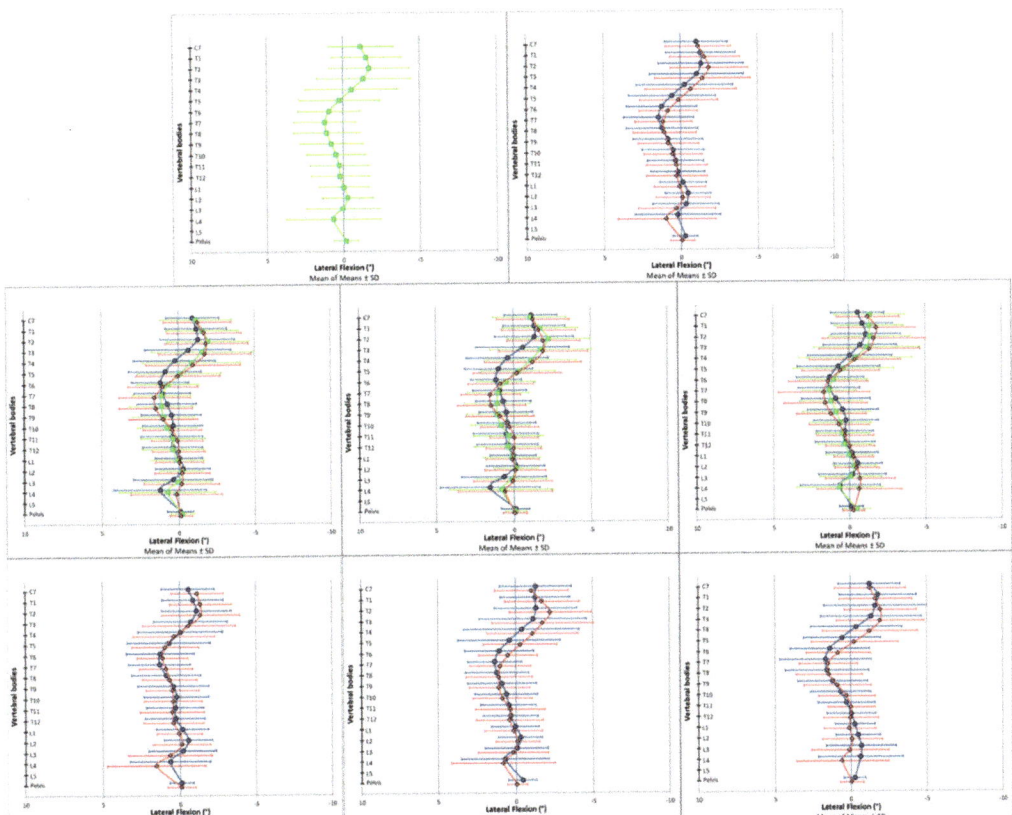

Figure 3. Vertebral body positions in the coronal plane. Positive values represent a tilt of the vertebral bodies to the left, and negative values represent a tilt of the vertebral bodies to the right. The scale of the *x*-axis is turned to enhance the intuitive visual interpretability of the results: (**Upper row**) (left picture: all participants (■, green); right picture: all female (♦, red) and all male (●, blue) participants). (**Middle row**) (left picture: all participants of the respective age cohorts: young (●, blue), middle (■, green) and old (♦, red); middle picture: all female participants of the respective age cohorts: young (●, blue), middle (■, green) and old (♦, red); right picture: all male participants of the respective age cohorts: young (●, blue), middle (■, green) and old (♦, red)). (**Lower row**) (left picture: all young female (♦, red) and all young male (●, blue) participants; middle picture: all middle-aged female (♦, red) and all middle-aged male (●, blue) participants; right picture: all old female (♦, red) and all old male (●, blue) participants.

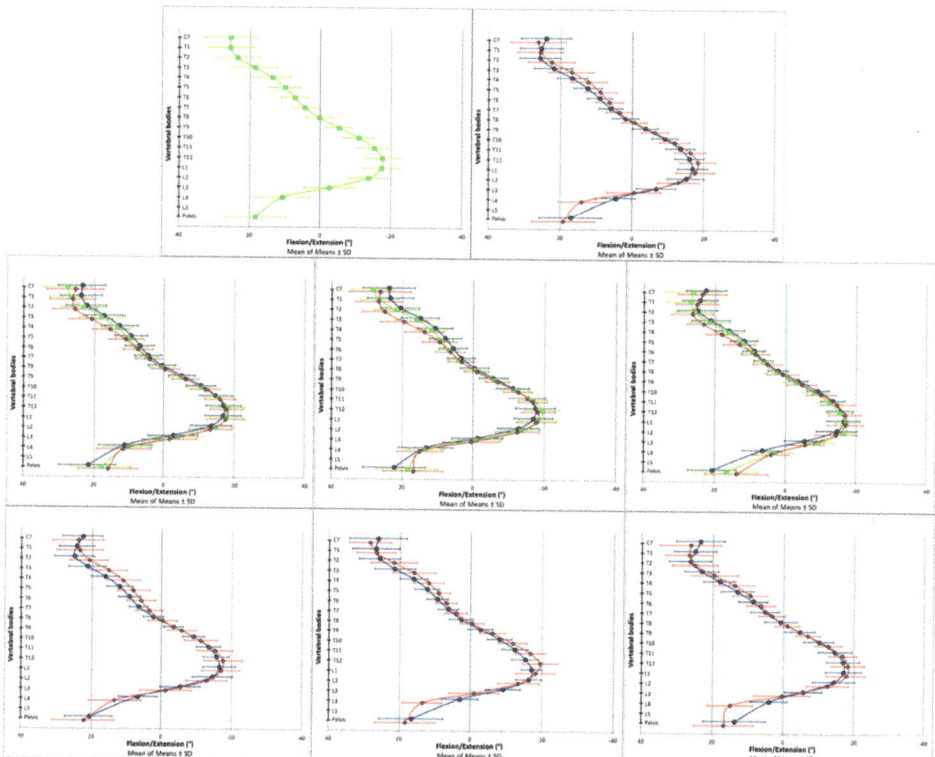

Figure 4. Vertebral body positions in the sagittal plane. Positive values represent a tilt of the vertebral bodies towards spinal flexion, and negative values represent a tilt of the vertebral bodies towards spinal extension. The scale of the *x*-axis is turned to enhance the intuitive visual interpretability of the results: (**Upper row**) (left picture: all participants (■, green); right picture: all female (♦, red) and all male (●, blue) participants). (**Middle row**) (left picture: all participants of the respective age cohorts: young (●, blue), middle (■, green) and old (♦, red); middle picture: all female participants of the respective age cohorts: young (●, blue), middle (■, green) and old (♦, red); right picture: all male participants of the respective age cohorts: young (●, blue), middle (■, green) and old (♦, red)). (**Lower row**) (left picture: all young female (♦, red) and all young male (●, blue) participants; middle picture: all middle-aged female (♦, red) and all middle-aged male (●, blue) participants; right picture: all old female (♦, red) and all old male (●, blue) participants.

3.2.1. Descriptive Data Analysis

In the transverse plane, the spine was not in a neutral rotary position. Instead, a systematic vertebral rotation to the right side was identified from T5 to L3 among all the investigated subgroups (Figure 2 and Table 2). In the coronal plane, a systematic deviation from the neutral centerline was also apparent. The vertebrae above T5 were laterally flexed to the right side, and around the fifth thoracic vertebrae, the side of lateral flexion changed in direction to the left (Figure 3 and Table 3). In the sagittal plane, T8 was found to be in an almost neutral position, indicating that it was the thoracic kyphosis apex (Figure 4 and Table 4). The vertebrae above (C7–T7) were tilted towards spinal flexion, while the vertebrae below were positioned in spinal extension (T9–~L3). The height of the lumbar lordosis apex, meaning the reverse change in direction from spinal extension to spinal flexion, differed between the analyzed subgroups but was systematically located between L2 and L4.

Table 5. Results of the explorative statistical analyses (one-sample Wilcoxon signed rank test and two-way analyses of variance) of the spinal parameters in all three planes of movement.

Table 5. *Cont.*

		Specific Parameters																			Global Parameters			
												Sagittal Plane												
		Sh (°)	C7 (°)	T1 (°)	T2 (°)	T3 (°)	T4 (°)	T5 (°)	T6 (°)	T7 (°)	T8 (°)	T9 (°)	T10 (°)	T11 (°)	T12 (°)	L1 (°)	L2 (°)	L3 (°)	L4 (°)	Pel (°)	Trunk Inclination (VP-DM) (°)	Trunk Inclination (VP-DM) (mm)	Thoracic Kyphosis (ICT-ITL) (°)	Lumbar Lordosis (ITL-ILS) (°)
AP vs. HM = 0 (One-Sample Wilcoxon Signed Rank Test)	Observed Median	-	25.01	25.24	23.95	19.04	13.65	10.36	7.91	4.83	0.23	−5.69	−10.98	−15.07	−17.42	−17.61	−14.08	−3.58	10.52	18.40	2.98	26.15	50.54	40.98
	Standardized Test Statistic	-	12.29	12.29	12.26	12.26	12.23	12.25	12.15	10.91	0.89	−11.74	−12.29	−12.26	−12.26	−12.26	−12.23	−4.97	11.74	12.27	11.84	11.84	12.26	12.29
	p-Value	-	**0.00 ***	**0.00 ***	**0.00 ***	**0.00 ***	**0.00 ***	**0.00 ***	**0.00 ***	**0.00 ***	0.38	**0.00 ***	**0.00 ***	**0.00 ***	**0.00 ***	**0.00 ***	**0.00 ***	**0.00 ***	**0.00 ***	**0.00 ***	**0.00 ***	**0.00 ***	**0.00 ***	**0.00 ***
Between-Subject Effects (two-way ANOVA)	Sex (Sig)	-	**0.05 ***	0.80	**0.00 ***	**0.00 ***	**0.00 ***	**0.00 ***	**0.00 ***	**0.00 ***	0.38	**0.00 ***	**0.00 ***	**0.00 ***	**0.00 ***	0.32	**0.01 ***	**0.00 ***	**0.00 ***	0.10	0.74	0.68	0.66	**0.00 ***
	Age Cohort (Sig)	-	**0.01 ***	**0.03 ***	**0.03 ***	**0.01 ***	**0.01 ***	**0.01 ***	0.19	0.47	0.30	0.14	0.11	0.13	0.20	0.42	0.59	0.33	0.13	0.31	**0.00 ***	0.85	0.80	**0.00 ***	0.70
	Sex *Age Cohort (Sig)	-	0.84	0.50	0.35	0.44	0.77	0.93	0.70	0.67	0.70	0.62	0.49	0.24	0.26	0.95	0.84	0.26	0.12	0.86	0.24	0.22	0.60	0.58
	Young vs. Old (Sig)	-	0.38	0.07	**0.01 ***	**0.00 ***	**0.00 ***	0.15	1.00	0.84	0.30	0.16	0.13	0.20	0.20	0.56	0.80	0.99	1.00	0.94	**0.00 ***	0.96	0.96	**0.00 ***	0.52
	Young vs. Middle (Sig)	-	**0.00 ***	**0.02 ***	0.80	0.84	0.75	0.70	0.47	0.82	0.98	1.00	0.96	0.78	0.38	0.58	0.66	1.00	1.00	0.60	**0.03 ***	0.88	0.84	0.06	0.80
	Middle vs. Old (Sig)	-	0.21	0.84	0.06	**0.01 ***	0.06	1.00	1.00	1.00	0.34	0.21	0.20	0.22	0.71	0.99	0.98	0.46	0.22	0.40	0.34	0.99	0.99	**0.02 ***	0.89

Bold and * = $p < 0.05$. Abbreviations: Sh = shoulder; Pel = pelvis; AP = group of all participants; HM = hypothetical median; Sig = significance.

The graphical data output of the specific spine parameters indicated systematic differences between the female and male participants and between the participants in the different age cohorts. In the transverse plane, these subgroup-dependent visual differences were present among almost all the investigated vertebral bodies. In the coronal plane, the differences seemed to be locally limited to the upper thoracic spine. In the sagittal plane, the curves of the analyzed subgroups ran more in parallel compared to the other two planes. In this regard, the differently scaled x-axes have to be considered.

3.2.2. Explorative Data Analysis

The graphically apparent deviations of the vertebral bodies from the symmetrical zero position in the transverse and the coronal planes could be confirmed by statistical data analyses. The deviations were significant from T5 to L3 in the transverse plane and from C7 to T4, from T6 to T12 and for the pelvis in the coronal plane when that data of the entire group were considered and tested versus a hypothetical median of zero. Likewise, all the global parameters in the two respective planes deviated significantly from the respective symmetrical spine position (Table 5). The visual differences between the analyzed subgroups, however, could not be statistically confirmed for the transverse and coronal plane data. Here, only the isolated parameters revealed statistical trends pointing towards a possible existing difference (for "Pelvis Rotation" between the young and middle participants ($p = 0.05$) and for "Right Side Apical Deviation VP-DM + max (mm)" ($p = 0.04$) between the female and male participants).

In the sagittal plane, systematic deviations from a straight upright spine position existed in all the vertebral bodies except for T8 (neutral vertebrae of the thoracic kyphosis) and all the global spine parameters. In contrast with the two other planes, the statistical analyses also revealed systematic trends pointing towards possible differences between the analyzed subgroups. The global parameter of "Lumbar Lordosis (ITL-ILS) (°)" differed between the female and male participants ($p < 0.001$), while the parameter of "Thoracic Kyphosis (ICT-ITL) (°)" indicated a trend towards a difference between the participants in the different age cohorts ($p < 0.001$). The systematic trend behind these findings becomes apparent when observing the specific spine parameters. Sex-specific differences could be found for all the specific parameters except for the two major turning points (meaning the most flexed (T1) and the most extended (L1) vertebrae). Differences between the age cohorts in the global parameter of "Thoracic Kyphosis (ICT-ITL) (°)" were also apparent at the level of the specific spine parameters. The systematic differences due to the participants' belonging to different age cohorts can be seen here in the isolated upper thoracic vertebrae (C7–T4) and the pelvis (Table 5).

3.3. Literature Comparison

Table 6 compares the results for the global spine parameters of the current study with those derived from previous publications using the same VRS measurement device [18–23]. Most of the results were found to be almost comparable; however, there was a trend towards slightly lower values derived from the current study for the parameters of the transverse and the coronal plane when compared to those of previous research.

Table 6. Comparison of the results for the global spine parameters from the current study with those of previous research.

			Transversal Plane					Coronal Plane					Sagittal Plane		
			Surface Rotation RMS (°)	Surface Rotation MAX (°)	(Right Side) Surface Rotation +Max (°)	(Left Side) Surface Rotation −Max (°)	Trunk Imbalance (VP-DM) (°)	Trunk Imbalance (VP-DM) (mm)	Apical Deviation RMS (mm)	Apical Deviation MAX (mm)	(Right Side) Apical Deviation (VP-DM) +Max (mm)	(Left Side) Apical Deviation (VP-DM) −Max (mm)	Trunk Inclination (VP-DM) (°)	Trunk Inclination (VP-DM) (mm)	Thoracic Kyphosis (ICT-ITL) (°)	Lumbar Lordosis (ITL-ILS) (°)
Current Study	All Participants	MoM	2.3	−1.9	1.5	−3.3	−0.2	−1.7	3.6	−1.8	3.2	−4.9	3.1	26.0	49.9	40.9
		SD	0.9	4.0	1.4	2.3	0.8	7.3	1.7	7.1	3.0	3.3	2.1	17.5	8.3	9.2
	Sex	All Females	MoM	2.2	−1.8	1.5	−3.2	−0.2	−1.6	3.5	−2.3	2.9	−4.9	3.1	25.6	50.1	44.0
		SD	0.9	4.0	1.4	2.3	0.9	7.7	1.7	6.7	2.8	3.3	2.1	17.6	8.2	8.5
		All Males	MoM	2.3	−2.1	1.4	−3.6	−0.2	−2.0	3.8	−0.8	3.8	−4.7	3.0	26.7	49.6	34.9
		SD	0.9	4.0	1.7	2.3	0.8	6.6	1.6	7.7	3.4	3.2	2.0	17.4	8.6	7.3
	Age Cohort "Young"	All Young Participants	MoM	2.3	−2.3	1.4	−3.5	−0.3	−2.5	3.5	−0.9	3.3	−4.4	2.9	24.8	46.5	40.1
		SD	0.9	3.6	1.2	2.2	0.8	6.5	1.6	7.0	2.9	3.1	2.2	18.4	7.1	8.9
		Young Females	MoM	2.4	−2.4	1.3	−3.5	−0.3	−2.6	3.4	−1.1	3.1	−4.4	2.8	22.6	46.9	43.0
		SD	0.9	3.8	1.3	2.3	0.8	6.7	1.6	7.2	2.7	3.1	2.1	17.5	6.9	8.7
		Young Males	MoM	2.2	−2.3	1.2	−3.6	0.8	−2.3	3.6	−0.4	3.8	−4.4	3.3	28.9	45.8	34.5
		SD	0.8	3.4	1.4	2.2	0.7	6.3	1.6	6.7	3.1	3.1	2.2	19.7	7.7	6.5
	Age Cohort "Middle"	All Middle Participants	MoM	2.1	−2.3	1.4	−3.4	−0.2	−1.9	3.8	−2.9	2.9	−5.3	3.2	27.0	49.7	41.0
		SD	1.0	3.6	1.4	2.2	0.8	7.0	1.8	7.0	3.2	3.3	2.0	17.0	7.7	9.0
		Middle Females	MoM	2.0	−2.2	1.3	−3.3	−0.2	−1.8	3.6	−3.3	2.8	−5.3	3.2	26.3	49.3	43.7
		SD	0.8	3.4	1.3	2.0	0.9	7.4	1.9	6.4	2.9	3.3	2.1	17.3	7.6	9.0
		Middle Males	MoM	2.3	−2.4	1.5	−3.6	−0.2	−2.2	4.1	−2.2	3.2	−5.4	3.2	28.3	50.5	35.7
		SD	1.1	3.8	1.4	2.6	0.7	6.2	1.7	8.0	3.7	3.4	1.9	16.7	7.9	6.2
	Age Cohort "Old"	All Old Participants	MoM	2.3	−1.1	1.8	−3.1	−0.1	−0.8	3.6	−1.5	3.3	−4.8	3.1	26.1	53.4	41.6
		SD	0.9	4.6	1.7	2.4	0.9	8.3	1.6	7.3	3.1	3.3	2.1	17.4	8.7	9.7
		Old Females	MoM	2.3	−0.9	1.8	−2.9	−0.2	−0.4	3.5	−2.4	2.8	−5.1	3.4	27.8	54.0	45.3
		SD	0.9	4.6	1.7	2.4	1.0	8.8	1.7	6.5	2.7	3.5	2.2	18.2	8.7	7.7
		Old Males	MoM	2.5	−1.4	1.8	−3.5	−0.1	−1.4	3.7	0.3	4.4	−4.3	2.6	22.8	52.4	34.4
		SD	0.9	4.8	1.7	2.3	0.9	7.4	1.6	8.5	3.6	3.0	1.8	15.5	8.7	9.1
Literature Comparison	Degenhardt et al., 2017 [22]	Young-Middle Participants	Mean	3.8	1.8	5.6	−4.6	0.1	1.0	5.6	3.6 ‡	7.9	−5.0	3.1	26.0	48.1	35.6
		SD	1.4	7.2	3.4	2.9	0.8	7.2	3.0	10.3 ‡	5.8	4.1	2.3	18.7	9.1	8.4
	Degenhardt et al., 2020 [23]	Young-Middle Participants	Mean	3.8	2.0	5.7	−4.5	0.2	1.3	5.4	4.3	8.0	−4.6	3.2	26.2	48.5	35.4
		SD	1.0	6.0	2.8	2.4	0.7	5.6	2.5	8.7	5.1	2.9	2.2	17.7	8.3	7.6
	Michalik et al., 2020 [19]	Young Females	Mean	3.6				−0.1		5.6				2.1		44.0 †	37.4 †
		SD	1.6						2.3				2.4		8.6 †	9.8 †
		Young Males	Mean	3.5				0.9		5.1				1.9		44.6 †	29.0 †
		SD	1.6												7.8 †	7.7 †
	Schröder et al., 2011 [20]	Young-Middle Females	Mean	3.6				1.0	6.9	2.1				1.9	12.3	47.1	42.7
		SD	1.8					4.6	5.5					17.9	8.6	8.2
		Young-Middle Males	Mean	3.1					7.7	2.3					10.3	49.2	35.8
		SD	1.5					7.2	5.8					16.4	9.3	6.6
	Schröder et al., 2014 [21]	Young Females	Mean	3.4					7.7	4.2				16.6 *		45.4	44.0
		SD	1.7					4.6	2.0				15.5 *		8.1	9.4
		Young Males	Mean	3.6					6.9	4.5				20.8 *		47.2	35.9
		SD	1.4					4.6	2.1				15.2 *		7.3	8.2
	Furian et al., 2013 [18]	Girls	Mean						5.7		4.9 ‡			2.6 *		42.1 †Δ	
		SD						0.7		0.7 ‡			0.7 *			
		Boys	Mean						7.4		4.7 ‡			3.0 *		47.1 †Δ	
		SD						0.8		0.4 ‡			0.2 *		7.5 †Δ	9.9 †Δ

Abbreviations: MoM = mean of means; SD = standard deviation; † = parameters differ slightly from those used in the current study ("Thoracic Kyphosis VP-T12", "Lumbar Lordosis T12-DM"); Δ = results are only available as one mean and SD for the entire group (n = 345) and not for the subgroups, respectively. [22]: n = 30 participants, age = 30.2 ± 9.8 years; [23]: n = 29 participants, age = 30.1 ± 10.1 years; [19]: n = 56 females, age = 23.6 ± 2.0 years and n = 65 males, age = 24.3 ± 2.2 years; [20]: n = 89 females, age = 26.4 ± 4.5 years and n = 88 males, age = 27.7 ± 4.4 years; [21]: n = 52 females, age = 26.1 ± 6.9 years and n = 51 males, age = 28.2 ± 7.4 years; [18]: n = 168 girls, age = 8.3 ± 1.3 years and n = 177 boys, age = 8.6 ± 1.2 years. ‡ = parameters could not be clearly assigned; * = values not comprehensible (unit of measurement questionable);

4. Discussion

Various studies have analyzed spinal posture and its possible adaptations to different spinal and other musculoskeletal pathologies using VRS [29–31]. However, reference values for the comparison of the possible pathological findings are only available for global spine parameters that mainly derived from children [18], younger adults [19–21], or young and middle-aged adults, but these are based on very small numbers of participants [22,23]. Systematically collected normative data, which differentiates between subgroups according to sex and age, which can be used to identify possible changes in spinal posture over the adult life span, were missing. One aim of this study was, therefore, to complement existing knowledge with a further reference dataset that meets those requirements. Spinal posture data were thus captured and analyzed based on 201 healthy participants according to sex and age over an adult life span of 18 to 70 years. A further aim was to expand the current knowledge by providing an additional reference dataset of specific spine parameters that contains three-dimensional posture data for every vertebral body (from C7 to L4 and the pelvis).

4.1. Global Spine Parameters

The results for the global spine parameters derived from the current study did not differ greatly from those of previous publications using the same VRS measurement device ([19–23]; Table 6). However, there seems to be a trend towards slightly lower measurement results for the parameters in the transverse and the coronal planes. Possible explanations for the deviation of the results could be, in addition to the different cohort compositions and cohort sizes, differences in the measurement protocol and data analysis. To obtain the most accurate data quality, we used a high standardization of the measurement protocol, the use of additional markers in the course of the vertebral column (~T3 and ~T12) and the systematic removal of extreme outliers from the raw dataset. Since the comparative studies do not provide corresponding information, the question regarding the reasons for the differences cannot be answered in a well-established manner.

In the current study, significant trends towards possible differences in several global spine parameters according to sex and age cohort were revealed through explorative data analyses. While these differences were not found to be systematic for the coronal plane parameter of the "(Right Side) Apical Deviation VP-DM + max (mm)", the results for the respective sagittal plane parameters were considered highly important. The "Lumbar Lordosis (ITL-ILS) (°)" angle revealed a trend towards a significant difference between the female and male participants, with females showing greater lordosis angles than their male counterparts. This is in accordance with previous publications using the same VRS measuring device [19–21]. These findings also match the results of a recent systematic review and meta-analysis describing age- and sex-based effects on the lumbar lordosis angles and the range of motion based on different clinically established measurement approaches (radiological and non-radiological). The authors also found significant differences according to sex, with females having greater lumbar lordosis angles than men, but in contrast to the current findings, they also revealed indications that age possibly affected the respective spine parameters [32]. Similar correlations between VRS- and X-ray-measured results were found for the sagittal plane parameter of "Thoracic Kyphosis". The current study found a trend towards significant differences between young and old ($p < 0.001$) and between middle and old ($p < 0.02$) participants, indicating an increase in the VRS-measured parameter with increasing age. Comparable results were published in a recent systematic review based on radiography-based Cobb angle calculations [33]. The authors described an increase in thoracic kyphosis with aging but did not find that sex affected the spine parameters.

These results confirm the importance of having VRS reference data that are not only distinguishable between subgroups according to sex, as has been the case thus far, but also according to different age cohorts. Without these data, changes in spinal posture that physiologically occur over a healthy life span could be falsely diagnosed as pathologic, resulting in troubling uncertainty for the affected patients in clinical practice.

4.2. Specific Spine Parameters

Apart from a previous sub-analysis of 100 female participants from the present study cohort, which was published by our own research group [24], this is the first paper to present systematic reference data for every vertebral body in all three dimensions for both sexes and for three different age cohorts, which were derived using the VRS "Formetric III 4D" measuring device. As already described, in contrast to the currently common clinical beliefs, the physiological spinal posture in the transverse and the coronal planes was not found to be straight and symmetric with regard to rotation and lateral flexion [24]. Instead, a systematic rotation of the mid- and lower thoracic and lumbar vertebrae towards the right side was observed and supported by explorative data analyses. This rotation was found to be more pronounced in males than females and in young compared to middle-aged and old participants. A pre-existing vertebral rotation in healthy participants was also previously described based on CT and MRI measurements [34]. In patients with a diagnosed situs inversus totalis, the side of the vertebral rotation changed, respectively [35]. These results suggest that the VRS findings of the current study are clinically comprehensible and that internal organ arrangement might be a possible physiological cause of the observed asymmetric spinal posture.

In the coronal plane, a lateral flexion to the right side was found in the case of the upper thoracic vertebrae, while the underlying vertebrae showed a systematic lateral flexion to the left. Contrary to the results for the spinal rotation, visually, the lateral flexion in the upper thoracic vertebrae seemed to be more pronounced in the female compared to the male participants, whereas no sex-specific differences were detectable in the mid- and lower thoracic or the lumbar vertebral body positions. According to age-related differences, the younger group visually seemed to demonstrate less lateral flexion than the middle-aged and old participants, specifically in the thoracic spinal region. Whether or not this might be caused by posture adaptations induced by normal degenerative changes in the spine remains unclear. However, Kilshaw et al. [36], who analyzed the lumbar spine retrospectively based on abdominal radiographs and found that deformities such as lumbar scoliosis, lateral listhesis and osteoarthritis in the coronal plane started to occur after the age of 50 and steadily increased with age, previously described such an effect, albeit in a different spinal section.

No unexpected outcomes for the vertebral positions were detected in the sagittal plane parameters. The apex of the VRS-measured thoracic kyphosis, meaning the least tilted vertebrae, appeared around T8. This is in accordance with recently published findings derived from radiographic data. Here, the thoracic apex was located between T7 and T9 [37,38]. In the current study, the lumbar lordosis apex appeared between the second and the fourth lumbar vertebrae, depending on the analyzed subgroup. As already described, a statistically significant trend towards a difference between the female and male participants was found for the global parameter of "Lumbar Lordosis (ITL-ILS) (°)". This difference according to sex was also apparent among almost all the specific spine parameters, except for the two major curvature turning points (the most flexed (T1) and the most extended (L1) vertebral body). In the thoracic spine, males showed a greater curvature in the upper thoracic spine, and females showed greater curvature in the lower thoracic spine. The authors assume that this difference between females and males canceled each other out, which is why the sex difference did not manifest in the global variable of "Thoracic Kyphosis (ICT-ITL) (°)". Nevertheless, the global parameter of "Thoracic Kyphosis (ICT-ITL) (°)" revealed significant differences between the analyzed age cohorts caused by the significant age differences in the respective specific parameters of the upper thoracic spine. Sex differences in spinopelvic alignment and in per-level vertebral inclination have also been reported in healthy participants based on upright low-dose digital biplanar X-ray analyses [39]. Similar to the current study, more dorsally inclined vertebrae were found in females than in males from T1 down to L2. In the current study, females showed more extended vertebral positions from T2 to L3 compared to their male counterparts. Even though the isolated raw values for vertebral inclination differed slightly between the two measurement approaches, the functional comparability of our results with those derived from X-ray analyses further supports the clinical importance of VRS as a non-invasive and simultaneously quick and easy assessment tool for spinal posture analysis in daily clinical routines.

However, despite the described functional agreement between the results based on the VRS and X-ray based measurements, the visual differences in the graphical data outputs between the analyzed subgroups could not be confirmed through statistical analyses for the specific spine parameters in the transverse or the coronal plane in the current study. One reason for this might be the large standard deviation identified in each of the analyzed variables. A normal spine anatomy also means that the results for the parameters in the transverse and the coronal planes are distribute naturally in a preferably narrow corridor reflecting an almost neutral spine position. No physiologically large differences are expected. Due to the high individuality displayed in the large standard deviation and those additional anatomical conditions, the analyzed sample of 201 healthy participants (and, partly, less than $n = 67$ in the respective subgroups) might have simply been too small to detect potential significant differences in the respective planes.

The fact that, in contrast, statistically significant trends in the possible differences between the analyzed subgroups were revealed for the parameters in the sagittal plane might be due to the presence of the two physiological major spinal curvatures, "thoracic kyphosis" and "lumbar lordosis". These anatomical conditions mean that there is a higher natural deviation from the neutral position throughout the whole vertebral column, making it easier to detect statistically significant deviations between the analyzed subgroups even in this "small" sample of 201 healthy participants.

The possibility that sagittal plane parameters will be suitable for detecting differences between subgroups and between different pathologies is in accordance with previously published research [40,41]. Artificial intelligence (AI)-driven analyses of VRS measurement results also found sagittal plane parameters to be one of the most important features with which to distinguish pathology-independent spinal posture data from healthy comparative datasets [41]. Similar results were found when dynamic VRS gait data were analyzed by AI-driven methods. Here, the parameters of the coronal and the sagittal planes were most relevant for the classifications between the sexes [40]. Whether or not sagittal spine parameters have the potential to systematically distinguish between physiological and pathological spinal postures and which parameters are specifically involved must be investigated further in the future. Nevertheless, the first results point in this direction.

4.3. Limitations

The manufacturer of the "Formetric III 4D" system recommends the use of reflective markers for spinal posture analysis only when the software is not able to identify the required visual landmarks (vertebra prominens (VP) and the two lumbar dimples (DM)) on its own. However, the use of three reflective markers for the landmarks is necessary for dynamic gait analysis. As this study is part of an overarching research project aiming to collect reference data for spinal posture in the habitual stance and when walking at four different walking speeds among the same healthy study cohort, it was necessary to mark all the participants with the three markers in order to render the stance and gait results comparable with each other. Software misinterpretations that arose in advance during the test measurements at the fast walking speeds, caused by the soft tissue and scapular motions of the participants' back surface, meant that the researchers decided to use two additional markers (~T3 and ~T12) to stabilize the systems' dynamic data analysis procedures. The researchers also decided to mark C7 and the PSIS instead of the VP and DM. This approach was chosen because marking C7 and the PSIS is recommended in cases where the VP and DM are not clearly identifiable on the surface of the participant's back.

In order to standardize the measuring procedure and to render the results as comparable to each other as possible, the marking of C7 and the PSIS was determined a priori for all the participants, even though this technique was definitely more prone to palpation bias [42,43]. Furthermore, only participants with a BMI of ≤30.0 kg/m^2 were included in the study due to data capture requirements. The procedures described enabled the collection of highly standardized data under controlled laboratory conditions. Nevertheless, the researchers are aware that this approach limits the external validity of the presented findings and, thus, their direct transferability to clinical practice.

The large number of parameters analyzed and the resulting high number of tested hypotheses also mean that the significant results have to be interpreted with caution. They are more suitable for showing trends in possible differences rather than real statistical significance. In this regard, it must also be mentioned that, retrospectively, the chosen sample size seemed to be too small to detect potential differences between the analyzed subgroups, especially for the specific spine parameters.

Finally, yet importantly, their radiation and contact-free nature mean that results derived from VRS measurements are calculated and based on mathematical algorithms. Even though their validity has been investigated in various publications, those studies mainly focused on comparisons between X-ray and VRS data captured from patients affected by different spinal pathologies (mainly scoliosis) [8,14,15,44,45]. For ethical reasons, no such comparative studies based on healthy participants are available. The results presented here, however, reveal a strong functional agreement with the results derived from clinically established measurement approaches, such as X-ray or MRI/CT scans, and VRS measurements [33,34,39]. This underlines the potential of VRS to serve as a non-invasive, quick and objective alternative for spinal posture analysis in clinical practice, especially when the therapeutic focus lies in function-orientated clinical outcomes and when pre-post measurements are required.

5. Conclusions

This study complements the existing VRS reference datasets for global spine parameters by adding normative values for different subgroups according to sex and age over an adult life span from 18 to 70 years. The closure of this gap, retrospectively, was found to be very important, because relevant changes over the life span in the isolated spine parameters became visible. Reference values for the specific spine parameters of every vertebral body from C7 to L4 in all three dimensions according to sex and age were presented and revealed visual but statistically non-significant differences between the analyzed subgroups. The sagittal plane parameters seem to have the greatest potential to detect differences between groups of participants. Whether or not those variations are possibly significant must be investigated in future studies by repeating the current project with an appropriate number of healthy participants.

The great variation in and individuality of the spinal posture displayed in the large standard deviation of the analyzed parameters, which was described previously by our research group using data derived from VRS measurements of asymptomatic female volunteers [24], were confirmed for the respective subgroups in the current study. Most importantly, and against widespread clinical expectations, the healthy human spine was found to be systematically asymmetric in the transverse and the coronal planes during upright habitual standing. There needs to be discussion in the therapeutic setting about whether approximations to an almost symmetrical spine in the respective planes are biomechanically desirable in any way [24].

Author Contributions: Conceptualization, J.H. and U.B.; methodology, J.H. and U.B.; software, J.K., C.W., R.W. and I.S.; validation, J.H., J.K., C.W., R.W. and I.S.; formal analysis, J.H., J.K., C.W., R.W. and I.S.; investigation, J.H.; resources, P.D. and U.B.; data curation, J.H., J.K., C.W., R.W. and I.S.; writing—original draft preparation, J.H.; writing—review and editing, J.K., C.W., R.W., I.S., P.D. and U.B.; visualization, J.H., J.K. and C.W.; supervision, J.K., P.D. and U.B.; project administration, J.K., P.D. and U.B. All authors have read and agreed to the published version of the manuscript.

Funding: This research received no external funding.

Institutional Review Board Statement: The study was conducted in accordance with the Declaration of Helsinki and was approved by the responsible ethics committee of the Rhineland-Palatinate Medical Association. The study is registered with the World Health Organization (WHO) (INT: DRKS00010834).

Informed Consent Statement: Informed consent was obtained from all subjects involved in the study.

Data Availability Statement: Due to ethical and privacy reasons, the data presented in this study are not publicly available.

Acknowledgments: The authors would like to express their gratitude to all the participants for their time and interest in participating in this study. Our colleagues are also acknowledged for their professional expertise and contributions to this project and their strong support during the participant recruitment process. Special thanks also go to Amira Basic and Kjell Heitmann (DIERS Company) for their technical support and assistance.

Conflicts of Interest: The authors declare no conflict of interest. Technical assistance was provided by staff members of the DIERS Company in preparation for the statistical data analysis process; however, there was no external influence on the design of the study; the collection, analysis, or interpretation of the data; the writing of the manuscript; or the decision to publish the results.

References

1. Dindorf, C.; Konradi, J.; Wolf, C.; Taetz, B.; Bleser, G.; Huthwelker, J.; Werthmann, F.; Drees, P.; Fröhlich, M.; Betz, U. Machine learning techniques demonstrating individual movement patterns of the vertebral column: The fingerprint of spinal motion. *Comput. Methods Biomech. Biomed. Eng.* **2021**, *25*, 821–831. [CrossRef] [PubMed]
2. Bundesärztekammer; Bundesvereinigung, K.; der Wissenschaftlichen, A.; Fachgesellschaften, M. *Nationale VersorgungsLeitlinie Nicht-spezifischer Kreuzschmerz—Langfassung*, 2nd ed.; Version 1; 2017; Available online: http://www.leitlinien.de/themen/kreuzschmerz (accessed on 11 December 2022). [CrossRef]
3. Fedorak, C.; Ashworth, N.; Marshall, J.; Paull, H. Reliability of the visual assessment of cervical and lumbar lordosis: How good are we? *Spine* **2003**, *28*, 1857–1859. [CrossRef] [PubMed]
4. Takatalo, J.; Ylinen, J.; Pienimäki, T.; Häkkinen, A. Intra- and inter-rater reliability of thoracic spine mobility and posture assessments in subjects with thoracic spine pain. *BMC Musculoskelet. Disord.* **2020**, *21*, 529. [CrossRef] [PubMed]
5. Mangone, M.; Paoloni, M.; Procopio, S.; Venditto, T.; Zucchi, B.; Santilli, V.; Paolucci, T.; Agostini, F.; Bernetti, A. Sagittal spinal alignment in patients with ankylosing spondylitis by rasterstereographic back shape analysis: An observational retrospective study. *Eur. J. Phys. Rehabil. Med.* **2020**, *56*, 191–196. [CrossRef] [PubMed]
6. Applebaum, A.; Ference, R.; Cho, W. Evaluating the role of surface topography in the surveillance of scoliosis. *Spine Deform.* **2020**, *8*, 397–404. [CrossRef] [PubMed]
7. Betsch, M.; Wild, M.; Rath, B.; Tingart, M.; Schulze, A.; Quack, V. Radiation-free diagnosis of scoliosis: An overview of the surface and spine topography. *Orthopade* **2015**, *44*, 845–851. [CrossRef] [PubMed]
8. Krott, N.L.; Wild, M.; Betsch, M. Meta-analysis of the validity and reliability of rasterstereographic measurements of spinal posture. *Eur. Spine J.* **2020**, *29*, 2392–2401. [CrossRef]
9. Drerup, B.; Hierholzer, E. Evaluation of frontal radiographs of scoliotic spines—Part I measurement of position and orientation of vertebrae and assessment of clinical shape parameters. *J. Biomech.* **1992**, *25*, 1357–1362. [CrossRef]
10. Drerup, B.; Hierholzer, E. Evaluation of frontal radiographs of scoliotic spines—Part II: Relations between lateral deviation, lateral tilt and axial rotation of vertebrae. *J. Biomech.* **1992**, *25*, 1443–1450. [CrossRef]
11. Drerup, B.; Hierholzer, E. Back shape measurement using video rasterstereography and three-dimensional reconstruction of spinal shape. *Clin. Biomech.* **1994**, *9*, 28–36. [CrossRef]
12. Drerup, B.; Ellger, B.; Meyer zu Bentrup, F.M.; Hierholzer, E. Functional rasterstereographic images. A new method for biomechanical analysis of skeletal geometry. *Orthopade* **2001**, *30*, 242–250. [CrossRef] [PubMed]
13. Drerup, B. Rasterstereographic measurement of scoliotic deformity. *Scoliosis* **2014**, *9*, 22. [CrossRef] [PubMed]
14. Mohokum, M.; Mendoza, S.; Udo, W.; Sitter, H.; Paletta, J.R.; Skwara, A. Reproducibility of rasterstereography for kyphotic and lordotic angles, trunk length, and trunk inclination: A reliability study. *Spine* **2010**, *35*, 1353–1358. [PubMed]
15. Mohokum, M.; Schülein, S.; Skwara, A. The validity of rasterstereography: A systematic review. *Orthop. Rev.* **2015**, *7*, 68–73. [CrossRef]
16. Schulte, T.L.; Hierholzer, E.; Boerke, A.; Lerner, T.; Liljenqvist, U.; Bullmann, V.; Hackenberg, L. Raster stereography versus radiography in the long-term follow-up of idiopathic scoliosis. *J. Spinal Disord. Tech.* **2008**, *21*, 23–28. [CrossRef]

17. Tabard-Fougere, A.; Bonnefoy-Mazure, A.; Hanquinet, S.; Lascombes, P.; Armand, S.; Dayer, R. Validity and Reliability of Spine Rasterstereography in Patients With Adolescent Idiopathic Scoliosis. *Spine* **2017**, *42*, 98–105. [CrossRef]
18. Furian, T.C.; Rapp, W.; Eckert, S.; Wild, M.; Betsch, M. Spinal posture and pelvic position in three hundred forty-five elementary school children: A rasterstereographic pilot study. *Orthop. Rev.* **2013**, *5*, e7. [CrossRef]
19. Michalik, R.; Hamm, J.; Quack, V.; Eschweiler, J.; Gatz, M.; Betsch, M. Dynamic spinal posture and pelvic position analysis using a rasterstereographic device. *J. Orthop. Surg. Res.* **2020**, *15*, 389. [CrossRef]
20. Schröder, J.; Stiller, T.; Mattes, K. Reference data for spine shape analysis. Approaching a majority norm and deviations for unspecific low back pain. *Man. Med.* **2011**, *49*, 161–166. [CrossRef]
21. Schröder, J.; Braumann, K.M.; Reer, R. Wirbelsäulenform- und Funktionsprofile. *Orthopäde* **2014**, *43*, 841–849. [CrossRef]
22. Degenhardt, B.F.; Starks, Z.; Bhatia, S.; Franklin, G.-A. Appraisal of the DIERS method for calculating postural measurements: An observational study. *Scoliosis Spinal Disord.* **2017**, *12*, 28. [CrossRef] [PubMed]
23. Degenhardt, B.F.; Starks, Z.; Bhatia, S. Reliability of the DIERS Formetric 4D Spine Shape Parameters in Adults without Postural Deformities. *Biomed. Res. Int.* **2020**, *2020*, 1796247. [CrossRef] [PubMed]
24. Wolf, C.; Betz, U.; Huthwelker, J.; Konradi, J.; Westphal, R.S.; Cerpa, M.; Lenke, L.; Drees, P. Evaluation of 3D vertebral and pelvic position by surface topography in asymptomatic females: Presentation of normative reference data. *J. Orthop. Surg. Res.* **2021**, *16*, 703. [CrossRef] [PubMed]
25. Bischoff, H.A.; Stahelin, H.B.; Monsch, A.U.; Iversen, M.D.; Weyh, A.; von Dechend, M.; Akos, R.; Conzelmann, M.; Dick, W.; Theiler, R. Identifying a cut-off point for normal mobility: A comparison of the timed 'up and go' test in community-dwelling and institutionalised elderly women. *Age Ageing* **2003**, *32*, 315–320. [CrossRef]
26. Bohannon, R.W.; Wang, Y.C.; Gershon, R.C. Two-minute walk test performance by adults 18 to 85 years: Normative values, reliability, and responsiveness. *Arch. Phys. Med. Rehabil.* **2015**, *96*, 472–477. [CrossRef]
27. Myklebust, M.; Magnussen, L.; Inger Strand, L. Back Performance Scale scores in people without back pain: Normative data. *Adv. Physiother.* **2009**, *9*, 2–9. [CrossRef]
28. Perry, J.; Burnfield, J.M. *Gait Analysis—Normal and Pathological Function*, 2nd ed.; SLACK Incorporated: Thorofare, NJ, USA, 2010.
29. Betsch, M.; Michalik, R.; Graber, M.; Wild, M.; Krauspe, R.; Zilkens, C. Influence of leg length inequalities on pelvis and spine in patients with total hip arthroplasty. *PLoS ONE* **2019**, *14*, e0221695. [CrossRef]
30. Schroeder, J.; Schaar, H.; Mattes, K. Spinal alignment in low back pain patients and age-related side effects: A multivariate cross-sectional analysis of video rasterstereography back shape reconstruction data. *Eur. Spine J.* **2013**, *22*, 1979–1985. [CrossRef]
31. Schulte, T.L.; Liljenqvist, U.; Hierholzer, E.; Bullmann, V.; Halm, H.F.; Lauber, S.; Hackenberg, L. Spontaneous correction and derotation of secondary curves after selective anterior fusion of idiopathic scoliosis. *Spine* **2006**, *31*, 315–321. [CrossRef]
32. Arshad, R.; Pan, F.; Reitmaier, S.; Schmidt, H. Effect of age and sex on lumbar lordosis and the range of motion. A systematic review and meta-analysis. *J. Biomech.* **2019**, *82*, 1–19. [CrossRef]
33. Zappalá, M.; Lightbourne, S.; Heneghan, N.R. The relationship between thoracic kyphosis and age, and normative values across age groups: A systematic review of healthy adults. *J. Orthop. Surg. Res.* **2021**, *16*, 447. [CrossRef] [PubMed]
34. Kouwenhoven, J.W.; Vincken, K.L.; Bartels, L.W.; Castelein, R.M. Analysis of preexistent vertebral rotation in the normal spine. *Spine* **2006**, *31*, 1467–1472. [CrossRef] [PubMed]
35. Kouwenhoven, J.W.; Bartels, L.W.; Vincken, K.L.; Viergever, M.A.; Verbout, A.J.; Delhaas, T.; Castelein, R.M. The relation between organ anatomy and pre-existent vertebral rotation in the normal spine: Magnetic resonance imaging study in humans with situs inversus totalis. *Spine* **2007**, *32*, 1123–1128. [CrossRef] [PubMed]
36. Kilshaw, M.; Baker, R.P.; Gardner, R.; Charosky, S.; Harding, I. Abnormalities of the lumbar spine in the coronal plane on plain abdominal radiographs. *Eur. Spine. J.* **2011**, *20*, 429–433. [CrossRef] [PubMed]
37. Sebaaly, A.; Silvestre, C.; Rizkallah, M.; Grobost, P.; Chevillotte, T.; Kharrat, K.; Roussouly, P. Revisiting thoracic kyphosis: A normative description of the thoracic sagittal curve in an asymptomatic population. *Eur. Spine J.* **2021**, *30*, 1184–1189. [CrossRef] [PubMed]
38. Lafage, R.; Steinberger, J.; Pesenti, S.; Assi, A.; Elysee, J.C.; Iyer, S.; Lenke, L.G.; Schwab, F.J.; Kim, H.J.; Lafage, V. Understanding Thoracic Spine Morphology, Shape, and Proportionality. *Spine* **2020**, *45*, 149–157. [CrossRef]
39. Janssen, M.M.; Drevelle, X.; Humbert, L.; Skalli, W.; Castelein, R.M. Differences in male and female spino-pelvic alignment in asymptomatic young adults: A three-dimensional analysis using upright low-dose digital biplanar X-rays. *Spine* **2009**, *34*, E826–E832. [CrossRef]
40. Dindorf, C.; Konradi, J.; Wolf, C.; Taetz, B.; Bleser, G.; Huthwelker, J.; Drees, P.; Fröhlich, M.; Betz, U. General method for automated feature extraction and selection and its application for gender classification and biomechanical knowledge discovery of sex differences in spinal posture during stance and gait. *Comput. Methods Biomech. Biomed. Eng.* **2020**, *24*, 299–307. [CrossRef]
41. Dindorf, C.; Konradi, J.; Wolf, C.; Taetz, B.; Bleser, G.; Huthwelker, J.; Werthmann, F.; Bartaguiz, E.; Kniepert, J.; Drees, P.; et al. Classification and Automated Interpretation of Spinal Posture Data Using a Pathology-Independent Classifier and Explainable Artificial Intelligence (XAI). *Sensors* **2021**, *21*, 6393. [CrossRef]
42. Cooperstein, R.; Hickey, M. The reliability of palpating the posterior superior iliac spine: A systematic review. *J. Can. Chiropr. Assoc.* **2016**, *60*, 36–46.

43. Póvoa, L.C.; Ferreira, A.P.A.; Zanier, J.F.C.; Silva, J.G. Accuracy of Motion Palpation Flexion-Extension Test in Identifying the Seventh Cervical Spinal Process. *J. Chiropr. Med.* **2018**, *17*, 22–29. [CrossRef] [PubMed]
44. Schülein, S.; Mendoza, S.; Malzkorn, R.; Harms, J.; Skwara, A. Rasterstereographic Evaluation of Interobserver and Intraobserver Reliability in Postsurgical Adolescent Idiopathic Scoliosis Patients. *J. Spinal. Disord. Tech.* **2013**, *26*, E143–E149. [CrossRef] [PubMed]
45. Tabard-Fougere, A.; Bonnefoy-Mazure, A.; Dhouib, A.; Valaikaite, R.; Armand, S.; Dayer, R. Radiation-free measurement tools to evaluate sagittal parameters in AIS patients: A reliability and validity study. *Eur. Spine J.* **2019**, *28*, 536–543. [CrossRef] [PubMed]

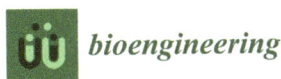

Article

Gait Initiation Impairment in Patients with Parkinson's Disease and Freezing of Gait

Chiara Palmisano [1,*], Laura Beccaria [1], Stefan Haufe [2], Jens Volkmann [1], Gianni Pezzoli [3] and Ioannis U. Isaias [1,3]

1. Department of Neurology, University Hospital and Julius-Maximilian-University, 97080 Würzburg, Germany
2. Uncertainty, Inverse Modeling and Machine Learning Group, Faculty IV Electrical Engineering and Computer Science, Technical University of Berlin, 10623 Berlin, Germany
3. Centro Parkinson, ASST Gaetano Pini-CTO, 20122 Milano, Italy
* Correspondence: palmisano_c@ukw.de

Abstract: Freezing of gait (FOG) is a sudden episodic inability to produce effective stepping despite the intention to walk. It typically occurs during gait initiation (GI) or modulation and may lead to falls. We studied the anticipatory postural adjustments (imbalance, unloading, and stepping phase) at GI in 23 patients with Parkinson's disease (PD) and FOG (PDF), 20 patients with PD and no previous history of FOG (PDNF), and 23 healthy controls (HCs). Patients performed the task when off dopaminergic medications. The center of pressure (CoP) displacement and velocity during imbalance showed significant impairment in both PDNF and PDF, more prominent in the latter patients. Several measurements were specifically impaired in PDF patients, especially the CoP displacement along the anteroposterior axis during unloading. The pattern of segmental center of mass (SCoM) movements did not show differences between groups. The standing postural profile preceding GI did not correlate with outcome measurements. We have shown impaired motor programming at GI in Parkinsonian patients. The more prominent deterioration of unloading in PDF patients might suggest impaired processing and integration of somatosensory information subserving GI. The unaltered temporal movement sequencing of SCoM might indicate some compensatory cerebellar mechanisms triggering time-locked models of body mechanics in PD.

Keywords: freezing of gait; gait initiation; Parkinson's disease; posture; segmental centers of mass; anthropometric measurement; base of support

---

Citation: Palmisano, C.; Beccaria, L.; Haufe, S.; Volkmann, J.; Pezzoli, G.; Isaias, I.U. Gait Initiation Impairment in Patients with Parkinson's Disease and Freezing of Gait. *Bioengineering* 2022, 9, 639. https://doi.org/10.3390/bioengineering9110639

Academic Editors: Christina Zong-Hao Ma, Zhengrong Li and Chen He

Received: 27 September 2022
Accepted: 15 October 2022
Published: 2 November 2022

Publisher's Note: MDPI stays neutral with regard to jurisdictional claims in published maps and institutional affiliations.

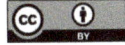

Copyright: © 2022 by the authors. Licensee MDPI, Basel, Switzerland. This article is an open access article distributed under the terms and conditions of the Creative Commons Attribution (CC BY) license (https://creativecommons.org/licenses/by/4.0/).

1. Introduction

Freezing of gait (FOG) is a dramatic phenomenon frequently affecting patients with Parkinson's disease (PD) [1], causing falls, mobility restrictions, and poor quality of life [2–4]. FOG is defined as a brief, episodic absence or marked reduction of forward progression of the feet despite the intention to walk [5], which typically occurs when initiating or modulating gait (e.g., turning, obstacle crossing, and so on).

Gait initiation (GI) is a highly challenging task for the balance control system and is of particular interest in the study of neural control of upright posture maintenance during whole-body movement [6]. Specifically, this task allows the precise assessment of anticipatory postural adjustments (APAs; i.e., muscular synergies that precede GI), aiming to destabilize the antigravity postural set by shifting the center of pressure (CoP) to generate a gravitational moment favoring the center of mass (CoM) forward acceleration [7]. APAs are considered a motor program controlled by feedforward mechanisms regulated by the supraspinal locomotor network [8–12]. The selection and scaling of appropriate APAs rely on the ability to use sensory information to determine the body positioning relative to the environment prior to step execution [13,14] and on the intended forthcoming movement (natural, slow, fast, obstacle, and so on) [7,15–17]. Striatal dopamine loss, a pathophysiological hallmark of PD, greatly impacts the production of APAs at GI and particularly the CoP displacement and velocity [12]. Only a few studies have specifically investigated the GI task in Parkinsonian patients with a history of FOG (PDF), non-implanted for deep brain stimulation (DBS), and after withdrawal of dopaminergic medication (meds-off state). The stimulation and medication condition should be carefully considered, as both DBS and dopaminergic drugs can variably influence posture and gait in PD [12,18–26]. Overall, these studies showed conflicting results, with APAs being reported as normal [27–29] or multiple and hypometric [10,30]. Several methodological discrepancies may account for such different findings, including a non-standardized meds-off state [27], imposed (pre-defined) feet positioning [29], cueing [10,29,30], and specific instructions on the execution of the GI task (e.g., to start walking as quickly as possible [30,31] or while performing a cognitive task [28]). All of these factors can significantly impact and alter APA expression at GI. Specifically, a cued start signal influences motor programming towards normalization, especially in PDF [9,18], similar to the improvements seen with the administration of levodopa for self-generated step initiation [18]. Moreover, the initial feet position [12,22,32] and posture [33–35] can significantly impact the biomechanical features of APAs at GI.

Postural changes in particular would have a detrimental impact on APA production. An altered representation of the body position (egocentric representation) may determine a functional re-organization of the supplementary motor area (SMA)-proper, hampering selection and re-scaling of APAs to adapt to the altered postural framework and bradykinetic stepping [33,34,36–38].

Our study aims to describe GI alteration in patients with PD and FOG, accounting for the influence of anthropometric measurements (AMs) and the base of support (BoS) and investigating their relationship with the initial posture. We have also addressed the relative timing and movement sequence of each body segment subserving GI.

2. Materials and Methods

2.1. Subjects

We recruited 23 patients with idiopathic PD (according to the U.K. Brain Bank criteria) and an unambiguous, previous history of FOG (PDF; i.e., patients reporting episodes of FOG on a daily basis prior to the experiment). On the day of the experiment, the presence of FOG was confirmed with a clinical evaluation by an experienced neurologist (I.U.I.). In addition, 20 patients with PD and no previous history of FOG (PDNF) and 23 healthy controls (HCs) were also included. HCs and PDNF patients were chosen to match in terms of demographic and clinical data with the PDF group. Subjects with neurological diseases other than PD, including cognitive decline (i.e., Mini-Mental State Examination score < 27), vestibular disorders, and orthopedic impairments that could interfere with gait were excluded. Disease severity was evaluated with the Unified Parkinson's Disease Rating Scale motor part (UPDRS-III).

2.2. Experimental Protocol

Patients were investigated in practical meds-off state, i.e., in the morning after overnight withdrawal (>12 h) of all dopaminergic drugs.

Kinematic data were recorded using an optoelectronic system with six cameras (sampling rate 60 Hz, SMART 1.10, BTS, Garbagnate Milanese, Italy) and a set of 29 markers placed on anatomical landmarks (temples, acromions, lateral humeral condyles, ulnar styloids, anterior superior iliac spines, middle thighs, lateral femoral condyles, fibula heads, tibial anterior side, lateral malleoli, Achilles tendon insertion, fifth metatarsal heads, halluxes, the seventh cervical vertebra [C7], point of maximum kyphosis, and middle point between the posterior superior iliac spines) [39,40]. Eight additional technical markers were placed on the trochanters, the medial condyles, the medial malleoli, and the first metatarsi for a short calibration trial, which allowed the computation of the AMs and BoS measurements [11,12,41]. Markers traces were filtered with a fifth-order lowpass Butterworth filter (cut-off frequency: 10 Hz [41]). Dynamic measurements were recorded with a force plate working at a sampling rate of 960 Hz (KISTLER 9286A, Winterthur, Switzerland). The resulting signal was low-pass filtered (fifth-order lowpass Butterworth filter) with a cut-off frequency of 30 Hz [11,42].

At the beginning of each trial, subjects stood upright on the force platform at a comfortable stance position for about 30 s. The initial stance position was not standardized to prevent modification of the subject's usual motor strategy to initiate gait [12].

Participants were instructed to start walking after a self-selected period from a verbal signal, in order to avoid any effect of cueing on GI. The instruction given was as follows: "Start walking at the moment of your choice". Subjects were not instructed on the stepping leg to use and they moved at their own pace until the end of the walkway. After a training session, at least three consecutive trials were recorded. The principal investigator supervised all participants during the experiment.

2.3. Biomechanical Measurements

2.3.1. Anthropometric Measurements and Base of Support

For each subject, we measured the following AMs (Table 1): body height, inter anterior-superior iliac spine distance, limb length, foot length, body mass, and body mass index. The AMs were recorded over a period of 5 s of standing using eight additional markers, as described in [12]. The AMs were used for the estimation of the CoM of each body segment (SCoM), according to the anthropometric tables and regression equations proposed by [43]. For each trial, the BoS area and BoS width were calculated. We also accounted for feet position asymmetry by measuring the foot alignment, the difference between feet extra-rotation angles, and the BoS opening angle [11,12].

Table 1. Biomechanical measurements. Abbreviations: AP, anteroposterior; C7, seventh cervical vertebra; CoM, center of mass; CoP, center of pressure; ML, mediolateral; PSIS, posterior superior iliac spine.

Description	Decomposition
Anthropometric measurements (AMs)	
Body Height [BH] (cm)	
Inter Anterior Superior Iliac Spine Distance [IAD] (cm)	
Limb Length [LL] (cm)	
Foot Length [FL] (cm)	
Body Mass [BM] (kg)	
Body Mass Index [BMI] (kg/cm^2)	
Base of support (BoS)	
BoS Area (cm^2): area of the polygon described by the markers placed on the heels, the lateral malleoli, the fifth metatarsal bones, and the hallux	
BoS Width (cm): distance between the ankle joint centers, estimated as the mid points between the lateral and medial malleoli	
Foot Alignment (cm): AP distance between the two markers placed on the heels	
$\beta\Delta$: Difference between the left (βL) and right (βR) feet extra-rotation angles (angles between the axis passing through the lateral and medial malleoli and the horizontal axis of the reference system of the laboratory) (°)	
β: BoS opening angle, sum of βL and βR (°)	
Postural angles	
Angle between the line connecting the markers on the middle point between the PSIS and the C7 and the laboratory vertical axis (°)	
Angle between the line connecting the knee and hip centers of rotation and the laboratory vertical axis (°)	
Angle between the line connecting the knee and ankle centers of rotation and the laboratory vertical axis (°)	

Table 1. Cont.

Description	Decomposition
GI measurements—Imbalance (IMB)	
IMB duration (s)	
IMB CoP displacement (mm)	AP, ML
IMB CoP average velocity (mm/s)	AP, ML
IMB CoP maximal velocity (mm/s)	AP, ML
CoM velocity at IMB end (m/s)	
CoM acceleration at IMB end (m/s^2)	
CoP–CoM distance at IMB end (m)	
Orientation of CoP–CoM vector with respect to the progression line at IMB end (°)	
GI measurements—Unloading (UNL)	
CoP distance from the line passing through the markers on the heels at swing heel off (mm)	AP
UNL duration (s)	
UNL CoP displacement (mm)	AP, ML
UNL CoP average velocity (mm/s)	AP, ML
UNL CoP maximal velocity (mm/s)	AP, ML
CoM velocity at UNL end (m/s)	
CoM acceleration at UNL end (m/s^2)	
CoP–CoM distance at UNL end (m)	
Slope of CoP–CoM vector at UNL end (°)	
GI measurements—Stepping phase	
CoP distance from the line passing through the markers on the heels at the swing foot toe-off (mm)	AP
CoM velocity at stance foot toe-off (m/s)	
CoM acceleration at stance foot toe-off (m/s^2)	
CoP–CoM distance at stance toe-off (m)	
First step length (m)	
First step average velocity (m/s)	
First step maximal velocity (m/s)	

2.3.2. Postural Profile

The standing postural profile was characterized by means of trunk, thigh, and shank sagittal angles (Figure 1) [20] computed shortly before the GI execution (during a 1 s window before the onset of the APAs). The trunk angle was defined as the inclination of the line passing through the markers placed on the middle point between the two posterior superior iliac spines and the seventh cervical vertebra with respect to the vertical axis of the laboratory. The thigh angle was calculated as the angle between the vector connecting the knee and hip center of rotation and the vertical axis of the laboratory. The shank angle was computed between the line connecting the joint centers of the knee and ankle and the vertical axis of the laboratory.

2.3.3. Anticipatory Postural Adjustments and Gait Initiation

GI variables were defined based on the displacement of the CoP, recorded by the force platform. The CoM was estimated as the weighted mean of the SCoM [44]. GI variables were calculated by dedicated algorithms in Matlab ambient (Matlab® R2018b, The MathWorks Inc., Natick, MA, USA) (as in [11,12]). All GI measurements computed in the study are listed and described in Table 1. Briefly, four reference instants were automatically identified on the CoP track and checked by visual inspection using an interactive software: the onset of the APAs, the heel-off of the swing foot (HO$_{SW}$), the toe-off of the swing foot (TO$_{SW}$), and the toe-off of the stance foot (TO$_{ST}$). The APA onset (APA$_{ONSET}$) was detected as the instant at which the CoP started moving consistently backward and toward the swing foot; HO$_{SW}$ was defined as the time at which CoP reached the most lateral position toward the swing foot; TO$_{SW}$ was defined as the moment at which the CoP shifted from lateral to anterior motion; and TO$_{ST}$ was defined as the last frame of the force platform signal

(Figure 2). The APAs were divided into two periods: the imbalance phase (IMB), from APA_{ONSET} to HO_{SW}, and the unloading phase (UNL), from HO_{SW} to TO_{SW} [12,20,40,45]. The following measurements were calculated for both the IMB and UNL periods: duration and anteroposterior and mediolateral CoP displacement, average velocity, and maximal velocity (Table 1). Of note, the mediolateral CoP displacement during the imbalance phase was considered positive when the shift of the CoP was towards the swing foot, while the mediolateral CoP displacement during the unloading phase was considered positive when the CoP was moving towards the stance foot. The IMB and UNL anteroposterior CoP displacement were both defined as positive when the CoP movement was oriented backwards. We additionally defined the stepping phase, from HO_{SW} to the subsequent heel contact of the swing foot, by means of markers placed on the feet. The first step was characterized in terms of step length and average and maximal velocity (Table 1). Velocity and acceleration of the CoM were defined at the end of the IMB and UNL phases and at the instant of TO_{ST}. Additionally, the position of the CoM with respect to the CoP and the inclination of the vector connecting the two points in the transversal plane were computed at the end of IMB and UNL and at the TO_{ST} (Table 1) [12].

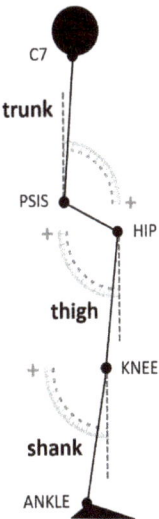

Figure 1. Scheme of the postural angles analyzed in the study. The trunk angle was defined as the inclination of the line passing through the markers placed on the middle point between the two posterior superior iliac spines and the seventh cervical vertebra with respect to the vertical axis of the laboratory. The thigh angle was calculated as the angle between the vector connecting the knee and hip center of rotation and the vertical axis of the laboratory. The shank angle was computed between the line connecting the joint centers of the knee and ankle and the vertical axis of the laboratory.

2.3.4. Segmental Centers of Mass

To describe the temporal pattern of segmental movements during GI, we computed the latency of movement onset of the following 16 SCoM: head, chest, abdomen, pelvis, swing arm, stance arm, swing forearm, stance forearm, swing hand, stance hand, swing thigh, stance thigh, swing shank, stance shank, swing foot, and stance foot (similarly to [46]). For each trial, the movement onset latency of each SCoM was computed as the movement time from the onset of the APAs and normalized for the total GI time (from APA_{ONSET} to the toe-off of the swing foot). For each subject, we rank-ordered the SCoM onset times and computed the following for each group: (i) the movement time from APA_{ONSET} normalized for the total GI time and (ii) the relative frequency of each SCoM onset time to appear as events 1–16 of GI. To improve the readability of the data, we repeated the analysis after combining the SCoM into six groups (upper trunk: head and chest; lower trunk: abdomen and pelvis; swing arm: swing arm, forearm, and hand; stance arm: stance arm, forearm, and hand; swing leg: swing thigh, shank, and foot; and stance leg: stance thigh, shank, and foot).

2.4. Statistical Analysis

For each subject, all measurements were averaged over GI trials executed with the same swing foot. Each participant performed at least three GI trials with the same swing foot. Single trials and average values were inspected and outliers were removed from further analyses based on the Mahalanobis distance [47,48].

First, we verified matching between groups for demographic, clinic, BoS, and AM features with a Mann–Whitney U-test (p-value set at 0.05). Before comparing the GI measurements across groups, we investigated their relationship with the BoS and AMs with two partial correlation analyses [12]. For each group, we correlated the GI measurements first with the BoS measurements controlling for the AMs, and then with the AMs controlling for the BoS. In agreement with [11], GI variables that significantly correlated (Spearman's $\rho > 0.5$ and p-value < 0.01) with the BoS in at least one group were excluded from further analyses. We opted for this conservative approach because the BoS was freely chosen by the subjects and may have been influenced by both the disease and compensatory mechanisms. The GI variables that correlated (Spearman's $\rho > 0.5$ and p-value < 0.01) with the AMs were instead corrected by means of the decorrelation normalization technique, as described by O'Malley [49]. This correction was applicable as AMs were not influenced by the disease (no patient had camptocormia, skeletal deformities, and so on).

GI variables not dependent on the BoS and decorrelated from the influence of the AMs were then compared between groups using a Dunn's test (p-value set at 0.05, adjusted with Bonferroni correction for multiple comparisons).

We then investigated alterations of the initial postural condition. As for the GI measurements, we assessed the correlation of the AMs and the BoS with the postural angles with partial correlation analyses (Spearman's $\rho > 0.5$ and p-value < 0.01), before comparing the postural angles across groups (Dunn's test, p-value set at 0.05, adjusted with Bonferroni correction for multiple comparisons).

As we found differences in the postural profiles across groups, we investigated whether altered GI measurements in the PD groups were related to postural changes rather than to impaired motor programming. We performed a partial correlation analysis between the GI outcome measurements and the postural angles correcting for the group variable. We considered a correlation significant when Spearman's $\rho > 0.5$ and p-value < 0.01.

Differences across groups in the SCoM movement onset were analyzed with a Dunn's test (p-value < 0.05, adjusted with Bonferroni correction for multiple comparisons).

All statistical analyses, except partial correlation analyses performed in Matlab, were performed with the JMP package (JMP® Pro 14.0.0, SAS Institute Inc., Cary, NC, USA).

3. Results

Demographic features, AM measurements, and BoS measurements did not significantly differ between groups (Table 2). Clinical data were similar between PDNF and PDF patients (Table 2).

Of note, none of the patients showed freezing episodes during GI recordings. Therefore, our results define primarily the impact of APA alterations and postural features in favoring FOG in PD and not a causal correlation with the occurrence of gait freezing episodes at GI.

3.1. Selection of GI Variables

The BoS did not correlate with most of the biomechanical measures of the IMB and stepping phases, but did correlate with the UNL. The results are consistent with our previous findings [12]. The GI variables that were independent from the BoS are listed in Table 3. The BoS and the AMs showed no correlations with the trunk, thigh, and shank angles.

Table 2. Demographic, clinical, anthropometric, and base of support features. Data are shown as mean (standard deviation). No statistically significant difference was found across groups (Mann–Whitney U-test, p-value set at 0.05). Abbreviations: HC, healthy controls; LEDD, levodopa equivalent daily dose; PDF, Parkinson's disease with freezing of gait; PDNF, Parkinson's disease with no freezing of gait; UPDRS-III, Unified Parkinson's Disease Rating scale, part III. Refer to Table 1 for a list of other abbreviations used.

		HC	PDNF	PDF
Demographic features	Gender (males/total)	14/23 (~61%)	10/20 (50%)	14/23 (~61%)
	Age (years)	61.17 (4.93)	63.32 (10.76)	63.83 (8.34)
Clinical data	Disease duration (years)	(-)	9.26 (3.89)	11.14 (3.47)
	Hoen and Yahr (I–V stage)	(-)	2.24 (0.42)	2.39 (0.50)
	UPDRS-III (0–108 score)	(-)	24.81 (9.43)	28.05 (9.96)
	LEDD (mg)	(-)	741.18 (221.26)	803.70 (358.33)
Anthropometric Measurements	BH (cm)	169.94 (10.53)	167.79 (11.05)	168.09 (11.44)
	LL (cm)	88.81 (5.37)	88.23 (7.81)	87.21 (5.84)
	FL (cm)	24.93 (1.66)	25.17 (1.58)	24.59 (1.65)
	BM (kg)	72.28 (11.11)	66.36 (13.01)	72.02 (14.83)
	BMI (kg/cm^2)	24.59 (3.02)	23.00 (3.99)	24.89 (5.18)
	IAD (cm)	27.76 (2.35)	27.89 (2.53)	27.42 (3.40)
Base of Support	BoS area (cm^2)	685.24 (91.56)	668.18 (75.19)	651.85 (114.90)
	BoS width (cm)	17.64 (4.10)	16.26 (2.78)	15.67 (2.59)
	Foot alignment (cm)	6.57 (3.36)	8.37 (4.54)	6.92 (3.76)
	Angle difference βΔ (°)	6.66 (3.29)	4.67 (2.58)	7.75 (4.98)
	BoS opening angle β (°)	40.67 (15.76)	37.25 (14.05)	43.56 (13.92)

Table 3. Gait initiation measurements: comparison between groups. Only biomechanical variables not correlated with the base of support are listed. Data are shown as mean (standard deviation). The mediolateral CoP displacement during imbalance and unloading was considered positive when the shift in the CoP was towards the swing and the stance foot, respectively. The anteroposterior CoP displacement during imbalance and unloading phase were both defined as positive when the CoP movement was oriented backwards. Abbreviations: HC, healthy controls; PDF, Parkinson's disease with freezing of gait; PDNF, Parkinson's disease with no freezing of gait; refer to Table 1 for a list of other acronyms used.

	HC	PDNF	PDF
IMB duration (s)	0.39 (0.08)	0.38 (0.08)	0.33 (0.09)
IMB displacement (mm)	61.23 [+] (20.32)	35.54 (19.71)	23.67 [+] (9.94)
IMB displacement ML (mm)	42.07 [#,+] (13.04)	24.04 [#] (13.61)	17.76 [+] (8.59)
IMB displacement AP (mm)	36.53 [+] (16.17)	18.79 (14.75)	9.16 [+] (5.93)
IMB average velocity (mm/s)	163.40 [#,+] (62.29)	90.79 [#] (47.29)	84.03 [+] (46.81)
IMB average velocity ML (mm/s)	110.94 [#] (34.90)	62.14 [#] (34.80)	67.53 (41.47)
IMB average velocity AP (mm/s)	103.36 [#,+] (53.78)	47.74 [#] (34.39)	40.19 [+] (30.45)
IMB maximal velocity (mm/s)	344.22 [#,+] (149.41)	189.88 [#] (113.54)	150.41 [+] (64.26)
IMB maximal velocity ML (mm/s)	238.29 [#,+] (77.82)	137.25 [#] (72.76)	124.97 [+] (56.96)
IMB maximal velocity AP (mm/s)	225.81 [+] (110.67)	124.78 (65.52)	101.41 [+] (55.74)
IMB end CoM velocity (m/s)	0.09 [+] (0.03)	0.06 (0.03)	0.04 [+] (0.02)
IMB end CoP–CoM distance (m)	0.07 [+] (0.02)	0.04 (0.02)	0.03 [+] (0.01)
UNL duration (s)	0.36 (0.08)	0.40 (0.08)	0.45 (0.19)
UNL displacement AP (mm)	−9.67 [+] (15.30)	−6.25 [*] (18.22)	14.69 [+,*] (14.70)
UNL average velocity (mm/s)	465.61 (162.21)	323.94 (131.02)	320.34 (150.20)
UNL average velocity ML (mm/s)	422.79 (148.96)	289.26 (121.24)	290.67 (140.81)
UNL average velocity AP (mm/s)	53.07 (20.97)	37.29 (17.16)	46.04 (34.21)
UNL maximal velocity AP (mm/s)	344.48 (154.35)	388.76 (169.88)	359.19 (178.76)
UNL end CoM velocity (m/s)	0.21 [+] (0.06)	0.16 (0.07)	0.11 [+] (0.04)

Table 3. Cont.

	HC	PDNF	PDF
UNL end CoM acceleration (m/s^2)	1.29 (0.33)	1.08 (0.41)	1.12 (0.25)
UNL end CoP–CoM distance (m)	0.08 (0.03)	0.07 (0.03)	0.07 (0.02)
ST toe-off CoM velocity (m/s)	0.86 #,+ (0.13)	0.63 # (0.24)	0.53 + (0.18)
ST toe-off CoM acceleration (m/s^2)	1.73 + (0.38)	1.28 (0.42)	1.08 + (0.33)
ST toe CoP–CoM distance (m)	0.48 (0.32)	0.51 (0.29)	0.34 (0.28)
First step length (m)	0.56 + (0.07)	0.43 (0.14)	0.33 + (0.13)

Dunn's test, significant p-value after Bonferroni correction: # HC vs. PDNF, + HC vs. PDF, * PDNF vs. PDF.

3.2. Postural Features

The trunk and thigh angles, but not the shank angle, were significantly altered in both PDNF and PDF patients compared with HCs (Table 4). Parkinsonian patients showed increased forward trunk bending associated with a reduced thigh angle. The trunk was more flexed in PDF patients than in PDNF patients, although this difference did not reach statistical significance. The thigh angle showed a negative average value only in the PDF group.

Table 4. Postural angles were computed shortly before the gait initiation execution (during a 1 s window before the onset of the anticipatory postural adjustments). Data are shown as mean (standard deviation). Abbreviations: HC, healthy controls; PDF, Parkinson's disease with freezing of gait; PDNF, Parkinson's disease with no freezing of gait.

	HC	PDNF	PDF
Trunk (°)	4.08 #,+ (2.43)	9.06 # (4.37)	12.58 + (5.65)
Thigh (°)	6.31 #,+ (2.69)	0.54 # (3.70)	−0.48 + (4.00)
Shank (°)	9.22 (2.93)	10.67 (2.77)	10.95 (2.47)

Dunn's test, significant p-value after Bonferroni correction: # HC vs. PDNF, + HC vs. PDF.

3.3. Effect of PD and History of FOG on GI

We observed significant alterations in the GI execution in both PDNF and PDF patients, with the latter group showing overall more severely altered APA measurements (Table 3, Figure 2).

The CoP displacement and velocity during IMB showed a progressive and significant reduction from HCs to PDNF to PDF groups along both the mediolateral and anteroposterior axes.

The UNL and stepping phases were also altered in PDNF and PDF patients (Table 3, Figure 2). Of most relevance, in PDF patients, the anteroposterior displacement of the CoP during UNL was backwards in most of the trials.

PDF patients had a significantly reduced first step length and both PD groups had a lower first step average velocity compared with HCs.

The CoM forward propulsion (velocity and acceleration) progressively decreased from HCs to PDNF to PDF.

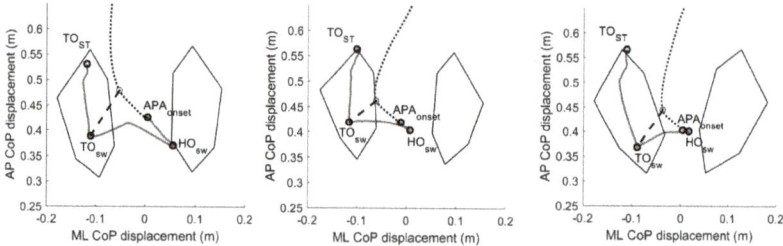

Figure 2. Two-dimensional center of pressure and center of mass trajectories during gait initiation.

Example of the pathway of the center of pressure (CoP, grey solid line) and center of mass (CoM, black dotted line) during a gait initiation trial of one healthy subject (left panel) and one Parkinsonian patient without (PDNF, central panel) and one patient with (PDF, right panel) a positive history of freezing of gait. We defined the imbalance (IMB) phase as the interval between the onset of the APAs (APAONSET) and the heel-off of the swing foot (HOSW), and the unloading phase (UNL) as the interval between the HOSW and the toe-off of the swing foot (TOSW). The black dashed line represents the CoP–CoM vector at the end of the unloading (UNL) phase. With respect to healthy controls, the CoP displacement during the IMB phase was reduced for both PD and PDF patients. The CoP displacement during the UNL phase was in most cases backwards for the PDF patients only. Please see Table 3 for further details. Abbreviations: APAs, anticipatory postural adjustments; AP, anterior–posterior; CoP, center of pressure; HC, healthy controls; HO, heel off; ML, mediolateral; PDF, Parkinson's disease with freezing of gait; PDNF, Parkinson's disease with no freezing of gait; TO, toe-off.

3.4. Relationship between the Standing Postural Profile and the GI

We did not find any significant correlation between the postural angles and the GI measurements. However, when not correcting for multiple comparisons, the shank angle was predictive for velocity variables of the IMB phase. The results are shown in Table 5.

Table 5. Correlation between the shank angle and gait initiation measurements. Only significant partial correlations between postural angles and gait initiation measurements corrected for the influence of the group variable are shown (Spearman's ρ, p-value < 0.05). No correlation was significant after Bonferroni correction for multiple comparisons.

		Spearman's ρ	p-Value
Shank (°)	IMB average velocity (mm/s)	0.32	0.014
	IMB average velocity AP (mm/s)	0.31	0.016
	IMB maximal velocity AP (mm/s)	0.38	0.003

3.5. Pattern of Movements during GI

The overall pattern of segmental movements during GI did not show clear differences between groups (Tables 6 and 7). However, PDF showed shorter times of movement onset for almost all ranked segments (Table 7), possibly suggesting tight inter-segmental coupling [50]. All groups started preferably with the swing or stance arm, especially the swing hand for HCs and PDNF and the stance hand for PDF (Figures S1 and S2). The abdomen was often the last body segment moved by HCs and PDNF, but not by PDF (Figure S1). Of note, we observed a remarkable inter-subject variability of SCoM onset times, especially for PD, as shown by the high value of the standard deviation (Table 6) and the large dispersion of the temporal order of SCoM movement onsets (Figure S1), which probably prevented us from capturing statistically significant differences.

Table 6. Onset of segmental movements at gait initiation. Data are shown as mean (standard deviation). Time of movement onset of each segmental center of mass was expressed as the percentage with respect to total gait initiation duration (i.e., from the onset of the anticipatory postural adjustments to the heel contact of the swing foot) and compared across groups (Dunn's test, no difference was significant after Bonferroni correction for multiple comparisons). Abbreviations: HC, healthy controls; PDF, Parkinson's disease with freezing of gait; PDNF, Parkinson's disease with no freezing of gait; ST: stance limb; SW: swing limb.

Segmental Center of Mass	HC	PDNF	PDF
Pelvis (%)	60.62 (9.27)	62.47 (13.74)	62.66 (21.69)
Thigh ST (%)	65.76 (10.75)	71.72 (20.13)	63.39 (19.97)
Shank ST (%)	71.17 (14.36)	68.57 (19.98)	65.73 (21.95)
Foot ST (%)	68.37 (10.46)	77.24 (22.53)	65.02 (22.87)

Table 6. Cont.

Segmental Center of Mass	HC	PDNF	PDF
Thigh SW (%)	62.67 (9.23)	64.75 (15.47)	55.85 (18.80)
Shank SW (%)	74.21 (13.85)	75.35 (24.26)	67.26 (19.36)
Foot SW (%)	69.15 (15.41)	64.63 (16.55)	59.20 (19.86)
Chest (%)	73.48 (14.29)	74.47 (26.12)	69.22 (19.85)
Abdomen (%)	79.50 (13.87)	81.57 (25.30)	57.88 (20.58)
Arm ST (%)	55.49 (18.27)	65.80 (26.63)	54.17 (19.98)
Arm SW (%)	62.71 (9.34)	65.08 (13.49)	56.57 (17.72)
Forearm ST (%)	38.98 (12.65)	53.73 (24.00)	39.40 (12.69)
Forearm SW (%)	51.34 (11.80)	62.57 (13.59)	47.26 (13.34)
Hand ST (%)	44.37 (19.82)	49.64 (21.32)	41.99 (30.95)
Hand SW (%)	34.36 (13.06)	46.93 (19.96)	47.71 (16.69)
Head (%)	54.33 (11.81)	58.15 (14.06)	60.06 (18.41)

Table 7. Onset of rank-ordered segmental movements at gait initiation. Data are shown as mean (standard deviation). Time of movement onset of rank-ordered segmental centers of mass was expressed as the percentage with respect to total gait initiation duration (i.e., from the onset of the anticipatory postural adjustments to the heel contact of the swing foot) and compared across groups (Dunn's test, no difference was significant after Bonferroni correction for multiple comparisons). Abbreviations: HC, healthy controls; PDF, Parkinson's disease with freezing of gait; PDNF, Parkinson's disease with no freezing of gait.

Rank-Ordered Segmental Center of Mass	HC	PDNF	PDF
1st segment (%)	27.88 (10.66)	35.42 (13.61)	26.51 (11.98)
2nd segment (%)	36.33 (10.40)	45.51 (15.10)	34.90 (13.48)
3rd segment (%)	42.62 (9.68)	50.70 (14.76)	41.43 (12.61)
4th segment (%)	46.70 (8.60)	54.47 (14.37)	44.29 (13.88)
5th segment (%)	50.58 (8.32)	57.41 (12.53)	46.68 (14.44)
6th segment (%)	54.40 (6.50)	59.49 (13.25)	49.54 (15.11)
7th segment (%)	57.49 (6.79)	61.70 (14.11)	51.87 (14.85)
8th segment (%)	59.71 (7.51)	64.81 (15.85)	54.13 (15.05)
9th segment (%)	61.31 (8.04)	66.18 (16.05)	55.93 (15.08)
10th segment (%)	62.94 (7.84)	67.59 (16.18)	58.10 (14.84)
11th segment (%)	65.75 (9.10)	68.86 (16.49)	60.79 (14.94)
12th segment (%)	67.89 (9.02)	70.65 (17.45)	62.66 (15.16)
13th segment (%)	70.64 (10.11)	72.32 (18.32)	65.83 (14.82)
14th segment (%)	73.91 (10.70)	74.85 (19.26)	68.93 (16.35)
15th segment (%)	78.42 (11.79)	78.81 (21.00)	74.20 (15.35)
16th segment (%)	84.95 (11.99)	83.19 (23.21)	82.42 (18.88)

4. Discussion

This study aimed to evaluate the specific biomechanical alterations of APAs at GI in PD patients with a positive history of FOG, accounting for known confounders such as medication condition, anthropometric measurements, base of support, and initial stance posture. The CoP displacement and velocity during the imbalance phase were altered in both PDNF and PDF patients, but more prominently in the latter group. The CoP displacement along the anteroposterior axis during the unloading phase was impaired only in PDF patients. The order of SCoM movements was unaltered in the two patient groups. The postural profile did not correlate with GI outcome measurements.

Our findings are in line with previous studies in PD that showed an impairment in APAs' production at GI [20,51]. However, a direct comparison with earlier works is limited because we aimed to minimize possible bias from cueing or imposed postural constraints that are known to affect the execution of the GI task [9,11,12,18,22,52–54].

We have now shown that there is a profound alteration of APA execution in PDF patients, which cannot be attributed to specific demographic or clinical features (such as disease severity and duration, medication dose, and efficacy) as the patient groups were matched for all of these features [55].

The IMB phase of APA execution was significantly altered in all PD patients, particularly in PDF (Table 3). Increasing evidence suggests that this GI phase is governed by centrally mediated feedforward signals and involves the cortico-basal ganglia loop, with the SMA-proper and the striatum chiefly contributing to the execution of these preprogrammed movements [6,8,9,11,12,56–60]. In PD, we have previously shown a detrimental effect of striatal dopamine loss in the IMB execution at GI [12]. Recent studies in Parkinsonian patients suggested that striatal dopamine may in part enable normal movement by encoding sensitivity to the energy cost of a movement [61–64]. Therefore, from the perspective of motor planning, especially of patterned and consolidated motor actions such as APAs, a reduced tonic dopaminergic activity could reframe the coding of the expected energetic costs and impair motor control [63].

In our study, we also showed a prominent alteration in the AP displacement of the CoP during the UNL phase in PDF patients. We interpret this result as a possible alteration, mainly of PDF patients, in the processing and integration of somatosensory information prior to stepping [6,14,65,66]. A chief contribution to integrate proprioceptive and voluntary components for a proper weight transfer during GI can be expected from the premotor–parietal–cerebellar loop [14,58,67–71]. An impaired ability to inhibit stance postural control and initiate stepping and poor set-shifting is also included in pathophysiological hypotheses of FOG in PD [5,10,57,72–77].

Despite impaired APA execution, the sequencing of the movement did not show major alterations in the PD groups. We speculate that additional inputs from the cerebellum could overcome impaired information processing by favoring internal movement timing [78]. The efficacy of an online compensatory role of the cerebellum [70,78] is suggested in our study by the relatively preserved SCoM temporal movement sequencing [79], which could have also prevented the appearance of any gait freezing episode during our acquisitions. Relative timing of segmental movements was also described as unaltered in patients with PD by Rosin and colleagues (1997), further suggesting a compensatory rather than detrimental role of the cerebellum in Parkinsonian patients with FOG and balance disturbances [60,78,80]. Of relevance, the high variability in the SCoM movement onsets might have prevented us from detecting differences across groups. Further studies with larger cohorts might further explore this aspect to definitively rule out the presence of PD-related alterations in the movement sequencing.

We envisioned a significant impact of postural abnormalities on GI in PD, but our results did not support this hypothesis. Interestingly, our findings instead confirmed previous physiological studies reporting no correlation between APA execution at GI and the natural inclination of the trunk [33] or of a forward leaning up to 30% of the maximum voluntary lean [35].

Our study suffers from some limitations. First, although we reduced as much as possible the influence of known confounders (i.e., initial feet position and posture, anthropometric parameters, and cues), we cannot fully exclude a residual influence of Parkinsonian symptoms such as bradykinesia and rigidity on the task performance [37]. However, in our previous work [12], we showed that levodopa intake, by improving bradykinesia and rigidity, increases the length and speed of the first step at GI, but does not affect the AP shift during UNL. We can thus hypothesize that the alterations in AP displacement during UNL in the PDF group are not related to akinetic-rigid symptoms, but to impairment of the motor program itself. Future studies are needed to better clarify this aspect. Second, the limited sample size and very stringent statistics may have limited the detection of differences between groups (e.g., SCoM onset times). Third, the lack of a brain imaging evaluation in this study prevents any firm conclusions about our pathophysiological interpretation of the kinematic and dynamic findings, but they match well with the brain metabolic activity changes [66,68] and network derangements [81–84] described during actual gait and gait freezing episodes in Parkinsonian patients.

In conclusion, our data demonstrate substantial impairment of feedforward motor programming mechanisms at GI in Parkinsonian patients. The deterioration of the UNL and stepping in PDF patients would suggest an additional impaired integration of postural and locomotor programs subserving gait initiation and modulation, which might be partly compensated by cerebellar mechanisms triggering time-locked models of body movement. Postural alterations seem to play a minor role in GI impairment in patients with PD. Last, but not least, our results suggest the potential clinical utility of recording the CoP displacement during GI, and particularly its AP shift during the UNL to identify patients at risk of FOG and to monitor the efficacy of therapeutic strategies. Future longitudinal studies may support this assumption.

Supplementary Materials: The following supporting information can be downloaded at https://www.mdpi.com/article/10.3390/bioengineering9110639/s1, Figure S1: Rank order of segmental CoM onset times; Figure S2: Rank order of onset times of groups of segmental CoM.

Author Contributions: Conceptualization, C.P. and I.U.I.; methodology, C.P. and I.U.I.; software, C.P. and S.H.; formal analysis, C.P., L.B., S.H. and I.U.I.; investigation, C.P. and I.U.I.; resources, C.P., G.P. and I.U.I.; data curation, C.P. and L.B.; writing—original draft preparation, C.P. and L.B.; writing—review and editing, J.V. and I.U.I.; visualization, C.P.; supervision, S.H., J.V. and I.U.I.; project administration, J.V. and I.U.I.; funding acquisition, J.V., G.P. and I.U.I. All authors have read and agreed to the published version of the manuscript.

Funding: The study was sponsored by the Deutsche Forschungsgemeinschaft (DFG, German Research Foundation)—Project-ID 424778381-TRR 295 and the Fondazione Grigioni per il Morbo di Parkinson. C.P. was supported by a grant from the German Excellence Initiative to the Graduate School of Life Sciences, University of Würzburg. L.B. was supported by a grant from New York University School of Medicine and The Marlene and Paolo Fresco Institute for Parkinson's and Movement Disorders, which was made possible with support from Marlene and Paolo Fresco. This publication was supported by the Open Access Publication Fund of the University of Würzburg.

Institutional Review Board Statement: The study was conducted in accordance with the Declaration of Helsinki and approved by the Ethics Committee of the Università degli Studi di Milano (5/16, 15.02.2016).

Informed Consent Statement: Informed consent was obtained from all subjects involved in the study.

Data Availability Statement: The data presented in this study are available upon request from the corresponding author. The data are not publicly available for privacy reasons.

Acknowledgments: We would like to thank all patients and caregivers for their participation. Our special thanks go to Paolo Cavallari for his help in conducting the study and to Monica Norcini for study management and administrative support. The study was sponsored by the Deutsche Forschungsgemeinschaft (DFG, German Research Foundation)—Project-ID 424778381-TRR 295 and the Fondazione Grigioni per il Morbo di Parkinson. C.P. was supported by a grant from the German Excellence Initiative to the Graduate School of Life Sciences, University of Würzburg. L.B. was supported by a grant from New York University School of Medicine and The Marlene and Paolo Fresco Institute for Parkinson's and Movement Disorders, which was made possible with support from Marlene and Paolo Fresco. This publication was supported by the Open Access Publication Fund of the University of Würzburg.

Conflicts of Interest: The authors declare no conflict of interest. The funders had no role in the design of the study; in the collection, analyses, or interpretation of data; in the writing of the manuscript; or in the decision to publish the results.

References

1. Perez-Lloret, S.; Negre-Pages, L.; Damier, P.; Delval, A.; Derkinderen, P.; Destée, A.; Meissner, W.G.; Schelosky, L.; Tison, F.; Rascol, O. Prevalence, Determinants, and Effect on Quality of Life of Freezing of Gait in Parkinson Disease. *JAMA Neurol.* **2014**, *71*, 884–890. [CrossRef] [PubMed]
2. Kerr, G.K.; Worringham, C.J.; Cole, M.H.; Lacherez, P.F.; Wood, J.M.; Silburn, P.A. Predictors of Future Falls in Parkinson Disease. *Neurology* **2010**, *75*, 116–124. [CrossRef] [PubMed]

3. Okada, Y.; Fukumoto, T.; Takatori, K.; Nagino, K.; Hiraoka, K. Abnormalities of the First Three Steps of Gait Initiation in Patients with Parkinson's Disease with Freezing of Gait. *Parkinsons. Dis.* **2011**, *2011*, 202937. [CrossRef] [PubMed]
4. Pelykh, O.; Klein, A.-M.; Bötzel, K.; Kosutzka, Z.; Ilmberger, J. Dynamics of Postural Control in Parkinson Patients with and without Symptoms of Freezing of Gait. *Gait Posture* **2015**, *42*, 246–250. [CrossRef]
5. Nutt, J.G.; Bloem, B.R.; Giladi, N.; Hallett, M.; Horak, F.B.; Nieuwboer, A. Freezing of Gait: Moving Forward on a Mysterious Clinical Phenomenon. *Lancet Neurol.* **2011**, *10*, 734–744. [CrossRef]
6. Yiou, E.; Caderby, T.; Delafontaine, A.; Fourcade, P.; Honeine, J.-L.L. Balance Control during Gait Initiation: State-of-the-Art and Research Perspectives. *World J. Orthop.* **2017**, *8*, 815–828. [CrossRef]
7. Crenna, P.; Frigo, C. A Motor Programme for the Initiation of Foroward-Oriented Movements in Humans. *J. Physiol.* **1991**, *437*, 635–653. [CrossRef]
8. Petersen, N.T.; Butler, J.E.; Marchand-Pauvert, V.; Fisher, R.; Ledebt, A.; Pyndt, H.S.; Hansen, N.L.; Nielsen, J.B. Suppression of EMG Activity by Transcranial Magnetic Stimulation in Human Subjects during Walking. *J. Physiol.* **2001**, *537*, 651–656. [CrossRef]
9. Hiraoka, K.; Matuo, Y.; Iwata, A.; Onishi, T.; Abe, K. The Effects of External Cues on Ankle Control during Gait Initiation in Parkinson's Disease. *Park. Relat. Disord.* **2006**, *12*, 97–102. [CrossRef]
10. Jacobs, J.V.; Nutt, J.G.; Carlson-Kuhta, P.; Stephens, M.; Horak, F.B. Knee Trembling during Freezing of Gait Represents Multiple Anticipatory Postural Adjustments. *Exp. Neurol.* **2009**, *215*, 334–341. [CrossRef]
11. Palmisano, C.; Todisco, M.; Marotta, G.; Volkmann, J.; Pacchetti, C.; Frigo, C.A.; Pezzoli, G.; Isaias, I.U. Gait Initiation in Progressive Supranuclear Palsy: Brain Metabolic Correlates. *NeuroImage Clin.* **2020**, *28*, 102408. [CrossRef]
12. Palmisano, C.; Brandt, G.; Vissani, M.; Pozzi, N.G.; Canessa, A.; Brumberg, J.; Marotta, G.; Volkmann, J.; Mazzoni, A.; Pezzoli, G.; et al. Gait Initiation in Parkinson's Disease: Impact of Dopamine Depletion and Initial Stance Condition. *Front. Bioeng. Biotechnol.* **2020**, *8*, 137. [CrossRef]
13. Inglis, J.T.; Horak, F.B.; Shupert, C.L.; Jones-Rycewicz, C. The Importance of Somatosensory Information in Triggering and Scaling Automatic Postural Responses in Humans. *Exp. Brain Res.* **1994**, *101*, 159–164. [CrossRef] [PubMed]
14. Mouchnino, L.; Fontan, A.; Tandonnet, C.; Perrier, J.; Saradjian, A.; Blouin, J.; Simoneau, M. Facilitation of Cutaneous Inputs during the Planning Phase of Gait Initiation. *J. Neurophysiol.* **2015**, *114*, 301–308. [CrossRef] [PubMed]
15. Brenière, Y.; Cuong Do, M.; Bouisset, S. Are Dynamic Phenomena Prior to Stepping Essential to Walking? *J. Mot. Behav.* **1987**, *19*, 62–76. [CrossRef] [PubMed]
16. Lepers, R.; Brenière, Y. The Role of Anticipatory Postural Adjustments and Gravity in Gait Initiation. *Exp. Brain Res.* **1995**, *107*, 118–124. [CrossRef] [PubMed]
17. Caderby, T.; Yiou, E.; Peyrot, N.; Begon, M.; Dalleau, G. Influence of Gait Speed on the Control of Mediolateral Dynamic Stability during Gait Initiation. *J. Biomech.* **2014**, *47*, 417–423. [CrossRef]
18. Burleigh-Jacobs, A.; Horak, F.B.; Nutt, J.G.; Obeso, J.A. Step Initiation in Parkinson's Disease: Influence of Levodopa and External Sensory Triggers. *Mov. Disord.* **1997**, *12*, 206–215. [CrossRef]
19. Frank, J.S.; Horak, F.B.; Nutt, J. Centrally Initiated Postural Adjustments in Parkinsonian Patients on and off Levodopa. *J. Neurophysiol.* **2000**, *84*, 2440–2448. [CrossRef]
20. Crenna, P.; Carpinella, I.; Rabuffetti, M.; Rizzone, M.; Lopiano, L.; Lanotte, M.; Ferrarin, M. Impact of Subthalamic Nucleus Stimulation on the Initiation of Gait in Parkinson's Disease. *Exp. Brain Res.* **2006**, *172*, 519–532. [CrossRef]
21. Liu, W.; McIntire, K.; Kim, S.H.; Zhang, J.; Dascalos, S.; Lyons, K.E.; Pahwa, R. Bilateral Subthalamic Stimulation Improves Gait Initiation in Patients with Parkinson's Disease. *Gait Posture* **2006**, *23*, 492–498. [CrossRef]
22. Rocchi, L.; Chiari, L.; Mancini, M.; Carlson-Kuhta, P.; Gross, A.; Horak, F.B. Step Initiation in Parkinson's Disease: Influence of Initial Stance Conditions. *Neurosci. Lett.* **2006**, *406*, 128–132. [CrossRef] [PubMed]
23. Chastan, N.; Do, M.C.; Bonneville, F.; Torny, F.; Bloch, F.; Westby, G.W.M.; Dormont, D.; Agid, Y.; Welter, M.L. Gait and Balance Disorders in Parkinson's Disease: Impaired Active Braking of the Fall of Centre of Gravity. *Mov. Disord.* **2009**, *24*, 188–195. [CrossRef] [PubMed]
24. Pötter-Nerger, M.; Volkmann, J. Deep Brain Stimulation for Gait and Postural Symptoms in Parkinson's Disease. *Mov. Disord.* **2013**, *28*, 1609–1615. [CrossRef]
25. Mazzone, P.; Paoloni, M.; Mangone, M.; Santilli, V.; Insola, A.; Fini, M.; Scarnati, E. Unilateral Deep Brain Stimulation of the Pedunculopontine Tegmental Nucleus in Idiopathic Parkinson's Disease: Effects on Gait Initiation and Performance. *Gait Posture* **2014**, *40*, 357–362. [CrossRef] [PubMed]
26. Curtze, C.; Nutt, J.G.; Carlson-Kuhta, P.; Mancini, M.; Horak, F.B. Levodopa Is a Double-Edged Sword for Balance and Gait in People With Parkinson's Disease. *Mov. Disord.* **2015**, *30*, 1361–1370. [CrossRef]
27. Nonnekes, J.; Geurts, A.C.H.; Nijhuis, L.B.O.; van Geel, K.; Snijders, A.H.; Bloem, B.R.; Weerdesteyn, V. Reduced StartReact Effect and Freezing of Gait in Parkinson's Disease: Two of a Kind? *J. Neurol.* **2014**, *261*, 943–950. [CrossRef]
28. de Souza Fortaleza, A.C.; Mancini, M.; Carlson-Kuhta, P.; King, L.A.; Nutt, J.G.; Chagas, E.F.; Freitas, I.F.; Horak, F.B. Dual Task Interference on Postural Sway, Postural Transitions and Gait in People with Parkinson's Disease and Freezing of Gait. *Gait Posture* **2017**, *56*, 76–81. [CrossRef]
29. Schlenstedt, C.; Mancini, M.; Nutt, J.; Hiller, A.P.; Maetzler, W.; Deuschl, G.; Horak, F. Are Hypometric Anticipatory Postural Adjustments Contributing to Freezing of Gait in Parkinson's Disease? *Front. Aging Neurosci.* **2018**, *10*, 36. [CrossRef]

30. Cohen, R.G.; Nutt, J.G.; Horak, F.B. Recovery from Multiple APAs Delays Gait Initiation in Parkinson's Disease. *Front. Hum. Neurosci.* **2017**, *11*, 60. [CrossRef]
31. Bayot, M.; Delval, A.; Moreau, C.; Defebvre, L.; Hansen, C.; Maetzler, W.; Schlenstedt, C. Initial Center of Pressure Position Prior to Anticipatory Postural Adjustments during Gait Initiation in People with Parkinson's Disease with Freezing of Gait. *Park. Relat. Disord.* **2021**, *84*, 8–14. [CrossRef] [PubMed]
32. Dalton, E.; Bishop, M.; Tillman, M.D.; Hass, C.J. Simple Change in Initial Standing Position Enhances the Initiation of Gait. *Med. Sci. Sports Exerc.* **2011**, *43*, 2352–2358. [CrossRef] [PubMed]
33. Leteneur, S.; Simoneau, E.; Gillet, C.; Dessery, Y.; Barbier, F. Trunk's Natural Inclination Influences Stance Limb Kinetics, but Not Body Kinematics, during Gait Initiation in Able Men. *PLoS ONE* **2013**, *8*, e55256. [CrossRef]
34. Fortin, A.P.; Dessery, Y.; Leteneur, S.; Barbier, F.; Corbeil, P. Effect of Natural Trunk Inclination on Variability in Soleus Inhibition and Tibialis Anterior Activation during Gait Initiation in Young Adults. *Gait Posture* **2015**, *41*, 378–383. [CrossRef] [PubMed]
35. Fawver, B.; Roper, J.A.; Sarmento, C.; Hass, C.J. Forward Leaning Alters Gait Initiation Only at Extreme Anterior Postural Positions. *Hum. Mov. Sci.* **2018**, *59*, 1–11. [CrossRef]
36. Yoshii, F.; Moriya, Y.; Ohnuki, T.; Ryo, M.; Takahashi, W. Postural Deformities in Parkinson's Disease–Mutual Relationships among Neck Flexion, Fore-Bent, Knee-Bent and Lateral-Bent Angles and Correlations with Clinical Predictors. *J. Clin. Mov. Disord.* **2016**, *3*, 1. [CrossRef]
37. Delafontaine, A.; Gagey, O.; Colnaghi, S.; Do, M.C.; Honeine, J.L. Rigid Ankle Foot Orthosis Deteriorates Mediolateral Balance Control and Vertical Braking during Gait Initiation. *Front. Hum. Neurosci.* **2017**, *11*, 214. [CrossRef]
38. Stansfield, B.; Hawkins, K.; Adams, S.; Church, D. Spatiotemporal and Kinematic Characteristics of Gait Initiation across a Wide Speed Range. *Gait Posture* **2018**, *61*, 331–338. [CrossRef]
39. Ferrari, A.; Benedetti, M.G.; Pavan, E.; Frigo, C.; Bettinelli, D.; Rabuffetti, M.; Crenna, P.; Leardini, A. Quantitative Comparison of Five Current Protocols in Gait Analysis. *Gait Posture* **2008**, *28*, 207–216. [CrossRef]
40. Isaias, I.U.; Dipaola, M.; Michi, M.; Marzegan, A.; Volkmann, J.; Roidi, M.L.R.; Frigo, C.A.; Cavallari, P. Gait Initiation in Children with Rett Syndrome. *PLoS ONE* **2014**, *9*, e92736. [CrossRef]
41. Palmisano, C.; Brandt, G.; Pozzi, N.G.; Alice, L.; Maltese, V.; Andrea, C.; Jens, V.; Pezzoli, G.; Frigo, C.A.; Isaias, I.U. Sit-to-Walk Performance in Parkinson's Disease: A Comparison between Faller and Non-Faller Patients. *Clin. Biomech.* **2019**, *63*, 140–146. [CrossRef]
42. Muniz, A.M.S.; Nadal, J.; Lyons, K.E.; Pahwa, R.; Liu, W. Long-Term Evaluation of Gait Initiation in Six Parkinson's Disease Patients with Bilateral Subthalamic Stimulation. *Gait Posture* **2012**, *35*, 452–457. [CrossRef]
43. Zatsiorsky, V.M. *Kinematics of Human Motion*; Human Kinetics: Champaign, IL, USA, 1998.
44. Dipaola, M.; Pavan, E.E.; Cattaneo, A.; Frazzitta, G.; Pezzoli, G.; Cavallari, P.; Frigo, C.A.; Isaias, I.U. Mechanical Energy Recovery during Walking in Patients with Parkinson Disease. *PLoS ONE* **2016**, *11*, e0156420. [CrossRef]
45. Martin, M.; Shinberg, M.; Kuchibhatla, M.; Ray, L.; Carollo, J.J.; Schenkman, M.L. Gait Initiation in Community-Dwelling Adults with Parkinson Disease: Comparison with Older and Younger Adults without the Disease. *Phys. Ther.* **2002**, *82*, 566–577. [CrossRef]
46. Rosin, R.; Topka, H.; Dichgans, J. Gait Initiation in Parkinson's Disease. *Mov. Disord.* **1997**, *12*, 682–690. [CrossRef]
47. Mahalanobis, P.C. On the Generalized Distance in Statistics. *Proc. Natl. Inst. Sci. India* **1936**, *2*, 49–55.
48. Farinelli, V.; Hosseinzadeh, L.; Palmisano, C.; Frigo, C. An Easily Applicable Method to Analyse the Ankle-Foot Power Absorption and Production during Walking. *Gait Posture* **2019**, *71*, 56–61. [CrossRef]
49. O'Malley, M.J. Normalization of Temporal-Distance Parameters in Pediatric Gait. *J. Biomech.* **1996**, *29*, 619–625. [CrossRef]
50. Crenna, P.; Carpinella, I.; Rabuffetti, M.; Calabrese, E.; Mazzoleni, P.; Nemni, R.; Ferrarin, M. The Association between Impaired Turning and Normal Straight Walking in Parkinson's Disease. *Gait Posture* **2007**, *26*, 172–178. [CrossRef]
51. Halliday, S.E.; Winter, D.A.; Frank, J.S.; Patla, A.E.; Prince, F. The Initiation of Gait in Young, Elderly, and Parkinson's Disease Subjects. *Gait Posture* **1998**, *8*, 8–14. [CrossRef]
52. Dibble, L.E.; Nicholson, D.E.; Shultz, B.; MacWilliams, B.A.; Marcus, R.L.; Moncur, C. Sensory Cueing Effects on Maximal Speed Gait Initiation in Persons with Parkinson's Disease and Healthy Elders. *Gait Posture* **2004**, *19*, 215–225. [CrossRef]
53. Plate, A.; Klein, K.; Pelykh, O.; Singh, A.; Bötzel, K. Anticipatory Postural Adjustments Are Unaffected by Age and Are Not Absent in Patients with the Freezing of Gait Phenomenon. *Exp. Brain Res.* **2016**, *234*, 2609–2618. [CrossRef]
54. Schlenstedt, C.; Mancini, M.; Horak, F.; Peterson, D. Anticipatory Postural Adjustment During Self-Initiated, Cued, and Compensatory Stepping in Healthy Older Adults and Patients With Parkinson Disease. *Arch. Phys. Med. Rehabil.* **2017**, *98*, 1316–1324.e1. [CrossRef]
55. Heilbron, M.; Scholten, M.; Schlenstedt, C.; Mancini, M.; Schöllmann, A.; Cebi, I.; Pötter-Nerger, M.; Gharabaghi, A.; Weiss, D. Anticipatory Postural Adjustmens Are Modulated by Substantia Nigra Stimulation in People with Parkinson's Disease and Freezing of Gait. *Park. Relat. Disord.* **2019**, *66*, 34–39. [CrossRef]
56. Lee, K.M.; Chang, K.H.; Roh, J.K. Subregions within the Supplementary Motor Area Activated at Different Stages of Movement Preparation and Execution. *Neuroimage* **1999**, *9*, 117–123. [CrossRef]
57. Jacobs, J.V.; Lou, J.S.; Kraakevik, J.A.; Horak, F.B. The Supplementary Motor Area Contributes to the Timing of the Anticipatory Postural Adjustment during Step Initiation in Participants with and without Parkinson's Disease. *Neuroscience* **2009**, *164*, 877–885. [CrossRef]

58. Bolzoni, F.; Bruttini, C.; Esposti, R.; Castellani, C.; Cavallari, P. Transcranial Direct Current Stimulation of SMA Modulates Anticipatory Postural Adjustments without Affecting the Primary Movement. *Behav. Brain Res.* **2015**, *291*, 407–413. [CrossRef]
59. Varghese, J.P.; Merino, D.M.; Beyer, K.B.; McIlroy, W.E. Cortical Control of Anticipatory Postural Adjustments Prior to Stepping. *Neuroscience* **2016**, *313*, 99–109. [CrossRef]
60. Richard, A.; Van Hamme, A.; Drevelle, X.; Golmard, J.L.; Meunier, S.; Welter, M.L. Contribution of the Supplementary Motor Area and the Cerebellum to the Anticipatory Postural Adjustments and Execution Phases of Human Gait Initiation. *Neuroscience* **2017**, *358*, 181–189. [CrossRef]
61. Morris, G.; Nevet, A.; Arkadir, D.; Vaadia, E.; Bergman, H. Midbrain Dopamine Neurons Encode Decisions for Future Action. *Nat. Neurosci.* **2006**, *9*, 1057–1063. [CrossRef]
62. Mazzoni, P.; Hristova, A.; Krakauer, J.W. Why Don't We Move Faster? Parkinson's Disease, Movement Vigor, and Implicit Motivation. *J. Neurosci.* **2007**, *27*, 7105–7116. [CrossRef]
63. Gepshtein, S.; Li, X.; Snider, J.; Plank, M.; Lee, D.; Poizner, H. Dopamine Function and the Efficiency of Human Movement. *J. Cogn. Neurosci.* **2014**, *26*, 645–657. [CrossRef]
64. Schultz, W. Multiple Dopamine Functions at Different Time Courses. *Annu. Rev. Neurosci.* **2007**, *30*, 259–288. [CrossRef]
65. Ruget, H.; Blouin, J.; Teasdale, N.; Mouchnino, L. Can Prepared Anticipatory Postural Adjustments Be Updated by Proprioception? *Neuroscience* **2008**, *155*, 640–648. [CrossRef]
66. Lhomond, O.; Teasdale, N.; Simoneau, M.; Mouchnino, L. Supplementary Motor Area and Superior Parietal Lobule Restore Sensory Facilitation Prior to Stepping When a Decrease of Afferent Inputs Occurs. *Front. Neurol.* **2018**, *9*, 1132. [CrossRef]
67. Picard, N.; Strick, P.L. Imaging the Premotor Areas. *Curr. Opin. Neurobiol.* **2001**, *11*, 663–672. [CrossRef]
68. Tard, C.; Delval, A.; Devos, D.; Lopes, R.; Lenfant, P.; Dujardin, K.; Hossein-Foucher, C.; Semah, F.; Duhamel, A.; Defebvre, L.; et al. Brain Metabolic Abnormalities during Gait with Freezing in Parkinson's Disease. *Neuroscience* **2015**, *307*, 281–301. [CrossRef]
69. Wolbers, T.; Hegarty, M.; Büchel, C.; Loomis, J.M. Spatial Updating: How the Brain Keeps Track of Changing Object Locations during Observer Motion. *Nat. Neurosci.* **2008**, *11*, 1223–1230. [CrossRef]
70. Hanakawa, T.; Fukuyama, H.; Katsumi, Y.; Honda, M.; Shibasaki, H. Enhanced Lateral Premotor Activity during Paradoxical Gait in Parkinson's Disease. *Ann. Neurol.* **1999**, *45*, 329–336. [CrossRef]
71. Voss, M.; Ingram, J.N.; Haggard, P.; Wolpert, D.M. Sensorimotor Attenuation by Central Motor Command Signals in the Absence of Movement. *Nat. Neurosci.* **2006**, *9*, 26–27. [CrossRef]
72. Jacobs, J.V.; Horak, F.B. External Postural Perturbations Induce Multiple Anticipatory Postural Adjustments When Subjects Cannot Pre-Select Their Stepping Foot. *Exp. brain Res.* **2007**, *179*, 29–42. [CrossRef]
73. Amboni, M.; Cozzolino, A.; Longo, K.; Picillo, M.; Barone, P. Freezing of Gait and Executive Functions in Patients with Parkinson's Disease. *Mov. Disord.* **2008**, *23*, 395–400. [CrossRef]
74. Naismith, S.L.; Shine, J.M.; Lewis, S.J.G. The Specific Contributions of Set-Shifting to Freezing of Gait in Parkinson's Disease. *Mov. Disord.* **2010**, *25*, 1000–1004. [CrossRef]
75. Heremans, E.; Nieuwboer, A.; Vercruysse, S. Freezing of Gait in Parkinson's Disease: Where Are We Now? Topical Collection on Movement Disorders. *Curr. Neurol. Neurosci. Rep.* **2013**, *13*, 350. [CrossRef]
76. Cohen, R.G.; Klein, K.A.; Nomura, M.; Fleming, M.; Mancini, M.; Giladi, N.; Nutt, J.G.; Horak, F.B. Inhibition, Executive Function, and Freezing of Gait. *J. Parkinsons. Dis.* **2014**, *4*, 111–122. [CrossRef]
77. Lira, J.L.O.; Ugrinowitsch, C.; Coelho, D.B.; Teixeira, L.A.; de Lima-Pardini, A.C.; Magalhães, F.H.; Barbosa, E.R.; Horak, F.B.; Silva-Batista, C. Loss of Presynaptic Inhibition for Step Initiation in Parkinsonian Individuals with Freezing of Gait. *J. Physiol.* **2020**, *598*, 1611–1624. [CrossRef]
78. Drucker, J.H.; Sathian, K.; Crosson, B.; Krishnamurthy, V.; McGregor, K.M.; Bozzorg, A.; Gopinath, K.; Krishnamurthy, L.C.; Wolf, S.L.; Hart, A.R.; et al. Internally Guided Lower Limb Movement Recruits Compensatory Cerebellar Activity in People with Parkinson's Disease. *Front. Neurol.* **2019**, *10*, 573. [CrossRef]
79. Avanzino, L.; Pelosin, E.; Vicario, C.M.; Lagravinese, G.; Abbruzzese, G.; Martino, D. Time Processing and Motor Control in Movement Disorders. *Front. Hum. Neurosci.* **2016**, *10*, 631. [CrossRef]
80. Isaias, I.U.; Brumberg, J.; Pozzi, N.G.; Palmisano, C.; Canessa, A.; Marotta, G.; Volkmann, J.; Pezzoli, G. Brain Metabolic Alterations Herald Falls in Patients with Parkinson's Disease. *Ann. Clin. Transl. Neurol.* **2020**, *7*, 579–583. [CrossRef]
81. Lipski, W.J.; Wozny, T.A.; Alhourani, A.; Kondylis, E.D.; Turner, R.S.; Crammond, D.J.; Richardson, R.M. Dynamics of Human Subthalamic Neuron Phase-Locking to Motor and Sensory Cortical Oscillations during Movement. *J. Neurophysiol.* **2017**, *118*, 1472–1487. [CrossRef]
82. Arnulfo, G.; Pozzi, N.G.; Palmisano, C.; Leporini, A.; Canessa, A.; Brumberg, J.; Pezzoli, G.; Matthies, C.; Volkmann, J.; Isaias, I.U. Phase Matters: A Role for the Subthalamic Network during Gait. *PLoS ONE* **2018**, *13*, e0198691. [CrossRef]
83. Georgiades, M.J.; Shine, J.M.; Gilat, M.; McMaster, J.; Owler, B.; Mahant, N.; Lewis, S.J.G. Hitting the Brakes: Pathological Subthalamic Nucleus Activity in Parkinson's Disease Gait Freezing. *Brain* **2019**, *142*, 3906–3916. [CrossRef]
84. Pozzi, N.G.; Canessa, A.; Palmisano, C.; Brumberg, J.; Steigerwald, F.; Reich, M.M.; Minafra, B.; Pacchetti, C.; Pezzoli, G.; Volkmann, J.; et al. Freezing of Gait in Parkinson's Disease Reflects a Sudden Derangement of Locomotor Network Dynamics. *Brain* **2019**, *142*, 2037–2050. [CrossRef]

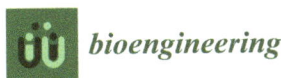

Article

The Influence of a Shoe's Heel-Toe Drop on Gait Parameters during the Third Trimester of Pregnancy

Xin Li [1], Zhenghui Lu [1], Dong Sun [1], Rongrong Xuan [2], Zhiyi Zheng [3],* and Yaodong Gu [1],*

[1] Faculty of Sports Science, Ningbo University, Ningbo 315211, China; 2011042028@nbu.edu.cn (X.L.); 2011042030@nbu.edu.cn (Z.L.); sundong@nbu.edu.cn (D.S.)
[2] The Affiliated Hospital of Medical School, Ningbo University, Ningbo 315211, China; fyxuanrongrong@nbu.edu.cn
[3] ANTA Sports Science Laboratory, ANTA (China) Co., Ltd., Xiamen 361008, China
* Correspondence: zhengzhiyi@anta.com (Z.Z.); guyaodong@nbu.edu.cn (Y.G.)

Abstract: Background: Changes in physical shape and body mass during pregnancy may increase the risk of walking falls. Shoes can protect and enhance the inherent function of the foot, helping to maintain dynamic and static stability. Methods: Sixteen women during the third trimester of pregnancy participated in this study to investigate the effect of negative heel shoes (NHS), positive heel shoes (PHS), and normal shoes (NS) on spatiotemporal parameters, ground reaction force (GRF), and stability. Differences in spatiotemporal parameter, GRF, and center of pressure (COP) between footwear conditions were examined using Statistical Parametric Mapping (SPM) and repeated measures analyses of variance (ANOVA). Results: The walking speed and step length increased with the increase in heel-toe drop. The anterior-posterior (AP)-COP in NHS decreased significantly ($p < 0.001$). When wearing NHS, peak posterior angles were significantly lower than NS and PHS ($p < 0.05$). Conclusions: The results show that changing the heel-toe drop can significantly affect the gait pattern of pregnant women. Understanding the gait patterns of pregnant women wearing shoes with different heel-toe drops is very important for reducing the risk of injury and equipment design.

Keywords: negative heel shoes; positive heel shoes; gait; pregnant women; OpenSim; IDEEA

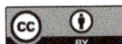

1. Introduction

Pregnancy induces tremendous changes in the body to accommodate a growing fetus [1]. During pregnancy, hormonal, anatomical, and physiological changes occur in the female body. These changes due to pregnancy include mass redistribution, an anterior shift in the center of gravity location, and increased joint and ligament flexibility [2–6]. These changes during pregnancy can cause physical pain and an increased risk of falls, especially in the third trimester [4,7]. During pregnancy, nearly a quarter of employed women sustain a fall [8]. This fall may result in musculoskeletal injury and maternal or fetal death [9–11].

Walking is the most commonly chosen type of physical activity during pregnancy [12]. The gait parameters, balance, and center of mass of pregnant women changes during walking and leads to a higher risk of falling [1,6,13,14]. The rate of falls during pregnancy is similar to that of women over 65 [6,8]. A decreased step length and cadence, increased base of support, and longer double support time are seen with the progression of pregnancy [15,16]; these changes provide a safer and more exploratory way for pregnant women to walk. However, results point toward excessive deviations from the optimal habitual spatiotemporal gait pattern as a pivotal factor that may contribute to falls in pregnant women [16]. Mei et al. studied pregnant women's gait biomechanics, which revealed lower limb kinematic and foot pressure alterations, and found that mean pressure in the forefoot increased. The center of pressure (COP) trajectory highlights a fall risk, particularly in the third trimester [4]. To improve their walking stability, pregnant women often use specially designed products, such as daily wearing shoes.

Shoes can protect and enhance the inherent function of the foot, helping to maintain dynamic and static stability [17,18]. Many previous studies have focused on changing the shape and materials of a shoe sole to reduce pregnant women's foot discomfort [19,20]. Jang et al. designed balanced incline shoes [21] and reported that the balanced incline shoes corrected the postures and stabilized the gait pattern.

Research about the effects of different heel-toe drop shoes on pregnant gait parameters is lacking. Heel-toe drop is the height difference between the heel and the forefoot of the shoe [22]. In positive heel shoes (PHS; Table 1 includes a description of abbreviations and acronyms used), the heel is higher than the toe part. In contrast, in the negative heel shoe (NHS), the toe part is higher than the heel [23]. Advocates of shoes with negative inclination believe that negative heel inclination decreases lumbar lordosis, causing the center of gravity to shift backwards [24,25]. As a result, back and hip pain can noticeably be reduced [19]. However, the American College of Obstetricians and Gynecologists (ACOG) recommends wearing positive heel shoes (PHS) to relieve back pain during pregnancy [26]. However, few studies have investigated the effect of different heel-toe drops on spatiotemporal parameters, ground reaction force (GRF), and the dynamic balance in the third trimester of pregnancy. It is necessary to know the effects of the different heel-toe drops to design maternity shoes and keep pregnant women healthy.

Table 1. List of abbreviations and acronyms used in this article.

Abbreviation	Explanation
PHS	Positive Heel Shoes
NHS	Negative Heel Shoes
NS	Normal Shoes
SPM	Statistical Parametric Mapping
ANOVA	Analyses of Variance
ACOG	American College of Obstetricians and Gynecologists
GRF	Ground Reaction Force
COP	Center of Pressure
AP	Anterior-Posterior
ML	Medial-Lateral

This study aimed to use a musculoskeletal simulation and Statistical Parametric Mapping (SPM)-based approach to investigate the effect of different heel-toe drops (negative 1.5 cm, 0 cm, positive 1.5 cm) on the spatiotemporal parameter, GRF, and dynamic balance during the third trimester of pregnancy. The results can provide a theoretical basis and ideas for the design of shoes for pregnant women in the third trimester.

2. Materials and Methods

2.1. Participants

Sixteen healthy third-trimester primigravid pregnant women (age: 28.4 ± 2.30 years and height: 1.63 ± 0.04 m and trimester: 33.43 ± 3.37 w) participated in the study. Exclusion criteria included the following medical conditions: lupus, rheumatoid arthritis, gestational diabetes mellitus, hypertension, musculoskeletal or neurologic abnormalities, and any other conditions affecting postural stability [5]. All participants understood the purpose and significance of the research and signed an informed consent form. This study with detailed guidelines for participants' safety and experiment protocols was approved by the Human Ethics Committee of Ningbo University.

2.2. Shoe Conditions

All participants conducted this study in shoes with a NHS, normal shoes (NS), and PHS (Figure 1b). The NS were commercially available walking shoes. The NHS and the PHS were self-fabricated based on the NS in our laboratory. For the three conditions, the shoes were identical models and designs in the upper and outsole.

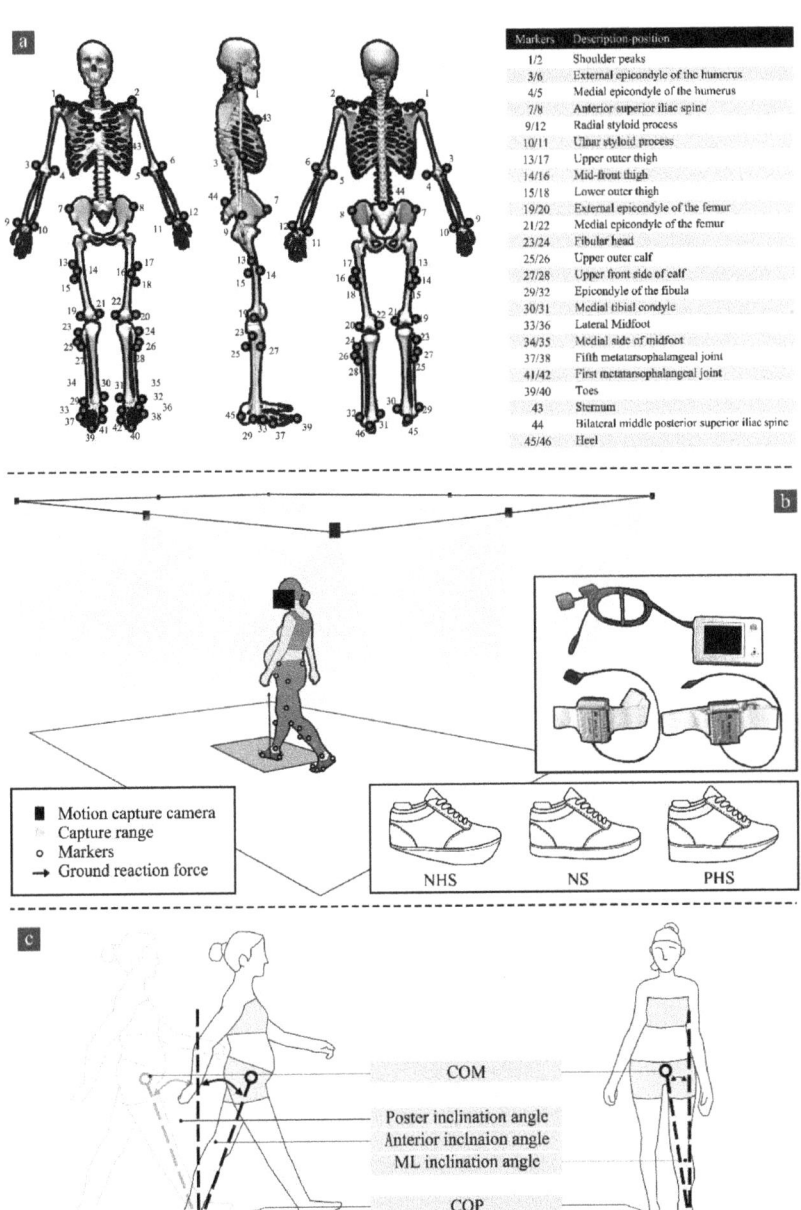

Figure 1. (a) Marking point paste location. (b) Experimental process, IDEEA position, and shoe conditions between NHS (negative 1.5 cm drop), NS (no drop), and PHS (1.5 cm drop). (c) Diagrammatic illustration of COM-COP inclination angles.

2.3. Testing Procedure

All participants walked with IDEEA (IDEEA, MiniSun, Fresno, CA, USA) on a 6.5 m walkway at their self-selected comfortable speed to present normal gait characters, striking their right foot on the force plate. Sensors were connected to a 32 Hz main recorder.

Previous studies have shown the reliability of IDEEA in measuring gait parameters [27–29]. Each footwear condition was collected with three successful trials for analysis. At the same time, an eight-camera Vicon motion capture system (Vicon Metrics Ltd., Oxford, UK) was used to capture the motion trajectory. The embedded AMTI force plates (AMTI, Watertown, MA, USA) recorded the GRF synchronously, with 200 Hz and 1000 Hz, respectively, as shown in Figure 1b. The camera system was calibrated to residual errors of 2.5 mm over a recording volume of approximately 6.5 m × 1.5 m × 1.80 m (L × W × H). The force plate was embedded in the middle of a 6.5-m walkway and covered with floor tiles to minimize participants' awareness of its presence. The original gait-2392 model in OpenSim was used for this study, with 23 degrees of freedom and 92 muscles (Figure 1a) [30].

2.4. Data Processing

Gait analyses were performed using a wearable intelligent analyzer (IDEEA, MiniSun, Fresno, CA, USA) equipped with accelerometers and gyroscopes, as shown in Figure 1b. The wearable intelligent analyzer consists of the main recorder and two secondary recorders. The gait data were collected and transmitted to the main recorder by the sensor affixed to the subject; each accelerometer used a proprietary algorithm [31]. The IDEEA was easy to wear and had almost no interference with normal walking. After the data acquisition was completed, the data were saved in the main recorder and downloaded to the computer. IDEEA Version 3.01 (IDEEA3, MiniSun, Fresno, CA, USA) was used for analysis [27]. The software equipped with the equipment can intercept the range of gait data needed and process it, and directly output walking speed, step frequency, stride length, and support time.

According to Winter's [32] description of the selected frequency for filtering biomechanical signals, the residual data analysis was carried out in subsets to determine the most appropriate signal-to-noise ratio. Marker trajectories and ground reaction forces were filtered by a zero-delay fourth-order Butterworth low-pass filter at 12 Hz and 30 Hz. A threshold of 20 N on the vertical GRF was applied to identify the initial foot contact and toe-off [33]. The magnitudes of each GRF component were normalized to the percentage of the participant's body weight, and the stance phase of each participant was normalized to 100% of their stance phase's duration [34]. The musculoskeletal model used was the generic OpenSim model Gait 2392 (Figure 1a), which has 23 degrees of freedom and 92 muscles [30] and calculates the center of mass (COM) in OpenSim.

2.5. Outcome Measures

The parameters evaluated in the study were: (1) Walking speed (m/s): the distance walked along the walkway per second. (2) Step frequency (steps/min): the number of steps per minute. (3) Stride length (m): the distance from one heel to the same heel touching the ground again during walking. (4) Double support time/single support time (%): double support time refers to the time taken by the use of biped support in a gait cycle, and single support time refers to the time spent using single foot support in a gait cycle. Double support time/single support time reflects the stability of the participants when walking, where the lower the ratio, the better the stability of the participants [27]. (5) Three-dimensional ground reaction forces (3D-GRF): GRF supports the body against gravity and accelerates the center of mass during walking. GRF is included in the vertical, anterior–posterior, and medial–lateral directions recorded from a three-dimensional force plate [35,36]. (6) The range of COP motion, including the medial–lateral range of the COP (ML-COP) and anterior–posterior range of the COP (AP-COP), were derived and averaged for all participants. (7) Center of mass (COM) and center of pressure (COP) inclination angles: we defined COM-COP inclination angles as the angle formed by the intersection of the line connecting the COP and COM with a vertical line through the COP [37], as shown in Figure 1c.

2.6. Data Analysis

Statistical analyses were performed using SPSS 16.0 (SPSS, Chicago, IL, USA) statistical analysis software. One-way repeated-measures analysis of variance (ANOVA) was performed to analyze the effects of different conditions on spatiotemporal parameters and peak COM-COP inclination angles. In the event of a significant main effect, post-hoc pairwise comparisons were conducted on all significant main effects, using a Bonferroni adjustment. Statistical parametric mapping based on the SPM1D package for Matlab (Mathworks, Natick, MA, USA) was used to compare the 3D GRF and COP statistically. In agreement with Patakt et al., SPM was implemented hierarchically, analogous to one-way repeated measures ANOVA (SPM F) with a post-hoc paired t-test [38]. The conditions NS vs. NHS, NS vs. PHS, and PHS vs. NHS were chosen to compare the 3D-GRF and COP waveforms [39,40]. The significance level was set at 0.05.

3. Results

3.1. Gait Spatiotemporal Parameters

Significant main effects were found for stride length and walking speed (Table 2). Post-hoc tests revealed significantly higher stride length for PHS compared with NHS. Furthermore, post-hoc tests revealed significantly lower walking speed for NHS when compared with NS and PHS. No significant differences were found in step frequency and double support time/single support time.

Table 2. Mean values, standard deviations, and results of the repeated measures ANOVA for spatiotemporal parameters.

Indexes (Unit)	NHS (Mean ± SD)	NS (Mean ± SD)	PHS (Mean ± SD)	F	p
Stride length (m)	0.99 ± 0.08 c	1.05 ± 0.07	1.11 ± 0.03 a	10.24	<0.001
Walking speed (m/s)	0.76 ± 0.11 bc	0.83 ± 0.16 a	0.90 ± 0.08 b	5.97	<0.001
Step frequency (step/s)	1.48 ± 0.13	1.56 ± 0.21	1.56 ± 0.14	1.51	0.25
Double support time/single support time (%)	0.32 ± 0.01	0.32 ± 0.02	0.31 ± 0.01	2.02	0.16

Note: NHS: negative heel shoes, NH: normal shoes, PHS: positive heel shoes. Post-hoc significant differences are marked with a (vs. NHS), b (vs. NS), c (vs. PHS).

3.2. GRF

SPM analysis with repeated measures ANOVA revealed a significant difference between shoe conditions in GRF (Figure 2). Post-hoc analysis shows the NHS's AP-GRF was smaller than NS at 77.1–90.3% and 94.6–100% of the stance phase ($p < 0.001$). The AP-GRF of NHS was smaller than PHS and was significant at 25–33.3%, 82.0–90.3%, and 94.6–100% of the stance phase ($p < 0.001$).

The post-hoc analysis results showed that the ML-GRF of NS was significantly larger than PNS during the stance phase (14.5–17.7%; 71.9–82.6%) ($p < 0.001$). At the 1.3–9.4% stance phases, the ML-GRF of NS was significantly more significant than the NHS ($p < 0.001$). At 1.3–4.6% and 8.8–10.3% of the stance phase, the ML-GRF PHS was significantly greater than NHS ($p < 0.05$).

The post-hoc analysis results showed that the vertical GRF of NHS in the third trimester of pregnancy was significantly larger than NS during the gait stance phase (91.8–100%) ($p < 0.001$). At 66.3–72.4% of the stance phase, PHS was significantly lower than the NS ($p < 0.001$). The vertical GRF of NHS was larger than that of PHS during 40–44%, 61–71.5%, and 92.5–100% of the stance phase ($p < 0.001$).

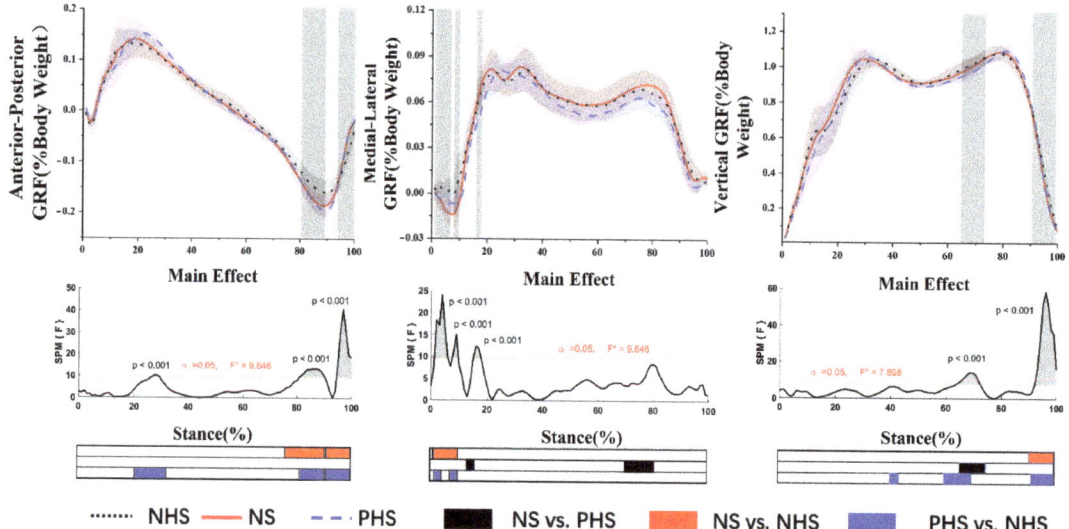

Figure 2. Ground reaction forces in anterior–posterior, medial–lateral and vertical directions (mean and SD) between NHS, NS, and PHS. The grey areas indicate significant differences between conditions, followed by the time-dependent F-values of the SPM. Colored bars beneath each plot indicate significant differences between waveforms, whereas the red, blue, and black bars represent significant differences for NS vs. NHS, NHS vs. PHS, and NS vs. PHS, respectively.

3.3. COP Trajectory

As shown in Figure 3, the results showed no difference in ML-COP between NHS, NS, and PHS. For AP-COP, there was a main effect. Post-hoc analysis showed that NHS demonstrated a significantly smaller range of AP-COP in NHS vs. NS for 19–90.5% and 93–100% of the stance phase. At 14.5–53.1%, 68.5–90% and 93.5–100% of the stance phase, the NHS posterior COP was significantly smaller than PHS ($p < 0.05$).

3.4. COM-COP Inclination Angles

No significant differences were found in step peak medial angles and peak anterior angles. Significant main effects were found for peak posterior angles (Table 3). Post-hoc tests revealed significantly lower peak posterior angles for NHS compared with NS and PHS.

Table 3. Mean values, standard deviations, and results of the repeated measures ANOVA for peak COM-COP inclination angle.

Indexes (Unit)	NHS (Mean ± SD)	NS (Mean ± SD)	PHS (Mean ± SD)	F	p
Peak medial angles (°)	3.28 ± 0.91	3.38 ± 0.70	3.14 ± 0.48	0.35	0.71
Peak anterior angles (°)	16.00 ± 1.79	15.90 ± 3.31	17.00 ± 1.61	1.22	0.30
Peak posterior angles (°)	12.82 ± 2.61 bc	15.22 ± 2.18 a	14.53 ± 1.72 a	16.52	<0.01

Note: NHS: negative heel shoes, NH: normal shoes, PHS: positive heel shoes. Post-hoc significant differences are marked with a (vs. NHS), b (vs. NS), and c (vs. PHS).

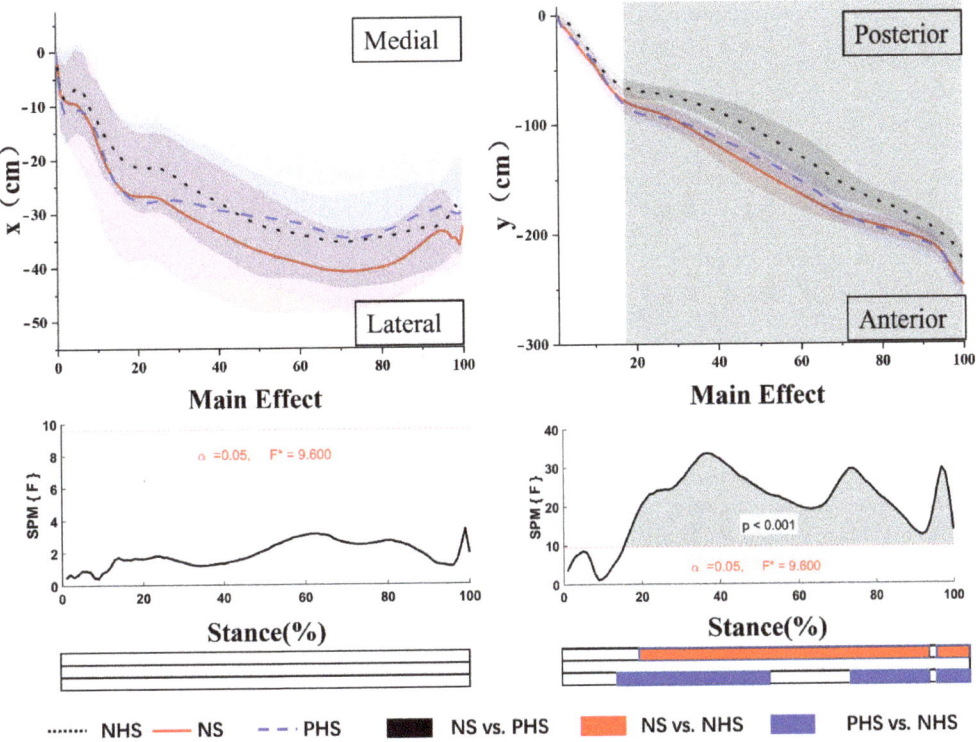

Figure 3. Mean cop trajectories in the x-time and y-time planes. The grey areas indicate significant differences between conditions, followed by the time-dependent F-values of the SPM. Colored bars beneath each plot indicate significant differences between waveforms, whereas the red, blue, and black bars represent significant differences for NS vs. NHS, NHS vs. PHS, and NS vs. PHS, respectively.

4. Discussion

The primary purpose of this study was to investigate the differences in gait spatiotemporal parameters, 3D-GRF, and COP of the condition of NHS, NS, and PHS in the third trimester of pregnancy. Compared with PHS and NS, pregnant women wearing NHS showed a more stable gait posture in the anterior–posterior direction, with slower walking speed and smaller peak posterior COM-COP inclination angles.

4.1. Gait Spatiotemporal Parameters

Gait parameters changed with different heel heights of shoes [41]. Although studies have shown that 2/3 of falls during pregnancy occur due to smooth surfaces, sudden acceleration, or moving objects [6,8], gait changes caused by pregnancy are still one of the critical causes of falls in pregnant women [16]. Therefore, it is necessary to understand the influence of shoes with different heels on the gait spatiotemporal parameters of pregnant women in the third trimester.

This study found that participants wearing NHS showed decreased stride length and speed compared to PHS. Similar to our results, Benz (1998) reported that the NHS's walking speed was significantly reduced due to a shorter stride length combined with an increased cadence [42]. Li et al. reported that walking with NHSs induced the upper body to tilt backward, which may have caused a disadvantage in the propulsion phase compared to walking with normal shoes [41]. This may be the reason for the decrease in stride length. PHS moved the center of gravity forward, and the forward tilt of the trunk assisted in moving the center of gravity outside the support area. There is more motivation during the duration of take-off [43,44], which may be the reason for the difference in stride length between NHS and PHS. Previous studies found that the habitual gait in the third trimester of pregnancy is characterized by slower speed and shorter step length, which may be caused by slow gait strategies [16]. Taking a shorter step during pregnancy reduced the gait's energy consumption and increased the gait's stability [16]. This change in stride length and speed may lead to changes in other gait parameters and may help increase gait stability in pregnant women. On the other hand, the decreased stride length may be due to unfamiliarity with NHS, which leads to anxiety about falls and a more conservative or unstable gait [16,45–47].

4.2. GRF

Ground reaction force (GRF), which can measure braking and propulsive forces during gait, is a summation of forces produced by all body segments [48]. Increases in magnitude and variability of the peaks of GRF during the weight acceptance and push-off phases are to be found in people with unstable locomotion [48]. Our result found that different heel-toe drops have no significant effect on the first and second peaks of vertical GRF. Therefore, it is reasonable to speculate that wearing NHS, NS, and PHS has little effect on the walking stability of pregnant women in the third trimester.

The results showed no significant change in the ML-GRF during the stance phase, except in the early stance phase, the ML-GRF of NHS was significantly smaller than PHS and NS. Previous studies have shown that in the early stages of the stance phase (0–6% stance phase), the maximum ground reaction of the supporting foot is directed laterally and increases significantly with increasing walking speed [49]. This is similar to the results of our research. Our research results show that with the increase in heel-toe drop, the velocity also increases, which may be the reason for the difference in ML-GRF. Less energy is expended when the body is stable on the inside. Therefore, NHS has a smaller ML-GRF, which may be evidence of reduced energy consumption in pregnant women wearing NHS.

The AP-GRF included braking and propulsion peaks [50]. Our study found that the AP-GRF of the NHS propulsion peak was significantly smaller than NS and PHS. At present, there is controversy about the change in AP-GRF during pregnancy. Some researchers believe that there is no significant difference in AP-GRF during pregnancy, and other studies have shown that the AP-GRF decreases during pregnancy [51]. This may be due to edema of the pregnant foot during pregnancy, which interferes with flexion by increasing the width of the foot, resulting in reduced thrust. Our study found that it may be due to the thickness of the front palm of the NHS, which leads to disturbance of the flexion of the metatarsophalangeal joints, which may be the reason for the small AP-GRF during the propulsion phase.

4.3. COP Trajectory

COP is used to describe the complex dynamic functions of the foot and foot-ground interface during gait [52]. The COP is not only used as a dynamic stability index and measured risk or consequence of various lower limb musculoskeletal disorders [52–55]. The lack of lateral stability is known to be a risk factor for falls [52,55]. The results showed no significant difference in the range of ML-COP in NHS, NS, and PHS, which is consistent with the previous study [56]. No significant differences in the range and velocity of ML-COP were found in the flat shoes, medium heel lift shoes (16 mm), heel lift shoes (25 mm), and heel lift shoes (34 mm) [56]. NHS and PHS may not pose a more significant biomechanical challenge to the medial–lateral control.

The AP-COP displacement measures the fluency of the stance phase during regular gait, with higher AP-COP displacement and gait line length indicating a more physiological gait pattern [57,58]. The results showed that the AP-COP of NHS is significantly smaller than NS and PHS. Previous studies have shown that AP-COP moves forward and decreases during the stance phase in pregnant women [13,14]. Reduced COP displacement in the AP direction could be linked to the waddling type of gait adopted by pregnant women [13]. Raymaks et al. found that the AP-COP increases with the increase in heel height, the AP-COP of NS is significantly smaller than that of PHS, and leg muscle activation increases when walking in high heels [59]. The results of our study may indicate that women in the third trimester of pregnancy have the lowest degree of muscle activation when walking with NHS.

4.4. COM-COP Inclination Angles

The medial COM-COP inclination angle may be a sensitive measure of gait stability [37]. Our study found that the ML-ROM and the peak medial COM-COP inclination angles were not significantly different under different conditions, and we inferred that changing heel-toe drop within a certain range does not change the ML stability of pregnant women in the third trimester of pregnancy. Our findings indicate that heel-toe drop affects the peak posterior COM-COP inclination angle in pregnant women in the third trimester and that NHS is significantly smaller in the peak posterior COM-COP inclination angle than NS., which may benefit the stability during the propulsion phase. Previous studies on NHS showed that foot contact angle and the angle of the ankle NHS are significantly larger than those of NS. This may indicate that wearing NHS may benefit stability in the front and rear directions. Of course, this change may be related to the slower walking speed of NHS, which has been shown to affect gait changes and COM movement [60–62].

4.5. Limitations

There are still some limitations. The acute effect of the footwear conditions was investigated, and no conclusions can be drawn for longer-term or habituation effects. We only investigated the impact of three different heel-toe drops on gait parameters. The study sample will be expanded in the future, and electromyography (EMG) data will be included to infer further what mechanisms are involved in the generation and change of force. Future studies should explore the effects of long-term different heel-toe drops on gait in pregnant women in different periods and the longer-term effects.

5. Conclusions

This study compared the gait spatiotemporal parameters, GRF, and balance of pregnant women wearing different heel-toe drop shoes in the third trimester of pregnancy. The results are as follows: (1) NHS reduced the walking speed of women in the third trimester of pregnancy by reducing the stride. (2) The results showed that the impact of a heel-toe drop on the AP-GRF during the propulsion phase was relatively large, which might be due to the various dorsiflexion of the ankle with different heel-toe drop conditions. We inferred that changing heel-toe drop within a certain range does not change the ML stability of pregnant women in the third trimester of pregnancy. (3) We found that peak posterior COM-COP inclination angles are significantly smaller, so NHS may increase the stability of the pregnant women's propulsion phase and help women maintain balance in the third trimester of pregnancy. Understanding the gait differences in NHS, NS, and PHS of pregnant women in the third trimester will provide information for future research, evidence for the design of shoes for pregnant women, and falls prevention.

Author Contributions: Conceptualization, X.L. and Z.L.; methodology, R.X. and Y.G.; software, X.L. and Z.L.; validation; formal analysis, X.L. and D.S.; data curation, D.S. and Z.Z.; writing original draft preparation, X.L.; writing—review and editing, Z.L. and Z.Z. supervision; R.X. and Z.Z.; project administration, Y.G. All authors have read and agreed to the published version of the manuscript.

Funding: This research was funded by the Key R&D Program of Zhejiang Province China (2021C03130), Zhejiang Province Science Fund for Distinguished Young Scholars (LR22A020002), Philosophy and Social Sciences Project of Zhejiang Province, China (22QNYC10ZD, 22NDQN223YB), Zhejiang Province Medical and Health Science and Technology Plan Project (2018KY710), Educational science planning project of Zhejiang Province (2021SCG083), Ningbo Public Welfare Science and Technology Plan Project (2019C50095), Public Welfare Science and Technology Project of Ningbo, China (2021S134),

Basic scientific research Funds of provincial Ningbo University (SJWY2022014) and K.C. Wong Magna Fund in Ningbo University.

Institutional Review Board Statement: The study was conducted according to the guidelines of the Declaration of Helsinki and approved by the Committee of Ningbo University (code RAGH20211106).

Informed Consent Statement: Written informed consent has been obtained from the participants to publish this paper.

Data Availability Statement: The data that support the findings of this study are available on reasonable request from the corresponding author. The data is not publicly available due to privacy or ethical restrictions.

Conflicts of Interest: The authors declare no conflict of interest.

References

1. Haddox, A.; Hausselle, J.; Azoug, A. Changes in segmental mass and inertia during pregnancy: A musculoskeletal model of the pregnant woman. *Gait Posture* **2020**, *76*, 389–395. [CrossRef] [PubMed]
2. Ren, S.; Gao, Y.; Yang, Z.; Li, J.; Xuan, R.; Liu, J.; Chen, X.; Thirupathi, A. The effect of pelvic floor muscle training on pelvic floor dysfunction in pregnant and postpartum women. *Phys. Act. Health* **2020**, *4*, 130–141. [CrossRef]
3. Gu, Y.D.; Li, J.S.; Lake, M.J.; Zeng, Y.J.; Ren, X.J.; Li, Z.Y. Image-based midsole insert design and the material effects on heel plantar pressure distribution during simulated walking loads. *Comput. Methods Biomech. Biomed. Engin.* **2011**, *14*, 747–753. [CrossRef] [PubMed]
4. Mei, Q.; Gu, Y.; Fernandez, J. Alterations of pregnant gait during pregnancy and post-partum. *Sci. Rep.* **2018**, *8*, 1–7.
5. Butler, E.E.; Colón, I.; Druzin, M.L.; Rose, J. Postural equilibrium during pregnancy: Decreased stability with an increased reliance on visual cues. *Am. J. Obstet. Gynecol.* **2006**, *195*, 1104–1108. [CrossRef]
6. Inanir, A.; Cakmak, B.; Hisim, Y.; Demirturk, F. Evaluation of postural equilibrium and fall risk during pregnancy. *Gait Posture* **2014**, *39*, 1122–1125. [CrossRef]
7. Kesikburun, S.; Güzelküçük, Ü.; Fidan, U.; Demir, Y.; Ergün, A.; Tan, A.K. Musculoskeletal pain and symptoms in pregnancy: A descriptive study. *Ther. Adv. Musculoskelet. Dis.* **2018**, *10*, 229–234. [CrossRef]
8. Dunning, K.; LeMasters, G.; Levin, L.; Bhattacharya, A.; Alterman, T.; Lordo, K. Falls in workers during pregnancy: Risk factors, job hazards, and high risk occupations. *Am. J. Ind. Med.* **2003**, *44*, 664–672. [CrossRef]
9. Dyer, I.; Barclay, D.L. Accidental trauma complicating pregnancy and delivery. *Am. J. Obstet. Gynecol.* **1962**, *83*, 907–929. [CrossRef]
10. Crosby, W.M. Traumatic injuries during pregnancy. *Clin. Obstet. Gynecol.* **1983**, *26*, 902–912. [CrossRef]
11. Fildes, J.; Reed, L.; Jones, N.; Martin, M.; Barrett, J. Trauma: The leading cause of maternal death. *J. Trauma* **1992**, *32*, 643–645. [CrossRef] [PubMed]
12. Connolly, C.P.; Conger, S.A.; Montoye, A.H.; Marshall, M.R.; Schlaff, R.A.; Badon, S.E.; Pivarnik, J.M. Walking for health during pregnancy: A literature review and considerations for future research. *J. Sport Health Sci.* **2019**, *8*, 401–411. [CrossRef]
13. Bertuit, J.; Leyh, C.; Rooze, M.; Feipel, F. Pregnancy-related changes in centre of pressure during gait. *Acta Bioeng. Biomech.* **2017**, *19*, 95–102.
14. Lymbery, J.K.; Gilleard, W. The stance phase of walking during late pregnancy: Temporospatial and ground reaction force variables. *J. Am. Podiatr. Med. Assoc.* **2005**, *95*, 247–253. [CrossRef]
15. Forczek, W.; Staszkiewicz, R. Changes of kinematic gait parameters due to pregnancy. *Acta Bioeng. Biomech.* **2012**, *14*, 113–119. [PubMed]
16. Błaszczyk, J.W.; Opala-Berdzik, A.; Plewa, M. Adaptive changes in spatiotemporal gait characteristics in women during pregnancy. *Gait Posture* **2016**, *43*, 160–164. [CrossRef] [PubMed]
17. Shi, Z.; Sun, D. Conflict between Weightlifting and Health? The Importance of Injury Prevention and Technology Assistance. *Phys. Act. Health* **2022**, *6*, 1–4. [CrossRef]
18. Nigg, B.; Hintzen, S.; Ferber, R. Effect of an unstable shoe construction on lower extremity gait characteristics. *Clin. Biomech.* **2006**, *21*, 82–88. [CrossRef]
19. Dimou, E.; Manavis, A.; Papachristou, E.; Kyratsis, P. A conceptual design of intelligent shoes for pregnant women. In Proceedings of the Workshop on Business Models and ICT Technologies for the Fashion Supply Chain, Florence, Italy, 20–22 April 2016; pp. 69–77.
20. Gimunová, M.; Zvonař, M.; Sebera, M.; Turčínek, P.; Kolářová, K. Special footwear designed for pregnant women and its effect on kinematic gait parameters during pregnancy and postpartum period. *PLoS ONE* **2020**, *15*, e0232901. [CrossRef]
21. Jang, S.I.; Lee, Y.R.; Kwak, H.S.; Moon, K.S.; Shin, J.-C.; Kim, J.-H. The effect of balanced incline shoes on walking and feet for the pregnant women. *Korean J. Obstet. Gynecol.* **2010**, *53*, 988–997. [CrossRef]
22. Mo, S.; Lam, W.-K.; Ching, E.C.; Chan, Z.Y.; Zhang, J.H.; Cheung, R.T. Effects of heel-toe drop on running biomechanics and perceived comfort of rearfoot strikers in standard cushioned running shoes. *Footwear Sci.* **2020**, *12*, 91–99. [CrossRef]

23. Li, J.X.; Hong, Y. Kinematic and electromyographic analysis of the trunk and lower limbs during walking in negative-heeled shoes. *J. Am. Podiatr. Med. Assoc.* **2007**, *97*, 447–456. [CrossRef] [PubMed]
24. Baaklini, E.; Angst, M.; Schellenberg, F.; Hitz, M.; Schmid, S.; Tal, A.; Taylor, W.R.; Lorenzetti, S. High-heeled walking decreases lumbar lordosis. *Gait Posture* **2017**, *55*, 12–14. [CrossRef] [PubMed]
25. Russell, B.S. The effect of high-heeled shoes on lumbar lordosis: A narrative review and discussion of the disconnect between Internet content and peer-reviewed literature. *J. Chiropr. Med.* **2010**, *9*, 166–173. [CrossRef] [PubMed]
26. Ferguson, B. ACSM's guidelines for exercise testing and prescription 9th Ed. 2014. *J. Can. Chiropr. Assoc.* **2014**, *58*, 328.
27. Lu, Z.; Sun, D.; Xu, D.; Li, X.; Baker, J.S.; Gu, Y. Gait Characteristics and Fatigue Profiles When Standing on Surfaces with Different Hardness: Gait Analysis and Machine Learning Algorithms. *Biology* **2021**, *10*, 1083. [CrossRef]
28. Sun, J.; Liu, Y.; Yan, S.; Wang, S.; Lester, D.K.; Zeng, J.; Miao, J.; Zhang, K. Clinical gait evaluation of patients with lumbar spine stenosis. *Orthop. Surg.* **2018**, *10*, 32–39. [CrossRef]
29. Zhang, H.H.; Yan, S.H.; Fang, C.; Zhang, K. To evaluate the operation effect of total hip arthroplasty with portable gait analyzer. *J. Med. Biomech.* **2015**, *6*, E361–E366.
30. Delp, S.L.; Anderson, F.C.; Arnold, A.S.; Loan, P.; Habib, A.; John, C.T.; Guendelman, E.; Thelen, D.G. OpenSim: Open-source software to create and analyze dynamic simulations of movement. *IEEE Trans. Biomed. Eng.* **2007**, *54*, 1940–1950. [CrossRef]
31. Saremi, K.; Marehbian, J.; Xiaohong, Y.; Regnaux, J.-P.; Elashoff, R.; Bussel, B.; Dobkin, B.H. Reliability and validity of bilateral thigh and foot accelerometry measures of walking in healthy and hemiparetic subjects. *Neurorehabilit. Neural Repair* **2006**, *20*, 297–305. [CrossRef]
32. Winter, D.A. *Biomechanics and Motor Control of Human Movement*; John Wiley & Sons: Hoboken, NJ, USA, 2009.
33. Xinyan, J.; Huiyu, Z.; Wenjing, Q.; Qiuli, H.; Baker, J.S.; Gu, Y. Ground Reaction Force Differences between Bionic Shoes and Neutral Running Shoes in Recreational Male Runners before and after a 5 km Run. *Int. J. Environ. Res. Public Health* **2021**, *18*, 9787.
34. Hasan, C.Z.C.; Jailani, R.; Tahir, N.M.; Ilias, S. The analysis of three-dimensional ground reaction forces during gait in children with autism spectrum disorders. *Res. Dev. Disabil.* **2017**, *66*, 55–63. [CrossRef]
35. Tucker, C.A. *Measuring Walking: A Handbook of Clinical Gait Analysis*; Mac Keith Press: London, UK, 2014.
36. Lin, Y.; Qichang, M.; Liangliang, X.; Wei, L.; Mohamad, N.I.; István, B.; Fernandez, J.; Yaodong, G. Principal Component Analysis of the Running Ground Reaction Forces With Different Speeds. *Front. Bioeng. Biotechnol.* **2021**, *9*, 629809.
37. Lee, H.J.; Chou, L.S. Detection of gait instability using the center of mass and center of pressure inclination angles. *Arch. Phys. Med. Rehabil.* **2006**, *87*, 569–575. [CrossRef] [PubMed]
38. Pataky, T.C.; Robinson, M.A.; Vanrenterghem, J. Vector field statistical analysis of kinematic and force trajectories. *J. Biomech.* **2013**, *46*, 2394–2401. [PubMed]
39. Buehler, C.; Koller, W.; De Comtes, F.; Kainz, H. Quantifying Muscle Forces and Joint Loading During Hip Exercises Performed With and Without an Elastic Resistance Band. *Front. Sports Act. Living* **2021**, 223. [CrossRef]
40. Pataky, T.C. One-dimensional statistical parametric mapping in Python. *Comput. Methods Biomech. Biomed. Eng.* **2012**, *15*, 295–301. [CrossRef]
41. Jing, L. Gait and metabolic adaptation of walking with negative heel shoes. *Res. Sports Med.* **2003**, *11*, 277–296.
42. Benz, D.A.; Stacoff, A.; Balmer, E.; Durrer, A.; Stuessi, E. Walking pattern with missing-heel shoes. *J. Biomech.* **1998**, *1001*, 132. [CrossRef]
43. Leroux, A.; Fung, J.; Barbeau, H. Postural adaptation to walking on inclined surfaces: I. Normal strategies. *Gait Posture* **2002**, *15*, 64–74.
44. Lange, G.W.; Hintermeister, R.A.; Schlegel, T.; Dillman, C.J.; Steadman, J.R. Electromyographic and kinematic analysis of graded treadmill walking and the implications for knee rehabilitation. *J. Orthop. Sports Phys. Ther.* **1996**, *23*, 294–301. [CrossRef] [PubMed]
45. Woollacott, M.H.; Tang, P.-F. Balance control during walking in the older adult: Research and its implications. *Phys. Ther.* **1997**, *77*, 646–660. [CrossRef] [PubMed]
46. Winter, D.A.; Patla, A.E.; Frank, J.S.; Walt, S.E. Biomechanical walking pattern changes in the fit and healthy elderly. *Phys. Ther.* **1990**, *70*, 340–347. [CrossRef] [PubMed]
47. Sudarsky, L. Gait disorders in the elderly. *N. Engl. J. Med.* **1990**, *322*, 1441–1446.
48. Hollman, J.H.; Brey, R.H.; Bang, T.J.; Kaufman, K.R. Does walking in a virtual environment induce unstable gait?: An examination of vertical ground reaction forces. *Gait Posture* **2007**, *26*, 289–294. [CrossRef]
49. John, C.T.; Seth, A.; Schwartz, M.H.; Delp, S.L. Contributions of muscles to mediolateral ground reaction force over a range of walking speeds. *J. Biomech.* **2012**, *45*, 2438–2443. [CrossRef]
50. Wannop, J.W.; Worobets, J.T.; Stefanyshyn, D.J. Normalization of ground reaction forces, joint moments, and free moments in human locomotion. *J. Appl. Biomech.* **2012**, *28*, 665–676. [CrossRef]
51. Moccellin, A.; Driusso, P. Adjustments in static and dynamic postural control during pregnancy and their relationship with quality of life: A descriptive study. *Fisioterapia* **2012**, *34*, 196–202. [CrossRef]
52. Sole, G.; Pataky, T.; Sole, C.C.; Hale, L.; Milosavljevic, S. Age-related plantar centre of pressure trajectory changes during barefoot walking. *Gait Posture* **2017**, *57*, 188–192. [CrossRef]
53. Winter, D.A. Human balance and posture control during standing and walking. *Gait Posture* **1995**, *3*, 193–214. [CrossRef]
54. Sims, K.; Brauer, S. A rapid upward step challenges medio-lateral postural stability. *Gait Posture* **2000**, *12*, 217–224. [CrossRef]

55. Maki, B.E.; McIlroy, W.E. Control of rapid limb movements for balance recovery: Age-related changes and implications for fall prevention. *Age Ageing* **2006**, *35*, ii12–ii18. [CrossRef] [PubMed]
56. Zhang, X.; Li, B. Influence of in-shoe heel lifts on plantar pressure and center of pressure in the medial–lateral direction during walking. *Gait Posture* **2014**, *39*, 1012–1016. [CrossRef] [PubMed]
57. Hesse, S.; Luecke, D.; Jahnke, M.; Mauritz, K. Gait function in spastic hemiparetic patients walking barefoot, with firm shoes, and with ankle-foot orthosis. *Int. J. Rehabil. Res.* **1996**, *19*, 133–141. [CrossRef] [PubMed]
58. Robain, G.; Valentini, F.; Renard-Deniel, S.; Chennevelle, J.; Piera, J. A baropodometric parameter to analyze the gait of hemiparetic patients: The path of center of pressure. *Ann. Readapt Med. Phys.* **2006**, *49*, 609–613. [CrossRef]
59. Nag, P.; Nag, A.; Vyas, H.; Shukla, P.S. Influence of footwear on stabilometric dimensions and muscle activity. *Footwear Sci.* **2011**, *3*, 179–188. [CrossRef]
60. Orendurff, M.S.; Segal, A.D.; Klute, G.K.; Berge, J.S.; Rohr, E.S.; Kadel, N.J. The effect of walking speed on center of mass displacement. *J. Rehabil. Res. Dev.* **2004**, *41*, 829–834. [CrossRef]
61. Xiang, L.; Mei, Q.; Wang, A.; Shim, V.; Fernandez, J.; Gu, Y. Evaluating function in the hallux valgus foot following a 12-week minimalist footwear intervention: A pilot computational analysis. *J. Biomech.* **2022**, *132*, 110941. [CrossRef]
62. Xu, D.; Quan, W.; Zhou, H.; Sun, D.; Baker, J.S.; Gu, Y. Explaining the differences of gait patterns between high and low-mileage runners with machine learning. *Sci. Rep.* **2022**, *12*, 2981. [CrossRef]

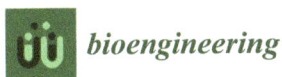

Article

Changes in Key Biomechanical Parameters According to the Expertise Level in Runners at Different Running Speeds

Cagla Fadillioglu [1,*,†], Felix Möhler [1,†], Marcel Reuter [2] and Thorsten Stein [1]

[1] BioMotion Center, Institute of Sports and Sports Science (IfSS), Karlsruhe Institute of Technology, 76131 Karlsruhe, Germany
[2] Department of Applied Training Science, German University of Applied Sciences for Prevention and Health Management (DHfPG), 66123 Saarbrücken, Germany
* Correspondence: cagla.fadillioglu@kit.edu
† These authors contributed equally to this work.

Abstract: Running has become increasingly popular worldwide. Among runners, there exists a wide range of expertise levels. Investigating the differences between runners at two extreme levels, that is novices and experts, is crucial to understand the changes that occur as a result of multiple years of training. Vertical oscillation of center of mass (CoM), stride frequency normalized to the leg length, and duty factor, which describes the step time relative to the flight time, are key biomechanical parameters that have been shown to be closely related to the running economy and are used to characterize the running style. The variability characteristics of these parameters may reveal valuable information concerning the control of human locomotion. However, how the expertise level and running speed affect the variability of these key biomechanical parameters has not yet been investigated. The aim of this study was to analyze the effects of expertise level (novice vs. expert) and running speed (10 km/h vs. 15 km/h) on these parameters and their variability. It was hypothesized that expert runners would have lower vertical oscillation of CoM, normalized stride frequency, and duty factor and show less variability in these parameters. The parameters' variability was operationalized by the coefficient of variation. The mean values and variability of these key biomechanical parameters according to expertise level and running speed were compared with rmANOVAs. The results showed that the experts had a lower duty factor and less variable vertical oscillation of CoM and normalized stride frequency, independently of the running speed. At a higher running speed, the variability of vertical oscillation of CoM was higher, whereas that of normalized stride frequency and duty factor did not change significantly. To the best of our knowledge, this is the first study analyzing the effects of expertise level and running speed on the variability of key biomechanical parameters.

Keywords: running economy; running style; duty factor; vertical oscillation; stride frequency

Citation: Fadillioglu, C.; Möhler, F.; Reuter, M.; Stein, T. Changes in Key Biomechanical Parameters According to the Expertise Level in Runners at Different Running Speeds. *Bioengineering* 2022, 9, 616. https://doi.org/10.3390/bioengineering9110616

Academic Editors: Christina Zong-Hao Ma, Zhengrong Li and Chen He

Received: 26 September 2022
Accepted: 23 October 2022
Published: 26 October 2022

Publisher's Note: MDPI stays neutral with regard to jurisdictional claims in published maps and institutional affiliations.

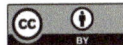

Copyright: © 2022 by the authors. Licensee MDPI, Basel, Switzerland. This article is an open access article distributed under the terms and conditions of the Creative Commons Attribution (CC BY) license (https://creativecommons.org/licenses/by/4.0/).

1. Introduction

Running is a sport that has been growing in popularity over the years [1]. Through multiple years of training, runners accomplish a variety of changes at different levels that include metabolic, neuromuscular, and biomechanical efficiency and ultimately result in improved running economy [2]. The changes in running economy play an important role in running performance, since a smaller energy expenditure at a given speed is beneficial, especially in disciplines that require running with submaximal speed for long distances. Therefore, not only cardiovascular and metabolic fitness (e.g., VO_2max) but also biomechanical and neuromuscular efficiency are crucial for individual running economy [2]. Even though VO_2max is typically used as a measure of running economy [3,4], studies that track the performance development of elite athletes for several years have reported improvements in performance without significant changes in VO_2max [5,6]. This emphasizes the importance of considering the whole scope of variables that are associated with running economy. Apart from factors such as age, gender, body temperature, and muscle fiber distribution, several biomechanical parameters as well as the running style have been shown to influence the running economy [7,8].

Positive correlations have been observed between isolated parameters and running economy. In particular, the vertical oscillation of the center of mass (osc_CoM) [2,8–10], step length (SL) [2,10], and step frequency (SF) [3,10] were identified as factors that influence the running economy in various running-related studies. The findings of these studies have indicated that an increase in running economy is associated with a lower osc_CoM [2,8,9,11] and a lower SF [3,10], whereas the results for SL have not been consistent across studies [10,12]. These varying results can be explained by the self-optimized SL/SF ratio [13,14]. On this basis, analyzing different running styles may be preferable to a comparison of isolated parameters when trying to understand the kinematic adaptations that occur as a result of training. However, the parameters used for the operationalization of the running style vary across the literature. Recently, in a study by van Overen et al. [13], it was suggested that the duty factor (DF), which is the ratio of stance to stride time, together with the SF normalized to the leg length (SF_norm) would be suitable to describe the running style and can be used for comparisons between individuals.

The expertise level is a major factor that influences various biomechanical parameters, including spatio-temporal parameters. Therefore, in studies that attempt to distinguish between groups of runners in terms of their expertise level and define them, several terms are used, including "expert", "novice", "elite", "amateur", and "good". In this study, the terms expert (to refer to elite runners), good, and novice (to refer to amateur runners) will be used to avoid confusion between terminologies. Such studies have reported that SF was found to increase with increase in experience, stride time was found to be unaffected [15–18], and DF was found to decrease [19]. In addition, the effects of running experience on running economy have been reported in various studies. Importantly, experts were shown to have a more efficient running style than novices [9,20]. In studies that compared the performance of expert and good distance runners, it was found that expert runners have a slightly lower osc_CoM and a better running economy than good runners [2].

Apart from the running experience, the running speed was also shown to influence the kinematic variables. Padulo et al. [21] showed that both for expert and for novice runners, SL and SF increased, while stance time decreased with an increase in running speed. A study by García-Pinillos et al. [22] investigated the alterations in spatiotemporal parameters in novice endurance runners and showed that stance time becomes shorter, while SL and flight time become longer, as speed increases. Furthermore, not only the mean values but also the variability in spatiotemporal parameters was found to change with an increasing speed. Jordan et al. [23] suggested that the variability in running gait is not random but manifests self-similarity depending on the gait speed and therefore, it may help to understand the control of human locomotion.

The term "movement variability" can refer to different aspects according to the context [24]. In sports, the main way to achieve the desired goal (e.g., hitting the basketball hoop) is to achieve consistency over multiple repetitions. On the other hand, a certain level of variability may increase the flexibility of the whole biological system and ultimately help to adapt to different conditions, such as fatigue and environmental changes, and may also help to reduce injuries [24]. It was suggested that the variability of a parameter, which is important as a movement goal, can be minimized over several movement repetitions, and thereby, variations in less important parameters may be allowed to a certain level so that their co-variation establishes a flexible but stable system [25–27]. However, in the case of sports such as running, it is difficult to definitively determine which parameters are prioritized by the central nervous system (CNS) in terms of control. Typically, runners aim to run as fast as possible for a given distance and, thereby, try to improve their running style to make it more energy-efficient [28]. Thereby, the goal is to ensure that the parameters that are crucial for this goal are kept stable, whereas the less important parameters may vary on a larger scale. For the analysis of running in terms of the variability and stability of biomechanical parameters, different methods exist (e.g., uncontrolled manifold approach and tolerance noise covariation) and were applied in several studies [29–31]. Even though these methods are ideal for investigating the structure of motor variability in redundant solution spaces, they are not useful for distinguishing a target parameter [27,29,30]. Analyzing the variability characteristics of biomechanical parameters may help to understand which parameters are of high priority for the CNS [27,32]. Despite its relevancy, only a few studies have analyzed the variability in running kinematics [22,33–36].

To sum up, three key biomechanical parameters, i.e., vertical oscillation of CoM, stride frequency, and duty factor, have been shown to be closely related to running economy and running style. However, the influence of expertise level and running speed on the variability of these key biomechanical parameters has only been partially researched, even though they may reveal valuable information regarding the control of human locomotion. Therefore, the goal of this study was to investigate the effects of expertise level on vertical oscillation of CoM, stride frequency, and duty factor, as well as their variabilities at two different running speeds. It was hypothesized that expert runners would show lower mean values and lower variability of the considered parameters compared with novice runners, regardless of the running speed.

2. Materials and Methods

The data used in the present study were analyzed with the uncontrolled manifold approach as in a previous study [37].

2.1. Participants

The participants of this study were all male and comprised two groups: one group of 13 expert runners (EXP: age, 23.5 ± 3.6 years; height: 1.80 ± 0.06 m; weight, 66.8 ± 5.4 kg) and one group of 12 novice runners (NOV: age, 23.9 ± 3.8 years; height: 1.83 ± 0.07 m; weight, 72.2 ± 6.6 kg). EXP included runners with a 10 km personal best time below 35 min (32:59 ± 01:19 min) who had been members of a running club for at least 2 years (7.2 ± 3.2 years) and ran a minimum of 50 km per week (duration: 6.5 ± 1.7 h/week). NOV included runners who participated in a maximum of two sport sessions per week, including a maximum of one running session (0.2 ± 0.2 h/week). Importantly, this group only included runners who had never prepared for a running event or trained in a running club. It was important for all participants to be free of recent injuries or pain in the lower limbs. They were asked not to perform any intense workout on the day preceding the measurement. All participants provided their written informed consent prior to participation. This study was approved by the ethics committee of the Karlsruhe Institute of Technology.

2.2. Protocol

The study was performed on a motorized treadmill (h/p/cosmos Saturn; Nussdorf-Traunstein, Germany), with participants wearing a safety harness that was connected to an emergency off button. Before the measurements, a total of 22 anthropometric measurements were taken manually for each participant, and 41 markers were attached on their body according to the guidelines of the ALASKA (Advanced Lagrangian Solver in kinetic Analysis) modelling system [38]. After a standardized session of treadmill familiarization (6 min of walking and 6 min of running, [39,40], the speed of the treadmill was accelerated up to 15 km/h and held for 15 s in order for the participants to experience the running speed that they would run at during the measurements. After a 2 min break, the participants performed runs at speeds of 10 and 15 km/h in a counterbalanced order. The participants ran for approximately 1 min at each of the two speeds. For each speed, 3D marker data for the 41 markers were recorded during 20 consecutive gait cycles using 11 Vicon MX cameras (Vicon Motion Systems; Oxford Metrics Group, Oxford, UK) that were capable of recording at 200 Hz. The two running speeds for the measurements, 10 and 15 km/h, were chosen based on previous comparable studies [16,22]. In the pre-tests for this experiment, the chosen running speeds were confirmed to be proper.

2.3. Data Processing

The marker data were post-processed using the Vicon Nexus software (V1.8.5) and filtered with a 10 Hz low-pass Butterworth filter using Matlab (The MathWorks, Natick, MA, USA). The gait cycles were segmented using the foot marker data [41]. The CoM was estimated with the ALASKA Dynamicus modelling system [38]. To calculate osc_CoM, the difference between the minimum and the maximum height of the CoM (Equation (1)) was calculated for each of the 20 gait cycles. SF_norm and DF were calculated using previously published formulae [13]. To calculate SF_norm, SF was calculated as 60 divided by the sum of stance time and flight time, and then it was normalized to the leg length (Equation (2)). To calculate DF, the stance time was divided by twice the sum of the stance and flight time (Equation (3)). The variability of these parameters was calculated as the coefficient of variation (CV). Their mean values were included in the analysis to compare the results with those published in the existing literature.

$$osc\_CoM = CoM_{Zmax} - CoM_{Zmin} \qquad (1)$$

$$SF\_norm = \frac{60}{\left(t_{stance} + t_{flight}\right) \cdot \sqrt{\frac{L_0}{g}}} \qquad (2)$$

$$DF = \frac{t_{stance}}{2 \cdot (t_{stance} + t_{flight})} \qquad (3)$$

2.4. Statistical Analysis

Shapiro–Wilk tests were conducted to confirm the normality of data distribution. The dependent variables were osc_CoM, SF_norm, and DF, as well as their variabilities (operationalized by CV). For each of these dependent variables, a 2 × 2 repeated-measures ANOVA (rmANOVA) was calculated with the factors expertise level (EXP and NOV) and speed (10 and 15 km/h). In total, six rmANOVAs were performed. The Bonferroni–Holm method was used to correct the results for multiple comparisons [42]. The significance level was set a priori to $p < 0.05$. Partial eta-squared (small effect: $\eta_p^2 < 0.06$; medium effect $0.06 \leq \eta_p^2 < 0.14$; large effect: $\eta_p^2 \geq 0.14$) was calculated as a measure of the effect size for rmANOVA.

3. Results

The results for the mean values and the variability are shown in Figure 1.

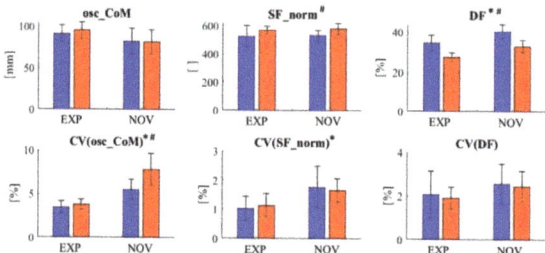

Figure 1. Mean value (**top row**) and coefficient of variation (CV) (**bottom row**) for the three parameters vertical oscillation of CoM (osc_CoM), normalized stride frequency (SF_norm), and duty factor (DF). The error bars show the standard deviation of the respective values. The values for the 10 km/h condition are shown in blue, and the values for the 15 km/h condition are shown in red; * significant effect for the factor expertise level, # significant effect for the factor speed.

3.1. Mean Value Changes in Vertical Oscillation, Normalized Frequency, and Duty Factor

The rmANOVA value for osc_CoM showed a non-significant main effect of the factor expertise level ($p = 0.33$, $\eta_p^2 = 0.189$) and a non-significant interaction effect of expertise level and speed, with a high effect size ($p = 0.576$, $\eta_p^2 = 0.142$). The main effect of the factor speed was also not significant ($p > 0.999$, $\eta_p^2 = 0.054$).

The rmANOVA for SF_norm showed a significant main effect of the factor speed, with a high effect size ($p = 0.018$, $\eta_p^2 = 0.438$) and a non-significant interaction between expertise level and speed ($p > 0.999$, $\eta_p^2 = 0.001$). The main effect of the factor expertise level was not significant ($p > 0.999$, $\eta_p^2 = 0.014$). In both groups, SF_norm increased from 10 to 15 km/h.

The rmANOVA for DF showed significant main effects of expertise level ($p = 0.018$, $\eta_p^2 = 0.502$) and speed ($p = 0.018$, $\eta_p^2 = 0.908$), with high effect sizes. However, the interaction effect of expertise level and speed was not significant ($p > 0.999$, $\eta_p^2 = 0.008$). In summary, DF decreased from 10 to 15 km/h and was overall higher for NOV than for EXP.

3.2. Changes in Variability according to the Expertise Level at Two Running Speeds

With regard to the CV of osc_CoM, rmANOVA showed significant main effects of expertise level ($p = 0.018$, $\eta_p^2 = 0.792$) and speed ($p = 0.018$, $\eta_p^2 = 0.408$), as well as non-significant interaction effects ($p = 0.084$, $\eta_p^2 = 0.279$), each with high effect sizes. This implies that the CV of osc_CoM was higher for NOV than for EXP. The CV of osc_CoM increased with an increase in speed.

The rmANOVA for the CV of SF_norm showed a significant effect of the factor expertise level, with a high effect size ($p = 0.018$, $\eta_p^2 = 0.435$). However, the effect of speed ($p > 0.999$, $\eta_p^2 < 0.001$) and the interaction effect of expertise level and speed ($p > 0.999$, $\eta_p^2 = 0.025$) were not significant. Accordingly, the results showed that the CV of SF_norm was higher for NOV than for EXP.

The rmANOVA for the CV of DF had no significant effects, but a high effect size was found for the factor expertise level ($p = 0.520$, $\eta_p^2 = 0.155$). In contrast, the effect sizes for speed ($p > 0.999$, $\eta_p^2 = 0.017$) and the interaction effect of expertise level and speed ($p > 0.999$, $\eta_p^2 < 0.001$) were low.

4. Discussion

The aim of this study was to analyze the effects of the expertise level on key biomechanical parameters and the variability of these parameters at two different running speeds. It was hypothesized that regardless of the running speed, expert runners are characterized by lower mean values and lower variability of all the considered parameters compared with their novice counterparts. The results indicated that the expert runners had a lower duty factor than the novices. Furthermore, the experts showed a significantly lower variability than the novices with regard to vertical oscillation of CoM and normalized stride frequency, independently of the running speed, but no differences in variability were observed for the duty factor. Based on the findings on this study, our hypotheses can be only partially accepted.

4.1. Lower Duty Factor for Expert Runners

EXP and NOV did not differ significantly in terms of osc_CoM (EXP, 10 km/h: 91.43 mm, 15 km/h: 95.06 mm; NOV, 10 km/h: 82.3 mm, 15 km/h: 81.36 mm). These findings are interesting, since more experienced runners are expected to have a better running economy [9,20], which was shown to be associated with a lower osc_CoM [2,8,9].

With regard to the results for SF_norm, they are in line with those of other studies [13,43], that is, an increased cadence was observed with an increase in speed. Based on these results, it can be suggested that SF_norm is not directly affected by the expertise level but, rather, is a function of the running speed.

DF, which describes the step time relative to the flight time, decreased with increasing speed in both groups in this study, and this finding is also in line with other published studies [8,44]. Furthermore, EXP showed an overall lower DF than NOV (10 km/h: 17.3% less; 15 km/h: 20.3% less); this indicates that EXP had a longer flight phase than NOV at a given stance time. The interpretation of the DF results is not straightforward, but an optimal level of DF seems to exist for runners. Even though a lower DF was shown to be associated with better running economy, a DF value that is too low could be uneconomical, given the high muscle activation that occurs over a very short stance time. Further, a DF value that is too high may indicate high start–stop accelerations and, therefore, a waste of mechanical work [45].

4.2. Lower Variability of Vertical Oscillation and Normalized Stride Frequency in Expert Runners

The results indicated that EXP had significantly lower variability in osc_CoM and SF_norm than NOV, independently of the running speed, whereas there were no significant changes in DF. In the time period over which a novice runner becomes an expert runner, a variety of changes occur in the runners' body that range from physiological to neuromuscular adaptations that are necessary for movement efficiency [9,46]. Ultimately, the running economy is improved to decrease the total energy need, since humans inevitably tend to conserve energy from an evolutionary perspective [47] and prefer an energy-optimal gait [48]. The lower variability in osc_CoM and SF_norm found in EXP could mean that after multiple years of training, the CNS tries to reduce the variability in these parameters because they are important for the running economy as well as for a consistent running style [2,9,13]. However, it is important to note that it is difficult to directly draw this conclusion from the findings of this study. Even though the variability in these two parameters was lower in the EXP, it is possible that the CNS primarily controls other parameters which consequently influence the variability of these key parameters.

Differences in variability between the two running speeds, that is 10 and 15 km/h, were only detected for osc_CoM. These findings imply that the expertise level plays a major role in terms of variability in these parameters, whereas the effects of speed were rather small. This could, however, be dependent on the choice of the running speed. To the best of our knowledge, there are very few studies whose results can be compared with those of this study. One such study [22] reported that amateur runners showed a higher variability in stance time and SL at running speeds of 15–16 km/h than at a speed of 10 km/h. However, it analyzed different parameters from those analyzed in this study and calculated the standard deviation (SD) instead of the CV. Therefore, it is difficult to compare their findings with the present findings. In this study, CV was preferred over SD, since it reflects changes in SD normalized to the mean value. It is also important to note that regardless of the research question, it is difficult to analyze the effects of the running speed in terms of running economy and running style, since humans seem to have an energy-optimal gait and prefer to move at this optimal speed, thus minimizing the energy requirement [48].

4.3. Limitations

Our study has some limitations that should be considered when interpreting the results. The first limitation is that the focus was on the running economy, even though it was not quantified by the parameters that are usually used for the operationalization of the running economy (e.g., VO_2 [12]). Rather, the key biomechanical parameters that have been shown to be strongly related to running economy and running style [2,8,9,13] were used. Another limitation of this study is that the measurements were conducted with a treadmill under laboratory conditions, which differ from the usual environment that most runners are exposed to. On the other hand, the use of a treadmill enabled a precise control of speed and, therefore, eliminated any confounding effects caused by a variable running speed. In addition, similar studies have also been performed under laboratory conditions [35,49]. The third limitation is that the sample size was chosen on the basis of comparable studies [20,50,51]. It might have been better to choose the sample size based on an a priori power analysis. The fourth and final limitation is that the chosen speeds were the same for all participants. It would have been preferable to choose individual speeds based on individual thresholds, since a connection between running speed and running economy in terms of VO_2 max has been demonstrated [9]. However, the interpretation of the results would have been much more complicated due to the addition of speed as an individually varying factor. Despite this, the results do indicate an overall lower variability among EXP than NOV, independent of the speed that they were running at.

5. Conclusions

The aim of this study was to investigate the effects of the expertise level on key biomechanical parameters and their variabilities at two different running speeds. The findings showed that, independently of the running speed, expert runners had a lower duty factor and showed less variable vertical oscillation of CoM and normalized stride frequency than novice runners, but the variation in duty factor did not differ between the two groups. At a higher running speed, the variability in vertical oscillation of CoM was higher, whereas the variability in the other two parameters did not change significantly, independently of the expertise level. Based on these results, it can be suggested that two of the three considered parameters, i.e., vertical oscillation of CoM and normalized stride frequency, are important parameters, whose variability decreased with the increase in the expertise level. A lower variability of these parameters found in expert runners may indicate that after multiple years of training, the CNS tries to reduce the variability in these parameters because they are important for the running economy as well as for a consistent running style. Further studies should address the variability of key biomechanical parameters in terms of running economy and running style in a more detailed manner to identify the parameters that are of high priority for the CNS.

Author Contributions: Conceptualization, C.F., F.M., M.R. and T.S.; methodology, C.F. and F.M.; software, F.M.; formal analysis, F.M.; investigation, C.F. and F.M.; resources, T.S.; data curation, F.M. writing—original draft preparation, C.F. and F.M.; writing—review and editing, C.F., F.M., M.R. and T.S.; supervision, T.S.; project administration, F.M.; funding acquisition, T.S. All authors have read and agreed to the published version of the manuscript.

Funding: This research received no external funding.

Institutional Review Board Statement: The study was conducted according to the guidelines of the Declaration of Helsinki and was approved by the ethics committee of the Karlsruhe Institute of Technology.

Informed Consent Statement: Informed consent was obtained from all subjects involved in the study.

Data Availability Statement: The data presented in this study are available on request from the corresponding author.

Acknowledgments: We acknowledge the support by the KIT-Publication Fund of the Karlsruhe Institute of Technology.

Conflicts of Interest: The authors declare no conflict of interest.

References

1. RaceMedicine. The State of Running. Available online: https://racemedicine.org/the-state-of-running-2019/ (accessed on 10 May 2022).
2. Barnes, K.R.; Kilding, A.E. Running economy: Measurement, norms, and determining factors. *Sport. Med. Open* **2015**, *1*, 8. [CrossRef] [PubMed]
3. Hunter, I.; Smith, G.A. Preferred and optimal stride frequency, stiffness and economy: Changes with fatigue during a 1-h high-intensity run. *Eur. J. Appl. Physiol.* **2007**, *100*, 653–661. [CrossRef] [PubMed]
4. Fuller, J.T.; Bellenger, C.R.; Thewlis, D.; Tsiros, M.D.; Buckley, J.D. The Effect of Footwear on Running Performance and Running Economy in Distance Runners. *Sport. Med.* **2015**, *45*, 411–422. [CrossRef] [PubMed]

5. Coyle, E.F. Improved muscular efficiency displayed as Tour de France champion matures. *J. Appl. Physiol.* **2005**, *98*, 2191–2196. [CrossRef] [PubMed]
6. Jones, A.M. The Physiology of the World Record Holder for the Women's Marathon. *Int. J. Sport. Sci. Coach.* **2006**, *1*, 101–116. [CrossRef]
7. Kyröläinen, H.; Belli, A.; Komi, P.V. Biomechanical factors affecting running economy. *Med. Sci. Sport. Exerc.* **2001**, *33*, 1330–1337. [CrossRef]
8. Folland, J.P.; Allen, S.J.; Black, M.I.; Handsaker, J.C.; Forrester, S.E. Running Technique is an Important Component of Running Economy and Performance. *Med. Sci. Sport. Exerc.* **2017**, *49*, 1412–1423. [CrossRef]
9. Saunders, P.U.; Pyne, D.B.; Telford, R.D.; Hawley, J.A. Factors-affecting-running-economy in trainer distance runners. *Sport. Med.* **2004**, *34*, 465–485. [CrossRef]
10. Tartaruga, M.P.; Brisswalter, J.; Peyré-Tartaruga, L.A.; Ávila, A.O.V.; Alberton, C.L.; Coertjens, M.; Cadore, E.L.; Tiggemann, C.L.; Silva, E.M.; Kruel, L.F.M. The relationship between running economy and biomechanical variables in distance runners. *Res. Q. Exerc. Sport* **2012**, *83*, 367–375. [CrossRef]
11. Moore, I.S.; Jones, A.; Dixon, S. The pursuit of improved running performance: Can changes in cushioning and somatosensory feedback influence running economy and injury risk? *Footwear Sci.* **2014**, *6*, 1–11. [CrossRef]
12. Barnes, K.R.; Kilding, A.E. Strategies to Improve Running Economy. *Sport. Med.* **2015**, *45*, 37–56. [CrossRef] [PubMed]
13. van Oeveren, B.T.; De Ruiter, C.J.; Beek, P.J.; Van Dieën, J.H. The biomechanics of running and running styles: A synthesis The biomechanics of running and running styles: A synthesis. *Sport. Biomech.* **2021**, 1–39. [CrossRef] [PubMed]
14. Hunter, I.; Lee, K.; Ward, J.; Tracy, J. Self-optimization of Stride Length Among Experienced and Inexperienced Runners. *Int. J. Exerc. Sci.* **2017**, *10*, 446–453. [PubMed]
15. Cavanagh, P.R.; Pollock, M.L.; Landa, J. A Biomechanical Comparison of Elite and Good Distance Runners. *Ann. New York Acad. Sci.* **1977**, *301*, 328–345. [CrossRef] [PubMed]
16. Gómez-Molina, J.; Ogueta-Alday, A.; Stickley, C.; Cámara, J.; Cabrejas-Ugartondo, J.; García-López, J. Differences in Spatiotemporal Parameters between Trained Runners and Untrained Participants. *J. Strength Cond. Res.* **2017**, *31*, 2169–2175. [CrossRef] [PubMed]
17. Nelson, R.C.; Gregor, R.J. Biomechanics of distance running: A longitudinal study. *Res. Q. Am. Alliance Heal. Phys. Educ. Recreat.* **1976**, *47*, 417–428. [CrossRef]
18. Slawinski, J.S.; Billat, V.L. Difference in mechanical and energy cost between highly, well, and nontrained runners. *Med. Sci. Sports Exerc.* **2004**, *36*, 1440–1446. [CrossRef]
19. Forrester, S.E.; Townend, J. The effect of running velocity on footstrike angle—A curve-clustering approach. *Gait and Posture* **2015**, *41*, 26–32. [CrossRef]
20. de Ruiter, C.J.; Verdijk, P.W.L.; Werker, W.; Zuidema, M.J.; de Haan, A. Stride frequency in relation to oxygen consumption in experienced and novice runners. *Eur. J. Sport Sci.* **2014**, *14*, 251–258. [CrossRef]
21. Padulo, J.; Annino, G.; Migliaccio, G.M.; D'Ottavio, S. Kinematics of Running at Different Slopes and Speeds. *J. Strength Cond. Res.* **2011**, *26*, 1331–1339. [CrossRef]
22. García-Pinillos, F.; Jerez-Mayorga, D.; Latorre-Román, P.; Ramirez-Campillo, R.; Sanz-López, F.; Roche-Seruendo, L.E. How do Amateur Endurance Runners Alter Spatiotemporal Parameters and Step Variability as Running Velocity Increases? A Sex Comparison. *J. Hum. Kinet.* **2020**, *72*, 39–49. [CrossRef] [PubMed]
23. Jordan, K.; Challis, J.H.; Cusumano, J.P.; Newell, K.M. Stability and the time-dependent structure of gait variability in walking and running. *Hum. Mov. Sci.* **2009**, *28*, 113–128. [CrossRef] [PubMed]
24. Cowin, J.; Nimphius, S.; Fell, J.; Culhane, P.; Schmidt, M. A Proposed Framework to Describe Movement Variability within Sporting Tasks: A Scoping Review. *Sport. Med. Open* **2022**, *8*, 85. [CrossRef] [PubMed]
25. Todorov, E. Optimality principles in sensorimotor control. *Nat. Neurosci.* **2004**, *7*, 907–915. [CrossRef] [PubMed]
26. Sternad, D. It's not (only) the mean that matters: Variability, noise and exploration in skill learning. *Curr. Opin. Behav. Sci.* **2018**, *20*, 183–195. [CrossRef]
27. Latash, M.L.; Scholz, J.P.; Schöner, G. Toward a new theory of motor synergies. *Mot. Control* **2007**, *11*, 276–308. [CrossRef]
28. Moore, I.S. Is There an Economical Running Technique? A Review of Modifiable Biomechanical Factors Affecting Running Economy. *Sport. Med.* **2016**, *46*, 793–807. [CrossRef]
29. Möhler, F.; Ringhof, S.; Debertin, D.; Stein, T. Influence of fatigue on running coordination: A UCM analysis with a geometric 2D model and a subject-specific anthropometric 3D model. *Hum. Mov. Sci.* **2019**, *66*, 133–141. [CrossRef]
30. Möhler, F.; Stetter, B.; Müller, H.; Stein, T. Stride-to-Stride Variability of the Center of Mass in Male Trained Runners After an Exhaustive Run: A Three Dimensional Movement Variability Analysis With a Subject-Specific Anthropometric Model. *Front. Sport. Act. Living* **2021**, *3*, 1–11. [CrossRef]
31. Möhler, F.; Fadillioglu, C.; Scheffler, L.; Müller, H.; Stein, T. Running-Induced Fatigue Changes the Structure of Motor Variability in Novice Runners. *Biology* **2022**, *11*, 942. [CrossRef]
32. Schöner, G.; Scholz, J.P. Analyzing variance in multi-degree-of-freedom movements: Uncovering structure versus extracting correlations. *Mot. Control* **2007**, *11*, 259–275. [CrossRef] [PubMed]
33. Möhler, F.; Fadillioglu, C.; Stein, T. Changes in spatiotemporal parameters, joint and CoM kinematics and leg stiffness in novice runners during a high-intensity fatigue protocol. *PLoS ONE* **2022**, *17*, e0265550. [CrossRef] [PubMed]

34. Padulo, J.; Ayalon, M.; Barbieri, F.A.; Di Capua, R.; Doria, C.; Ardigò, L.P.; Dello Iacono, A. Effects of Gradient and Speed on Uphill Running Gait Variability. *Sport. Health A Multidiscip. Approach* **2022**, 194173812110677. [CrossRef] [PubMed]
35. Nakayama, Y.; Kudo, K.; Ohtsuki, T. Variability and fluctuation in running gait cycle of trained runners and non-runners. *Gait Posture* **2010**, *31*, 331–335. [CrossRef] [PubMed]
36. Möhler, F.; Fadillioglu, C.; Stein, T. Fatigue-Related Changes in Spatiotemporal Parameters, Joint Kinematics and Leg Stiffness in Expert Runners During a Middle-Distance Run. *Front. Sport. Act. Living* **2021**, *3*, 634258. [CrossRef]
37. Möhler, F.; Marahrens, S.; Ringhof, S.; Mikut, R.; Stein, T. Variability of running coordination in experts and novices: A 3D uncontrolled manifold analysis. *Eur. J. Sport Sci.* **2020**, *20*, 1187–1196. [CrossRef]
38. Härtel, T.; Hermsdorf, H. Biomechanical modelling and simulation of human body by means of DYNAMICUS. *J. Biomech.* **2006**, *39*, 549. [CrossRef]
39. Matsas, A.; Taylor, N.; McBurney, H. Knee joint kinematics from familiarised treadmill walking can be generalised to overground walking in young unimpaired subjects. *Gait Posture* **2000**, *11*, 46–53. [CrossRef]
40. Lavcanska, V.; Taylor, N.F.; Schache, A.G. Familiarization to treadmill running in young unimpaired adults. *Hum. Mov. Sci.* **2005**, *24*, 544–557. [CrossRef]
41. Leitch, J.; Stebbins, J.; Paolini, G.; Zavatsky, A.B. Identifying gait events without a force plate during running: A comparison of methods. *Gait Posture* **2011**, *33*, 130–132. [CrossRef]
42. Holm, S. A Simple Sequentially Rejective Multiple Test Procedure. *Scand. J. Stat.* **1979**, *6*, 65–70.
43. García-Pinillos, F.; Cartón-Llorente, A.; Jaén-Carrillo, D.; Delgado-Floody, P.; Carrasco-Alarcón, V.; Martínez, C.; Roche-Seruendo, L.E. Does fatigue alter step characteristics and stiffness during running? *Gait Posture* **2020**, *76*, 259–263. [CrossRef] [PubMed]
44. Burns, G.T.; Gonzalez, R.; Zendler, J.M.; Zernicke, R.F. Bouncing behavior of sub-four minute milers. *Sci. Rep.* **2021**, *11*, 10501. [CrossRef] [PubMed]
45. Usherwood, J.R. The muscle-mechanical compromise framework: Implications for the scaling of gait and posture. *J. Hum. Kinet.* **2016**, *52*, 107–114. [CrossRef]
46. Preece, S.J.; Bramah, C.; Mason, D. The biomechanical characteristics of high-performance endurance running. *Eur. J. Sport Sci.* **2019**, *19*, 784–792. [CrossRef]
47. Bramble, D.M.; Lieberman, D.E. Endurance running and the evolution of Homo. *Nature* **2004**, *432*, 345–352. [CrossRef]
48. Selinger, J.C.; Hicks, J.L.; Jackson, R.W.; Wall-Scheffler, C.M.; Chang, D.; Delp, S.L. Running in the wild: Energetics explain ecological running speeds. *Curr. Biol.* **2022**, *32*, 2309–2315.e3. [CrossRef]
49. Floría, P.; Sánchez-Sixto, A.; Harrison, A.J.; Ferber, R. The effect of running speed on joint coupling coordination and its variability in recreational runners. *Hum. Mov. Sci.* **2019**, *66*, 449–458. [CrossRef]
50. Apte, S.; Prigent, G.; Stöggl, T.; Martínez, A.; Snyder, C.; Gremeaux-Bader, V.; Aminian, K. Biomechanical Response of the Lower Extremity to Running-Induced Acute Fatigue: A Systematic Review. *Front. Physiol.* **2021**, *12*, 646042. [CrossRef]
51. Garciá-Pinillos, F.; Garciá-Ramos, A.; Ramírez-Campillo, R.; Latorre-Román, P.; Roche-Seruendo, L.E. How Do Spatiotemporal Parameters and Lower-Body Stiffness Change with Increased Running Velocity? A Comparison between Novice and Elite Level Runners. *J. Hum. Kinet.* **2019**, *70*, 25–38. [CrossRef]

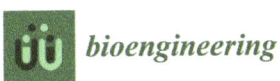

Systematic Review

Intracycle Velocity Variation in Swimming: A Systematic Scoping Review

Aléxia Fernandes [1], José Afonso [1], Francisco Noronha [1], Bruno Mezêncio [2], João Paulo Vilas-Boas [1] and Ricardo J. Fernandes [1,*]

[1] Centre of Research, Education, Innovation and Intervention in Sport and Porto Biomechanics Laboratory, Faculty of Sport, University of Porto, 4200-450 Porto, Portugal
[2] Biomechanics Laboratory, School of Physical Education and Sport, University of São Paulo, São Paulo 05508-030, Brazil
* Correspondence: ricfer@fade.up.pt

Abstract: Intracycle velocity variation is a swimming relevant research topic, focusing on understanding the interaction between hydrodynamic propulsive and drag forces. We have performed a systematic scoping review to map the main concepts, sources and types of evidence accomplished. Searches were conducted in the PubMed, Scopus and Web of Science databases, as well as the Biomechanics and Medicine in Swimming Symposia Proceedings Book, with manual searches, snowballing citation tracking, and external experts consultation. The eligibility criteria included competitive swimmers' intracycle velocity variation assessment of any sex, distance, pace, swimming technique and protocol. Studies' characteristics were summarized and expressed in an evidence gap map, and the risk of bias was judged using RoBANS. A total of 76 studies, corresponding to 68 trials involving 1440 swimmers (55.2 and 34.1% males and females), were included, with only 20 (29.4%) presenting an overall low risk of bias. The front crawl was the most studied swimming technique and intracycle velocity variation was assessed and quantified in several ways, leading to extremely divergent results. Researchers related intracycle velocity variation to coordination, energy cost, fatigue, technical proficiency, velocity, swimming techniques variants and force. Future studies should focus on studying backstroke, breaststroke and butterfly at high intensities, in young, youth and world-class swimmers, as well as in IVV quantification.

Keywords: biomechanics; competitive swimming; performance; velocity fluctuations

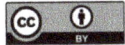

1. Introduction

Intracycle velocity variation (IVV) is a biomechanical variable that reflects the velocity fluctuation within a swimming cycle and was one of the first swimming-related research topics [1,2] aiming to better understand performance evolution constraints. IVV depends on the interaction between propulsive and resistive forces for each upper limb cycle, with the interaction between these accelerations and decelerations considered an efficiency estimator [3,4]. The first attempt to evaluate this variable was made for the backstroke, breaststroke and front crawl [1], and concluded that common stopwatches could not adequately assess swimming velocity (changes were observed within an s or an m). Velocity was measured with a natograph (recording the distance travelled every 1/5 of an s), and its variation was observed in each studied swimming technique (with front crawl being the fastest due to its smoothness). At that time, swimming was associated with motor cars' mechanics since, if driving with a variable speed would be wasteful, the same should occur in the human machine. This study provided important insights and investigation lines for the current topic.

Afterwards, the natograph was improved [2,5–7], with several mechanical devices beginning to be used (cable speedometers [8,9], accelerometers [10], and other gadgets [11]), all characterized by a mechanical connection to a swimmer's anatomical point. Despite the incapacity to monitor the swimmer's bodily inertia due to the constant change in the position of the centre of mass, these methods were very interactive and relevant to training due to the immediate output availability. Cinematography was also very common for evaluating IVV [12–14], qualitatively and quantitatively assessing the movements in a three-dimensional nature with (at least) two cameras. These image-based methods, usually involving the digitisation of film or video images, presented similar issues related to the body inertia capture, as well as image distortions, water bobbles and waves, parallax, digitising and calibration errors, and reduced interactivity (due to the delay between data collection and the swimmer feedback as a result of image processing).

Methods dealing with the centre of mass motion have the abovementioned problems but are even more time-consuming and complex. Nowadays, depending on the aims of IVV investigation, researchers are divided between using an anatomical fixed point or the centre of mass [15–17]. Considering the accessibility of mechanical methods, the agreement between these measures was evaluated, but the centre of mass reference was constantly overestimated, and it is axiomatically considered a gold standard in those comparisons [17–19]. Due to the current approach to this issue, forward hip movements were considered a good estimate of the swimmers' horizontal velocity and displacement, being relevant for diagnostic purposes but not representing the movement of the centre of mass [15,16,20]. Hip error magnitude should also be considered because it overestimates swimming velocity and, consequently, the IVV of the four conventional swimming techniques [17–19].

Despite the above-referenced methodological concerns, the association between swimming IVV and performance continues to be investigated even though the findings are quite divergent. Increases in velocity were associated with lower [3,21], stable [22–33] and higher IVV [34,35] in different swimming techniques. Better propulsive continuity in front crawl and lower swimming economy in breaststroke and butterfly (due to elevated resistive forces and amount of work) are the suggested explanations. In addition, when comparing competitive swimming levels for the same pace and swimming technique, better swimmers were observed to have higher [36,37], lower [10,21,23,33,34,38,39] or similar IVV [40,41] values compared to their counterparts. Regarding conventional swimming techniques, breaststroke presents the highest IVV values, followed by butterfly, backstroke and front crawl [3], although alternative techniques' scores are very similar [42].

Considering the IVV research background and its significance to assess biomechanical development in swimming, the aim of the current study wa to accomplish a systematic scoping review of IVV in competitive swimming regarding the four conventional techniques, assessment and quantification methods, participants' information (sex, competitive level and age category), protocols, and association with swimming economy and hydrodynamic drag. The closest work to a review about IVV is a book chapter [43] addressing it as a relevant variable to assess swimming biomechanical and coordinative development, as well as its association with swimmers' technique, exercise intensity, economy and fatigue.

2. Materials and Methods

The current systematic scoping review protocol was designed according to PRISMA 2020 [44] and Prisma-ScR guidelines [45], as well as Cochrane recommendations [46]. The protocol was created and pre-registered as an OSF project on 6 July 2022 (https://osf.io/m43pj, accessed on 23 December 2022).

2.1. Eligibility Criteria

Original peer-reviewed articles and texts from the Proceedings Book of the Biomechanics and Medicine in Swimming, published in any language or date, were included in the current study. Letters, editorials, meetings abstracts, commentaries, and reviews were excluded. The eligibility criteria were defined by the Population, Exposition, Comparator, Outcomes and Study (PECOS) design model, in accordance with PRISMA guidelines:

(i) population (competitive swimmers of any sex, with no injuries, excluding triathletes, divers and Paralympic athletes and artistic and open-water swimmers); (ii) exposure (IVV assessments at any swimming distance, pace, technique and protocol); (iii) comparison (not mandatory if intervention was performed); (iv) outcome (IVV was the primary outcome, with the secondary outcomes being described in the 2.6. data items subsection and not used as inclusion/exclusion criteria) and (v) study design (no limitations for the study strategy).

2.2. Information Sources

Searches were conducted until 6 July 2022, in the PubMed, Scopus and Web of Science literature databases, as well as in the Proceedings Books of the Biomechanics and Medicine in Swimming Symposia (no filters were applied). After the automated searches, the reference lists of the included studies were screened and prospective snowballing citation tracking was performed in PubMed, Scopus and Web of Science databases. Two external experts (holding a PhD in Sport Sciences and having considerable published research on the topic) were consulted to provide further suggestions of potentially relevant studies. Included studies' errata, corrections, corrigenda and retractions were sought [46].

The International Symposia for Biomechanics and Medicine in Swimming have been held every four years since 1970 and are considered the most prestigious international aquatic-oriented scientific congresses. These meetings have provided the swimming science community with some of the most outstanding contributions books and collections (Available at https://www.iat.uni-leipzig.de/datenbanken/iks/bms/ accessed on 6 July 2022), as sought and valuable as some of the available studies published in high-impact, peer-reviewed journals. All submissions go through a peer review process, leading to a collection of peer-reviewed scientific papers, serving as a valuable resource for all who are interested in keeping up to date with aquatic research. Relevant pioneering works were published in the 13 editions of the Symposium, adding relevant information to the current review.

2.3. Search Strategy

The general search strategy used free text terms applied to the title or abstracts: swim* AND intracycl* OR "intra-cycl*" OR IVV AND velocity OR speed* OR accelera* OR quick*. The full search strategy for each database is shown in Table 1.

Table 1. Full search strategies for PubMed, Scopus, Web of Science databases, and Biomechanics and Medicine in Swimming Symposia.

Database	Observations	Search Strategy
PubMed	Nothing to report	(((((((swim*[Title/Abstract]) AND (intracycl*[Title/Abstract])) OR ("intra-cycl*"[Title/Abstract])) OR (IVV[Title/Abstract])) AND (velocity[Title/Abstract])) OR(speed*[Title/Abstract])) OR (accelera*[Title/Abstract])) OR (quick*[Title/Abstract])
Scopus	The search for title and abstract also includes keywords	((swim*[Title/Abstract]) AND (intracycl*[Title/Abstract] OR "intra-cycl*"[Title/Abstract] OR IVV[Title/Abstract])) AND (velocity[Title/Abstract] OR speed*[Title/Abstract] OR accelera*[Title/Abstract] OR quick*[Title/Abstract])
Web of Science	Title/abstract is not available in this database. The option "Topic" includes title, abstract and keywords, and was used instead	swim* (Topic) AND intracycl* OR "intra-cycl*" OR IVV (Topic) AND velocity OR speed* OR accelera* Or quick* (Topic)
Biomechanics and Medicine in Swimming Symposia	Title/abstract was not available in this database. The option "All Fields" was used instead	(All Fields:swim*) AND (All Fields:intracycl* OR "intra-cycl*" OR IVV) AND (All Fields:velocity OR speed* OR accelera* OR quick*)

2.4. Selection Process

Two authors (AF and JA) independently screened all the database records and performed the manual searches, as well as snowballing citation tracking, with disagreements decided by a third author (RJF). Automated removal of duplicates was performed using EndNote™ 20.3 (Clarivate™, Philadelphia, PA, USA), but manual duplicate removal was required.

2.5. Data Collection Process

Two authors (AF and BM) independently collected data, and, in the case of disagreements, a third author (RJF) provided arbitrage. No automation tools were used, and a specifically tailored Excel worksheet was created for the extraction of raw data.

2.6. Data Items

The current study's primary outcome was IVV assessment in the four conventional swimming techniques (according to the above-referred defined eligibility criteria). Velocity assessment methodologies, IVV quantification, participant and protocol information, and associations with swimming economy or hydrodynamic drag were the secondary outcomes. Velocity can be assessed by mechanical, image-based and mixed methods, and IVV can be quantified by the (i) difference between maximal and minimum instantaneous velocity (dv); (ii) ratio of the mean velocity/difference between the maximal and minimum instantaneous velocity; (iii) ratio of the minimum and maximum velocities/intracycle mean velocity (dv/v); (iv) coefficient of variation (CV); and (v) other.

Regarding participants' characteristics, we have included studies with samples of female, male or both sexes and young (<14), youth (between 15–16), junior (between 17–18), senior (>19) or master (>25 years) swimmers (following the World of Aquatics stratification). Aiming for a homogeneous classification of competitive level, two authors (AF and JA) applied the Participant Caliber Framework [47] using training volume and performance metrics to classify participants as sedentary, recreational, trained, highly trained, elite and world class. Swimming paces were established according to the intensity training zones, with maximal corresponding to sprint (25–50 m), extreme to anaerobic power (100 m), severe to anaerobic capacity (200 m), heavy to aerobic power (400 m), moderate to aerobic capacity (800 m) and low to prolonged aerobic capacity (>1500 m). Studies were conducted in swimming pool and in swimming flume conditions, and information was gathered regarding the included studies that associated swimming economy or hydrodynamic drag with IVV.

2.7. Studies' Risk of Bias Assessment

Risk of bias in individual studies was judged using Cochrane's Risk of Bias Assessment for Non-randomized studies (RoBANS; [48]), evaluating six domains: (i) the participant selection; (ii) confounding variables; (iii) the exposure measurement; (iv) the outcome assessments blinding; (v) incomplete outcome data; and (vi) selective outcome reporting.

2.8. Effect Measures

IVV mean ± SD or median ± IQR values were calculated, and, when needed, two authors (AF and BM) independently extracted data from graphs using the WebPlotDigitizer v4.5 (Pacifica, CA, USA) [49].

2.9. Synthesis Methods

A narrative synthesis of the main findings was performed and supplemented with an interactive evidence gap map (generated by EPPI-Mapper v.2.2.3, London, UK, powered by EPPI Reviewer and created by the Digital Solution Foundry team). This map can be accessed online, providing interactive ways to visualize the current review's included studies (including authors, abstracts and keywords) and the primary and secondary outcomes.

3. Results

The initial search identified 227 potentially relevant articles, with 126 being duplicates, which were consequently removed (Figure 1). Following the titles and abstract screening, 17 and 10 studies were excluded by eligibility criteria and article type (respectively). After the seventy-four full texts were screened, one was excluded by type [50], six by exposure [51–56], seven by outcomes [57–63] and one by participant [64] eligibility criteria. Reference list analysis revealed 31 studies on the topic as potentially meeting the inclusion criteria, with full-text analysis excluding 10 articles by type [65–74], 2 by exposure [75,76] and 8 by outcomes [18,77–83]. Seven additional studies from snowballing citation tracking process were deemed eligible for inclusion, and all were included [29,84–89]. Expert consultations did not yield any new studies, so the combined total sample was n = 76 corresponding to 68 trials. Studies from the same trial were grouped for the analysis [4,22,25–27,29–31,33,39,90–93].

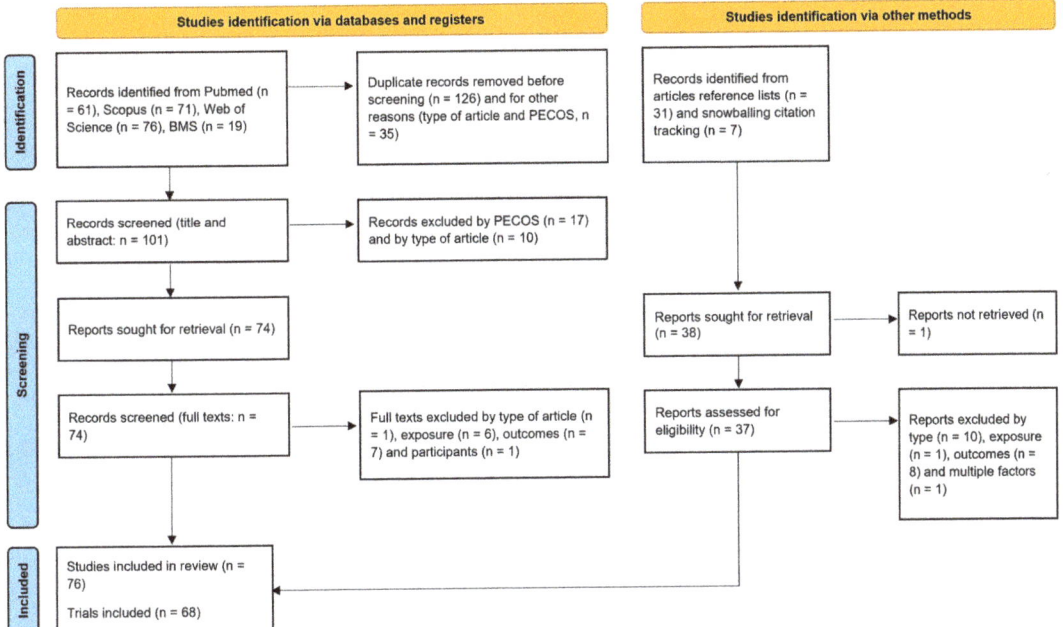

Figure 1. Search and screening processes used in the current study displayed as a PRISMA 2020 flow diagram.

3.1. Studies Risk of Bias Assessment

Sixty-eight trials were considered for judging risk of bias, with 20 [6,20,28,36,37,40, 41,87–89,94–103] and 48 considered as having overall low and high risk (respectively). The selection of participants showed a low risk of bias for 79% of the trials due to the overall purpose of evaluating competitive swimmers (Figure 2). However, 19% of the trials presented high risk due to the unbalanced number of females versus males [7,104,105], heterogeneity of participants [86,92,106,107], lack of information [10,92,108], or the non-competitive or inexperienced participation in the trials [84,109–111]. Two studies [26,27] were judged unclear because of the uncertainty of how swimmers were analysed. Fifty-one percent of the trials had a high risk of bias in the domain of confounding variables due to participant-related problems (lack of information [10,23,26,27,108–110,112], swimmers with different characteristics mixed in the same group [15,17,24,85,86,92,104,107,111,113–115], swimmers experience [3,84,116,117] and specialty [118]) and protocol-related problems (snorkel use [4,21,25,30,34,35,42,90,91,105,119,120], possible fatigue effect [32,121] and different evaluation conditions [122]).

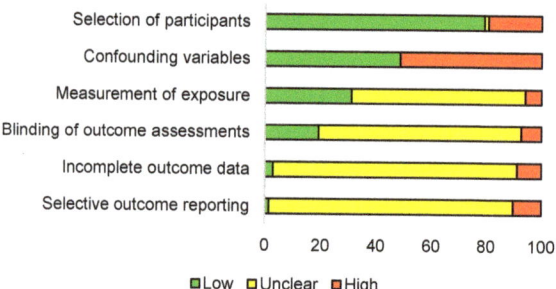

Figure 2. Percentage for each risk-of-bias domain regarding the included trials.

Considering that no data were provided concerning the validity and reliability of the software used or whether the process was fully automated in the different studies analysed, exposure measurement was judged unclear for 63% of the trials. High risk was evaluated for 6% of the trials with specific measurement issues; in particular, (i) the electrical resistance variation method had not been previously validated, with authors not providing proof of its reliability [104]; (ii) the preparation procedures and the evaluation protocol were performed for different swimming techniques [123]; (iii) various devices were used for different swimmers, and the evaluation frequency varied substantially in a retrospective study [124], raising questions concerning the actual measurement exposure consistency; and (iv) evaluations did not respect the same time period from the main competitions [125].

Many trials (74%) did not mention outcome assessment blinding and it was unclear if video analysis was fully automated (probably interfering with the measurements). High risk was attributed to 7% of the trials due to no blinding and to the inexistence of data concerning the reliability of the automated process [4,16,25,30,31,90,91,93,116,124]. Due to an absence of information on whether the selected swimmers were part of a larger sample, incomplete outcome data were judged unclear for 88% of the trials, except for a case study [125] and a trial that included an a priori sample-power analysis [109]. High risk was evaluated for 9% of the trials due to missing data, given that this could influence the study outcomes [4,19,25,29,30,39,90,91,111,126,127]. Eighty-eight percent of the trials had no pre-registered protocol to compare to, with the selective outcome reporting unclear. High risk was judged for the trials belonging to the same study [4,22,25–27,29–31,33,39,90,91,93] and for those that did not fully report the pre-defined primary outcomes [19,104].

3.2. Studies Characteristics

The included trials' main characteristics are presented in Table 2. Across the 68 trials, 1440 swimmers were evaluated for IVV (55.2% male and 10.7% missing information), with n = 1–126 sample sizes and 11.7 ± 0.8–42.5 ± 9.5 years of age. Some trials did not present information regarding IVV [16,19,111,120], female swimmers' participation [10, 23,26,27,92,102,112], competitive level [104,110], age category [7,10,21,104], or protocol intensity [111]. Thirty-nine trials assessed IVV as the main study purpose, of which three analysed and described the swimming cycles curves [7,104,118]; nine related IVV with coordination [22,23,26,27,30–33,103], six with swimming economy [21,30,34,35,90,105,123], six with fatigue [26,27,84,107,108,112], six with technique [4,36,41,107,111,113] and five with velocity [3,6,37,41,124]; three analysed different swimming techniques variants [35,106,126]; two related to force [94,99]; six were methodological [10,17,19,20,86,87]; one was a dynamical systems approach [40]; and one was a training intervention [88].

Table 2. List of included trials and respective main characteristics (including the evaluated swimming technique, the participants characteristics, the used methodology, the conflicts of interests and the corresponding funding).

Study	Swimming Technique	Participants	Assessment	Protocol	Conflicting Interest and Funding
Miyashita [7]	Front crawl	Eight highly trained male and 1 sedentary female swimmers	Cable speedometer	100 m at best effort	Unreported
Holmer [10]	Breaststroke, front crawl	1 elite, 1 trained and 1 recreational swimmer	Accelerometer	1–2 min each at several different velocities up to their maximal velocity	Unreported
Craig, et al. [118]	Breaststroke	Twelve trained male swimmers (19 years)	Cable speedometer	5 repeated swims using a range of 20–30 upper limbs cycles per minute for the slowest swims up to his maximal velocity (50–60 stroke rate)	Unreported
Loetz, et al. [104]	Backstroke, breaststroke, butterfly, front crawl	1 male and 8 female swimmers	Electrical impedance	Sprint	Unreported
Manley and Atha [6]	Breaststroke	4 highly trained male and 4 trained female swimmers (14–16 years)	Swimming tachometer	12 m maximum, 12 m 50% maximum and 12 m acceleration from 50 to 100%	Unreported
Ungerechts [111]	Breaststroke	13 male and 9 female highly trained swimmers (14.5–20.5 years)	3D	Unreported	Unreported
Vilas-Boas [35]	Breaststroke	Thirteen highly trained male swimmers (15.8 ± 2.2 years)	Photo-optical method	3 × 200 m: 2 at submaximal velocities, 1 maximal effort	Unreported
Colman, et al. [126]	Breaststroke	25 male (19.9 ± 2.6) and 20 female (17.9 ± 3.07) elite swimmers	2D	25 m at 100 m competitive pace	Unreported
D'Acquisto and Costill [94]	Breaststroke	7 male (19.7 ± 1.5) and 8 female (19.0 ± 1.1 years) trained swimmers	Cable speedometer, 2D	Two all-out 15 yards (22.86 m)	Unreported
Alberty, et al. [26] Alberty, et al. [27]	Front crawl	Seventeen highly trained swimmers (21 ± 3 years)	Cable speedometer	2 × 25 submaximal with 4 × 50 m max in between to induce fatigue and 25 m front crawl test at maximal velocity 30 min before 200 and just after 200 m	Unreported
Barbosa, et al. [19]	Butterfly	Seven highly trained and elite male swimmers (18.4 ± 1.9 years)	3D	3 sets of 3 × 25 m as fast as possible	Unreported
Kjendlie, et al. [110]	Front crawl	10 children (11.7 ± 0.8) and 13 adults (21.4 ± 3.7 years)	2D	4 × 25 m front crawl at submaximal velocities	Unreported
Takagi, et al. [127]	Breaststroke	46 male and 35 female world-class swimmers	2D	25 m of 50, 100 and 200 m breast	Unreported
Barbosa, et al. [34]	Butterfly	3 male (17.6 ± 2.9) and 2 female highly trained swimmers (15.0 ± 1.4 years)	3D	3 × 200 m butterfly: 2 submaximal (75 and 85%), one maximal	Unreported

115

Table 2. Cont.

Study	Swimming Technique	Participants	Assessment	Protocol	Conflicting Interest and Funding
Balonas, et al. [123]	Backstroke, breaststroke, butterfly, front crawl	Twelve elite male swimmers (19.8 ± 3.5 years)	3D	Test until exhaustion	Unreported
Barbosa, et al. [21]	Backstroke, breaststroke, butterfly, front crawl	12 male and 5 female elite swimmers	3D	Incremental set of n × 200 m	Unreported
Novais, et al. [105]	Breaststroke	2 male (17.0 ± 0.0) and 2 female elite swimmers (17.5 ± 2.1)	3D	Incremental set of n × 200 m	Unreported
Schnitzler, et al. [22] Schnitzler, et al. [33]	Front crawl	6 male (22.3 ± 4) and 6 female (21.0 ± 2.4 years) elite swimmers	2D	5 × 25 m at paces of 3000, 400, 200, 100 and 50 m	Unreported
Tella, et al. [108]	Front crawl	10 male and 7 female highly trained swimmers (between 14–16 years)	Cable speedometer	2 × 25 m and 100 m at maximum velocity	Unreported
Leblanc, et al. [36]	Breaststroke	9 elite male (19.9 ± 2.3) and 9 trained swimmers (15.1 ± 0.9 years)	Cable speedometer	3 × 25 m trials at 200, 100 and 50 m race pace	Unreported
Barbosa, et al. [113]	Butterfly	Ten international male swimmers (18.4 ± 1.9 years)	3D	2 × 25 m at high velocity	Unreported
Tella, et al. [112]	Front crawl	Sixteen trained and highly trained swimmers (17.0 ± 0.8 years)	Accelerometer	2 × 25 m front crawl sprint	No conflicts of interest Funded by University of Valencia (UV-AE-20041029)
Figueiredo, et al. [16]	Front crawl	Eight highly trained male swimmers (20.3 ± 2.8 years)	3D	25 m near maximum	Unreported conflicting interest Funded by Portuguese Science and Technology Foundation (SFRH/BD/38462/2007)
Psycharakis and Sanders [20]	Front crawl	Ten highly trained and elite male swimmers (16.9 ± 1.2 years)	3D	One maximum swim	Unreported conflicting interest Funded by Greek State's Scholarship Foundation
Arellano, et al. [106]	Front crawl	5 male and 8 female trained and highly trained swimmers (19.6 ± 2.2 years)	Cable speedometer	25 m as fast as possible	Unreported conflicting interest Funded by Secretary of State for Research, Ministry of Science and Innovation. Ref. DEP2009-08411. University of Granada, Physical Education and Sports Department and Research Group of Physical Activity and Sports on Aquatic Environment [CTS.527]

Table 2. *Cont.*

Study	Swimming Technique	Participants	Assessment	Protocol	Conflicting Interest and Funding
Psycharakis, et al. [37]	Front crawl	Eleven junior and senior elite and highly trained swimmers (16.9 ± 1.2 years)	3D	200 m race pace	Unreported
Schnitzler, et al. [32]	Front crawl	10 elite/highly trained swimmers (22.5 ± 3.6) and 12 trained swimmers (23.0 ± 1.7 years)	Cable speedometer	Four swim trials at 100, 80–90, 70–80 and 60–70%	Unreported
De Jesus, et al. [128]	Butterfly	Seven trained female swimmers (17.6 ± 2.0 years)	2D	2 × 100 m butterfly swim: one at submaximal and one at maximal velocity	Unreported
Fernandes, et al. [15]	Front crawl	Sixteen highly trained and trained swimmers (29.2 ± 10.3 years)	3D	Intermittent protocol with increments of 0.05 m/s each step and 30 s rest intervals	Unreported conflicting interest Funded by PTDC/DES/101124/2008 [FCOMP-01-0124-FEDER-009577]
Ferreira, et al. [120]	Front crawl	Nine male highly trained swimmers (18.0 ± 2.3 years)	3D	200 and 400 m race pace	Unreported conflicts of interest Funded by Portuguese Science and Technology Foundation [POCI/DES/58362/2004]
Figueiredo, et al. [90] Figueiredo, et al. [4] Figueiredo, et al. [91] Figueiredo, et al. [25] Figueiredo, et al. [30]	Front crawl	Ten male highly trained swimmers (21.6 ± 2.4 years)	3D	200 m race pace	No conflicts of interest Funded by Portuguese Science and Technology Foundation [SFRH/BD/38462/2007] and [PTDC/DES/101124/2008—FCOMP-01-0124-FEDER-009577]
Barbosa, et al. [3]	Backstroke, breaststroke, butterfly, front crawl	23 male and 22 female highly trained and trained swimmers (12.8 ± 1.2 years)	Cable speedometer	Maximal 4 × 25 m	Unreported
Feitosa, et al. [87]	Breaststroke, butterfly	12 male (14.4 ± 1.2) and 11 female highly trained and trained swimmers (12.7 ± 0.8 years)	Cable speedometer	Maximal 2 × 25 m	Unreported
Gourgoulis, et al. [31] Gourgoulis, et al. [93]	Front crawl	Nine female highly trained swimmers (18.4 ± 4.9 years)	3D	25 m trials at different paces	No conflicts of interest No funding
Morais, et al. [117]	Front crawl	62 male (12.8 ± 0.7) and 64 female highly trained and trained swimmers (12.0 ± 0.9 years)	Cable speedometer	3 × 25 m	Unreported conflicting interest Funded by Portuguese Science and Technology Foundation (SFRH/BD/76287/2011)

Table 2. Cont.

Study	Swimming Technique	Participants	Assessment	Protocol	Conflicting Interest and Funding
Figueiredo, et al. [92]	Front crawl	Thirteen trained swimmers (27.8 ± 10.9 years)	3D	30 min	Unreported
Komar, et al. [95]	Breaststroke	11 male and 7 female elite (20.8 ± 2.1) and recreational swimmers (20.4 ± 1.5 years)	3D	2 × 25 at maximal velocity + 4 × 25 m: 2 at 90 and 2 at 70% of the maximal velocity	Unreported conflicting interest Funded by CPER/GRR1880 Logistic Transport and Information Treatment 2007–2013
Matsuda, et al. [23]	Front crawl	7 elite (20.9 ± 0.9) and 9 highly trained swimmers (20.2 ± 1.6 years)	2D	30 m front crawl at 4 velocities: maximal velocity (Vmax) and 75, 85, and 95% Vmax	Unreported
Seifert, et al. [102]	Breaststroke	Seven highly trained swimmers (17.5 ± 2.2 years)	3D	3 × 200 m at 70% of their breast 200 m personal best	No conflicts of interest Unreported funding
Soares, et al. [107]	Front crawl	15 male (18.8 ± 2.4) and 13 female (16.5 ± 2.4 years) trained swimmers	Cable speedometer	50 m all-out	Unreported
Sanders, et al. [89]	Breaststroke	Two male elite swimmers (18 years)	3D	S1: 4 × 25 m front crawl maximal sprint. S2: 4 × 50 m front and back sprints	No conflicts of interest Unreported funding
Barbosa, et al. [85]	Backstroke, breaststroke, butterfly, front crawl	34 male (17.1 ± 4.1) and 34 female elite swimmers (15.0 ± 3.0 years)	Cable speedometer	Maximal 4 × 25 m	No conflicts of interest Funded by NIE acrf grant (RI11/13TB)
Dadashi, et al. [24]	Front crawl	13 and 5 female swimmers, 9 highly trained (19.3 ± 1.8) and 9 trained swimmers (16.0 ± 1.8 years)	Accelerometer	3 × 300 m at 70, 80 and 90% of their front-crawl 400 m personal best time with 6 min rest between trials	No conflicts of interest Unreported funding
De Jesus, et al. [28]	Front crawl	Ten male highly trained swimmers (19.8 ± 4.3 years)	3D	Intermittent incremental protocol of 7 × 200 m with increments of 0.05 m/s and 30 s resting intervals between steps	No conflicts of interest Funded by PTDC/DES/101224/2008 (FCOMP-01-0124-FEDER-009577) and CAPES /543110-7/2011
Figueiredo, et al. [116]	Front crawl	51 male and 52 female highly trained and trained swimmers (11.8 ± 0.8 years)	2D	25 m front crawl at a 50 m front crawl race pace	Unreported
Morais, et al. [98]	Front crawl	12 male (13.6 ± 0.7) and 15 female (13.2 ± 0.9 years) highly trained and trained swimmers	Cable speedometer	Maximal 3 × 25 m	Unreported

Table 2. Cont.

Study	Swimming Technique	Participants	Assessment	Protocol	Conflicting Interest and Funding
Seifert, et al. [101]	Front crawl	Five male elite swimmers (20.8 ± 3.2 years)	Cable speedometer	Three front crawl variants (with steps of 200, 300 and 400 m distances) incremental step test until exhaustion (with a 48 h rest period in-between)	Unreported Funded by PTDC/DES/101224/2008 (FCOMP-01-0124-FEDER-009577), CAPES/543110-7/2011 and Séneca Foundation 19615/EE/14.
Barbosa, et al. [114]	Backstroke, breaststroke, butterfly, front crawl	21 male and 4 female elite (15.7 ± 1.5), 11 male and 14 female highly trained (15.7 ± 3.6) and 18 male and 7 female recreational swimmers (22.9 ± 3.4 years)	Cable speedometer	Maximal 4 × 25 m	Unreported conflicts of interest Funded by NIE acrf grant (RI11/13TB)
Costa, et al. [109]	Backstroke, front crawl	Sixteen recreational swimmers (19.8 ± 1.1 years)	Cable speedometer	2 × 25 m	Unreported
Van Houwelingen, et al. [103]	Breaststroke	14 male and 12 female (20.0 ± 3.3 years) highly trained swimmers	2D	10 × 50 m (70% of the maximal velocity)	No conflicts of interest Funded by Stichting voor de Technische Weteschappen, grant number 12868
Barbosa, et al. [84]	Front crawl	12 male and 12 female recreational swimmers (22.4 ± 1.7 years)	Cable speedometer	All out 25 m freestyle pre (rest) and post (fatigue) test	No conflicts of interest Funded by NIE acrf grant (RI11/13TB)
Bartolomeu, et al. [122]	Backstroke, breaststroke, butterfly, front crawl	24 male and 25 highly trained and trained swimmers (14.2 ± 1.7 years)	Cable speedometer	Maximal 4 × 25 m	No conflicts of interest Funded by European Regional Development Fund [POCI-01-0145-FEDER-006969]; Portuguese Science and Technology Foundation [UID/DTP/04045/2013]
Gonjo, et al. [42]	Backstroke, front crawl	Ten male highly trained swimmers (17.5 ± 1.0 years)	3D	300 m at VO2 steady state	No conflicts of interest Funded by YAMAHA Motor Foundation for Sports (YMFS) International Sport Scholarship
Gourgoulis, et al. [17]	Breaststroke	Nine male trained swimmers (21.6 ± 4.2 years)	3D	25 m at maximal intensity	No conflicts of interest No funding

Table 2. *Cont.*

Study	Swimming Technique	Participants	Assessment	Protocol	Conflicting Interest and Funding
Morouço, et al. [88]	Front crawl	Nine male recreational swimmers (42.5 ± 9.5 years)	Cable speedometer	25 m at maximal intensity	Unreported conflicts of interest Funded by Portuguese Science and Technology Foundation (pest-OE/EME/UI4044/2013).
Morouço, et al. [99]	Front crawl	Twenty-two male highly trained swimmers (18.6 ± 2.4 years)	Cable speedometer	50 m time-trial	Unreported conflicts of interest Funded by Portuguese Science and Technology Foundation (UID/Multi/04044/2013)
Krylov, et al. [96]	Front crawl	Nine male elite swimmers (18.0–24.0 years)	2D	3 × 25 m self-selected pace at 100, 200 and 1500 m	No conflicts of interest Unreported funding
Silva, et al. [39] Silva, et al. [29]	Front crawl	Twenty-three male and 26 female trained swimmers (15.7 ± 0.8 and 14.5 ± 0.8 years)	3D	50 m at maximal velocity	No conflicts of interest Funded by Portuguese Science and Technology Foundation (SFRH/BD/87780/2012)
Correia, et al. [119]	Front crawl	Fourteen trained male swimmers (23.0 ± 5.0 years)	3D	200 simulating 400 m	No conflicts of interest Unreported funding
dos Santos, et al. [121]	Front crawl	Twenty trained swimmers (18.5 ± 3.9 years)	2D	Repeated 50 m maximum performance with 10 s interval	Unreported conflicts of interest No funding
Ruiz-Navarro, et al. [100]	Front crawl	Sixteen male trained swimmers (19.6 ± 3.3 years)	Cable speedometer	25, 50 and 100 m	Unreported conflicts of interest Funded by Ministry of Economy, Industry and Competitiveness (Spanish Agency of Research) and the European Regional Development Fund (ERDF); DEP2014-59707-P. Spanish Ministry of Education, Culture and Sport: FPU17/02761
Barbosa, et al. [124]	Front crawl	Fourteen male elite swimmers (25.7 ± 6.4 years)	Cable speedometer	25 m maximal sprint	No conflicts of interest Funded by Swedish Research Council
Barbosa, et al. [125]	Butterfly	One world-class male swimmer (26 years)	Cable speedometer	25 m maximal sprint	No conflicts of interest No funding
Engel, et al. [86]	Breaststroke	4 male (16 ± 0.7) and 6 female trained swimmers (14.9 ± 0.9 years)	Accelerometer	100 m moderate intensity	No conflicts of interest Funded by Federal Institute for Sports Science (ZMVI4-070804/19-21)

Table 2. Cont.

Study	Swimming Technique	Participants	Assessment	Protocol	Conflicting Interest and Funding
Morais, et al. [97]	Butterfly	10 male (15.4 ± 0.2) and 10 female (14.4 ± 0.2 years) highly trained swimmers	Cable speedometer	Three all outs	No conflicts of interest Funded by Portuguese Foundation for Science and Technology (UIDB/DTP/04045/2020)
Neiva, et al. [115]	Front crawl	16 male and 6 female recreational swimmers (39.9 ± 6.1 years)	Cable speedometer	2 × 25 m at maximal velocity	No conflicts of interest Funded by Portuguese Foundation for Science and Technology (UIDB04045/2020)
Fernandes, et al. [40]	Backstroke	12 male and 9 female swimmers, 16 elite (16.2 ± 1.0) and 15 trained (15.7 ± 1.3 years)	Cable speedometer	25 m at maximal velocity	No conflicts of interest Funded by Portuguese Science and Technology Foundation (2020.06799.BD)
Fernandes, et al. [41]	Front crawl	10 male (16.2 ± 1.8) and 17 female elite swimmers (18.3 ± 3.5 years)	Cable speedometer	25 m at maximal velocity	No conflicts of interest Funded by Portuguese Science and Technology Foundation (DFA/BD/6799/2020)

IVV was not the primary outcome in 31 trials but was included in a larger analysis, being described [127] and analysed together with anthropometric, kinematic, energetic, coordinative neuromuscular activity and other biomechanical variables [25,30,39,91,97,110,117,119]. Trials also related IVV with coordination [28,29,95], swimming economy [42,92], fatigue [28,29,95,121,128], technique [24,93,120] and velocity [125]. Thus, IVV was included in methodological approaches [15,16,89,96,100], dynamical systems approaches [85,102,114,122] and training interventional trials [29,98,101,109,115]. No conflicting interests were declared or were not addressed by 34 and 66% of the trials. Funding information was not reported by 54% of the trials, while 40% had financial support. Trials dissemination was growing over time (records were published every year) and 2016 was the year with the most publications (seven records).

3.3. Evidence Synthesis

The evaluation of the evidence gap map and trials' risk of bias can be accessed through the Supplementary File S1. IVV was assessed in 46 front crawl, 10 backstroke, 24 breaststroke and 14 butterfly-related trials, most of them focusing on mixed and male-only groups regarding swimmers' sex (56 and 39%, respectively). High-level swimmers were the most studied, followed by elite and trained, recreational, world-class and sedentary swimmers (37, 25, 26, 9, 3 and 1%, respectively), from which senior, youth and junior, young and master swimmers participated (50, 18, 18, 10 and 5%, respectively). Regarding the protocol intensity, most trials focused on swimming at sprint and severe intensities (36 and 19%), and fewer implemented incremental protocols that include other intensities (extreme, heavy, moderate and low: 11, 11, 12 and 11%, respectively). Trials conducted in swimming pool conditions were used 99% of the time.

Image- (47 and 53% in two and three dimensions) and mechanical-based methods were used (56 and 41%, respectively), with speedometers being mostly selected (82%). Velocity was calculated using an anatomical fixed point as a reference, most of the time with the hip chosen (and only twice selecting the head/neck) rather than the centre of mass (71 and 29%, respectively). The coefficient of variation was preferred regarding IVV quantification versus the difference between the maximum and minimum instantaneous velocity (dv; 61 and 7%, respectively), the ratio maximum and minimum instantaneous velocity difference/intracycle mean velocity (dv/v; 7%), the ratio of the mean velocity/difference between the maximal and minimum instantaneous velocity (3%) and other methods (such as cycle characterization, curves acceleration and dynamic indexes; 23%). Twenty-five trials reported variables associated with swimming economy (such stroke length and stroke index) and only two reported hydrodynamic drag related variables.

Front-crawl-related trials almost covered all secondary outcomes, even though gaps were identified for the four conventional swimming techniques. No trials were conducted with world-class swimmers focused on extreme, heavy, moderate and low intensities; used accelerometers; or quantified IVV with overall methods. Young swimmers were not used as samples in trials that were conducted at extreme and low swimming intensities, accelerometers were employed, and, when characterizing these age group IVV, its quantification was performed using only three methods. Master swimmers were not called to participate in protocols with extreme intensity and were not evaluated using accelerometers, while IVV quantification in this population was conducted only through the coefficient of variation. Trials using youth/junior, world-class, elite, highly trained and trained swimmers did not have associated IVV and hydrodynamic drag.

3.4. Study Results

Higher-level swimmers presented superior mean velocities for the same swimming intensity, but IVV was not related to swimming competitive levels or to the mean velocities regarding the four swimming techniques (Table 3). Except for front crawl, studies were mostly interested in analysing IVV when swimmers were performing at maximal intensity. IVV was not related to mean velocity in front crawl or backstroke [37,40,41,100], even if a non-linear relationship was also observed (with the velocity increase leading to a IVV decrease in young swimmers in the four swimming techniques [3] and in the swimmers with high-level front crawl [4]). Data gathered from so many swimmers and diverse samples should be cautiously analysed. Some outputs were obtained from a single trial performed at a specific swimming intensity, while others were gathered by averaging the data available. In addition, in some studies, swimmers from different competitive levels were pooled, and data were presented as a single group.

Table 3. Mean ± SD or median ± IQR mean velocity and IVV values obtained in the swimming trials included in the current study.

Swimming Technique	Competitive Level	Sprint	Extreme	Severe	Heavy	Moderate	Low
Backstroke	World class	-	-	-	-	-	-
	Elite	1.54 ± 0.11 m/s 13.18 ± 3.67%	-	1.29 ± 0.09 m/s 18.49 ± 2.44%	-	-	-
	Highly trained	1.19 ± 0.1 m/s 11.02 ± 4.17%	-	-	-	-	-
	Highly trained/trained	1.11 ± 0.63 m/s 6.99 ± 2.77%	-	-	-	-	-
	Recreational	0.96 ± 0.16 m/s 12.99 ± 4.94%	-	-	-	-	-
Breaststroke	World class	-	-	-	-	-	-
	Elite	1.23 ± 0.11 m/s 39.72 ± 4.47% 0.76 ± 0.18 m/s	-	1.04 ± 0.09 m/s 20.75 ± 4.8%	-	-	-
	Highly trained	1.35 ± 0.11 m/s 26.93 ± 3.38% 1.46 ± 0.33 m/s	-	-	-	-	0.92 ± 0.08 m/s 1.18 ± 0.22%
	Highly trained/trained	0.94 ± 0.11 m/s 45.34 ± 3.25% 0.81 ± 0.07 m/s	-	-	-	-	-
	Recreational	0.75 ± 0.20 m/s 41.19 ± 6.69%	-	-	-	-	-
Butterfly	World class	1.78 m/s 24.32%	-	-	-	-	-
	Elite	1.75 ± 0.09 m/s 21.86 ± 4.33%	-	1.21 ± 0.12 m/s 29.71 ± 7.54%	-	-	1.03–1.48 m/s 39.20 ± 11.50%
	Highly trained	1.15 (1.06–1.34) m/s 25.68 ± 14.72%	-	-	-	-	-
	Highly trained/trained	1.06 ± 0.16 m/s 26.98 ± 9.69%	-	-	-	-	-
	Trained	1.31 ± 0.10 m/s 27.87 ± 14.68%	1.29 ± 1.31 m/s 19.92 ± 22.48%	-	-	-	-
	Recreational	32.44 ± 6.92%	-	-	-	-	-
Front crawl	World Class	-	-	-	-	-	1.28 ± 0.11 m/s
	Elite	1.84 ± 0.06 m/s 12.30 ± 2.39%	1.52 ± 0.11 m/s 5.23 ± 1.77%	1.43 ± 0.54 m/s 11.76 ± 4.01%	1.53 ± 0.12 m/s 9.70 ± 3.49%	12%	6.87 ± 2.91%
	Elite/highly trained	1.80 ± 0.10 m/s 14.30 ± 2.40%	-	1.60 ± 0.10 m/s 14.10 ± 1.80%	1.40 ± 0.20 m/s 14.50 ± 1.60%	-	1.20 ± 0.20 m/s 14.30 ± 2.10%
	Highly trained	1.51 ± 0.16 m/s 6.99 ± 2.18%	1.74 ± 0.06 m/s 2.44 ± 0.74%	1.43 ± 0.13 m/s 8.62 ± 1.60%	1.40 ± 0.05 m/s 4.51 ± 0.2%	1.08 ± 0.06 m/s 0.17 ± 0.01%	1.11 ± 1.13 m/s 8.74 ± 15.67%
	Highly trained/trained	1.41 ± 0.14 m/s 5.24 ± 1.77%	-	1.06 ± 0.29 m/s 22 ± 6.50%	-	-	-
	Trained	1.36 ± 0.20 m/s 8.36 ± 2.28%	1.50 ± 0.08 m/s 9.20 ± 1.27%	1.30 ± 0.14 m/s 13.73 ± 2.89%	1.16 ± 0.11 m/s 9.25 ± 1.67%	1.06 ± 0.14 m/s 23 ± 5%	0.94 ± 0.76 m/s 15.83 ± 8.94%
	Recreational	1.28 ± 0.19 m/s 2.42 ± 0.78%	-	-	-	-	-

Legend: IVV quantified by dv/v is presented in the breaststroke row.

In breaststroke, IVV is usually quantified by dv/v (m/s), as presented in Equation (1), with vmax,LL as the maximum centre of mass's velocity achieved at the end of lower limb propulsion; vmin,LL as the first minimum peak of the centre of mass's velocity following upper and lower limbs recovery (corresponding to the beginning of lower limb propulsion); vmax,UL as the maximum centre of mass's velocity at the end of the upper limb propulsion; and vmin,T as the minimum centre of mass's velocity during the transition between upper and lower limb propulsion (corresponding to the centre of mass's velocity during gliding).

$$IVV = \frac{v_{max,LL} - v_{min,LL} + v_{max,UL} - v_{max,T}}{v_{mean}} \quad (1)$$

Some trials showed periodic velocity fluctuations related to the upper limbs' actions and the rate and the number of peaks per cycle, with a higher IVV range in lower- than in higher-level swimmers [7,104,118,127]. Furthermore, successful swimmers were able to more effectively combine intracycle peak velocity with relatively longer cycle periods [6]. When a front crawl technical training intervention period was conducted, IVV decreased [29,88,109] or did not change [98,115]. Although propulsive and drag forces were higher in swimmers of superior level, larger index of coordination values for front crawl were also presented even if IVV did not change across intensities [10,21,23,33,34,38,39], suggesting that better propulsive continuity allows a stable IVV [22,24–33]. Conversely, IVV increased throughout paces in less skilled swimmers [23]. IVV for highly trained swimmers was lower than for trained counterparts at all front crawl swimming velocities (in both senior and youth age groups) [23,39] but in backstroke, IVV did not differ between elite and highly trained swimmers [40].

IVV was directly related to swimming economy in the four swimming techniques [21,34,35,105,123,126] even though, in one study, no association between these variables was reported [90]. However, front crawl and backstroke IVV did not differ; nonetheless, lower energy cost values for front crawl vs. backstroke were observed [42], and they showed a tendency to decrease in a maximal lactate steady-state test [92]. Similarly, swimmers maintained their IVV values when performing at submaximal intensity, but IVV rose at maximal intensity [84,107,108,112,123,128], even though others described no changes [26,27,121]. This IVV increase with effort is probably justified by the progressive increase in fatigue, resulting in swimmers becoming less mechanically efficient. Swimmers with higher intracycle force variation also presented higher IVV values, leading to a progressive decrease in performance [94,99].

Methodological trials mainly assessed the relationship between the hip and the centre-of-mass kinematics to provide simpler methods to quantify IVV in swimming. It seems consensual that the hip does not adequately represent the centre of mass in intracycle variation in butterfly, breaststroke and front crawl. Some authors clearly state that this anatomic point should not be used in this kind of assessment [16,19,20] because it greatly overestimates the swimmer's real variation in velocity [15,17]. Other trials aimed to validate methods to quantify and express IVV [10,86,87,89,96]. When applying dynamical system approaches to swimming, nonlinear properties can be observed [114], with their magnitude differing according to the swimming technique and the swimmer's level. The breaststroke and butterfly techniques displayed more complex (but predictable) patterns [85,114,122] and elite vs. non-elite swimmers' performances were more unstable and complex (even though their IVV did not differ) [40].

4. Discussion

The current systematic scoping review focused on the IVV assessment in swimming that is retrospectively available for almost a century. The IVV-related trials' main interest is in the interactions between the cyclical propulsive and drag forces, which help understand the cyclic effectiveness of the upper and lower limbs while swimming and, consequently, swimmers' technical efficiency. In the first studies on IVV, breaststroke was the most studied swimming technique due to the simultaneity between the movements of the upper and lower limbs (which allowed researchers to easily identify when these movements were occurring) [6,118]. Then, new methodologies were developed, with researchers focusing their attention on the four conventional techniques, but our results showed that front crawl aroused greater interest. It is now accepted that the techniques with simultaneous movements (butterfly and breaststroke) present higher IVV than those with alternated movements (front crawl and backstroke) due to the mechanical impulses applied to the swimmer's body [3,114,122]. Furthermore, the alternated techniques' IVVs are very similar due to the biomechanical similarities between the front and back crawl (an "old" term used to designate backstroke) [42].

From the analysed trials, we could observe that male swimmers were the most studied even though mixed groups were also used due to the interest in checking differences between female and male swimmers (particularly regarding anthropometric characteristics [39,117], mechanical power output [6,33], technical proficiency and hydrodynamic profile [33,126]). Researchers focused their attention on trained, highly trained and elite swimmers, with the most elevated competitive levels being preferred for analysis. Most trials focused on senior swimmers, displaying strong confidence in results due to their experience. The same was not observed for trials conducted in master swimmers, with considerable gaps found, probably due to their heterogeneity of age and competitive level. Swimmers were mainly evaluated using maximal-intensity protocols to assess the kinematics directly related to the competitive events with the most participation (the 50 and 100 m distances). The 200 m distance was also often investigated, since its metabolic characteristics are important determinants of the kinematic variables' behaviour during these mixed aerobic–anaerobic events [4,37]. Few studies have focused on the backstroke, breaststroke and butterfly techniques at heavy, severe and extreme intensities.

The included trials used distinct evaluation protocols, with some analysing non-breathing cycles [15,24,26,27,31,32,85,93,96,104,105,119–121,127] and other not reporting the breathing condition or the inclusion of a specific space in which the participants were not allowed to breathe [3,6,10,16,17,19,21–25,30,31,33,36,37,42,85,87,88,90,91,93,95,104,107, 108,111,112,115,116,122,124,126,127]. Even though breathing was shown to lead to coordination asymmetry [129], upper-limb-cycle kinematics with individual breathing patterns presented IVV similarities to those in apnoea [41]. Data from trials that used a snorkel for assessing oxygen consumption should be carefully analysed [4,25,30,34,35,42,86,89–91,102,105,107,108,119,123]. Concerning the use of the hip vs. the centre of mass for assessing IVV, it was clear that the latter was the most reliable method to measure kinematical variables, although some authors still consider hip movements to provide a good IVV estimate [3,15]. These methods were previously compared with the hypothesis that the hip represented the centre of mass (and not the opposite), which was considered a priori the best methodology [15–17,19,20]. Future studies should clarify why the centre of mass is the gold standard considering the complexity of evaluation.

As a consequence of specific front crawl intervention protocols, IVV decreased or remained stable due to better swimming technique [6,102,106,111,113]. This also might have happened in other swimming techniques, with butterfly IVV decreasing when the hands' velocity at the end of the underwater path and the vertical velocity during the lower limbs' actions increased, and the velocity during the hands' entry decreased [111,113]. The hands, trunk and lower limbs role are also fundamental for lowering IVV [4,6,93,126]. Even though it is widely accepted that lower IVV should be achieved for enhanced performance, IVV has no standardized values and is highly variable according to the studied population and the methods used. Therefore, it would be very useful to implement more frequent intervention programs with strategies to upgrade swimmers' technique and overall performance.

Researchers have started to characterize swimming cycles' shape and number of peaks, developing quantification methods such as the absolute average velocity, root mean square [10], coefficient of variation and range of maximum and minimum velocities in a cycle [130]. Unfortunately, only one work compared these measurements [131], concluding that the coefficient of variation was the only approach sensitive to the mean swimming velocity and to the instantaneous velocity dispersion during the cycle. Mathematically, it is the more accurate method for IVV quantification but it may overestimate its value in breaststroke (due to this technique's complexity regarding mechanical impulses and coordination). Nevertheless, even this measure does not reflect the hydrodynamic drag characteristics, and it may be helpful to develop a new method of IVV determination.

Swimmers at a higher level present higher IVV values due to their capacity to generate and sustain the highest velocities (rather than being more economical), displaying larger amplitude of velocity [36,124]. However, breaststrokers eliminated in the preliminaries of a World Swimming Championships displayed higher IVV values than those that qualified for the semi-finals [127], probably as a result of a very low minimal instantaneous velocity (and not necessarily related to the maximal velocity value achieved within a cycle). In short distances, depending on the swimming technique, better swimmers find solutions to improve technical proficiency, producing high mechanical power to generate superior propulsive forces, reducing hydrodynamic drag, and adopting greater propulsive continuity [33,34,38,41], which will cause different IVV.

The quality of the trials included in the current study can be questioned due to the lack of detailed information and uncertainty of the evidence provided (being indeterminate whether it would result in a high or low risk of bias). Disregarding the already mentioned factors that influenced a high risk of bias, most variables were unclear because it the validity and reliability of the exposure measurement were not mentioned, nor were the blinding of the outcome assessment or even the information about whether swimmers belonged to a larger sample. In the scope of swimming, experimental protocols aim to replicate swimmers' performance and are not usually registered in databases. Furthermore, the current scoping review included trials since 1971 that were not as concerned about the studies' quality as is dictated today.

5. Study Limitations

The number of included trials highlighted the importance and utility of performing a systematic scoping review in swimming IVV. We believe that including the Proceedings Books of the Biomechanics and Medicine in Swimming Symposia strengthened our work, since this book series contains several important documents that added relevant information to the current review. This research aimed to provide an overall representation of the IVV scope of competitive swimming, but we recognize that considering IVV calculations in conditions such as using snorkelling or swimming with/without breathing could affect its interpretation. For sake of the clarity, those studies were properly identified.

6. Conclusions

The current study compiles the studies available on the topic of the swimming IVV in the most respected and well-known literature databases. We have described the literature gaps and the most interesting IVV-related topics within almost the past century. IVV was often used in front-crawl-related studies, involving mixed samples and senior swimmers that performed at sprint intensity in swimming pools and were evaluated with cable speedometer using an anatomical fixed point as a reference and that quantified IVV using the coefficient of variation. There is a clear need for investigating backstroke, breaststroke and butterfly swimming techniques performed at heavy, severe and extreme intensities. Since these paces correspond to the characteristics of the official competitive events, it would be imperative to assess them more often. Young and youth swimmers were less studied, even though their performance development in swimming is important in their training process throughout their careers. It would be very helpful to evaluate world-class swimmers as well to acknowledge the top-level performers' behaviour. Although there is no proof that the coefficient of variation is the best measure to assess IVV, researchers generally agreed that it best reflects the velocity fluctuations in swimming.

7. Future Directions

Future investigations should cover the gaps found in the current study to allow for meaningful results and possible comparisons. IVV measurements should be revised, and a new approach that accounts for hydrodynamic characteristics is welcome to standardize results according to these factors. Future research should strive to reduce the risk of bias by (i) attending to a balance between female and male swimmers, looking for better sample homogeneity; (ii) providing important personal characteristics; (iii) controlling the evaluation conditions; (iv) providing the software validity and reliability; (v) blinding the outcome evaluators; (vi) providing data on the inter-evaluator reliability of outcome measurement or measures of error for the methodologies used (when applicable); (vii) providing information about whether swimmers are part of larger samples; and (viii) pre-registering the research protocols.

Supplementary Materials: The following supporting information can be downloaded at: https://www.mdpi.com/article/10.3390/bioengineering10030308/s1, File S1: Evidence Gap Map.

Author Contributions: Conceptualization, A.F., J.A., F.N., B.M., J.P.V.-B. and R.J.F.; Methodology, A.F., J.A. and B.M.; Formal analysis and investigation A.F., J.A., F.N., B.M. and R.J.F.; Resources, J.P.V.-B. and R.J.F.; Writing—original draft preparation, A.F.; Writing—review and editing, A.F., J.A., F.N., B.M., J.P.V.-B. and R.J.F.; Supervision B.M., J.P.V.-B. and R.J.F.; Project administration, A.F., J.P.V.-B. and R.J.F.; Funding acquisition, J.P.V.-B. and R.J.F. All authors have read and agreed to the published version of the manuscript.

Funding: This research was funded by Fundação para a Ciência e Tecnologia, grant number 2020.06799.BD.

Institutional Review Board Statement: The study was conducted in accordance with the Declaration of Helsinki and approved by the Ethics Committee of Faculty of Sport of University of Porto (CEFADE 24 2020, 11 November 2020).

Informed Consent Statement: Not applicable.

Data Availability Statement: Not applicable.

Acknowledgments: We would like to acknowledge the support of Daniel Daly and Flávio Castro for their role as external experts. They verified our eligibility criteria and our list of included studies, suggesting additional potentially relevant studies. This acknowledgement was consented by them.

Conflicts of Interest: The authors declare no conflict of interest.

References

1. Karpovich, P.V. Swimming Speed Analyzed. *Sci. Am.* **1930**, *142*, 224–225. [CrossRef]
2. Kent, M.R.; Atha, J. A device for the on-line measurement of instantaneous swimming velocity. *Int. Ser. Sport Sci.* **1975**, *2*, 58–63.
3. Barbosa, T.M.; Morouço, P.G.F.; Jesus, S.; Feitosa, W.G.; Costa, M.J.; Marinho, D.A.; Silva, A.J.; Garrido, N.D. The interaction between intra-cyclic variation of the velocity and mean swimming velocity in young competitive swimmers. *Int. J. Sport. Med.* **2013**, *34*, 123–130. [CrossRef]
4. Figueiredo, P.; Kjendlie, P.L.; Vilas-Boas, J.P.; Fernandes, R.J. Intracycle velocity variation of the body centre of mass in front crawl. *Int. J. Sport. Med.* **2012**, *33*, 285–290. [CrossRef]
5. Karpovich, P.V.; Karpovich, G.P. Magnetic Tape Natograph. *Res. Q Am. Assoc. Health Phys. Educ.* **1970**, *41*, 119–122. [CrossRef]
6. Manley, P.; Atha, J. Intra-stroke velocity fluctuations in paced breastsroke swimming. In *Biomechanics and Medicine in Swimming. Swimming Science VI*; Taylor & Francis Group: Abingdon, UK, 1992; pp. 151–160.
7. Miyashita, M. An analysis of fluctuations of swimming speed. In Proceedings of the First International Symposium on "Biomechanics and Swimming, Waterpolo and Diving", Bruxelles, Belgien, 14–16 September 1970; pp. 53–58.
8. Costill, D.; Lee, G.; D'Acquisto, L.J. Video-computer assisted analysis of swimming technique. *J. Swim. Res.* **1987**, *3*, 5–9.
9. Craig, A.B., Jr.; Pendergast, D.R. Relationships of stroke rate, distance per stroke, and velocity in competitive swimming. *Med. Sci. Sport.* **1979**, *11*, 278–283. [CrossRef]
10. Holmer, I. Analysis of acceleration as a measure of swimming proficiency. In *Proceedings of the International Symposium of Biomechanics in Swimming, Edmonton, AB, Canada*; University Park Press: Baltimore, MD, USA, 1979; pp. 118–124.
11. Boicev, K.; Tzvetkov, A. Instrumentation and methods for the complex investigations of swimming. *Int. Ser. Sport. Sci.* **1975**, *2*, 80–89.
12. Dal Monte, A. Presenting an apparatus for motion picture, television and scan shots of the movement of swimming. In *Swimming I*; Lewillie, L., Clarys, J.P., Eds.; Université Libre de Bruxelles: Bruxelles, Belgium, 1971; pp. 127–128.
13. Mcintyre, D.R.; Hay, J.G. Dual media cinematography. In *Swimming II*; Clarys, J.P., Lewillie, L., Eds.; University Park Press: Baltimore, MD, USA, 1975; pp. 51–57.
14. Vertommen, L.; Fauvart, H.; Clarys, J.P. *A Simple System for Underwater Video Filming*; Human Kinetics Publishers: Champaign, IL, USA, 1983; Volume 14, pp. 120–122.
15. Fernandes, R.; Ribeiro, J.; Figueiredo, P.; Seifert, L.; Vilas-Boas, J. Kinematics of the hip and body center of mass in front crawl. *J. Hum. Kinet.* **2012**, *33*, 15–23. [CrossRef]
16. Figueiredo, P.; Vilas Boas, J.P.; Maia, J.; Gonçalves, P.; Fernandes, R.J. Does the hip reflect the centre of mass swimming kinematics? *Int. J. Sport. Med.* **2009**, *30*, 779–781. [CrossRef]
17. Gourgoulis, V.; Koulexidis, S.; Gketzenis, P.; Tzouras, G. Intracyclic velocity variation of the center of mass and hip in breaststroke swimming with maximal intensity. *J. Strength Cond. Res.* **2018**, *32*, 830–840. [CrossRef] [PubMed]
18. Maglischo, C.W.; Maglischo, E.W.; Santos, T.R. The relationship between the forward velocity of the centre of gravity and the hip in the four competitive strokes. *J. Swim. Res.* **1987**, *3*, 11–17.

19. Barbosa, T.; Santos Silva, V.; Sousa, F.; Vilas-Boas, J.P. Comparative study of the response of kinematical variables from the hip and the center of mass in butterfliers. In Proceedings of the IXth International World Symposium on Biomechanics and Medicine in Swimming, Saint Etiénne, France, 21–22 June 2002; Université de Saint Etiénne: Saint Etiénne, France, 2003; pp. 93–98.
20. Psycharakis, S.G.; Sanders, R.H. Validity of the use of a fixed point for intracycle velocity calculations in swimming. *J. Sci. Med. Sport.* **2009**, *12*, 262–265. [CrossRef] [PubMed]
21. Barbosa, T.M.; Lima, F.; Portela, A.; Novais, D.; Machado, L.; Colaço, P.; Goncalves, R.F.; Keskinen, K.L.; Vilas-Boas, J.P. Relationships between energy cost, swimming velocity and speed fluctuation in competitive swimming strokes. In *Proceedings of the Biomechanics and Medicine in Swimming X*; Porto Faculdade de Desporto da Universidade do Porto: Porto, Portugal, 2006; pp. 192–194.
22. Schnitzler, C.; Ernwein, V.; Seifert, L.; Chollet, D. Use of index of coordination to assess optimal adaptation: A case study. In *Proceedings of the Biomechanics and Medicine in Swimming X*; Porto Faculdade de Desporto da Universidade do Porto: Porto, Portugal, 2006; pp. 257–259.
23. Matsuda, Y.; Yamada, Y.; Ikuta, Y.; Nomura, T.; Oda, S. Intracyclic velocity variation and arm coordination for different skilled swimmers in the front crawl. *J. Hum. Kinet.* **2014**, *44*, 67–74. [CrossRef]
24. Dadashi, F.; Millet, G.P.; Aminian, K. Front-crawl stroke descriptors variability assessment for skill characterization. *J. Sport. Sci.* **2016**, *34*, 1405–1412. [CrossRef]
25. Figueiredo, P.; Sousa, A.; Gonçalves, P.; Suzana, P.; Susana, S.; Vilas-Boas, J.P.; Fernandes, R.J. Biophysical analysis of the 200m front crawl swimming: A case study. In Proceedings of the XIth International Symposium for Biomechanics and Medicine, Oslo, Norway, 16–19 June 2010; pp. 79–81.
26. Alberty, M.; Sidney, M.; Hespel, J.M.; Dekerle, J. Effects of an exhaustive exercise on upper limb coordination and intracyclic velocity variations in front crawl stroke. In *Proceedings of the IXth World Symposium on Biomechanics and Medicine in Swimming*; Université de Saint-Etienne: Saint-Etienne, France, 2003; pp. 81–85.
27. Alberty, M.; Sidney, M.; Huot-Marchand, F.; Hespel, J.M.; Pelayo, P. Intracyclic velocity variations and arm coordination during exhaustive exercise in front crawl stroke. *Int. J. Sport. Med.* **2005**, *26*, 471–475. [CrossRef]
28. De Jesus, K.; Sanders, R.; De Jesus, K.; Ribeiro, J.; Figueiredo, P.; Vilas-Boas, J.P.; Fernandes, R.J. The effect of intensity on 3-dimensional kinematics and coordination in front-crawl swimming. *Int. J. Sport. Physiol. Perform.* **2016**, *11*, 768–775. [CrossRef]
29. Silva, A.F.; Figueiredo, P.; Vilas-Boas, J.P.; Fernandes, R.J.; Seifert, L. The Effect of a Coordinative Training in Young Swimmers' Performance. *Int. J. Environ. Res. Public Health* **2022**, *19*, 7020. [CrossRef]
30. Figueiredo, P.; Toussaint, H.M.; Vilas-Boas, J.P.; Fernandes, R.J. Relation between efficiency and energy cost with coordination in aquatic locomotion. *Eur. J. Appl. Physiol.* **2013**, *113*, 651–659. [CrossRef]
31. Gourgoulis, V.; Aggeloussis, N.; Boli, A.; Michalopoulou, M.; Toubekis, A.; Kasimatis, P.; Vezos, N.; Mavridis, G.; Antoniou, P.; Mavrommatis, G. Inter-arm coordination and intra-cyclic variation of the hip velocity during front crawl resisted swimming. *J. Sport. Med. Phys. Fit.* **2013**, *53*, 612–619.
32. Schnitzler, C.; Seifert, L.; Alberty, M.; Chollet, D. Hip velocity and arm coordination in front crawl swimming. *Int. J. Sport. Med.* **2010**, *31*, 875–881. [CrossRef] [PubMed]
33. Schnitzler, C.; Seifert, L.; Ernwein, V.; Chollet, D. Arm coordination adaptations assessment in swimming. *Int. J. Sport. Med.* **2008**, *29*, 480–486. [CrossRef] [PubMed]
34. Barbosa, T.M.; Keskinen, K.L.; Fernandes, R.; Colaço, P.; Lima, A.B.; Vilas-Boas, J.P. Energy cost and intracyclic variation of the velocity of the centre of mass in butterfly stroke. *Eur. J. Appl. Physiol.* **2005**, *93*, 519–523. [CrossRef] [PubMed]
35. Vilas-Boas, J.P. Speed fluctuations and energy cost of different breaststroke techniques. In *Proceedings of the Biomechanics and Medicine in Swimming VII*; Routledge: Liverpool, UK, 1996; pp. 167–171.
36. Leblanc, H.; Seifert, L.; Tourny-Chollet, C.; Chollet, D. Intra-cyclic distance per stroke phase, velocity fluctuations and acceleration time ratio of a breaststroker's hip: A comparison between elite and nonelite swimmers at different race paces. *Int. J. Sport. Med.* **2007**, *28*, 140–147. [CrossRef]
37. Psycharakis, S.G.; Naemi, R.; Connaboy, C.; McCabe, C.; Sanders, R.H. Three-dimensional analysis of intracycle velocity fluctuations in frontcrawl swimming. *Scand. J. Med. Sci. Sport.* **2010**, *20*, 128–135. [CrossRef]
38. Alves, F.; Gomes Pereira, J.; Pereira, F. Determinants of energy cost of front crawl and backstroke swimming and competitive performance. In *Proceedings of the Biomechanics and Medicine in Swimming VII*; Routledge: Liverpool, UK, 1996; pp. 185–191.
39. Silva, A.F.; Ribeiro, J.; Vilas-Boas, J.P.; Figueiredo, P.; Alves, F.; Seifert, L.; Fernandes, R.J. Integrated analysis of young swimmers' sprint performance. *Mot. Control.* **2019**, *23*, 354–364. [CrossRef]
40. Fernandes, A.; Goethel, M.; Marinho, D.A.; Mezencio, B.; Vilas-Boas, J.P.; Fernandes, R.J. Velocity Variability and Performance in Backstroke in Elite and Good-Level Swimmers. *Int. J. Env. Res. Public Health* **2022**, *19*, 6744. [CrossRef]
41. Fernandes, A.; Mezêncio, B.; Soares, S.; Duarte Carvalho, D.; Silva, A.; Vilas-Boas, J.P.; Fernandes, R.J. Intra- and inter-cycle velocity variations in sprint front crawl swimming. *Sport. Biomech.* **2022**, 1–14. [CrossRef]
42. Gonjo, T.; McCabe, C.; Sousa, A.; Ribeiro, J.; Fernandes, R.J.; Vilas-Boas, J.P.; Sanders, R. Differences in kinematics and energy cost between front crawl and backstroke below the anaerobic threshold. *Eur. J. Appl. Physiol.* **2018**, *118*, 1107–1118. [CrossRef]
43. Vilas-Boas, J.P.; Fernandes, R.J.; Barbosa, T.M. Intra-cycle velocity variations, swimming economy, performance, and training in swimming. In *The World Book of Swimming: From Science to Performance*; Nova Science Publishers, Hauppauge: New York, NY, USA, 2011; pp. 119–134.

44. Page, M.J.; McKenzie, J.E.; Bossuyt, P.M.; Boutron, I.; Hoffmann, T.C.; Mulrow, C.D.; Shamseer, L.; Tetzlaff, J.M.; Akl, E.A.; Brennan, S.E.; et al. The PRISMA 2020 statement: An updated guideline for reporting systematic reviews. *BMJ* **2021**, *372*, n71. [CrossRef]
45. Tricco, A.C.; Lillie, E.; Zarin, W.; O'Brien, K.K.; Colquhoun, H.; Levac, D.; Moher, D.; Peters, M.D.J.; Horsley, T.; Weeks, L.; et al. PRISMA Extension for Scoping Reviews (PRISMA-ScR): Checklist and Explanation. *Ann. Intern. Med.* **2018**, *169*, 467–473. [CrossRef] [PubMed]
46. Higgins, J.; Thomas, J.; Chandler, J.; Cumpston, M.; Li, T.; Page, M.; Welch, V. *Cochrane Handbook for Systematic Reviews of Interventions*; Wiley Online Library: Hoboken, NJ, USA, 2019. [CrossRef]
47. McKay, A.K.A.; Stellingwerff, T.; Smith, E.S.; Martin, D.T.; Mujika, I.; Goosey-Tolfrey, V.L.; Sheppard, J.; Burke, L.M. Defining Training and Performance Caliber: A Participant Classification Framework. *Int. J. Sport. Physiol. Perform.* **2022**, *17*, 317–331. [CrossRef]
48. Kim, S.Y.; Park, J.E.; Lee, Y.J.; Seo, H.J.; Sheen, S.S.; Hahn, S.; Jang, B.H.; Son, H.J. Testing a tool for assessing the risk of bias for nonrandomized studies showed moderate reliability and promising validity. *J. Clin. Epidemiol.* **2013**, *66*, 408–414. [CrossRef] [PubMed]
49. Rohatgi, A. *WebPlotDigitizer*, version 4.5; Pacifica, CA, USA, 2021.
50. de Jesus, K.; de Jesus, K.; Figueiredo, P.A.; Goncalves, P.; Vilas-Boas, J.P.; Fernandes, R.J. Kinematical Analysis of Butterfly Stroke: Comparison of Three Velocity Variants. In Proceedings of the Biomechanics and Medicine in Swimming XI, Oslo, Norway, 16–19 June 2010; p. 92.
51. Buchner, M.; Reischle, K. Measurements of the horizontal intracyclical acceleration in competitive swimming with a newly developed accelometer-goniometer-device. In Proceedings of the Biomechanics and Medicine in Swimming IX, Saint-Etienne, France, 21–23 June 2002; pp. 57–62.
52. Dominguez-Castells, R.; Izquierdo, M.; Arellano, R. An updated protocol to assess arm swimming power in front crawl. *Int. J. Sport. Med.* **2013**, *34*, 324–329. [CrossRef]
53. Kovalchuk, V.; Mospan, M.; Smoliar, I.; Tolkunova, I.; Adyrkhaeva, L.; Kolumbet, A. Optimization of the process of technical fitness management of highly skilled swimmers. *J. Phys. Educ. Sport.* **2021**, *21*, 2507–2514. [CrossRef]
54. Seifert, L.; Toussaint, H.; Schnitzler, C.; Alberty, M.; Chavallard, F.; Lemaitre, F.; Vantorre, J.; Chollet, D. Effect of velocity increase on arm coordination, active drag and intra-cyclic velocity variations in front crawl. In *The Book of Proceedings of the 1st International Scientific Conference of Aquatic Space Activities*; University of Tsukuba: Tsukaba, Japan, 2008; pp. 254–259.
55. Seifert, L.; Toussaint, H.M.; Alberty, M.; Schnitzler, C.; Chollet, D. Arm coordination, power, and swim efficiency in national and regional front crawl swimmers. *Hum. Mov. Sci.* **2010**, *29*, 426–439. [CrossRef] [PubMed]
56. Tsunokawa, T.; Nakashima, M.; Takagi, H. Use of pressure distribution analysis to estimate fluid forces around a foot during breaststroke kicking. *Sport. Eng.* **2015**, *18*, 149–156. [CrossRef]
57. Alberty, M.; Sidney, M.; Pelayo, P.; Toussaint, H.M. Stroking characteristics during time to exhaustion tests. *Med. Sci. Sport. Exerc.* **2009**, *41*, 637–644. [CrossRef]
58. Cohen, R.C.Z.; Cleary, P.W.; Mason, B.R.; Pease, D.L. Studying the effects of asymmetry on freestyle swimming using smoothed particle hydrodynamics. *Comput. Methods Biomech. Biomed. Engin.* **2020**, *23*, 271–284. [CrossRef]
59. Ruiz-Navarro, J.J.; Cano-Adamuz, M.; Andersen, J.T.; Cuenca-Fernández, F.; López-Contreras, G.; Vanrenterghem, J.; Arellano, R. Understanding the effects of training on underwater undulatory swimming performance and kinematics. *Sport. Biomech.* **2021**, 1–16. [CrossRef]
60. Schnitzler, C.; Ernwein, V.; Seifert, L.; Chollet, D. Intracyclic velocity signal as a tool to evaluate propulsive phase duration. In *Proceedings of the Biomechanics and Medicine in Swimming X*; Porto Faculdade de Desporto da Universidade do Porto: Porto, Portugal, 2006; pp. 88–90.
61. Seifert, L.; Leblanc, H.; Chollet, D.; Delignières, D. Inter-limb coordination in swimming: Effect of speed and skill level. *Hum. Mov. Sci.* **2010**, *29*, 103–113. [CrossRef] [PubMed]
62. Strzala, M.; Krezalek, P.; Glab, G.; Kaca, M.; Ostrowski, A.; Stanula, A.; Tyka, A.K. Intra-Cyclic Phases of Arm-Leg Movement and Index of Coordination in Relation to Sprint Breaststroke Swimming in Young Swimmers. *J. Sport. Sci. Med.* **2013**, *12*, 690–697.
63. Valkoumas, I.; Gourgoulis, V.; Aggeloussis, N.; Antoniou, P. The influence of an 11-week resisted swim training program on the inter-arm coordination in front crawl swimmers. *Sport. Biomech.* **2020**. [CrossRef]
64. Dos Santos, K.B.; Lara, J.P.R.; Rodacki, A.L.F. Reproducibility and Repeatability of Intracyclic Velocity Variation in Front Crawl Swimming from Manual and Semi-Automatic Measurement. *Hum. Mov. Sci.* **2017**, *18*, 55–59. [CrossRef]
65. Barbosa, T.; Costa, M.; Morais, J.; Jesus, S.; Marques, M.; Batista, J.; Gonçalves, J. Conception, development and validation of a software interface to assess human's horizontal intra-cyclic velocity with a mechanical speedo-meter. In Proceedings of the XXIIIrd Congress of the International Society of Biomechanics, Brussels, Belgium, 3–7 July 2011.
66. Mosunov, D.F. The method of application analysis of intracyclic speed in swimming. *Adapt. Fiz. Kul'tura* **2013**, *4*, 56–64.
67. Fujishima, M.; Miyashita, M. Velocity degradation caused by its fluctuation in swimming and guidelines for improvement of average velocity. In *Proceedings of the Biomechanics and Medicine in Swimming VIII*; University of Jyvaskyla: Jyväskylä, Finland, 1999; pp. 41–45.
68. Gonjo, T.; Olstad, B. Body wave characteristics and variability of an international and a regional swimmer in 50 m butterfly swimming. *ISBS Proc. Arch.* **2020**, *38*, 200.

69. Ichikawa, H.; Ohgi, Y.; Miyaji, C. Analysis of stroke of the freestyle swimming using accelerometer. In *Proceedings of the Biomechanics and Medicine in Swimming VIII*; University of Jyvaskyla: Jyväskylä, Finland, 1999; pp. 159–164.
70. Kornecki, S.; Bober, T. Extreme velocities of a swimming cycle as a technique criterion. In *Swimming Medicine IV*; Erifsson, B., Furberg, B., Eds.; University Park Press: Baltimore, MD, USA, 1978; pp. 402–407.
71. Krylov, A.; Boutov, A.; Wendt, G. Natatometer. Real-Time Intra-Cycle Velocity Data for Swimming Stroke Correction. *Uchenye Zap. Univ. Im. P.F. Lesgafta* **2014**, *113*, 109–113. [CrossRef]
72. Krylov, A.; Butov, A.; Vinogradov, E. Metrological analysis of method "natatometry" at the study of inside cycle speed of swimming. *Uchenye zapiski universiteta imeni P.F. Lesgafta* **2018**, 156–162. Available online: https://cyberleninka.ru/article/n/metrologicheskiy-analiz-metoda-natatometriya-pri-izuchenii-vnutritsiklovoy-skorosti-plavaniya/viewer (accessed on 23 December 2022).
73. Martins-Silva, A.; Alves, F. Determinant factors to variation in butterfly velocity. In Proceedings of the XVIII International Symposium on Biomechanics in Sports—Swimming, Hong Kong, China, 25–30 June 2000; Faculty of Education of the University of Edinburgh,: Edinburg, UK, 2000; pp. 73–74.
74. Vilas-Boas, J.P.; Cunha, P.; Figueiras, T.; Ferreira, M.; Duarte, J. Movement analysis in simultaneous swimming techniques. In *Proceedings of the Cologne Swimming Symposium*; Sport-Fahnemann: Bockenem, Germany, 1997; pp. 95–103.
75. Barbosa, T.; Costa, M.; Morais, J.; Jesus, S.; Silva, A.; Batista, J.; Gonçalves, J. Validation of an integrated system to assess horizontal intra-cyclic velocity with a mechanical speedo-meter. *Rev. Port. Cien. Desp.* **2011**, *11*, 833–835.
76. Tourny, C.; Chollet, D.; Micallef, J.P.; Macabies, J. Comparative analysis of studies of speed variations within a breaststroke cycle. In *Proceedings of the Biomechanics and Medicine in Swimming VI*; London E & FN Spon: London, UK, 1992; pp. 161–166.
77. Bideault, G.; Herault, R.; Seifert, L. Data modelling reveals inter-individual variability of front crawl swimming. *J. Sci. Med. Sport.* **2013**, *16*, 281–285. [CrossRef]
78. Dadashi, F.; Crettenand, F.; Millet, G.P.; Aminian, K. Front-crawl instantaneous velocity estimation using a wearable inertial measurement unit. *Sensors* **2012**, *12*, 12927–12939. [CrossRef]
79. Ganzevles, S.; Beek, P.J.; Daanen, H.A.M.; Coolen, B.M.A.; Truijens, M.J. Differences in swimming smoothness between elite and non-elite swimmers. *Sport. Biomech.* **2019**. [CrossRef] [PubMed]
80. Huot-Marchand, F.; Nesi, X.; Sidney, M.; Alberty, M.; Pelayo, P. Variations of stroking parameters associated with 200 m competitive performance improvement in top-standard front crawl swimmers. *Sport. Biomech.* **2005**, *4*, 89–99. [CrossRef] [PubMed]
81. McCabe, C.B.; Psycharakis, S.; Sanders, R. Kinematic differences between front crawl sprint and distance swimmers at sprint pace. *J. Sport. Sci.* **2011**, *29*, 115–123. [CrossRef] [PubMed]
82. Morouço, P.; Lima, A.B.; Semblano, P.; Fernandes, D.; Gonçalves, P.; Sousa, F.; Fernandes, R.; Barbosa, T.M.; Correia, M.V.; Vilas-Boas, J.P. Validation of a cable speedometer for butterfly evaluation. *Rev. Port. Cien. Desp.* **2006**, *6*, 236–239.
83. Sanders, R.H.; Button, C.; McCabe, C.B. Variability of upper body kinematics in a highly constrained task—Sprint swimming. *Eur. J. Sport. Sci.* **2019**, *20*, 624–632. [CrossRef] [PubMed]
84. Barbosa, T.M.; Chen, S.; Morais, J.E.; Costa, M.J.; Batalha, N. The changes in classical and nonlinear parameters after a maximal bout to elicit fatigue in competitive swimming. *Hum. Mov. Sci.* **2018**, *58*, 321–329. [CrossRef]
85. Barbosa, T.M.; Goh, W.X.; Morais, J.E.; Costa, M.J.; Pendergast, D. Comparison of Classical Kinematics, Entropy, and Fractal Properties as Measures of Complexity of the Motor System in Swimming. *Front. Psychol.* **2016**, *7*, 1566. [CrossRef]
86. Engel, A.; Ploigt, R.; Mattes, K.; Schaffert, N. Intra-cyclic analysis of the breaststroke swimming technique using an inertial measurement unit. *J. Sport. Hum. Perform.* **2021**, *9*, 33–50. [CrossRef]
87. Feitosa, W.G.; Costa, M.J.; Morais, J.E.; Garrido, N.M.d.F.; Silva, A.J.; Lima, A.B.; Barbosa, T.M. A mechanical speedo-meter to assess swimmer's horizontal intra-cyclic velocity: Validation at front-crawl and backstroke. In Proceedings of the International Society of Biomechanics, Natal, Brazil, 4–9 August 2013.
88. Morouço, P.; Ribeiro, J.; Soares, S.; Fernandes, R.; Abraldes, J.A. Efeitos de um mesociclo de treino na velocidade média e variação intracíclica da velocidade de nadadores masters. *Rev. Port. De Ciências Do Desporto* **2018**, *18*, 58–69. [CrossRef]
89. Sanders, R.H.; Gonjo, T.; McCabe, C.B. Reliability of Three-Dimensional Linear Kinematics and Kinetics of Swimming Derived from Digitized Video at 25 and 50 Hz with 10 and 5 Frame Extensions to the 4(th) Order Butterworth Smoothing Window. *J. Sport. Sci. Med.* **2015**, *14*, 441–451.
90. Figueiredo, P.; Barbosa, T.M.; Vilas-Boas, J.P.; Fernandes, R.J. Energy cost and body centre of mass' 3D intracycle velocity variation in swimming. *Eur. J. Appl. Physiol.* **2012**, *112*, 3319–3326. [CrossRef]
91. Figueiredo, P.; Pendergast, D.R.; Vilas-Boas, J.P.; Fernandes, R.J. Interplay of Biomechanical, Energetic, Coordinative, and Muscular Factors in a 200 m Front Crawl Swim. *Biomed. Res. Int.* **2013**, *2013*, 897232. [CrossRef] [PubMed]
92. Figueiredo, P.; Nazario, R.; Sousa, M.; Pelarigo, J.G.; Vilas-Boas, J.P.; Fernandes, R. Kinematical analysis along maximal lactate steady state swimming intensity. *J. Sport. Sci. Med.* **2014**, *13*, 610–615.
93. Gourgoulis, V.; Boli, A.; Aggeloussis, N.; Toubekis, A.; Antoniou, P.; Kasimatis, P.; Vezos, N.; Michalopoulou, M.; Kambas, A.; Mavromatis, G. The effect of leg kick on sprint front crawl swimming. *J. Sport. Sci.* **2014**, *32*, 278–289. [CrossRef] [PubMed]
94. D'Acquisto, L.J.; Costill, D.L. Relationships between intracyclic linear body velocity fluctuations, power, and sprint breaststroke performance. *J. Swim. Res.* **1998**, *13*, 8–14.

95. Komar, J.; Sanders, R.H.; Chollet, D.; Seifert, L. Do qualitative changes in interlimb coordination lead to effectiveness of aquatic locomotion rather than efficiency? *J. Appl. Biomech.* **2014**, *30*, 189–196. [CrossRef]
96. Krylov, A.I.; Gorelov, A.A.; Tretyakov, A.A. Integral indicators of the swimming techniques effectiveness of highly qualified crawl-stroke swimmers. *Pedagog. Psychol. Med.-Biol. Probl. Phys. Train. Sport.* **2019**, *23*, 169–175. [CrossRef]
97. Morais, J.; Barbosa, T.M.; Lopes, V.P.; Marques, M.C.; Marinho, D.A. Propulsive Force of Upper Limbs and its Relationship to Swim Velocity in the Butterfly Stroke. *Int. J. Sport. Med.* **2021**, *42*, 1105–1112. [CrossRef] [PubMed]
98. Morais, J.E.; Silva, A.J.; Marinho, D.A.; Marques, M.C.; Barbosa, T.M. Effect of a specific concurrent water and dry-land training over a season in young swimmers' performance. *Int. J. Perform. Anal. Sport.* **2016**, *16*, 760–775. [CrossRef]
99. Morouço, P.G.; Barbosa, T.M.; Arellano, R.; Vilas-Boas, J.P. Intracyclic variation of force and swimming performance. *Int. J. Sport. Physiol. Perform.* **2018**, *13*, 897–902. [CrossRef]
100. Ruiz-Navarro, J.J.; Morouço, P.G.; Arellano, R. Relationship between tethered swimming in a flume and swimming performance. *Int. J. Sport. Physiol. Perform.* **2020**, *15*, 1087–1094. [CrossRef] [PubMed]
101. Seifert, L.; Jesus, K.; Komar, J.; Ribeiro, J.; Abraldes, J.A.; Figueiredo, P.; Vilas-Boas, J.P.; Fernandes, R.J. Behavioural variability and motor performance: Effect of practice specialization in front crawl swimming. *Hum. Mov. Sci.* **2016**, *47*, 141–150. [CrossRef] [PubMed]
102. Seifert, L.; Komar, J.; Crettenand, F.; Millet, G. Coordination pattern adaptability: Energy cost of degenerate behaviors. *PLoS ONE* **2014**, *9*, e107839. [CrossRef] [PubMed]
103. Van Houwelingen, J.; Roerdink, M.; Huibers, A.V.; Evers, L.L.W.; Beek, P.J. Pacing the phasing of leg and arm movements in breaststroke swimming to minimize intra-cyclic velocity fluctuations. *PLoS ONE* **2017**, *12*, e0186160. [CrossRef] [PubMed]
104. Loetz, C.; Reischle, K.; Schmitt, G. The evaluation of highly skilled swimmers via quantitative and qualitative analysis. In *Swimming Science V*; Human Kinetics Books: Champaign, IL, USA, 1988; pp. 361–367.
105. Novais, D.; Carmo, C.; Gonçalves, P.; Sousa, F.; Lima, A.B.; Barbosa, T.M.; Santos, P.; Machado, L.; Keskinen, K.L.; Fernandes, R.J.; et al. Energy cost and intra-cyclic variation of the velocity of the centre of mass in front crawl. *Rev. Port. Cien. Desp.* **2006**, *6*, 107–109.
106. Arellano, R.; Dominguez-Castells, R.; Perez-Infantes, E.; Sanchez, E. Effect of stroke drills on intra-cycle hip velocity in front crawl. In Proceedings of the Biomechanics and Medicine in Swimming XI, Oslo, Norway, 16–19 June 2010; pp. 45–47.
107. Soares, S.M.; Fernandes, R.J.; Machado, J.L.; Maia, J.A.; Daly, D.J.; Vilas-Boas, J.P. Assessment of fatigue thresholds in 50-m all-out swimming. *Int. J. Sport. Physiol. Perform.* **2014**, *9*, 959–965. [CrossRef]
108. Tella, V.; Llop, F.; Jorda, J.; Madera, J.; Benavent, J. Intracyclic speed and coordination vs. fatigue in swimming. In *Proceedings of the Biomechanics and Medicine in Swimming X*; Porto Faculdade de Desporto da Universidade do Porto: Porto, Portugal, 2006; pp. 105–107.
109. Costa, M.J.; Barbosa, T.M.; Morais, J.E.; Miranda, S.; Marinho, D.A. Can concurrent teaching promote equal biomechanical adaptations at front crawl and backstroke swimming? *Acta Bioeng. Biomech.* **2017**, *19*, 81–88. [CrossRef]
110. Kjendlie, P.L.; Ingjer, F.; Stallman, R.K.; Stray-Gundersen, J. Factors affecting swimming economy in children and adults. *Eur. J. Appl. Physiol.* **2004**, *93*, 65–74. [CrossRef]
111. Ungerechts, B.E. The interrelation of hydrodynamic forces and swimming speed in breaststroke. In *Biomechanics and Medicine in Swimming. Swimming Science VI*; Taylor & Francis Group: London, UK, 1992; pp. 69–74.
112. Tella, V.; Toca-Herrera, J.L.; Gallach, J.E.; Benavent, J.; González, L.M.; Arellano, R. Effect of fatigue on the intra-cycle acceleration in front crawl swimming: A time-frequency analysis. *J. Biomech.* **2008**, *41*, 86–92. [CrossRef]
113. Barbosa, T.M.; Fernandes, R.J.; Morouco, P.; Vilas-Boas, J.P. Predicting the intra-cyclic variation of the velocity of the centre of mass from segmental velocities in butterfly stroke: A pilot study. *J. Sport. Sci. Med.* **2008**, *7*, 201–209.
114. Barbosa, T.M.; Goh, W.X.; Morais, J.E.; Costa, M.J. Variation of linear and nonlinear parameters in the swim strokes according to the level of expertise. *Mot. Control.* **2017**, *21*, 312–326. [CrossRef] [PubMed]
115. Neiva, H.P.; Fernandes, R.J.; Cardoso, R.; Marinho, D.A.; Abraldes, J.A. Monitoring master swimmers' performance and active drag evolution along a training mesocycle. *Int. J. Environ. Res. Public Health* **2021**, *18*, 3569. [CrossRef] [PubMed]
116. Figueiredo, P.; Silva, A.; Sampaio, A.; Vilas-Boas, J.P.; Fernandes, R.J. Front crawl sprint performance: A cluster analysis of biomechanics, energetics, coordinative, and anthropometric determinants in young swimmers. *Mot. Control.* **2016**, *20*, 209–221. [CrossRef]
117. Morais, J.E.; Garrido, N.D.; Marques, M.C.; Silva, A.J.; Marinho, D.A.; Barbosa, T.M. The Influence of Anthropometric, Kinematic and Energetic Variables and Gender on Swimming Performance in Youth Athletes. *J. Hum. Kinet.* **2013**, *39*, 203–211. [CrossRef] [PubMed]
118. Craig, A.B.; Boomer, W.L.; Skehan, P.L. Patterns of velocity in competitive breaststroke swimming. In *Swimming Science V*; Champaign Human Kinetics Books: Champaign, IL, USA, 1988; pp. 73–77.
119. Correia, R.A.; Feitosa, W.G.; Figueiredo, P.; Papoti, M.; Castro, F.A.S. The 400-m Front Crawl Test: Energetic and 3D Kinematical Analyses. *Int. J. Sport. Med.* **2020**, *41*, 21–26. [CrossRef]
120. Ferreira, M.I.; Silva, A.J.; de Oliveira, D.R.; Garrido, N.D.; Barbosa, T.M.; Marinho, D.A.; Reis, V.M. Analysis of the determinant kinematical parameters for performance in the 200-m freestyle swimming event. *Motriz* **2012**, *18*, 366–377. [CrossRef]
121. dos Santos, K.B.; Bento, P.C.B.; Payton, C.; Rodacki, A.L.F. Kinematic Parameters after Repeated Swimming Efforts in Higher and Lower Proficiency Swimmers and Para-swimmers. *Res. Q. Exerc. Sport.* **2020**, *91*, 574–582. [CrossRef]

122. Bartolomeu, R.F.; Costa, M.J.; Barbosa, T.M. Contribution of limbs' actions to the four competitive swimming strokes: A nonlinear approach. *J. Sport. Sci.* **2018**, *36*, 1836–1845. [CrossRef]
123. Balonas, A.; Goncalves, P.; Silva, J.; Marinho, D.; Moreira, P.; Lima, A.; Barbosa, T.; Keskinen, K.L.; Fernandes, R.; Vilas-Boas, J.P. Time limit at the minimum velocity of VO2max and intracyclic variation of the velocity of the centre of mass. In *Proceedings of the Biomechanics and Medicine in Swimming X*; Porto Faculdade de Desporto da Universidade do Porto: Porto, Portugal, 2006; pp. 189–192.
124. Barbosa, A.C.; Barroso, R.; Gonjo, T.; Rossi, M.M.; Paolucci, L.A.; Olstad, B.H.; Andrade, A.G.P. 50 m freestyle in 21, 22 and 23 s: What differentiates the speed curve of world-class and elite male swimmers? *Int. J. Perform. Anal. Sport.* **2021**, *21*, 1055–1065. [CrossRef]
125. Barbosa, A.C.; Barroso, R.; Olstad, B.H.; Andrade, A.G. Long-term changes in the speed curve of a world-class butterfly swimmer. *J. Sport. Med. Phys. Fit.* **2021**, *61*, 152–158. [CrossRef]
126. Colman, V.; Persyn, U.; Daly, D.; Stijnen, V. A comparison of the intra-cyclic velocity variation in breaststroke swimmers with flat and undulating styles. *J. Sport. Sci.* **1998**, *16*, 653–665. [CrossRef]
127. Takagi, H.; Sugimoto, S.; Nishijima, N.; Wilson, B. Differences in stroke phases, arm-leg coordination and velocity fluctuation due to event, gender and performance level in breaststroke. *Sport. Biomech.* **2004**, *3*, 15–27. [CrossRef] [PubMed]
128. De Jesus, K.; De Jesus, K.; Figueiredo, P.A.; Goncalves, P.; Vilas-Boas, J.P.; Fernandes, R.J. Effects of fatigue on kinematical parameters during submaximal and maximal 100-m butterfly bouts. *J. Appl. Biomech.* **2012**, *28*, 599–607. [CrossRef] [PubMed]
129. Seifert, L.; Chehensse, A.; Tourny-Chollet, C.; Lemaitre, F.; Chollet, D. Effect of breathing pattern on arm coordination symmetry in front crawl. *J. Strength Cond. Res.* **2008**, *22*, 1670–1676. [CrossRef]
130. Miyashita, M. Method of Calculating Mechanical Power in Swimming the Breast Stroke. *Res. Q. Am. Alliance Health Phys. Educ. Recreat.* **1974**, *45*, 128–137. [CrossRef]
131. Figueiredo, P.; Marques, E.A.; Vilas-Boas, J.P.; Fernandes, R.J. Methods of intracycle velocity variation assessment in front crawl. In Proceedings of the International Society of Biomechanics, Natal, Brazil, 4–9 August 2013.

Disclaimer/Publisher's Note: The statements, opinions and data contained in all publications are solely those of the individual author(s) and contributor(s) and not of MDPI and/or the editor(s). MDPI and/or the editor(s) disclaim responsibility for any injury to people or property resulting from any ideas, methods, instructions or products referred to in the content.

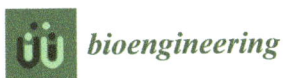

Article

Continuous Shoulder Activity Tracking after Open Reduction and Internal Fixation of Proximal Humerus Fractures

Michiel Herteleer [1], Armin Runer [2,3], Magdalena Remppis [4], Jonas Brouwers [1], Friedemann Schneider [2], Vasiliki C. Panagiotopoulou [4], Bernd Grimm [5], Clemens Hengg [2], Rohit Arora [2], Stefaan Nijs [1,6] and Peter Varga [4,*]

1 Department of Trauma Surgery, University Hospitals Leuven, 3000 Leuven, Belgium
2 University Hospital for Orthopaedics and Traumatology, Medical University Innsbruck, 6020 Innsbruck, Austria
3 Orthopaedic Sports Medicine, Klinikum Rechts der Isar, Technical University of Munich, 80333 Munich, Germany
4 AO Research Institute Davos, 7270 Davos, Switzerland
5 Department of Precision Health, Luxembourg Institute of Health, 1445 Strassen, Luxembourg
6 Utrecht Medical Centre Utrecht, 3584 CX Utrecht, The Netherlands
* Correspondence: peter.varga@aofoundation.org

Abstract: Postoperative shoulder activity after proximal humerus fracture treatment could influence the outcomes of osteosynthesis and may depend on the rehabilitation protocol. This multi-centric prospective study aimed at evaluating the feasibility of continuous shoulder activity monitoring over the first six postoperative weeks, investigating potential differences between two different rehabilitation protocols. Shoulder activity was assessed with pairs of accelerometer-based trackers during the first six postoperative weeks in thirteen elderly patients having a complex proximal humerus fracture treated with a locking plate. Shoulder angles and elevation events were evaluated over time and compared between the two centers utilizing different standard rehabilitation protocols. The overall mean shoulder angle ranged from 11° to 23°, and the number of daily elevation events was between 547 and 5756. Average angles showed longitudinal change <5° over 31 ± 10 days. The number of events increased by 300% on average. Results of the two clinics exhibited no characteristic differences for shoulder angle, but the number of events increased only for the site utilizing immediate mobilization. In addition to considerable inter-patient variation, not the mean shoulder angle but the number of elevations events increased markedly over time. Differences between the two sites in number of daily events may be associated with the different rehabilitation protocols.

Keywords: shoulder activity; sensor; rehabilitation protocol; proximal humerus fracture

1. Introduction

Proximal humeral fractures are common fractures in the elderly and affecting up to 111 per 100,000 persons per year [1]. In displaced three- or four-part fractures, open reduction and internal fixation (ORIF) aims at the best possible restoration of shoulder anatomy and thus shoulder function [2–4]. Shoulder function after ORIF mainly improves between 3 and 12 months after surgery but acute loss of reduction usually happens within 6 weeks after surgery [5–8]. In addition to other factors such as the donor's age and sex, bone stock quality, complexity and reduction quality of the fracture, comorbidities, fixation type and augmentation, the rehabilitation protocol may contribute to these early failures [9–18]. There are differences in rehabilitation programs after ORIF whereas some surgeons stimulate an immediate functional non-weight bearing rehabilitation program, while others have a less aggressive approach and prefer an initial physiotherapist assisted rehabilitation program [19]. It remains unclear what impact these different rehabilitation programs have on postoperative patient satisfaction, return to function, complications and failures [20]. Moreover, it remains challenging to capture the frequency and extent of shoulder activity

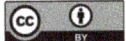

performed by a patient throughout the day. Technological advancements allow recording patient activity via trackers and motion capture sensors, allowing continuous assessment of activities of daily life for periods ranging from a few days up to several weeks [21,22].

The goal of this pilot study was threefold. The first aim was to evaluate the feasibility of continuously monitoring shoulder activity over a period of several weeks. The second aim was to describe the evolution of shoulder activity within the first six postoperative weeks in proximal humerus fracture patients treated with locked plate osteosynthesis. The third aim was to evaluate potential differences in the degree of postoperative shoulder activity between two different rehabilitation protocols.

2. Materials and Methods

This multi-centric prospective study investigated shoulder activity with accelerometer-based trackers during the first six postoperative weeks in elderly patients with a complex proximal humerus fracture treated with the PHILOS plate (DePuy Synthes, Zuchwil, Switzerland). The two study centers were the University Hospitals Leuven and Medical University Innsbruck. Note that the study sites will be referred to in an anonymized manner below. The study was approved by the local ethical committees (approval numbers S62376 and 1281/2018, respectively).

2.1. Patient Recruitment

Inclusion criteria were age $\geq$ 50 years, displaced or unstable three- or four-part fracture of the proximal humerus (except isolated displaced fractures of the greater or lesser tuberosity) treated with a plate and screw osteosynthesis (PHILOS locking plate—with or without screw augmentation) within 10 days after injury, ability to understand the content of the study and the patient consent form and voluntary signed informed consent.

Exclusion criteria were previous proximal humerus fracture on the ipsilateral limb, humeral head impression/splitting fracture, fibula grafting, bone block or any other non-cement augmentation of the PHILOS locking plate fixation, associated nerve or vessel injury, serious fracture fixation issues such as too long screw, screw perforation through the humeral head, or a broken screw or implant recognized directly on the first postoperative X-ray. Other exclusion criteria were severe systematic diseases rated in class 4 and higher of the American Society of Anesthesiologists (ASA) physical status classification, substance abuse, prisoner, participation in another medical device or product study in the past month that could affect this study, pregnancy, or pacemaker.

Patient data including age, gender, height, weight, residential status, injury side, arm dominance and fracture type were collected at recruitment.

2.2. Postoperative Protocol

The two university hospitals used different postoperative rehabilitation protocols according to their standard of care. In hospital H1, the patients were treated with a sling for 3 weeks and were only allowed passive and active-assisted mobilization under supervision of a physiotherapist for the first 3 weeks. Patients in hospital H2 were treated without a sling and allowed to mobilize without restrictions immediately. Physiotherapy was started immediately postoperatively and prescribed 2–3 times per week in both hospitals.

2.3. Activity Tracking Apparatus and Procedure

Accelerometer sensors (AX3, Axivity Ltd., Newcastle upon Tyne, UK) [23] (Figure 1, left) were used to measure shoulder activity continuously (24/7) for 6 weeks after the operation in two consecutive 3-week periods. The length of the measurement period was determined by the sensor's battery and memory capacities. The first period started at the latest 4 days postoperatively and ended at 21 $\pm$ 3 days, the second period started at the same visit and ended at 42 $\pm$ 3 days. Two sensors were used for each patient and period. One sensor was attached to the upper arm of the treated side, and another was located at the chest and served as a reference (Figure 1, right), allowing evaluation of the shoulder angle as the orientation difference between both devices. Data recording was performed at 50 Hz frequency within ±4 g limits that were deemed suitable in a pilot evaluation. The sensors were attached to the skin using a dedicated certified medical-grade adhesive tape (3M 4077, 3M Medical Materials & Technologies, Oakdale, CA, USA). Attachment (directly postoperatively and at the 3-week follow-up visit) and detachment (at the 3-week and 6-week follow-up visits) were performed by trained study personnel according to standard operating procedures to ensure consistent sensor location and alignment. The start and end time points of a given period were marked by knocking five times synchronously at both arm and chest sensors. The patients were allowed to follow their normal daily activities including showering with the attached device. At the end of the measurement periods and after detachment, sensor data were downloaded using the Open Movement GUI software (Open Movement project).

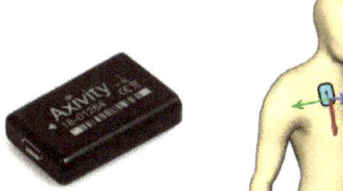 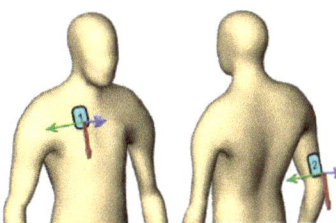

Figure 1. Accelerometer sensors (Axivity AX3, (**left**), source: https://axivity.com/) were attached to the patients (illustrated on the (**right**)), on the chest ("1") and on the back of the upper arm on the treated side ("2"). Each sensor had its own coordinate system, indicated with the red–green–blue arrows.

2.4. Data Processing

The raw data of the sensors were corrected, filtered, synchronized, and evaluated using Matlab (R2020b, MathWorks, Natick, MA, USA) as follows. Calibration was performed to compensate for imperfections in magnitude and directional errors of each sensor such that the acceleration was measured in stationary position equal to 1.0 g (gravity, i.e., 9.81 m/s^2 acceleration) in each direction, and the orientation of the measured vector is perpendicular to the planar sides of the sensor's housing when resting on a horizontal flat surface [24]. The detailed description of these calibrations is provided in Appendix A. The quantified imperfections were used to correct the raw data.

Since the arm and chest sensors were recording independently, their data needed to be synchronized in time. This required shifting and scaling operations based on the time landmarks defined by the knocking events at attachment and detachment. Shifting was achieved based on the starting point of the activity assessment, which was dictated by five knocking events on both sensors directly after attachment. Scaling was evaluated and corrected based on the lengths of the measurement periods of the two sensors determined by the time difference of the initial and final knocking events; interpolation ensured that the data were available at the same time points for both sensors.

The measurement noise of the raw data was alleviated using a combination of a low-pass Butterworth filter with a cut-off of 5 Hz to remove high-frequency noise, which was followed by a smoothing step using a moving average filter utilizing quadratic regression with a window size of 60 ms.

Shoulder angle was calculated as the rotational difference between the coordinate systems of the arm sensor versus the chest sensor (Figure 1, right). The calculation method was validated in an experimental setup to ensure <2° accuracy in the angles between the two sensors. The 0° angle was defined at the initial knocking event performed directly after sensor attachment, at neutral position of the shoulder with the patient being in an upright position. Due to the limitation that accelerometer sensors can determine their orientation only with respect to the gravity vector in steady states, it was not possible to discriminate the different anatomical components of shoulder rotation. Thus, only a single shoulder angle integrating components of flexion–extension and adduction–abduction could be determined. Large acceleration events, i.e., >1.5 g, were excluded to ensure reliable orientation assessment for the sensors. Moreover, the part of the data related to the sleeping and resting periods of the patients was excluded, as these periods were not of primary interest and could not be reliably assessed due to the technical limitations of accelerometers and their attachment to the skin. Therefore, the final evaluation was restricted to periods when the upper body posture was between $-30°$ and $+30°$, as assessed by the chest sensor.

Shoulder elevations, referred to below as "events", were determined as peaks between increasing and subsequent decreasing angle in the shoulder activity data with a minimum prominence of $10°$.

The average magnitude of shoulder angles and number of shoulder elevation events were evaluated for each post-operative day. Additionally, the changes compared to the direct postoperative status; i.e., the average of the 2–5 postoperative days were evaluated for both the average shoulder angle and number of elevation events. These relative values allowed for a more direct comparison between patients. The two different rehabilitation protocols were compared by averaging the data of all patients per hospital and comparing the outcomes of the hospitals.

3. Results

This feasibility study included 14 patients (11 women and 3 men), with seven patients treated in each hospital H1 and H2 (Table 1). One patient from hospital H2 had to be excluded from follow-up because of discomfort wearing the activity trackers. Mean age at time of surgery for the remaining thirteen patients was 63 ± 8 years. Five patients were living alone. The injured and tracked arm was the dominant arm in eight patients. Sling removal time was 23 ± 4.5 days and 2 ± 1.5 days in hospitals H1 and H2, respectively.

Table 1. Demographic data, shoulder angles and number of daily shoulder elevation events of the patients involved in the study. Sex: F = female and M = male. SD refers to standard deviation.

Patient ID	Age in Years	Sex	Shoulder Angle in °		Number of Daily Events	
			Mean	SD	Mean	SD
H1_P01	79	F	14	6.9	1325	357
H1_P02	60	F	18	9.7	3170	554
H1_P03	52	F	17.9	12.1	5756	1440
H1_P05	58	M	12	7.9	3267	693
H1_P06	72	F	11	8	547	159
H1_P07	58	F	23	9.9	4073	1305
H2_P01	61	F	16.4	4.8	3942	2016
H2_P01	76	F	11.8	4.6	1996	1450
H2_P03	63	F	14.8	6.2	5407	1558
H2_P04	56	F	16.3	9.3	4109	1684
H2_P05	69	F	11.3	7.1	3421	1468
H2_P06	54	M	18.6	9.2	3385	1434
H2_P07	58	M	15.3	8.1	2517	1040

The total recording time was on average 31 ± 10 days (mean $\pm$ standard deviation (SD)). Ten patients had measurements in both first and second 3-weeks periods. Two patients had mild adverse event in form of skin irritation or reactions at the sensor attachment site during the first recording period and could not complete the second period. All adverse events were fully resolved by three months. Another four patients experienced mildly irritated, red skin but were able to take part in the second recording period.

The tracker of four patients ran out of battery before the end of the measurement period, and thus, the collected data were not complete. A single sensor broke and did not allow the data to be accessed. Six patients reported incidents of tape detachment; these were reattached by the patients themselves. Wherever possible, the date and time of de- and reattachments were assessed by the patient and the study personnel. Analysis of the sensor data allowed to identify and correct or exclude these parts of the data.

The overall mean shoulder angle ranged between 11° and 23° in all patients (Table 1). The evolution of daily average of shoulder angle over time showed no longitudinal change for most patients (Figure 2 top and middle). This trend was confirmed by the evolution of the relative change of shoulder angle compared to the direct postoperative days, remaining smaller than 5° (Figure 2, bottom).

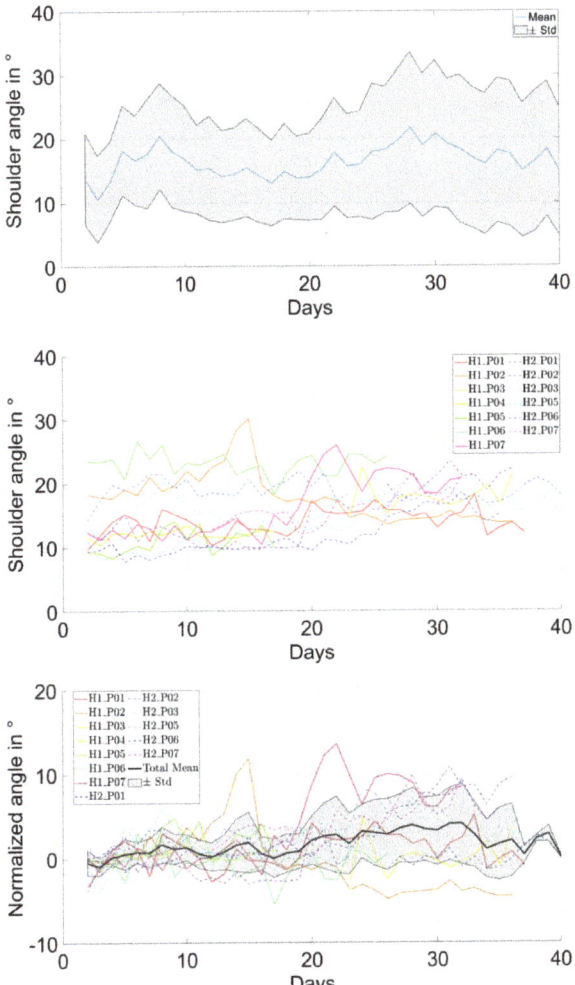

Figure 2. Daily average shoulder angle results. (**Top**): the mean (blue line) and standard deviation (gray zone) of shoulder angle for each postoperative day of a patient (H2_P04). The overall mean ± standard deviation of shoulder angle for the entire tracking period of this patient was 16.3 ± 9.3°. (**Middle**): absolute daily average of the shoulder angles for each patient. (**Bottom**): normalized (compared to the direct postoperative state) daily average of the shoulder angles for each patient. Note that the data were not available throughout the entire six-week period for some patients.

The overall average number of daily shoulder elevation events ranged between 547 and 5756 in all patients (Table 1). The number of daily events increased for most but not all patients (Figures 3 and 4, top). The relative change of daily event numbers compared to the direct postoperative days showed an increasing trend over time, reaching up to 300% increase (Figure 4, bottom).

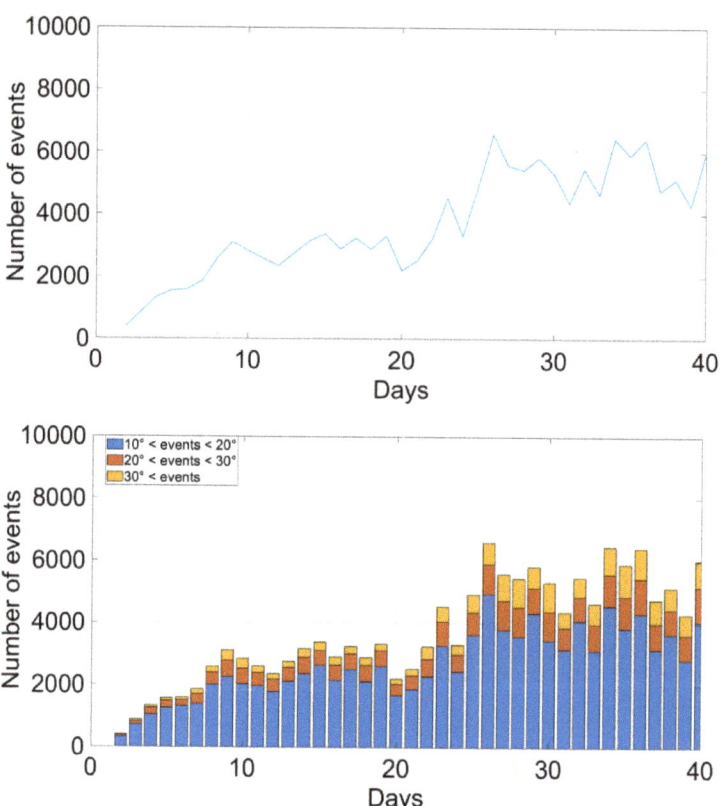

Figure 3. Number of shoulder elevation events of one patient (H2_P04). (**Top**): evolution of the number of shoulder elevation events throughout the tracking period. (**Bottom**): evolution of the number of shoulder elevation events throughout the tracking period categorized into three ranges according to the maximum shoulder angle reached. The daily mean ± standard deviation of shoulder elevation events of this patient was 4109 ± 1684.

There were no characteristic differences between the two clinical sites, i.e., rehabilitation protocols, in terms of the longitudinal evolution of the change in the average shoulder angle (Figure 5). However, the evolution of the percentile changes in the number of events relative to the postoperative period was increasing for H2 but not for H1, and the differences between sites became more pronounced for higher elevation thresholds (Figure 6).

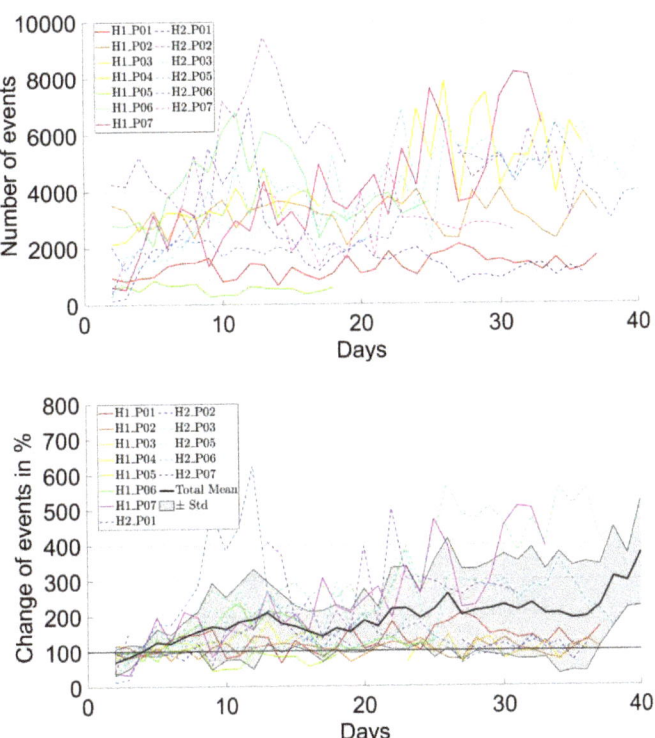

Figure 4. Absolute (**top**) and relative ((**bottom**), compared to the direct postoperative state) number of daily shoulder elevations larger than 10°, shown for each patient. Note that the data were not available throughout the entire six-week period for some patients.

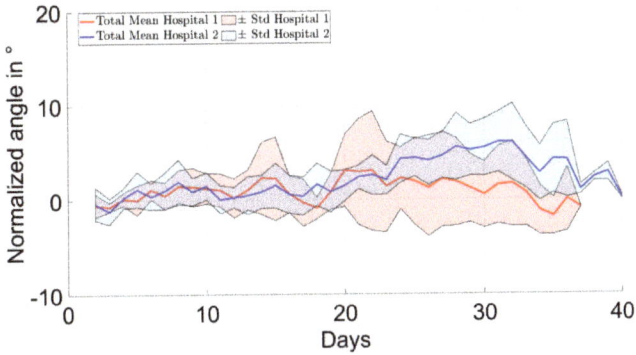

Figure 5. Comparison of the average results of the two clinical sites, i.e., rehabilitation protocols, in terms of the change in the shoulder angle compared to the direct postoperative period.

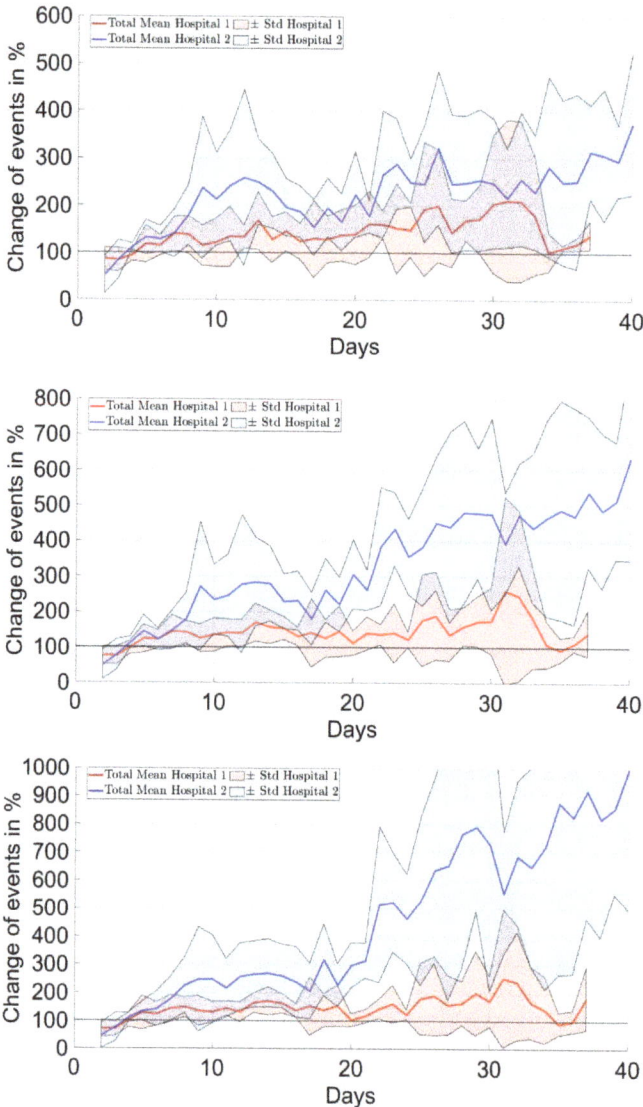

Figure 6. Comparison of the average results of the two clinical sites, i.e., rehabilitation protocols, in terms of the change in the total number of shoulder elevation events over time. The sub-figures show the data for shoulder elevation events beyond 10° (**top**), 20° (**middle**) and 30° (**bottom**).

4. Discussion

The primary findings of this study were that in patients after proximal humerus fracture undergoing ORIF, the mean shoulder angle varied up to a factor 2 between individuals, but it hardly increases in the first six weeks. The number of events exhibited a 10-fold difference between subjects, and the time evolution of event numbers showed an increasing trend. The comparison of the two hospitals indicated that the rehabilitation protocol might affect the number of daily shoulder elevation events with patients following an immediate functional non-weight bearing rehabilitation program having a higher number of events, especially for large shoulder angles.

Postoperative rehabilitation protocols after proximal humerus ORIF vary substantially between different hospitals and surgical centers ranging from strict immobilization using a shoulder sling to a more progressive, functional non-weight-bearing approach without sling immobilization [25]. If immobilized, the duration of postoperative sling usage ranged from none to eight weeks [25]. A recent review summarizing five comparative studies did not find any benefit of longer sling immobilization compared to early functional therapy. While exercise and early functional mobilization is clearly advised, the amount and influence of postoperative mobilization and its effect on clinical and subjective outcomes as well as revision and failure rates are still unknown [26,27].

When recording physical activity or joint motion, wearable activity trackers are frequently used, and single day data acquisition was our method of choice [28]. While this might be less burdensome for the patient in comparison to long-term recording, the informative value of these data is limited and long-term recordings are recommended. To the best of the authors' knowledge, the present work represents the first study providing detailed insights into the longitudinal evolution of postoperative shoulder activity of surgically treated patients with proximal humerus fracture. The relevance of long-term measurement was underlined by the time evolution of the assessed parameters. Although the average daily shoulder angles remained fairly constant over time, the number of shoulder angles showed an increasing trend over time, exhibiting important differences between patients, especially after three weeks postoperatively and in particular for large shoulder angle events. These may be related to the different rehabilitation protocols adopted by both investigation sites. While in the first two weeks, there is no difference with regard to the total number of elevation events >10°, an increased number of events for patients following the unrestricted, i.e., non-weight bearing, rehabilitation protocol was recorded thereafter. For non-operatively treated proximal humerus fractures, early active rehabilitation yields equal complications and shoulder functions as prolonged sling immobilization and restricted rehabilitation [26,29]. Similarly, the present data suggest a potential benefit of early active rehabilitation in terms of faster return to motion and function compared to a more restricted rehabilitation protocol. Nevertheless, the influence of a patients' preoperative activity level on the amount of shoulder activity in the early postoperative phase is still unknown, and therefore, caution is needed when interpreting these results.

Recording detailed postoperative shoulder activity, using wearables is challenging, and little high-quality knowledge exists. Van de Kleut et al. investigated daily shoulder activity before and after reverse Total Shoulder Arthroplasty (rTSA) using Inertial Measurement Units (IMUs) [30]. Their results showed an increased frequency of arm elevations to higher angles but no difference in the amount of time spent in the elevation. Moreover, shoulder elevation accounted for less than 1% of daily shoulder motion, and even after one year postoperatively, patients spent more than 95% of the day in shoulder angles below 60° [30]. These results compare to the present work, where patients spent 94% of the time in shoulder angles below 40°. The initial increase in shoulder events seen in the present study may be due to postoperative physiotherapy, which is in line with previously reported data showing a significant increase in events only in the early postoperative period but not thereafter [30]. This can be explained by the fact that physiotherapy is adapted to the state of the patient starting with simple exercises that become more challenging over time. Therefore, it is more likely to see a general increase in activity over time which is the case in the present work. Furthermore, physiotherapy is performed only during a limited amount of time during the day and might therefore have only a limited effect on daily shoulder activity. In general, the present data show that after open reduction and internal fixation, the shoulder activity level of patients is low and that the early return to full range of motion is not seen in the first weeks.

This study has some limitations. The small number of patients included into this pilot study did not allow for meaningful statistical analysis to be performed, but the indicated trends can be used to design more specific and focused investigations. Moreover, the feasibility of long-term tracking was assessed, providing novel insights and highlighting potential pitfalls. Technical limitations included the issue that the battery of the activity trackers did not always last for the desired time window of three weeks. Since for the calculation of the shoulder angle, the recordings of both activity trackers are necessary, the analysis could only be conducted as long as both activity trackers were functional. Detachment of the tape fixing the sensors occurred due to the loss of adhesion to the skin or ruptures of the material, causing a partial unavailability of data until reattachment. The assessed shoulder angles were not validated against optical tracking techniques. However, the method for calculating the shoulder angle used here was similar to the one applied by Chapman et al. [31], who validated their results against a laboratory motion capture system and reported errors smaller than 2° for abduction, forward flexion, internal and external rotation. In addition, over the long-term, i.e., days to weeks, activity monitoring application with thousands of events, the accuracy of a single event is less critical as the focus is on behavioral change and the large data sample compensates for a potentially lower accuracy compared to what would be needed during a single functional test. Shoulder activity monitoring by counting events beyond certain joint angle thresholds may be affected by the lifestyle of the subject. Thus, correct interpretation of the absolute number of events would require a pre-trauma reference. With the latter being hardly possible, in future studies, the unaffected shoulder could be monitored simultaneously for an intra-subject reference and potential transfer of activities during the rehabilitation phase.

5. Conclusions

Activity tracker-based continuous shoulder activity assessment in patients with a complex proximal humerus fracture treated with a locking plate was feasible and revealed that the mean value of the shoulder angle had up to two times differences between individuals but hardly increased during the first 6 postoperative weeks for most patients. Up to 10-fold differences in the daily shoulder elevation events between patients could be seen. There was a considerable difference in the number of shoulder elevation events > 10° between patients of both hospitals, which may be due to different rehabilitation protocols. Event counts above a functionally demanding threshold seemed to be the most sensitive digital mobility parameter monitoring post-traumatic recovery and may streamline wearable sensor data analysis in future studies as well as establish comparability between trials. These observations require confirmation by future studies including a larger cohort. When applied to a larger group of patients, the presented methods could be used in future studies to objectively and functionally evaluate the effect of postoperative activity on the outcomes of proximal humerus fracture fixation and to assess patient compliance. The resulting data could serve as the basis for developing improved and potentially personalized rehabilitation protocols and guidance for the patient.

Author Contributions: Conceptualization: V.C.P., B.G., S.N. and P.V.; investigation: M.H., A.R., J.B., F.S., C.H. and S.N.; resources: M.H., A.R., J.B., F.S., C.H. and S.N.; methodology: M.R., V.C.P., B.G. and P.V.; software: M.R.; validation: M.R. and P.V.; formal analysis: M.R. and P.V.; data curation: M.R. and P.V.; writing—original draft preparation: M.H., A.R. and P.V.; writing—review and editing: M.R., J.B., F.S., V.C.P., B.G., C.H., R.A. and S.N.; visualization: M.R. and P.V.; supervision: C.H., R.A., S.N. and P.V.; project administration: V.C.P. and P.V.; funding acquisition: P.V. All authors have read and agreed to the published version of the manuscript.

Funding: This research was funded by AO Foundation via the AOTRAUMA Network, grant number AR 2018/01.

Institutional Review Board Statement: The study was conducted in accordance with the Declaration of Helsinki and approved by the Ethics Committees of University Hospitals Leuven (protocol code S62376, date of approval: 24 April 2019) and Medical University Innsbruck (protocol code 1281/2018, date of approval: 24 April 2019).

Informed Consent Statement: Informed consent was obtained from all subjects involved in the study.

Data Availability Statement: Not applicable.

Acknowledgments: The authors thank Jérôme Schlatter for his assistance with the illustrations.

Conflicts of Interest: The authors declare no conflict of interest. The authors, their immediate families, and any research foundations with which they are affiliated have not received any financial payments or other benefits from any commercial entity related to the subject of this article.

Appendix A. Sensor Data Processing

Magnitude calibration of the activity sensors was performed by calculating a correction factor to rescale the vector magnitude in stationary periods to the value of 1 g (9.81 m/s^2) in numerous directions. The sensor was mounted to a special vise allowing angulations in two directions, and acceleration data were recorded for 20 s of stationary periods. This was repeated for different orientations covering a sphere with steps on 10°. Imperfections in the offset (eccentricity) and magnitude (scaling) were corrected via iterative closest point fitting of the measured points to the target unit sphere (Figure A1). The resulting correction factors were used to correct the recorded data.

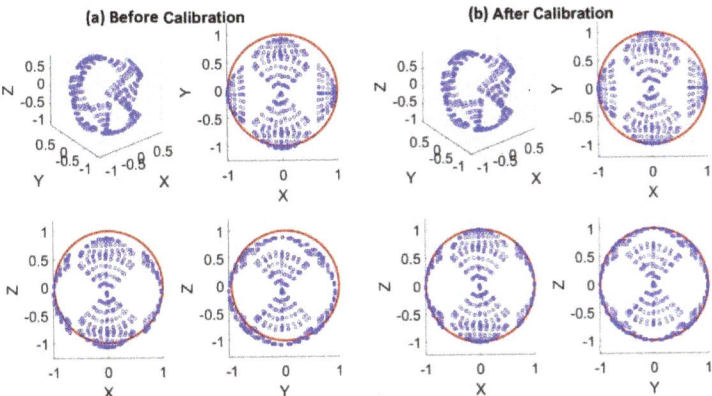

Figure A1. Illustration of the accelerometer's magnitude calibration. Data points shown in blue represent accelerations in units of gravity measured in different directions for stationary periods, and the red circle shows the target unit sphere with a radius of 1 g. Imperfections before calibration (**a**) are resolved by the corrections after calibration (**b**).

Directional calibration of the sensors aimed to correct for potential obliqueness of the sensor positioning within the housing. Acceleration data were recorded for 10 s of stationary periods while positioning the housing with one of its sides on a horizontal surface. Correction was then applied to match recorded data with the target unit vector of 1 g length for each side.

References

1. Dauwe, J.; Danker, C.; Herteleer, M.; Vanhaecht, K.; Nijs, S. Proximal Humeral Fracture Osteosynthesis in Belgium: A Retrospective Population-Based Epidemiologic Study. *Eur. J. Trauma Emerg. Surg.* **2020**, *48*, 4509–4514. [CrossRef] [PubMed]
2. Robinson, C.M.; Stirling, P.H.C.; Goudie, E.B.; Macdonald, D.J.; Strelzow, J.A. Complications and Long-Term Outcomes of Open Reduction and Plate Fixation of Proximal Humeral Fractures. *J. Bone Jt. Surg.-Am. Vol.* **2019**, *101*, 2129–2139. [CrossRef]
3. Baker, H.P.; Gutbrod, J.; Strelzow, J.A.; Maassen, N.H.; Shi, L. Management of Proximal Humerus Fractures in Adults-A Scoping Review. *J. Clin. Med.* **2022**, *11*, 6140. [CrossRef] [PubMed]
4. Südkamp, N.; Bayer, J.; Hepp, P.; Voigt, C.; Oestern, H.; Kääb, M.; Luo, C.; Plecko, M.; Wendt, K.; Köstler, W.; et al. Open Reduction and Internal Fixation of Proximal Humeral Fractures with Use of the Locking Proximal Humerus Plate. Results of a Prospective, Multicenter, Observational Study. *J. Bone Jt. Surg. Am.* **2009**, *91*, 1320–1328. [CrossRef] [PubMed]
5. Panagiotopoulou, V.C.; Varga, P.; Richards, R.G.; Gueorguiev, B.; Giannoudis, P.V. Late Screw-Related Complications in Locking Plating of Proximal Humerus Fractures: A Systematic Review. *Injury* **2019**, *50*, 2176–2195. [CrossRef]

6. Kralinger, F.; Blauth, M.; Goldhahn, J.; Kach, K.; Voigt, C.; Platz, A.; Hanson, B. The Influence of Local Bone Density on the Outcome of One Hundred and Fifty Proximal Humeral Fractures Treated with a Locking Plate. *J. Bone Jt. Surg. Am.* **2014**, *96*, 1026–1032. [CrossRef] [PubMed]
7. Agudelo, J.; Schürmann, M.; Stahel, P.; Helwig, P.; Morgan, S.J.; Zechel, W.; Bahrs, C.; Parekh, A.; Ziran, B.; Williams, A.; et al. Analysis of Efficacy and Failure in Proximal Humerus Fractures Treated with Locking Plates. *J. Orthop. Trauma* **2007**, *21*, 676–681. [CrossRef]
8. Oldrini, L.M.; Feltri, P.; Albanese, J.; Marbach, F.; Filardo, G.; Candrian, C. PHILOS Synthesis for Proximal Humerus Fractures Has High Complications and Reintervention Rates: A Systematic Review and Meta-Analysis. *Life* **2022**, *12*, 311. [CrossRef]
9. Krappinger, D.; Bizzotto, N.; Riedmann, S.; Kammerlander, C.; Hengg, C.; Kralinger, F.S. Predicting Failure after Surgical Fixation of Proximal Humerus Fractures. *Injury* **2011**, *42*, 1283–1288. [CrossRef]
10. Koeppe, J.; Katthagen, J.C.; Rischen, R.; Freistuehler, M.; Faldum, A.; Raschke, M.J.; Stolberg-Stolberg, J. Male Sex Is Associated with Higher Mortality and Increased Risk for Complications after Surgical Treatment of Proximal Humeral Fractures. *J. Clin. Med.* **2021**, *10*, 2500. [CrossRef]
11. Schnetzke, M.; Bockmeyer, J.; Porschke, F.; Studier-Fischer, S.; Grützner, P.-A.; Guehring, T. Quality of Reduction Influences Outcome After Locked-Plate Fixation of Proximal Humeral Type-C Fractures. *J. Bone Jt. Surg. Am.* **2016**, *98*, 1777–1785. [CrossRef] [PubMed]
12. Hättich, A.; Harloff, T.J.; Sari, H.; Schlickewei, C.; Cramer, C.; Strahl, A.; Frosch, K.-H.; Mader, K.; Klatte, T.O. Influence of Fracture Reduction on the Functional Outcome after Intramedullary Nail Osteosynthesis in Proximal Humerus Fractures. *J. Clin. Med.* **2022**, *11*, 6861. [CrossRef] [PubMed]
13. Porschke, F.; Bockmeyer, J.; Nolte, P.-C.; Studier-Fischer, S.; Guehring, T.; Schnetzke, M. More Adverse Events after Osteosyntheses Compared to Arthroplasty in Geriatric Proximal Humeral Fractures Involving Anatomical Neck. *J. Clin. Med.* **2021**, *10*, 979. [CrossRef] [PubMed]
14. Schuetze, K.; Boehringer, A.; Cintean, R.; Gebhard, F.; Pankratz, C.; Richter, P.H.; Schneider, M.; Eickhoff, A.M. Feasibility and Radiological Outcome of Minimally Invasive Locked Plating of Proximal Humeral Fractures in Geriatric Patients. *J. Clin. Med.* **2022**, *11*, 6751. [CrossRef] [PubMed]
15. Laux, C.J.; Grubhofer, F.; Werner, C.M.L.; Simmen, H.-P.; Osterhoff, G. Current Concepts in Locking Plate Fixation of Proximal Humerus Fractures. *J. Orthop. Surg. Res.* **2017**, *12*, 137. [CrossRef] [PubMed]
16. Hengg, C.; Nijs, S.; Klopfer, T.; Jaeger, M.; Platz, A.; Pohlemann, T.; Babst, R.; Franke, J.; Kralinger, F. Cement Augmentation of the Proximal Humerus Internal Locking System in Elderly Patients: A Multicenter Randomized Controlled Trial. *Arch. Orthop. Trauma Surg.* **2019**, *139*, 927–942. [CrossRef] [PubMed]
17. Hristov, S.; Visscher, L.; Winkler, J.; Zhelev, D.; Ivanov, S.; Veselinov, D.; Baltov, A.; Varga, P.; Berk, T.; Stoffel, K.; et al. A Novel Technique for Treatment of Metaphyseal Voids in Proximal Humerus Fractures in Elderly Patients. *Medicina* **2022**, *58*, 1424. [CrossRef] [PubMed]
18. Biermann, N.; Prall, W.C.; Böcker, W.; Mayr, H.O.; Haasters, F. Augmentation of Plate Osteosynthesis for Proximal Humeral Fractures: A Systematic Review of Current Biomechanical and Clinical Studies. *Arch. Orthop. Trauma Surg.* **2019**, *139*, 1075–1099. [CrossRef]
19. Patch, D.A.; Reed, L.A.; Hao, K.A.; King, J.J.; Kaar, S.G.; Horneff, J.G.; Ahn, J.; Strelzow, J.A.; Hebert-Davies, J.; Little, M.T.M.; et al. Understanding Postoperative Rehabilitation Preferences in Operatively Managed Proximal Humerus Fractures: Do Trauma and Shoulder Surgeons Differ? *J. Shoulder Elb. Surg.* **2022**, *31*, 1106–1114. [CrossRef]
20. Bruder, A.M.; Shields, N.; Dodd, K.J.; Taylor, N.F. Prescribed Exercise Programs May Not Be Effective in Reducing Impairments and Improving Activity during Upper Limb Fracture Rehabilitation: A Systematic Review. *J. Physiother.* **2017**, *63*, 205–220. [CrossRef]
21. Anglin, C.; Wyss, U.P. Review of Arm Motion Analyses. *Proc. Inst. Mech. Eng. H* **2000**, *214*, 541–555. [CrossRef] [PubMed]
22. Braun, B.J.; Grimm, B.; Hanflik, A.M.; Richter, P.H.; Sivananthan, S.; Yarboro, S.R.; Marmor, M.T. Wearable Technology in Orthopedic Trauma Surgery—An AO Trauma Survey and Review of Current and Future Applications. *Injury* **2022**, *53*, 1961–1965. [CrossRef] [PubMed]
23. Available online: https://axivity.com/product/ax3 (accessed on 1 January 2023).
24. Doherty, A.; Jackson, D.; Hammerla, N.; Plötz, T.; Olivier, P.; Granat, M.H.; White, T.; van Hees, V.T.; Trenell, M.I.; Owen, C.G.; et al. Large Scale Population Assessment of Physical Activity Using Wrist Worn Accelerometers: The UK Biobank Study. *PLoS ONE* **2017**, *12*, e0169649. [CrossRef] [PubMed]
25. Handoll, H.; Brealey, S.; Rangan, A.; Keding, A.; Corbacho, B.; Jefferson, L.; Chuang, L.-H.; Goodchild, L.; Hewitt, C.; Torgerson, D. The ProFHER (PROximal Fracture of the Humerus: Evaluation by Randomisation) Trial—A Pragmatic Multicentre Randomised Controlled Trial Evaluating the Clinical Effectiveness and Cost-Effectiveness of Surgical Compared with Non-Surgical Treatment for Proxi. *Health Technol. Assess* **2015**, *19*, 1–280. [CrossRef] [PubMed]
26. Handoll, H.H.; Elliott, J.; Thillemann, T.M.; Aluko, P.; Brorson, S. Interventions for Treating Proximal Humeral Fractures in Adults. *Cochrane Database Syst. Rev.* **2022**, *6*, CD000434. [CrossRef] [PubMed]
27. Hodgson, S. Proximal Humerus Fracture Rehabilitation. *Clin. Orthop. Relat. Res.* **2006**, *442*, 131–138. [CrossRef]
28. Carnevale, A.; Longo, U.G.; Schena, E.; Massaroni, C.; Lo Presti, D.; Berton, A.; Candela, V.; Denaro, V. Wearable Systems for Shoulder Kinematics Assessment: A Systematic Review. *BMC Musculoskelet. Disord.* **2019**, *20*, 546. [CrossRef]

29. Martínez, R.; Santana, F.; Pardo, A.; Torrens, C. One Versus 3-Week Immobilization Period for Nonoperatively Treated Proximal Humeral Fractures: A Prospective Randomized Trial. *J. Bone Jt. Surg. Am.* **2021**, *103*, 1491–1498. [CrossRef]
30. Van de Kleut, M.L.; Bloomfield, R.A.; Teeter, M.G.; Athwal, G.S. Monitoring Daily Shoulder Activity before and after Reverse Total Shoulder Arthroplasty Using Inertial Measurement Units. *J. Shoulder Elb. Surg.* **2021**, *30*, 1078–1087. [CrossRef]
31. Chapman, R.M.; Torchia, M.T.; Bell, J.E.; Van Citters, D.W. Assessing Shoulder Biomechanics of Healthy Elderly Individuals During Activities of Daily Living Using Inertial Measurement Units: High Maximum Elevation Is Achievable but Rarely Used. *J. Biomech. Eng.* **2019**, *141*, 0410011–0410017. [CrossRef]

Disclaimer/Publisher's Note: The statements, opinions and data contained in all publications are solely those of the individual author(s) and contributor(s) and not of MDPI and/or the editor(s). MDPI and/or the editor(s) disclaim responsibility for any injury to people or property resulting from any ideas, methods, instructions or products referred to in the content.

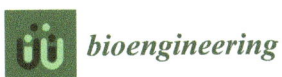

Article

Evaluation of a Locking Autocompression Screw Model in Pauwels Type-3 Femoral Neck Fracture: In Vitro Analysis

Vincenzo Giordano [1,*], Anderson Freitas [2,3], Robinson Esteves Pires [4], Leonardo Rigobello Battaglion [5], Mariana de Oliveira Lobo [3] and William Dias Belangero [6]

1. Orthopedics and Traumatology Service Prof. Nova Monteiro, Hospital Municipal Miguel Couto, Rua Mario Ribeiro, 117, Rio de Janeiro 22430-160, RJ, Brazil
2. Home Hospital Ortopédico e Medicina Especializada, SGAS Quadra 613-Conjunto C-Asa Sul, Brasília 70200-730, DF, Brazil
3. Orthopedics and Traumatology Service, Hospital Regional do Gama, Área Especial No. 01, Brasília 72405-901, DF, Brazil
4. Department of the Locomotive Apparatus, Universidade Federal de Minas Gerais (UFMG), Av. Pres. Antônio Carlos, 6627, Belo Horizonte 31270-901, MG, Brazil
5. Ribeirão Preto School of Medicine, Universidade de São Paulo (FMRP-USP), Av. Dr. Arnaldo, 455, Ribeirão Preto 01246-903, SP, Brazil
6. Department of Orthopedics and Traumatology, Faculty of Medical Sciences, Universidade Estadual de Campinas (UNICAMP), Rua Vital Brasil, 80, Campinas 13083-888, SP, Brazil
* Correspondence: v_giordano@me.com; Tel.: +55-21-997516859

Citation: Giordano, V.; Freitas, A.; Pires, R.E.; Battaglion, L.R.; Lobo, M.d.O.; Belangero, W.D. Evaluation of a Locking Autocompression Screw Model in Pauwels Type-3 Femoral Neck Fracture: In Vitro Analysis. *Bioengineering* 2022, 9, 464. https://doi.org/10.3390/bioengineering9090464

Academic Editors: Christina Zong-Hao Ma, Zhengrong Li and Chen He

Received: 31 August 2022
Accepted: 6 September 2022
Published: 12 September 2022

Publisher's Note: MDPI stays neutral with regard to jurisdictional claims in published maps and institutional affiliations.

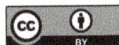

Copyright: © 2022 by the authors. Licensee MDPI, Basel, Switzerland. This article is an open access article distributed under the terms and conditions of the Creative Commons Attribution (CC BY) license (https://creativecommons.org/licenses/by/4.0/).

Abstract: Femoral neck fractures in young adults are uncommon, resulting from high-energy trauma. Despite their infrequency in this population, there is higher rate of complications, especially in the more vertical fracture line, classified by Pauwels as a type-3 femoral neck fracture. The implant type is of paramount importance for maintaining anatomical reduction, since it must resist the deforming forces that act on the fracture. We comparatively evaluated two constructions of the novel locking autocompression implant (X-PIN and X-PIN+P) using the finite element method and previously established methods for treating Pauwels type-3 femoral neck fractures. Six fixation models were developed for the study: a dynamic hip screw (DHS), a DHS with an anti-rotation screw (DHS+P), the inverted triangle multiple cannulated screws construction (ASNIS), the multiple cannulated screws in an L-configuration (L), and the two models of the novel locking autocompression screw (X-PIN and X-PIN+P). Under the same conditions with a load of 2100 N, the following parameters were evaluated using SIMLAB® software: the main maximum (Max P), main minimum (Min P), localized maximum P1 (Max P1), localized maximum P2 (Max P2), total displacement, localized displacement, rotation displacement, and von Mises stress. Compared to the DHS+P and ASNIS models, the X-PIN+P model presented, respectively, increases of 51.6% and 64.7% for Max P, 85% and 247% for Min P, and 18.9% and 166.7% for von Mises stress. Max P1 did not differ between the models, but Max P2 was 55% and 50% lower for X-PIN+P than ASNIS and L, respectively. All displacement values were lower for X-PIN+P than the other models. In this FEM testing, the X-PIN+P was superior to the other models, which was due to improvement in all parameters of stress distribution, displacement, and von Mises stress compared to models using a lateral plate (DHS and DHS+P) or not (ASNIS and L).

Keywords: femoral neck fracture; internal fixation; intramedullary fixation; finite element analysis

1. Introduction

Femoral neck fractures (FNF) in young adults are uncommon, accounting for 3% of all hip fractures, and usually result from high-energy trauma [1,2]. Treatment is focused on preserving the proximal extremity of the femur through anatomical reduction and stable internal fixation [3,4]. Despite their infrequency in the younger population, there is higher rate of femoral head osteonecrosis and nonunion, which directly contribute to a poor outcome and uneventfully are associated with reoperations and salvage procedures [2]. Although many factors have been shown to play a significant role in preventing these devastating complications, the quality of the reduction and its maintenance are the main recognized factors in reducing the risk of avascular necrosis of the head and nonunion of the femoral neck [2,4]. Epidemiological studies have shown up to a 59% nonunion incidence in FNF and from 12–86% avascular necrosis incidence in young patients after femoral neck fracture [2,5–7], with implant failure occurring in approximately 10% of cases in young patients [8].

The implant type is of paramount importance for maintaining anatomical reduction, since it must resist the deforming forces that act on the fracture focus [9]. The more unstable the fracture plane, the more critical this becomes, e.g., in Pauwels type-3 (P3) fractures, in which a dominant shear force is inherent to the fracture pattern, resulting in a higher rate of failure and nonunion [2,8–10]. The deformities often seen are varus angulation and inferior translation of the proximal femoral neck/head fragment, with failure often resulting after a non-anatomic reduction and inadequate fixation [2]. Thus, the search for effective methods of internal fixation has become the focus of scientific research over the years, resulting in the development of numerous implants that combine intra- and extramedullary characteristics [10–14].

Currently, the sliding hip screw, combined or not with an anti-rotation (or erotational) screw, is considered the standard implant in P3 FNF [7,10]. Several authors have shown that the sliding hip screw has less inferior femoral head displacement, less shearing displacement, and a greater load to failure when compared to multiple cannulated cancellous screws [9–13]. Bonnaire and Weber [15] observed that the sliding hip screw with the derotational screw presents the best mechanical environment for this challenging fracture pattern. Although the sliding hip screw has been found to be very effective in treating Pauwels type-3 femoral neck fractures, care should be taken in significantly comminuted fractures in a vertical orientation [16,17].

Despite the sliding hip screw's superior mechanical strength to other extramedullary implants, problems related mainly to its inability to control rotation, especially when an additional derotational screw is not used, with varus subsidence and femoral neck shortening, which alter hip offset, have been reported in the literature [18]. This is mainly because the cephalic screw gradually slides, causing impaction of the fracture focus, which is greater in a malreduced fracture and in cases where the anti-rotation screw is not used. Thus, our hypothesis was that an implant which retained the main characteristics of existing systems (such as the cephalic screw and an intra- or extramedullary anchorage stop) but prevented the progressive collapse of the femoral neck during the healing process could minimize the rate of complications observed in young adult FNF. Indeed, some authors showed a reduced load-to-failure with the fixed-angle proximal femoral locking plate (PFLP), potentially minimizing femoral neck shortening and other complications [16,19,20]. Liporace et al. reported a nonunion rate of 8% for Pauwels type-3 FNF treated a PFLP, compared with 19% in those treated with multiple cannulated screws [20].

The main objective of this study is to evaluate the biomechanical behavior of a locking autocompression screw, called X-PIN, and a variant (X-PIN+P) in P3 FNF using a finite element model (FEM). The secondary objective was to compare the results of this model with clinically established fixation methods for FNF.

2. Materials and Methods

A fourth generation 3908 virtual model of the femur (Sawbones, Seattle, WA, USA) was used, which corresponds to a physical model with 17 pounds per cubic foot and characterizes the model as a young adult femur [21]. A full section was performed in the middle third of the femoral neck at an angle of 70° to the ground, which is considered a P3 fracture. Although some controversy still exists over the exact interpretation of Pauwels' original description, current accepted interpretation is that type III fractures contain a fracture line oriented 70 degrees from the horizontal, which is considered inherently biomechanically unstable due to the shearing displacement [17]. No coefficient of friction value was added to the fracture surface (Figure 1).

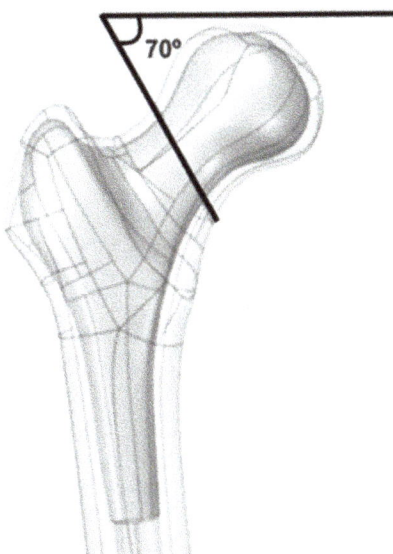

Figure 1. Representation of a Pauwels type-3 neck fracture. Note that the fracture line is oriented 70 degrees from the horizontal.

The X-PIN model features a main screw with 12.7 mm of distal diameter and 13 mm of proximal diameter, both extremities with threads of different pitches and areas, allowing compression between the fractured fragments, and a 4.7 mm locking screw that crosses the main screw through a smooth hole and anchors bicortically. The only change in the X-PIN+P model was a fully threaded 4.7 mm screw, positioned from posterior to anterior along the femoral neck, transfixing the fracture without a sliding tunnel, thus acting as a position screw (Figure 2).

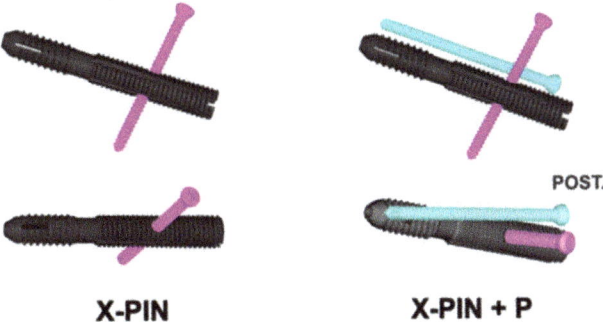

Figure 2. Representation of the X-PIN (left side) and the X-PIN+P. Observe that both extremities of the main screw have threads of different pitches and areas, allowing compression between the fractured fragments. A 4.7 mm locking screw (represented in pink) crosses the main screw from superior to inferior through a smooth hole and anchors bicortically. In the X-PIN+P model, a third screw (a fully threaded 4.7 mm screw, represented in blue) acts as a position screw from posterior to anterior along the femoral neck, transfixing the fracture without a sliding tunnel.

For biomechanical comparison, we used a 135° dynamic hip screw (DHS) and a 7.0 mm cannulated screw, both manufactured by Hexagon Ltd. (São Paulo, SP, Brazil), in conformity with models approved for clinical use by the Brazilian National Regulatory Agency (ANVISA—Agência Nacional de Vigilância Sanitária).

The models were abbreviated according to implant type: DHS, DHS with anti-rotation screw (DHS+P), inverted triangle multiple cannulated screws (ASNIS), multiple cannulated screws in an L-configuration (L), and X-PIN and X-PIN+P (the new autocompression system) (Figure 3).

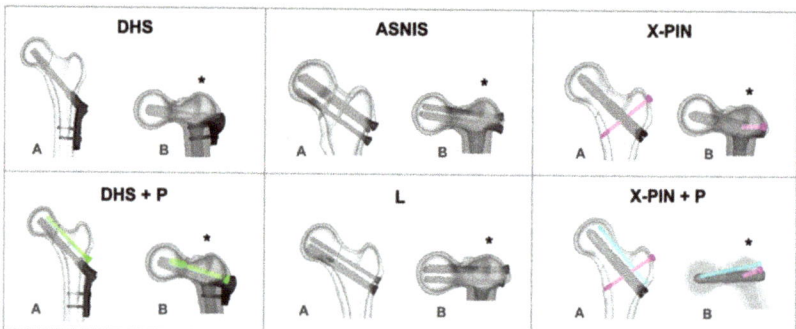

Figure 3. Illustrations of the included synthesis models. (*): posterior region; (**A**) coronal view of the proximal femur; (**B**) axial view of the proximal femur.

For the simulations, the material properties, modulus of elasticity, and Poisson's coefficient of each of the parts of the digital models (cortical bone, trabecular bone, and steel alloy) were previously defined. All metallic models in this study shared a common alloy (Table 1).

Table 1. Material properties.

Material	Material Properties	
	Modulus of Elasticity (MPa)	Poisson's Coefficient (V)
Cortical bone	16,350	0.26
Trabecular bone	137	0.30
Syntheses (steel)	200,000	0.33

After controlling the meshes of each part to certify perfect contact between the different structures, the regions of load application in the X, Y, and Z axes were selected. For the study, a 2100 N load was applied in the Z axis (which corresponds to the stress applied to the femur of a young adult weighing 70 kg in single-leg stance); no loads were applied to both the X and Y axes. Subsequently, the movement restriction regions (fixations) were delimited, marked in all directions of the X, Y, and Z axes to guarantee the stability of the system. A tetrahedral mesh formation was adopted for the meshes, and the models were tested with a 10° inclination in the Z axis (lateral) and a 9° inclination in the Y axis (posterior), with the load applied perpendicular to the ground in the superior region of the femoral head (Figure 4). The decision to adopt a single-leg stance was based on the observation that the bulk of the body weight mainly relies on the hip joint in this position, thus adequately representing the related forces acting around this joint when the whole body is standing on one foot [22].

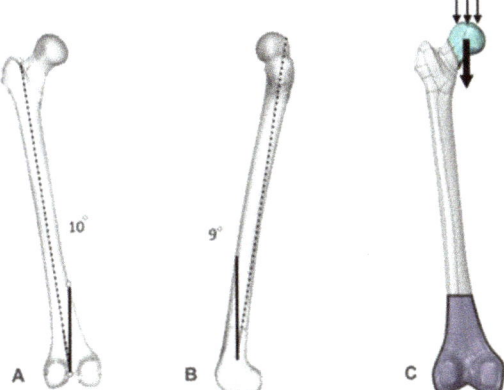

Figure 4. (**A**,**B**) Model of the virtual femur representing the inclination used in the tests; (**C**) the conditions and contours used during the test: load application area (blue with small arrows), load direction (larger arrow) and attachment area (purple).

Data on the displacement and stress in the FEM were collected, including the total principal maximum (Max P), localized maximum P1 (Max P1: area of greatest tension in the upper region of the femoral neck), localized maximum P2 (Max P2: area of greatest tension in the lateral peri-implant region of the femur), total principal minimum (Min P), presented as a negative value to represent the application axis, total displacement, localized displacement (displacement of the fracture focus), rotation deviation, and distribution of von Mises stress.

The Max P1 and P2 values were calculated using the mean tension obtained in the nodes of the most affected region for each group. The rotation displacement was calculated by observing two coincident elements on opposite sides of the fracture before and after loading to evaluate their displacement (Figure 5).

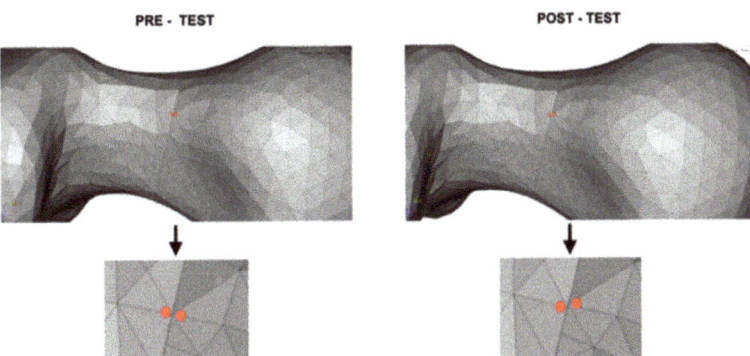

Figure 5. Upper left, nodes on the anterior face of the femoral neck selected for rotation deviation assessment (pre-test). Upper right, skewed nodes (post-test). In the two lower images, the pre- and post-test nodes at higher magnification. Observe that nodes are shown in red color in both figures.

The von Mises stress was captured in the synthesis material of the models and all the results are presented in absolute values and percentiles between the models.

3. Results

All results are presented for the DHS, DHS+P, ASNIS, L, X-PIN, and XPIN+P models in Table 2.

Table 2. Results for each model.

Analysis	Models					
	X-PIN	X-PIN+P	DHS	DHS+P	ASNIS	L
Max total (MPa)	582	1078	607	711	654.3	501
Min total (MPa)	−856	−959	−765	−517	−276	−597
Max P1 (MPa)	28	25	29	24	23	19
Max P2 (MPa)	31	21	36	27	47	42
Total displacement. (mm)	9	2.41	8.4	7.1	9.2	8.7
Local displacement (mm)	2.6	0.8	2.1	1.2	2	1.7
Rotational displacement (mm)	4.1	1.1	3.5	1.5	2.6	2.3
Von Mises stress (MPa)	988	1195	859	1005	448	393

Max P1: localized maximum P1 (area of greatest tension in the upper region of the femoral neck); Max P2: localized maximum P2 (area of greatest tension in the lateral peri-implant region of the femur).

The Max P values were 607, 711, 654.3, 501, 582, and 1078 MPa (Figure 6). The X-Pin+P model results were 51.6% and 64.7% higher than the DHS+P and ASNIS models, respectively.

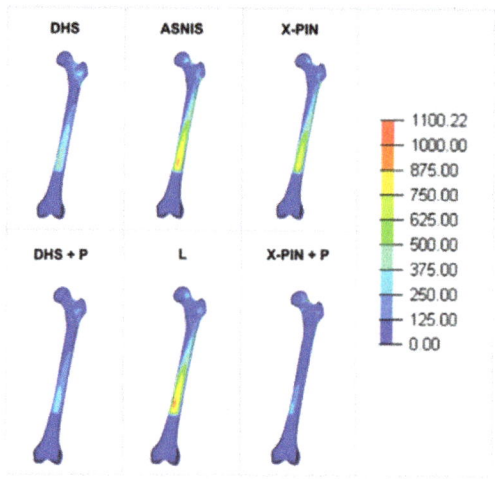

Figure 6. Maximum principal tension in the models.

The Min P values were "−765", "−517", "−276", "−597", "−856", and "−959" MPa (Figure 7), with the X-PIN+P results 85% and 247% higher than DHS+P and ASNIS, respectively.

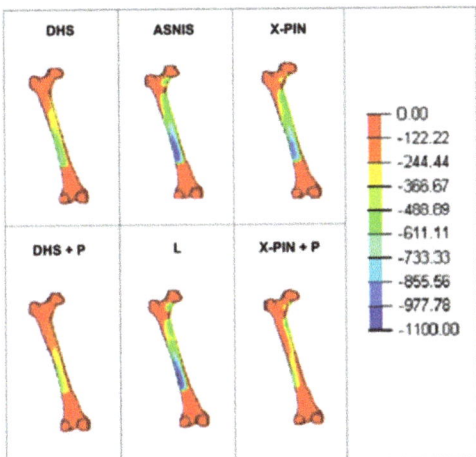

Figure 7. Minimum principal tension in the models.

The Max P1 values were 29, 24, 23, 19, 28, and 25 MPa (Figure 8A). The models were balanced except for the L model, which had a lower value. The Max P2 values were 36, 27, 47, 42, 31, and 21 MPa (Figure 8B), with the X-PIN+P results 55% and 50% lower than ASNIS and L (the multiple cannulated screw models), respectively.

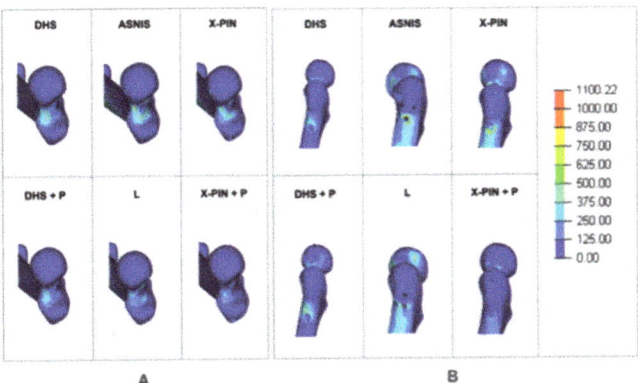

Figure 8. (**A**) Maximum local tension P1; (**B**) maximum local tension P2.

The total displacement values were 8.4, 7.1, 9.2, 8.7, 9.0, and 2.4 mm. (Figure 9A), with the X-PIN+P results 66% and 73% lower than DHS+P and ASNIS, respectively. The localized displacement values were 2.1, 1.2, 2.0, 1.7, 2.6, and 0.8 mm (Figure 9B), while those of rotation deviation were 3.5, 1.5, 2.6, 2.3, 4.1, and 1.1 mm, with X-PIN+P lower than the other models.

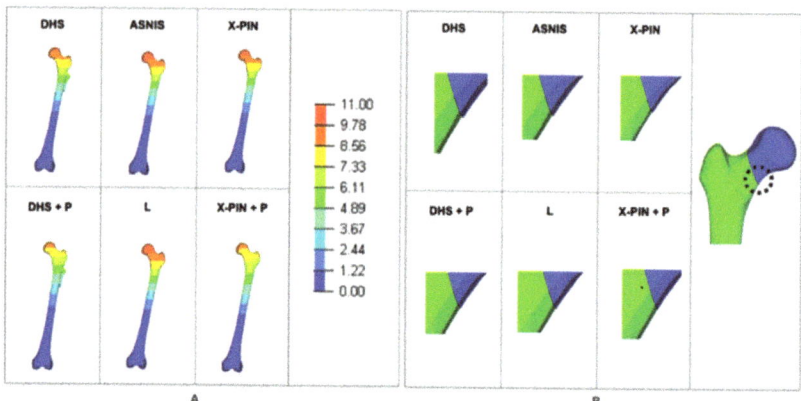

Figure 9. (**A**) Total displacement for each model; (**B**) localized displacement for each model.

Finally, the von Mises values were 859, 1005, 448, 393, 955, and 1195 MPa, with the X-PIN+P results 18% and 166% higher than DHS+P and ASNIS, respectively (Figure 10).

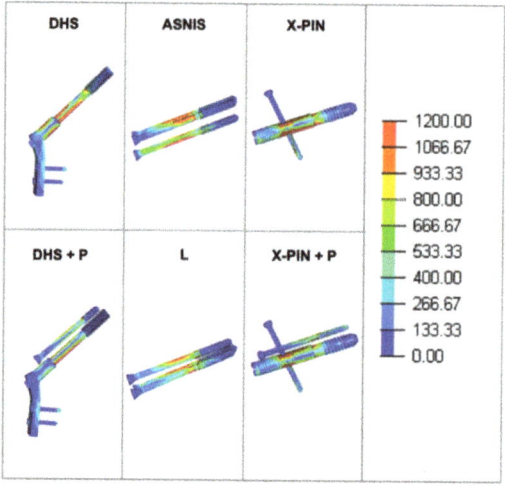

Figure 10. Von Mises stress in each group.

4. Discussion

FNF in young adults have been the subject of several studies, especially P3 femoral neck fractures, due to the inherent instability of the vertical fracture line. Although the sliding hip screw is considered standard for this fracture pattern, the mechanical and biological failure rates are still not very acceptable. In addition, a large amount of bone is removed making later reconstructions difficult if required and there is a higher possibility of damaging the femoral head blood supply if the implant is imperfectly placed or there is a mechanical failure with varus collapse of the head [2]. Thus, it is necessary to study new designs and implant configurations for P3 FNF to mechanically improve the fixation, reducing or avoiding the deforming forces acting at the proximal extremity of the femur.

In this scenario, the X-PIN model was developed and tested in vitro using FEM, a fundamental tool for biomechanical investigations in orthopedics [23,24]. FEM verification focuses on the mathematical aspects, determining if the solution that has been computed is accurate, which has been validated in a number of studies for this purpose [14,21,25–27].

By allowing implant design projects and experimental tests, FEM provides understanding of the biomechanics of the bone synthesis material, effectively and efficiently evaluating several variables, such as implant variations and surgical techniques, to optimize not only the design, but also screening, prediction, and treatment in orthopedics [23]. In the present study, the new X-PIN device, especially when combined with an anti-rotation screw (X-PIN+P), was biomechanically superior to all other implants tested (DHS, DHS+P, ANIS, and L). In particular, the von Mises stress was higher and the total displacement was lower in the X-PIN+P group than in the other groups, which translates into greater stress absorption, especially when the values of these two measurements are observed together. The lower von Mises stress on the main screw of the X-PIN+P compared to the X-PIN was chiefly due to its function as a position screw, which acted to protect the main cephalic screw of the X-PIN. The position screw in X-PIN+P generally led to better stress distribution than the X-PIN in all analyses. In a certain way, this is observed with the sliding hip screw when used with an anti-rotation screw [15].

Recently, other systems in which the sliding screw is locked by another screw have been biomechanically and clinically investigated. Moon et al. [28] compared the stability of proximal fragment fixation and the mechanical characteristics in proximal femur models of a basicervical femoral neck fracture fixed by the new Femoral Neck System (FNS) vs. a sliding hip screw (the DHS). They used 20 composite femurs whose density was customized to young adult characteristics and a Pauwels type 2 femur neck fracture. No significant differences were found in the mean values of axial stiffness, rotation in the X, Y, and Z axes, cranial and axial migration of screws within the femoral head, or failure under vertical load. They concluded that a femoral neck system provides comparable biomechanical stability to the DHS for treating displaced femoral neck fractures in young adults. Unfortunately, their conclusion cannot be extrapolated to the more vertical P3 FNF. Davidson et al. [29] conducted a multicenter retrospective cohort analysis of patients treated with a femoral neck system, including 102 patients with a mean follow-up of 7 months. The fractures were classified according to the Garden system rather than Pauwels system. Overall, the revision rate was 9.2% (14 patients with implant cut-out, 10 with osteonecrosis of the femoral head, 8 with nonunion, and 8 requiring implant removal). The authors concluded that the femoral neck system is a safe treatment option for FNF, with failure rates comparable to those reported for other frequently used implants for this fracture type. Although we have not tested the femoral neck system, our findings cannot, even indirectly, be compared to those of these authors, since they did not use the Pauwels system.

Regarding distribution of the main maximum stresses in our study, the X-PIN+P was similar to the DHS and the DHS+P, but with better distribution. One hypothesis for this is the different cephalic screw locking system, with a screw inserted obliquely, more medially, and bicortically. Freitas et al. [30] found the same behavior in a similar study with a metaphyseal nailing system. Similarly, it can be interpreted that the oblique bicortical locking screw acts as a buttress mechanism, allowing angular stability and preventing proximal and distal migration of the cephalic screw.

It is interesting to note that the lack of a lateral plate on the femur (ASNIS and L) increased the load on this cortex, producing local weakness that is normally observed in clinical studies using only screws to fix P3 FNFs [31–33]. This could be a critical point in the new X-PIN system, since there is no lateral plate. However, the peri-implant stress in X-PIN and X-PIN+P was lower than that of the ASNIS and L models, showing that the lateral cortex of the femur is not weakened with the new system. Furthermore, the localized and rotation displacements were similar in the DHS+P and X-PIN+P groups, with lower values than the other groups. Finally, regarding distribution of the main maximum stresses, the X-PIN+P was similar to the DHS and the DHS+P, but with better distribution.

The main limitation of our study is the comparison between our findings with those of other biomechanical benchtop and clinical studies that did not use previous FEM analysis, which could be subject to several types of bias. The results of FEM can be influenced by several factors, such as the software, the types of meshes and elements, the minimum differences in conditions, and the contours. On the other hand, the results of benchtop tests have not always matched the clinical experience and a computer simulation might be indicated instead of idealized, simple models often used in experimental tests [34]. Augat et al. [34] stated that biomechanical studies typically have a higher sensitivity to detect a true difference between groups in a timely and cost-effective manner compared with clinical studies. Moreover, "if research precedes implant design, the results can lead to innovative solutions in a systematic, evidence-based strategy" [34]. Nevertheless, although our findings look promising for the X-PIN system, especially when combined with an anti-rotation screw (X-PIN+P), we strongly recommend extrinsic comparison to make sure that the biomechanical characteristics of these implants are reproducible under different conditions, such as benchtop tests or even clinical application in P3 FNF. In continued FEM analysis, we are formatting prototypes and conducting bench tests to be tested in other in vitro experiments under controlled conditions. Finally, as this is a controlled FEM analysis, we cannot assess the technical difficulty of placing the implant in a clinical situation. Future studies that will be carried out in phase 3 (clinical studies) will be able to show more assertively the step by step process of the X-PIN operative technique.

The main strength of our study is that stress distribution was better in X-PIN+P than DHS or DHS+P and, thus, was apparently superior to implants developed to treat the difficult condition of P3 FNF in young adults. Although we have not compared the X-PIN and X-PIN+P with the more contemporary implants such as the Synthes Femoral Neck System, the Rotationally Stable Screw-Anchor (RoSA) and the InterTan nail, biomechanical studies have shown that both mean axial stiffness and mean torsional stiffness of these implants were comparable to that of the DHS, especially when fractures were stabilized using the sliding hip screw system with a blade [35–37].

5. Conclusions

In FEM testing, the X-PIN+P was superior to the other models, which was due to improvement in all parameters of stress distribution, displacement, and von Mises stress compared to models using a lateral plate (DHS and DHS+P) or not (ASNIS and L).

Author Contributions: Conceptualization, A.F. and V.G.; methodology, A.F., V.G., R.E.P. and W.D.B.; software, L.R.B.; validation, A.F., V.G., R.E.P., L.R.B., M.d.O.L. and W.D.B.; formal analysis, A.F., V.G., R.E.P. and W.D.B.; investigation, A.F., V.G., R.E.P., L.R.B., M.d.O.L. and W.D.B.; resources, A.F., V.G., R.E.P., L.R.B., M.d.O.L. and W.D.B.; data curation, A.F., V.G., R.E.P. and W.D.B.; writing—original draft preparation, A.F.; writing—review and editing, V.G., R.E.P., L.R.B., M.d.O.L., W.D.B. and A.F.; visualization, V.G., A.F. and M.d.O.L.; supervision, A.F., V.G., R.E.P. and W.D.B.; project administration, A.F.; funding acquisition, A.F. All authors have read and agreed to the published version of the manuscript.

Funding: This study received funding from HEXAGON Ltd. to acquire the virtual Sawbone model, perform the finite element testing, and publish this article.

Institutional Review Board Statement: Not applicable.

Informed Consent Statement: Not applicable.

Data Availability Statement: All relevant data are presented in the paper.

Acknowledgments: To Paulo Cesar Rigolo and Felipe de Morais Machado for technically and financially supporting this study.

Conflicts of Interest: The authors received no financial support for researching and/or authoring this study. The authors received financial support from HEXAGON Ltd. to acquire the virtual Sawbone model, perform the finite element testing, and publish this article.

References

1. Hoskins, W.; Rayner, J.; Sheehy, R.; Claireaux, H.; Bingham, R.; Santos, R.; Bucknill, A.; Griffin, X.L. The effect of patient, fracture and surgery on outcomes of high energy neck of femur fractures in patients aged 15–50. *Hip Int.* **2019**, *29*, 77–82. [CrossRef] [PubMed]

2. Ly, T.V.; Swiontkowski, M.F. Management of femoral neck fractures in young adults. *Indian J. Orthop.* **2008**, *42*, 3–12. [CrossRef] [PubMed]
3. Shen, M.; Wang, C.; Chen, H.; Rui, Y.F.; Zhao, S. An update on the Pauwels classification. *J. Orthop. Surg. Res.* **2016**, *11*, 161. [CrossRef] [PubMed]
4. Parker, M.J. Results of internal fixation of Pauwels type-3 vertical femoral neck fractures. *J. Bone Jt. Surg.* **2009**, *91*, 490–491.
5. Haidukewych, G.J.; Rothwell, W.S.; Jacofsky, D.J.; Torchia, M.E.; Berry, D.J. Operative treatment of femoral neck fractures in patients between the ages of fifteen and fifty years. *J. Bone Jt. Surg.* **2004**, *86*, 1711–1716. [CrossRef] [PubMed]
6. Bartonicek, J. Pauwels' classification of femoral neck fractures: Correct interpretation of the original. *J. Orthop. Trauma* **2001**, *15*, 358–360. [CrossRef] [PubMed]
7. Cha, Y.H.; Yoo, J.I.; Hwang, S.Y.; Kim, K.J.; Kim, H.Y.; Choy, W.S.; Hwang, S.C. Biomechanical evaluation of internal fixation of pauwels type III femoral neck fractures: A systematic review of various fixation methods. *Clin. Orthop. Surg.* **2019**, *11*, 1–14. [CrossRef]
8. Slobogean, G.P.; Sprague, S.A.; Scott, T.; Bhandari, M. Complications following young femoral neck fractures. *Injury* **2015**, *46*, 484–491. [CrossRef]
9. Panteli, M.; Rodham, P.; Giannoudis, P.V. Biomechanical rationale for implant choices in femoral neck fracture fixation in the non-elderly. *Injury* **2015**, *46*, 445–452. [CrossRef]
10. Giordano, V.; Alves, D.D.; Paes, R.P.; Amaral, A.B.; Giordano, M.; Belangero, W.; Freitas, A.; Koch, H.A.; do Amaral, N.P. The role of the medial plate for Pauwels type III femoral neck fracture: A comparative mechanical study using two fixations with cannulated screws. *J. Exp. Orthop.* **2019**, *6*, 18. [CrossRef]
11. Imren, Y.; Gurkan, V.; Bilsel, K.; Desteli, E.E.; Tuna, M.; Gurcan, C.; Tuncay, I.; Sen, C. Biomechanical comparison of dynamic hip screw, proximal femoral nail, cannulated screw, and monoaxial external fixation in the treatment of basicervical femoral neck fractures. *Acta Chir. Orthop. Traumatol. Cech.* **2015**, *82*, 140–144. [CrossRef]
12. Roderer, G.; Moll, S.; Gebhard, F.; Claes, L.; Krischak, G. Side plate fixation vs. intramedullary nailing in an unstable medial femoral neck fracture model: A comparative biomechanical study. *Clin. Biomech.* **2011**, *26*, 141–146. [CrossRef]
13. Rupprecht, M.; Grossterlinden, L.; Ruecker, A.H.; de Oliveira, A.N.; Sellenschloh, K.; Nuchtern, J.; Puschel, K.; Morlock, M.; Rueger, J.M.; Lehmann, W. A comparative biomechanical analysis of fixation devices for unstable femoral neck fractures: The Intertan versus cannulated screws or a dynamic hip screw. *J. Trauma Acute Care Surg.* **2011**, *71*, 625–634. [CrossRef]
14. Giordano, V.; Paes, R.P.; Alves, D.D.; Amaral, A.B.; Belangero, W.D.; Giordano, M.; Freitas, A.; Koch, H.A. Stability of L-shaped and inverted triangle fixation assemblies in treating Pauwels type II femoral neck fracture: A comparative mechanical study. *Eur. J. Orthop. Surg. Traumatol.* **2018**, *28*, 1359–1367. [CrossRef]
15. Bonnaire, F.A.; Weber, A.T. Analysis of fracture gap changes, dynamic and static stability of different osteosynthetic procedures in the femoral neck. *Injury* **2002**, *33* (Suppl. 3), 24–32. [CrossRef]
16. Chan, D.S. Femoral neck fractures in young patients: State of the art. *J. Orthop. Trauma* **2019**, *33*, S7–S11. [CrossRef]
17. Davidovitch, R.I.; Jordan, C.J.; Egol, K.A.; Vrahas, M.S. Challenges in the treatment of femoral neck fractures in the nonelderly adult. *J. Trauma Acute Care Surg.* **2010**, *68*, 236–242. [CrossRef]
18. Swiontkowski, M.F. Intracapsular fractures of the hip. *J. Bone Jt. Surg. Am.* **1994**, *76*, 129–138. [CrossRef]
19. Aminian, A.; Gao, F.; Fedoriw, W.W.; Zhang, L.Q.; Kalainov, D.M.; Merk, B.R. Vertically oriented femoral neck fracture: Mechanical analysis of four fixation techniques. *J. Orthop. Trauma* **2007**, *21*, 544–548. [CrossRef]
20. Liporace, F.; Gaines, R.; Collinge, C.; Haidukewych, G.J. Results of internal fixation of Pauwels type-3 vertical femoral neck fractures. *J. Bone Jt. Surg. Am.* **2008**, *90*, 1654–1659. [CrossRef]
21. Gardner, M.P.; Chong, A.C.; Pollock, A.G.; Wooley, P.H. Mechanical evaluation of large-size fourth-generation composite femur and tibia models. *Ann. Biomed. Eng.* **2010**, *38*, 613–620. [CrossRef]
22. Okolie, O.; Stachurek, I.; Kandasubramanian, B.; Njuguna, J. Material challenges and opportunities in 3D printing for hip implant applications. *Recent Prog. Mater.* **2022**, *4*, 004. [CrossRef]
23. Pfeiffer, F.M. The use of finite element analysis to enhance research and clinical practice in orthopedics. *J. Knee Surg.* **2016**, *29*, 149–158. [CrossRef]
24. Oefner, C.; Herrmann, S.; Kebbach, M.; Lange, H.E.; Kluess, D.; Woiczinski, M. Reporting checklist for verification and validation of finite element analysis in orthopedic and trauma biomechanics. *Med. Eng. Phys.* **2021**, *92*, 25–32. [CrossRef]
25. Ye, Y.; Hao, J.; Mauffrey, C.; Hammerberg, E.M.; Stahel, P.F.; Hak, D.J. Optimizing stability in femoral neck fracture fixation. *Orthopedics* **2015**, *38*, 625–630. [CrossRef]
26. Noda, M.; Saegusa, Y.; Takahashi, M.; Tezuka, D.; Adachi, K.; Naoi, K. Biomechanical study using the finite element method of internal fixation in pauwels type III vertical femoral neck fractures. *Arch. Trauma Res.* **2015**, *4*, e23167. [CrossRef]
27. Samsami, S.; Saberi, S.; Sadighi, S.; Rouhi, G. Comparison of three fixation methods for femoral neck fracture in young adults: Experimental and numerical investigations. *J. Med. Biol. Eng.* **2015**, *35*, 566–579. [CrossRef]
28. Moon, J.K.; Lee, J.I.; Hwang, K.T.; Yang, J.H.; Park, Y.S.; Park, K.C. Biomechanical comparison of the femoral neck system and the dynamic hip screw in basicervical femoral neck fractures. *Sci. Rep.* **2022**, *12*, 7915. [CrossRef] [PubMed]
29. Davidson, A.; Blum, S.; Harats, E.; Kachko, E.; Essa, A.; Efraty, R.; Peyser, A.; Giannoudis, P.V. Neck of femur fractures treated with the femoral neck system: Outcomes of one hundred and two patients and literature review. *Int. Orthop.* **2022**, *46*, 2105–2115. [CrossRef] [PubMed]

30. Freitas, A.; Barin, F.R.; Battaglion, L.R.; da Costa, H.I.; Santos, E.D.; Rosado, H.A.; Giordano, M.; Giordano, V.; Shimano, A.C. Proposal for a new fixation method for pauwels type III femoral neck fracture-metaphyseal stem: A finite-element analysis. *Indian J. Orthop.* **2021**, *55*, 378–384. [CrossRef] [PubMed]
31. Freitas, A.; Toledo Junior, J.V.; Ferreira Dos Santos, A.; Aquino, R.J.; Leao, V.N.; Pericles de Alcantara, W. Biomechanical study of different internal fixations in Pauwels type III femoral neck fracture—A finite elements analysis. *J. Clin. Orthop. Trauma* **2021**, *14*, 145–150. [CrossRef]
32. Lim, E.J.; Shon, H.C.; Cho, J.W.; Oh, J.K.; Kim, J.; Kim, C.H. Dynamic hip screw versus cannulated cancellous screw in pauwels Type II or Type III femoral neck fracture: A systematic review and meta-analysis. *J. Pers. Med.* **2021**, *11*, 1017. [CrossRef]
33. Zeng, W.; Liu, Y.; Hou, X. Biomechanical evaluation of internal fixation implants for femoral neck fractures: A comparative finite element analysis. *Comput. Methods Programs Biomed.* **2020**, *196*, 105714. [CrossRef]
34. Augat, P.; Hast, M.W.; Schemitsch, G.; Heyland, M.; Trepczynski, A.; Borgiani, E.; Russow, G.; Märdian, S.; Duda, G.N.; Hollensteiner, M.; et al. Biomechanical models: Key considerations in study design. *OTA Int.* **2021**, *4*, e099. [CrossRef]
35. Knobe, M.; Altgassen, S.; Maier, K.J.; Gradl-Dietsch, G.; Kaczmarek, C.; Nebelung, S.; Klos, K.; Kim, B.S.; Gueorguiev, B.; Horst, K.; et al. Screw-blade fixation systems in Pauwels three femoral neck fractures: A biomechanical evaluation. *Int. Orthop.* **2018**, *42*, 409–418. [CrossRef]
36. Stoffel, K.; Zderic, I.; Gras, F.; Sommer, C.; Eberli, U.; Mueller, D.; Oswald, M.; Gueorguiev, B. Biomechanical evaluation of the Femoral Neck System in unstable Pauwels III femoral neck fractures: A comparison with the Dynamic Hip Screw and cannulated screws. *J. Orthop. Trauma* **2017**, *31*, 131–137. [CrossRef]
37. Wang, Z.; Yang, Y.; Feng, G.; Guo, H.; Chen, Z.; Chen, Y.; Jin, Q. Biomechanical comparison of the femoral neck system versus InterTan nail and three cannulated screws for unstable Pauwels type III femoral neck fracture. *BioMed. Eng. OnLine* **2022**, *21*, 34. [CrossRef]

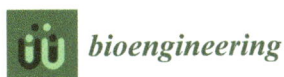

Article

Optimization of Spinal Reconstructions for Thoracolumbar Burst Fractures to Prevent Proximal Junctional Complications: A Finite Element Study

Chia-En Wong [1,†], Hsuan-Teh Hu [2,3,†], Yu-Heng Huang [2] and Kuo-Yuan Huang [4,*]

1. Section of Neurosurgery, Department of Surgery, National Cheng Kung University Hospital, College of Medicine, National Cheng Kung University, Tainan 704, Taiwan
2. Department of Civil Engineering, National Cheng Kung University, Tainan 701, Taiwan
3. Department of Civil and Disaster Prevention Engineering, National United University, Miaoli 360, Taiwan
4. Department of Orthopedics, National Cheng Kung University Hospital, College of Medicine, National Cheng Kung University, Tainan 704, Taiwan
* Correspondence: hkyuan@mail.ncku.edu.tw
† These authors contributed equally to this work.

Abstract: The management strategies of thoracolumbar (TL) burst fractures include posterior, anterior, and combined approaches. However, the rigid constructs pose a risk of proximal junctional failure. In this study, we aim to systemically evaluate the biomechanical performance of different TL reconstruction constructs using finite element analysis. Furthermore, we investigate the motion and the stress on the proximal junctional level adjacent to the constructs. We used a T10-L3 finite element model and simulated L1 burst fracture. Reconstruction with posterior instrumentation (PI) alone (U2L2 and U1L1+(intermediate screw)) and three-column spinal reconstruction (TCSR) constructs (U1L1+PMMA and U1L1+Cage) were compared. Long-segment PI resulted in greater global motion reduction compared to constructs with short-segment PI. TCSR constructs provided better stabilization in L1 compared to PI alone. Decreased intradiscal and intravertebral pressure in the proximal level were observed in U1L1+IS, U1L1+PMMA, and U1L1+Cage compared to U2L2. The stress and strain energy of the pedicle screws decreased when anterior reconstruction was performed in addition to PI. We showed that TCSR with anterior reconstruction and SSPI provided sufficient immobilization while offering additional advantages in the preservation of physiological motion, the decreased burden on the proximal junctional level, and lower risk of implant failure.

Keywords: finite element; proximal junctional failure; spinal reconstruction; thoracolumbar

1. Introduction

Burst fractures in the thoracolumbar (TL) spine are biomechanically characterized by the compression and failure of the anterior and middle spinal columns [1]. The management of TL burst fractures remains challenging, and different treatment strategies are available. These include posterior instrumentation (PI), anterior reconstruction, and three-column spinal reconstruction (TCSR) with combined PI and anterior reconstruction having been reported and deliberated on in the literature [2–4]. Among the different approaches, TCSR combined PI and anterior reconstruction with PMMA augmentation or titanium strut graft has been shown to provide immediate stabilization and restore spinal integrity in highly comminuted burst fractures [2]. Clinical studies have reported the advantages of TCSR over stand-alone PI or anterior-only surgery, including better neurological improvement, stability, restoration of sagittal balance, and less implant failure [2–4].

However, the rigid nature of the constructs increases the risk of adjacent segment complications. Adjacent compression fractures or adjacent disc degeneration at the proximal junctional level are devastating and result in proximal junctional failure (PJF) [5]. PJF can

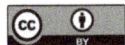

lead to spinal cord compression, spinal instability, and kyphotic deformity, which often require a second surgery. Reported risk factors for PJF include osteoporosis, older age, greater preoperative sagittal imbalance, and longer-segment fixation [6,7].

Compared to conventional long-segment PI (LSPI), which involves instrumentation at two levels above and below the index level, short-segment PI (SSPI) had less stiffness and less increase in stress on the adjacent levels but was associated with an increased risk of implant failure [8,9]. In contrast, other studies advocated that SSPI could provide sufficient stabilization [10]. Given the incongruent results, controversy remains in the choice of posterior fixation techniques [11,12]. Moreover, the complexity of TL reconstruction was increased by the different anterior vertebral column reconstruction materials, including Polymethyl methacrylate (PMMA) cement and titanium cages, which have both been widely used in vertebral body reconstruction [13]. Although previous studies have demonstrated similar clinical and radiographical outcomes between PMMA and titanium cages in TL reconstruction [14], their effects on the proximal junctional level and the biomechanics of PMMA and titanium cage-based reconstruction constructs have not been evaluated. Since PI resulted in the redistribution of the spinal loading between the anterior vertebral graft and the pedicle screw-rod construct [15], TCSR constructs involving combined anterior and posterior instrumentation should be evaluated as a whole. Given the biomechanical complexity of the TL region and the paucity of clinical and biomechanical evidence, the decision-making of selecting an optimal spinal reconstruction strategy remains controversial but appears to be important.

To address the knowledge gap, we designed a finite element (FE) study to investigate the biomechanical performance of different TCSR constructs. Furthermore, we thought to find the optimal strategy to reduce the burden on the proximal junctional level. We established FE models of T10-L3 TL segments and the simulated failure of the L1 vertebral body to represent a burst fracture. Reconstructions with PI and TCSR constructs were simulated and compared. The range of motion (ROM) in flexion, extension, lateral bending, and axial rotation of the whole model and the reconstructed vertebra was analyzed. The mechanical burden of each construct on the reconstructed level, proximal junctional vertebra, disc, facets, and the construct itself was also compared. The objective of this study was aimed to compare and optimize the design of thoracolumbar reconstruction constructs by systematically investigating their biomechanical properties and how they affect the proximal junctional level. The knowledge gained from this study can provide help spine surgeons select an optimal TL reconstruction construct to minimize proximal junctional complications.

2. Materials and Methods

2.1. Generation of T10-L3 Finite Element Model

A three-dimensional FE model of the T10-L3 thoracolumbar spine was created using 1 mm thin-cut axial computed tomography images obtained from a resin cast of an Asian male cadaver without spinal deformities or abnormalities (Figure 1). The images were imported into the software 3D-DOCTOR (Able Software Corp.) to reconstruct the geometric structure of the T10-L3 TL spine, and the corresponding mesh was prepared using the preprocessing software Patran (MSC Software). The mesh generation was performed with software Hypermesh (Altair Technologies Inc), and the FE models were imported into Abaqus 6.12 (Simulia Inc) to solve. In this study, we assumed linear and isotropic material properties for cancellous bone, cortical bone, posterior bony elements, endplate, and disc structures including annulus fiber layers, annulus ground substance, nucleus pulposus, and implant materials (Table 1). The material properties used in the present study were derived from the previous studies by Shin et al. and Wilcox et al. [16,17].

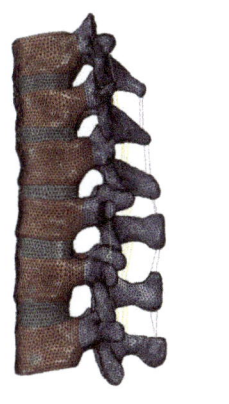 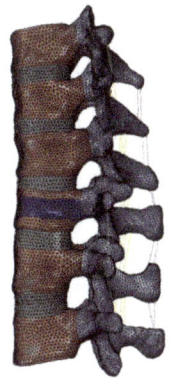

Intact   **Simulated L1 failure**

Figure 1. Finite element model of T10-L3 TL spine and simulation of L1 failure. The present finite element model of the intact spine (**left**) and simulated L1 failure (**right**). The weakened materials were indicated in blue.

Table 1. Material properties and mesh types of the FE model.

Component	Young's Modulus (MPa)	Poisson's Ratio	Element Type
Annulus Fibers			
Inner Laminate: Inner Layer	360	0.30	
Inner Laminate: Middle Layer	385	0.30	
Inner Laminate: Outer Layer	420	0.30	Shell (STRI3)
Outer Laminate: Inner Layer	440	0.30	
Outer Laminate: Middle Layer	495	0.30	
Outer Laminate: Outer Layer	550	0.30	
Annulus Ground Substance	4.2	0.30	Tetrahedron (C3D4)
Cancellous Bone	100	0.20	Tetrahedron (C3D4)
Cancellous Bone (L1 failure)	10		
Cortical Bone	12,000	0.30	Shell (S3R)
Cortical Bone (L1 failure)	1200		
Posterior Bony Elements	3500	0.25	Tetrahedron (C3D4)
Endplate	12,000	0.30	Shell (S3R)
Nucleus Pulposus	1	0.49	Tetrahedron (C3D4)
ALL/PLL/LF/ISL/SSL	20/20/20/10/15	0.25	Truss (T3D2)
Titanium screw/rod/cage	110,000	0.30	Tetrahedron (C3D4)
PMMA	2900	0.30	Tetrahedron (C3D4)

The model for a vertebra consisted of a vertebral body and a posterior element. For the vertebral body, a closed surface was first generated, consisting of cortical bones and endplates assigned to three-node shell elements (S3R). Considering the structures of the cortical bone and endplates of the vertebra, which cover the outer surface of the vertebral body and surround the cancellous bone, it is more reasonable to use shell elements than tetrahedral elements to represent the geometry of the cortex and endplates, and this modeling strategy was also reported in previous FE studies [18,19]. The thicknesses of the cortical bone and endplate were assigned as 0.35 mm and 0.5 mm, according to previous studies [20–22]

The interior of the cortical surface contained cancellous bone assigned to C3D4 continuum elements. The posterior element and the facet were modeled according to the original geometry using C3D4 tetrahedron elements as previously described [23,24]. A three-dimensional surface-to-surface contact with friction was assigned to simulate the facet contact behavior with a finite sliding interaction defined to allow random motions, including sliding, rotation, and separation. The friction characteristic was modeled with a classic isotropic Coulomb friction model with a friction coefficient of 0.1 [25].

The intervertebral discs (IVDs) were modeled with three different components: annulus fibers, annulus ground substance, and nucleus pulposus [25,26]. The IVDs were generated with the superior and inferior boundaries assigned to the endplates of the adjacent vertebra, and the outer boundaries of the IVDs were generated according to the scanned geometry. The annulus was constructed as a ring-shaped structure between the outer and inner annulus fibers. The annulus fibers were modeled with six layers of shell elements with a thickness of 1.5 mm. The annulus ground substance was defined between the two annulus fiber layers and was modeled by solid tetrahedral elements (C3D4). The nucleus pulposus was modeled by non-compressible solid tetrahedral linear elements (C3D4) inside the inner annulus fiber.

The ligamentous complex, including anterior longitudinal ligaments (ALL), posterior longitudinal ligaments (PLL), ligamentum flavum (LF), interspinous ligaments (ISL), and supraspinous ligaments (SSL), were modeled using hyperelastic, tension-only Truss elements (T3D2). The properties of the ligaments were adopted from Goel et al. [27]. The element types and number of elements used in the components of the spine are listed in Table 2.

Table 2. Element count and mesh type of the present intact model.

Component	Element Type	No. of Elements					
		T10	T11	T12	L1	L2	L3
Cortical bone	S3R	2581	2401	2511	2789	2892	3098
Cancellous bone	C3D4	15,144	17,500	18,509	21,312	23,452	19,079
Endplate	S3R	1905	1780	1796	2145	2010	2268
Posterior elements	C3D4	17,472	16,613	16,820	19,951	20,628	21,503
		T10/11	T11/12	T12/L1	L1/L2	L2/L3	
Nucleus pulposus	C3D4	4513	3840	3076	5206	4565	
Annulus fiber	STRI3	1025	812	732	1336	1436	
Annulus ground substance	C3D4	5374	4937	3929	6479	5703	
Ligaments		ALL	PLL	LF	ISL	SSL	
No. of elements	T3D2	25	25	20	15	10	

2.2. Simulation of TCSR Models

L1 burst fracture and vertebral body failure were simulated by weakening the material property of the middle 30% of the L1 vertebral body, according to the previously described method with some modifications (Figure 1) [28]. The Young's modulus of the affected cortical and cancellous bone was decreased by 90% (Table 1).

For anterior reconstruction with PMMA, the surgery model was created by replacing the weakened elements in the L1 vertebral body with PMMA modeled by solid tetrahedral elements (C3D4) (Figure 2). For reconstruction with a titanium cage, an L1 corpectomy was simulated by removing the entire L1 vertebral body and the adjacent intervertebral discs at T12-L1 and L1-L2, and a titanium cage implant was simulated (Figure 2). The three-dimensional structures of the screws, rods, and titanium cage were created in the software Patran (MSC Software). The primary dimensions (diameter, length) of the pedicle screws for the thoracic and lumbar vertebrae were 5.5 mm × 45 mm and 6.5 mm × 45 mm, respectively. The diameter of the rods was 6 mm. The outer diameter, thickness, and height of the titanium cage were 14 mm, 2 mm, and 60 mm, respectively. The pedicle screws, rods, and cage were composed of titanium. The material properties of the implants were shown in Table 1. Mesh structures were prepared using the software Hypermesh 11.0 (Altair Technologies Inc., Fremont, CA, USA) and imported into Abaqus 6.12 (Simulia Inc., Johnston, RI, USA) to solve.

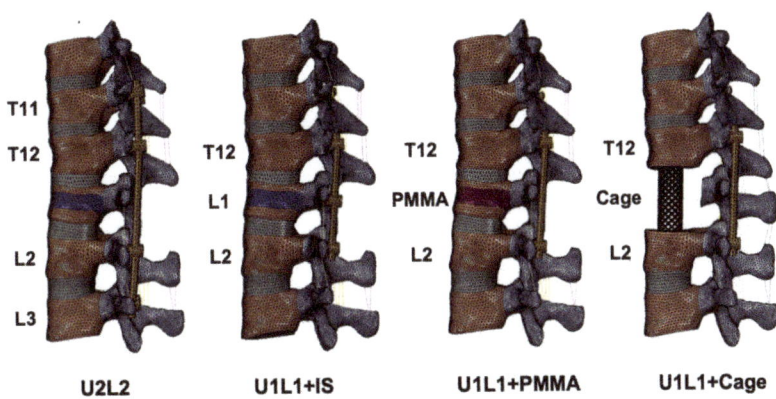

Figure 2. Different spinal reconstruction constructs. Four spinal reconstruction constructs simulated in this study including long-segment instrumentation (U2L2), short-segment instrumentation with intermediate screw (U1L1+IS), and TCSR constructs (U1L1+PMMA and U1L1+Cage). The weakened materials were indicated in blue, and PMMA was indicated in red.

Four surgery models were simulated in the present study, including (1) posterior fixation with LSPI alone (U2L2); posterior fixation with SSPI and intermediate pedicle screw at the L1 level (U1L1+IS); (3) TCSR with PMMA and SSPI (U1L1+PMMA); (4) TCSR with a titanium cage and SSPI (U1L1+Cage) (Figure 2).

2.3. Loading and Boundary Conditions

The preload was set to 150 N and applied evenly using the follower load technique on the T10 superior endplate to simulate the weight of the upper body. For the simulation of the upper body weight, a preload ranging from 100–200 N was used in the literature, and a 150 N preload was chosen in the present study [29]. A 10 Nm moment was applied in the sagittal, coronal, and transverse plane to create motions in flexion–extension, lateral bending, and axial rotation, respectively. The boundary condition of the simulations was set with the nodes on the inferior endplate of L3 constrained in all directions. The interfaces between the bone, pedicle screws, PMMA, and titanium cage were assigned with tie constraints.

2.4. Convergence Test

Convergence tests were performed on the intact model. First, the displacement of a reference point at the center of the T10 superior endplate was measured under a 150 N axial preload. Four different amounts of elements, 190,432, 208,776, 309,217, and 555,384, were compared for the displacements. By setting the displacement of the T10 superior endplate in a model consisting of 1,199,183 elements as the reference value, the errors of the simulations with the total number of elements reduced were all within 4.9 percent. Next, the maximum von Mises stress in posterior elements under a 150 N axial preload was compared. Compared to the reference model, the error of the four models with the total number of elements reduced were all within 7.9 percent. For material stress, it is generally expected that the error may be greater than displacement in FE models [30]. In the present model, we selected the model consisting of 309,217 elements for the intact model based on the small relative displacement error of 2.84% and a von Mises stress error of 4.18%, with the element size ranging from 1.0 to 2.0 mm. The convergence tests were performed on the implant models, including the pedicle screws and titanium cage. For the titanium cage, a final model consisting of 134,203 elements with mesh sizes ranging from 0.4 to 0.6 mm was selected. The error was 3.96% compared to the reference model with 220,141 elements. For the pedicle screw, a final model with 13,927 elements and element size ranging from 0.1 to 1.0 mm was selected. The error was 0.92% compared to the 23,550 element reference.

3. Results

3.1. Model Validation

To validate the finite element model, the simulated ROM and IVD stress in the present intact T10-L3 model were compared with the literature. First, the ROM of the intact thoracolumbar model in flexion-extension, lateral bending, and axial rotation were compared with three in vitro experiments by Chin et al., Rustenburg et al., and Obid et al. [31–33]. The global ROM of the present intact model was as follows: flexion–extension, 6.86 degrees; lateral bending, 3.04 degrees; and axial rotation, 1.54 degrees. Compared with the literature, the results were all within one standard deviation (SD) (Figure 3A). Next, the intact model was also compared with the in vitro intradiscal pressure measurements at L2/L3 IVD conducted by Cunningham et al., Brinckmann et al., and Wilke et al. [34–36]. The maximal IVD stress of this model under sagittal flexion and extension was 0.49 Mpa, which was within one SD compared to the results of Cunningham et al. and Wilke et al. but slightly larger (1.24 SD) than the result reported by Brinckmann et al. (Figure 3B). An extended explanation of the differences is given in the Discussion section.

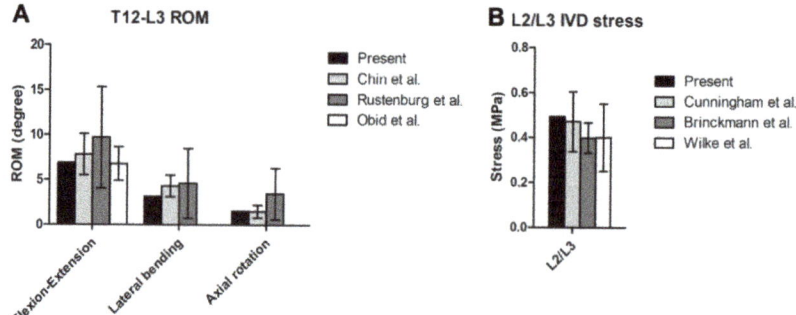

Figure 3. Validation of the present FE model. Comparisons between the (**A**) ROM and (**B**) IVD pressure of the present intact model with the literature [31–36] (presented in mean and standard deviation).

3.2. Global Range of Motion in the TL Spine

The global flexion, extension, lateral bending, and axial rotation ROMs of the intact and surgical models were shown in Figure 4A. The failure of the L1 vertebra resulted in 7.4, 10.1, 18.0, and 11.5% increases in motion under flexion, extension, lateral flexion, and axial rotation, respectively. All four surgical constructs reduced the global ROM in all directions. The LSPI (U2L2) had the most significant reductions in global ROM in the flexion, extension, lateral flexion, and axial rotation of 88.6, 70.7, 81.1, and 40.7%, respectively. The comparison among U1L1+IS, U1L1+PMMA, and U1L1+Cage showed that TCSR with a titanium cage (U1L1+Cage) results in a slightly larger reduction in ROM than the other two structures (U1L1+IS and U1L1+PMMA), but the differences between each other were all less than 0.5 degrees in all motions.

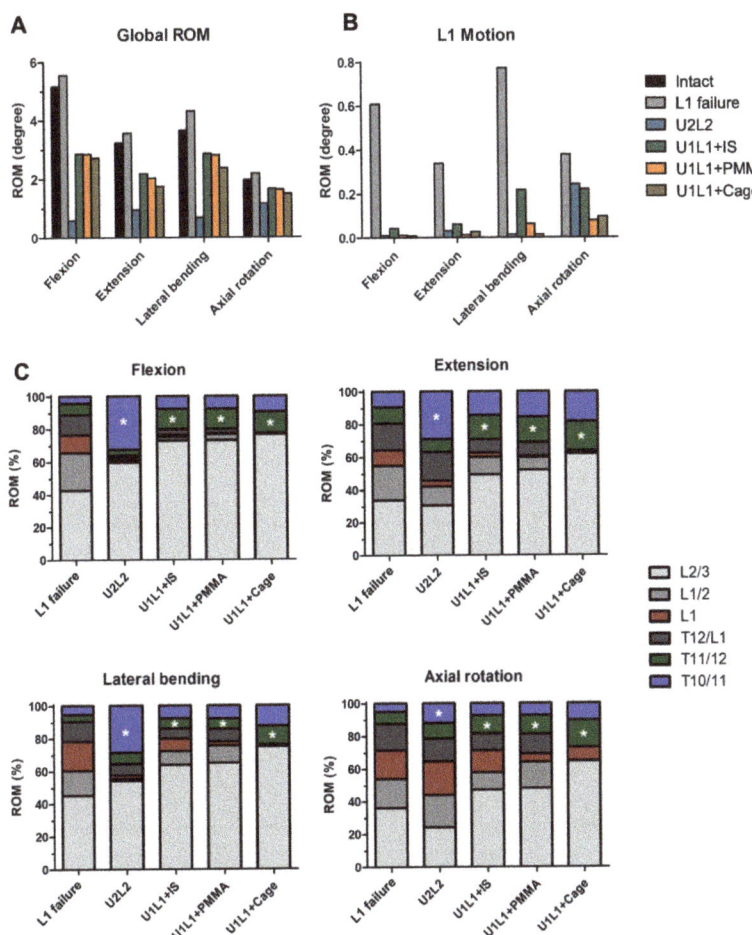

Figure 4. The global ROM, ROM in L1, and ROM distributions. The simulated global ROM (**A**) and the pathological ROM in the L1 vertebra (**B**). ROM distributions (**C**) among the T10–L3 levels. The pathological motion in L1 was indicated in red. * The asterisks indicate the motions in the supradjacent levels.

3.3. Motion in the Fractured L1 Vertebral Body and Motion Distributions

Our simulations showed that failure of the anterior and middle spinal column resulted in increased motion in the affected L1 vertebra. The pathological intravertebral motion within the failed L1 was shown in Figure 4B. The largest motion was observed in lateral bending with 0.77 degrees, followed by 0.61, 0.38, and 0.34 degrees in flexion, axial rotation, and extension, respectively. Comparisons between the constructs revealed that TCSR constructs (U1L1+PMMA and U1L1+Cage) had a greater percentage of motion reduction than PI alone. In flexion and lateral bending, U1L1+Cage had the most ROM reduction by 98.6 and 98.1%, respectively. In extension and axial rotation, U1L1+PMMA had the best ROM reduction by 94.9 and 79.1%, respectively.

The ROM distribution was shown in Figure 4C. The pathological motion in L1 was indicated in red and the motions in the supradjacent levels were indicated by the asterisks. In flexion, extension, and lateral bending, all constructs reduced the percentage of motion in L1. Comparisons of the surgical models showed U2L2 had increased ROM distributed in the supradjacent level. In axial rotation, U2L2 had an increased percentage of motion in L1 while other constructs had decreased percentages of motion in L1. The difference in the percentage of the supradjacent ROM in the axial rotation was not significant.

3.4. The Effect of PI and TCSR on the Proximal Junctional Level

The maximum von Mises stresses exerted on the vertebral body immediately proximal to the constructs (T10 vertebra in U2L2; T11 vertebra in U1L1+IS, U1L1+PMMA, and U1L1+Cage) were shown in Figure 5A. For all constructs, the maximum stress at the proximal junctional vertebra ranged from 0.95 to 5.04 MPa. The highest stress occurred in lateral bending (4.80–5.04 Mpa) in all constructs, followed by flexion (2.77–3.81 Mpa). The greatest differences in stress at the proximal vertebra between the constructs occurred in flexion, in which U2L2 resulted in larger stresses by 1.04, 0.92, and 0.88 Mpa than U1L1+IS, U1L1+Cage, and U1L1+PMMA, respectively. The differences in stress at the proximal vertebra in extension, lateral bending, and axial rotation were all less than 0.5 MPa.

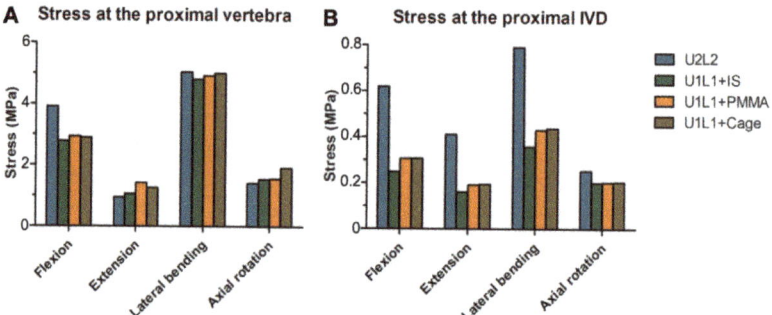

Figure 5. The maximum von Mises stress in the proximal junctional level. The maximum von Mises stress in the proximal vertebral body (**A**) and the proximal junctional IVD (**B**) in flexion, extension, lateral bending, and axial rotation.

The maximum von Mises stresses exerted on the IVD immediately proximal to the constructs (T10/11 disc in U2L2; T11/12 disc in U1L1+IS, U1L1+PMMA, and U1L1+Cage) were shown in Figure 5B. Comparison between the constructs showed a similar trend in all motions, with U2L2 having the largest stress at the proximal IVD and U1L1+IS having the smallest stress at the proximal IVD. The differences in the proximal IVD stresses between U1L1+PMMA and U1L1+Cage were all within 0.01 MPa.

3.5. The Effect of PI and TCSR on the Proximal Articular Facets

The maximum contact force exerted on articular facets immediately proximal to the constructs (T10/11 facets in U2L2; T11/12 facets in U1L1+IS, U1L1+PMMA, and U1L1+Cage) were shown in Figure 6. In flexion, U2L2 had 2.8, 2.7, and 2.7 N less contact forces on the proximal facet joints compared to U1L1+IS, U1L1+PMMA, and U1L1+Cage, respectively. In extension, U2L2 had 5.6, 5.5, and 5.4 N more contact forces on the proximal facet joints compared to U1L1+IS, U1L1+PMMA, and U1L1+Cage, respectively. The differences in the proximal facet contact forces in lateral bending and axial rotation were all less than 1.2 N.

3.6. Von Mises Stress and Strain Energy Density on the Screw and Rod Construct

The maximum von Mises stress and strain energy density of the pedicle screws in each construct were presented in Table 3. The maximum stress of the pedicle screws occurred in axial rotation in all constructs. U2L2 had the highest pedicle screw stress of 27.98 MPa, followed by 27.31, 24.01, and 16.78 MPa in U1L1+PMMA, U1L1+IS, and U1L1+Cage, respectively. The maximum stress was observed at L2 in constructs involving PI alone (U2L2 and U1L1+IS) but was observed at T12 in TCSR constructs (U1L1+PMMA and U1L1+Cage). The stress distributions were shown in Figure 7. The maximum strain energy density of the pedicle screws occurred in axial rotation in U2L2, U1L1+IS, and U1L1+PMMA, while U1L1+Cage had the highest strain energy density in flexion. U2L2 had the highest strain energy density of 12.41 mJ/mm^3, followed by 8.05, 5.72, and 4.55 mJ/mm^3 in U1L1+IS, U1L1+PMMA, and U1L1+Cage, respectively.

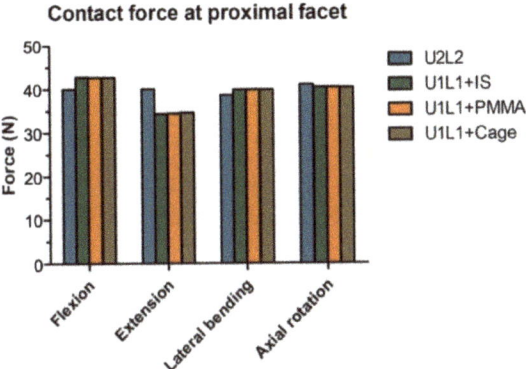

Figure 6. The maximum contact force at the proximal articular facets. The maximum facet contact force in the proximal level in flexion, extension, lateral bending, and axial rotation.

Table 3. Maximum von Mises stress and strain energy in the pedicle screws.

	Maximum Stress in the Pedicle Screws			
construct	U2L2	U1L1+IS	U1L1+PMMA	U1L1+Cage
Stress (MPa)	27.98	24.01	27.31	16.78
level	L2	L2	T12	T12
motion	rotation	rotation	rotation	rotation
	Maximum Strain Energy Density in the Pedicle Screws			
construct	U2L2	U1L1+IS	U1L1+PMMA	U1L1+Cage
Energy (mJ/mm^3)	12.41	8.05	5.72	4.55
Motion	rotation	rotation	rotation	flexion

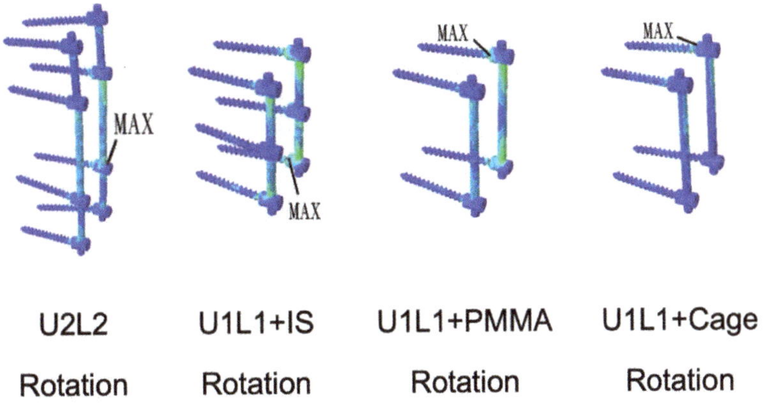

U2L2	U1L1+IS	U1L1+PMMA	U1L1+Cage
Rotation	Rotation	Rotation	Rotation

Figure 7. The stress distributions of the pedicle screw and rod constructs in the motions of maximum von Mises stress detected.

4. Discussion

In the present study, we systemically evaluate the biomechanical performance of different TL reconstruction constructs using FE analysis. Our results showed that TCSR constructs provided better stabilization in the fracture of L1 compared to PI alone. Further, there were decreased intradiscal and intravertebral pressures in the proximal level in U1L1+IS, U1L1+PMMA, and U1L1+Cage compared to U2L2. The stress and strain energy of the pedicle screws were lower in TCSR constructs than in PI alone. We showed that TCSR with anterior reconstruction and SSPI provided sufficient immobilization while offering additional advantages in the preservation of physiological motion, a decreased burden on the proximal junctional level, and lower mechanical stress and strain in the implants.

TCSR with PI and anterior vertebral augmentation or intermediate screw fixation has been shown to provide the immediate stabilization and restoration of spinal integrity [2]. Although previous studies have reported the advantages of TCSR in terms of better neurological improvement, stability, restoration of sagittal balance, and fewer implant failures [2–4], the rigid constructs in the TL region pose a significant risk for PJF [5], and the ideal strategy for TL reconstruction remains controversial. This study evaluated and compared the biomechanics of different reconstruction strategies using FE analysis.

The T10-L3 FE model in this study was validated against previously published in vitro measurements of the ROM and intradiscal pressure. The majority of our simulation results remained compatible and within one SD compared to the literature [31–34,36]. Some differences were noted in the intradiscal pressure between our results and previous experiments by Brinckmann et al. (1.24 SD) [35]. Factors such as the anatomical variation between the present model and the cadavers in the literature could result in the differences. Moreover, the location where the intradiscal pressure was measured in the cadaveric experiments could also contribute to the difference since the pressure measured at the periphery of a degenerated disc tends to be greater than the pressure in the center [37,38]. Further, the assumption of isotropic material properties in the present FE model and the difference in the loading application technique might also contribute to the differences since the mechanical responses of the spine to moments in different planes may not be the same. Despite these variations, the difference between our results and that of Brinckmann et al. remained small and within 1.24 SD [35].

To achieve adequate immobilization at the failure level and prevent PJF, the present analysis was aimed to optimize TL reconstruction constructs to minimize motion in the failed L1 level as well as lessen the impact or burden of the constructs on the proximal junctional level. The relation between excessive motion and pseudarthrosis has been established, especially in the TL area, where T12–L2 is susceptible to premature micromotion due to its transitional biomechanics [39,40]. Our current analysis showed that although all constructs successfully reduced the pathological motion at L1, TCSR constructs were shown to provide better ROM reduction compared to PI alone. This is consistent with the clinical results showing better clinical satisfaction, improved fusion rates, and reduced segmental kyphosis in patients receiving TCSR [41]. In addition, the construct of TCSR with SSPI can also provide sufficient stability to the fractured vertebral body, thereby reducing the number of fixed vertebral segments compared to conventional LSPI. As demonstrated in our study and in the literature, this configuration provides the additional advantage of preserving more vertebral motion segments with better physiologic motion and less overall ROM reduction [24].

The present study highlighted the effect of TL constructs on the proximal junctional level by investigating the intravertebral pressure, intradiscal pressure, and facet contact force of the proximal level adjacent to the fixation. PJF remained a significant complication after TL fusion, with associated neurological injury reported in 11-19% of patients [5,42,43]. A major risk factor for PJF was an excessively long fixed spinal motion segment, which is consistent with our results that U2L2 had a higher risk than (U1L1+IS, U1L1+PMMA, and U1L1+cage) [6,7]. We found a reduced intradiscal pressure at the supradjacent disc in all motions and a decreased intravertebral pressure in the supradjacent vertebra in flexion in the constructs with SSPI (U1L1+IS, U1L1+PMMA, and U1L1+Cage) compared to U2L2. It is important to note that although the stimulation of the highest intravertebral pressure occurs in lateral bending, the orientation of the thoracic facet joints and the presence of the ribs and thoracic cage limit the lateral motion of the thoracic segment. Therefore, intravertebral pressure exerted during flexion may be more clinically relevant than lateral bending, so most PJFs are associated with compression and kyphosis in the sagittal plane [5,6].

In addition to investigating the disc and facet joint pressures at the proximal junction near the spinal fixation device for TL burst fractures, this study also investigated the maximum von Mises stress and strain energy of pedicle screws since one of the main problems of SSPI is increased pedicle screw stress, which may contribute to the risk of early implant failure [44]. Since material failure occurs when the von Mises stress surpasses the tensile yield [45], the maximum von Mises stress in the pedicle screws is associated with the risk of acute screw breakage. However, since the tensile yield stress of titanium is approximately 880 MPa and the maximum stress in the present analysis was 29.78 MPa in U2L2, acute screw breakage is unlikely unless there is major trauma. On the other hand, cyclic strain energy during repetitive motion is related to material fatigue, so the strain energy density in pedicle screws may be an indicator of the constructs' susceptibility to implant failure due to long-term wear [46]. Our result showed that the strain energy of U1L1+PMMA and U1L1+Cage is lower than that of U2L2 and U1L1+IS, while U1L1+Cage has the least strain energy of 4.55 mJ/mm^3. A plausible explanation for this finding is the effect of stress shielding [47], where part of the axial load is transferred to the anteriorly reconstructed constructs of the PMMA or titanium cage. These results suggested that the TCSR constructs might have a lower risk of implant failure than PI alone and that the titanium cage may provide better stress shielding than PMMA. Further, among the PI constructs, our result also showed that the addition of IS to SSPI also lowers the strain energy density in pedicle screws, but the effect was less compared to TCSR constructs. Taken together, our biomechanical assessments demonstrate that TCSR with SSPI provides adequate stability for an A3 burst fracture at L1 with additional advantages in the preservation of more physiologic motion and reducing the burden on the proximal junctional level to the spinal fixation. Anterior reconstruction with PMMA or a titanium cage also provides stress shielding for pedicle screws, which may lower the risk of screw loosening or wear.

There are some limitations in the present study. First, since the transitional anatomy of the thoracolumbar junction between the rigid thoracic spine and mobile lumbar spine featured unique biomechanics, changing the level of the construct was likely to alter the biomechanical response of the TL segments. With this in mind, considering burst fracture was one of the most common indications requiring thoracolumbar reconstruction, we selected the level with the highest incidence of burst fracture, L1, for simulation [48]. A different location of burst fracture would yield different outcomes in our model. Second, the simplification of the material properties including the assumption of linear isotropic materials might not reflect the real-world behavior of the tissues and the surgical constructs. Third, the position and configuration of the implants including the pedicle screws, PMMA cement, and titanium cage are likely to have variations. Changes in the position and orientation of the implants may vary the motion and stress; however, this is very challenging to simulate since multiple real-world factors including anatomical variation, surgical approach, and surgeon's preference could all influence the positioning of the hardware. In addition, the bone quality of the spine as well as the decision on whether spinal canal decompression would be performed may also be important issues that affect the overall success of internal fixation surgery. The assumption of the thickness of the cortical bone and endplate might also influence the simulation results. Previous studies have shown that aging and degeneration resulted in decreased endplate thickness [20], and their effect that spinal biomechanics requires future studies to investigate. It should be noted that in the present FE model, convergence tests were performed separately on the spinal model and implant models, and the instrumented model was built based on modifications of the intact model after the convergence tests were performed and the mesh size was reduced. This approach of performing convergence tests prior to the addition of implants was also utilized in previous FE publications [49–52] and had an advantage in the consistency among the FE models since only part of the model was modified in each surgical construct and the other parts remained unaltered. Finally, perfect contact with tie constraints was achieved between implants and bone. However, the main conclusions of this study were based on comparisons among the surgical construct models. The above-mentioned model simplifications were equally applied to all models, yet their impacts may artificially influence the comparative analyses.

5. Conclusions

In this study, we utilized a validated FE model to investigate the biomechanics of different thoracolumbar reconstruction strategies for TL burst fracture and compared their effect on the proximal junctional level. Our results showed that TCSR constructs provided better stabilization in the fracture L1. Further, there were decreased intradiscal and intravertebral pressures in the proximal level in U1L1+IS, U1L1+PMMA, and U1L1+Cage compared to U2L2. The stress and strain energy of the pedicle screws were lower in TCSR constructs than in PI alone. We showed that TCSR with anterior reconstruction and SSPI provided sufficient immobilization while offering additional advantages in the preservation of physiological motion, the decreased burden on the proximal junctional level, and lower mechanical stress and strain in the implants. The knowledge gained from this study can provide help spine surgeons select an optimal TL reconstruction construct to minimize proximal junctional complications.

Author Contributions: Conceptualization, C.-E.W. and K.-Y.H.; methodology, H.-T.H. and K.-Y.H.; software, H.-T.H. and Y.-H.H.; validation, C.-E.W. and K.-Y.H.; formal analysis, C.-E.W.; investigation, C.-E.W.; resources, H.-T.H.; data curation, C.-E.W. and Y.-H.H.; writing—original draft preparation, C.-E.W.; writing—review and editing, C.-E.W. and K.-Y.H.; visualization, C.-E.W.; supervision, H.-T.H. and K.-Y.H.; project administration, H.-T.H. and K.-Y.H. All authors have read and agreed to the published version of the manuscript.

Funding: This research was funded by the Ministry of Science and Technology (Taiwan) under grant numbers MOST 110-2314-B-006-020 and MOST 108-2314-B-006-048-MY2.

Institutional Review Board Statement: Not applicable.

Informed Consent Statement: Not applicable.

Data Availability Statement: The datasets generated during and/or analyzed during the current study are available from the corresponding author upon reasonable request.

Conflicts of Interest: The authors declare no conflict of interest.

References

1. Denis, F. The Three Column Spine and Its Significance in the Classification of Acute Thoracolumbar Spinal Injuries. *Spine (Phila Pa 1976)* **1983**, *8*, 817–831. [CrossRef]
2. Xu, R.; Garcés-Ambrossi, G.L.; McGirt, M.J.; Witham, T.F.; Wolinsky, J.P.; Bydon, A.; Gokaslan, Z.L.; Sciubba, D.M. Thoracic Vertebrectomy and Spinal Reconstruction via Anterior, Posterior, or Combined Approaches: Clinical Outcomes in 91 Consecutive Patients with Metastatic Spinal Tumors—Clinical Article. *J. Neurosurg. Spine* **2009**, *11*, 272–284. [CrossRef] [PubMed]
3. Shannon, F.J.; DiResta, G.R.; Ottaviano, D.; Castro, A.; Healey, J.H.; Boland, P.J. Biomechanical Analysis of Anterior Poly-Methyl-Methacrylate Reconstruction Following Total Spondylectomy for Metastatic Disease. *Spine (Phila Pa 1976)* **2004**, *29*, 2096–3012. [CrossRef] [PubMed]
4. Lai, O.; Hu, Y.; Yuan, Z.; Sun, X.; Dong, W.; Zhang, J.; Zhu, B. Modified One-Stage Posterior/Anterior Combined Surgery with Posterior Pedicle Instrumentation and Anterior Monosegmental Reconstruction for Unstable Denis Type B Thoracolumbar Burst Fracture. *Eur. Spine J.* **2017**, *26*, 1499–1505. [CrossRef] [PubMed]
5. Nguyen, N.-L.M.; Kong, C.Y.; Hart, R.A. Proximal Junctional Kyphosis and Failure-Diagnosis, Prevention, and Treatment. *Curr. Rev. Musculoskelet. Med.* **2016**, *9*, 299–308. [CrossRef]
6. Park, S.-J.; Lee, C.-S.; Chung, S.-S.; Lee, J.-Y.; Kang, S.-S.; Park, S.-H. Different Risk Factors of Proximal Junctional Kyphosis and Proximal Junctional Failure Following Long Instrumented Fusion to the Sacrum for Adult Spinal Deformity: Survivorship Analysis of 160 Patients. *Neurosurgery* **2017**, *80*, 279–286. [CrossRef]

7. Kim, J.S.; Phan, K.; Cheung, Z.B.; Lee, N.; Vargas, L.; Arvind, V.; Merrill, R.K.; Gidumal, S.; di Capua, J.; Overley, S.; et al. Surgical, Radiographic, and Patient-Related Risk Factors for Proximal Junctional Kyphosis: A Meta-Analysis. *Glob. Spine J.* **2019**, *9*, 32–40. [CrossRef]
8. Wang, W.; Pei, B.; Pei, Y.; Shi, Z.; Kong, C.; Wu, X.; Wu, N.; Fan, Y.; Lu, S. Biomechanical Effects of Posterior Pedicle Fixation Techniques on the Adjacent Segment for the Treatment of Thoracolumbar Burst Fractures: A Biomechanical Analysis. *Comput. Methods Biomech. Biomed. Eng.* **2019**, *22*, 1083–1092. [CrossRef]
9. McDonnell, M.; Shah, K.N.; Paller, D.J.; Thakur, N.A.; Koruprolu, S.; Palumbo, M.A.; Daniels, A.H. Biomechanical Analysis of Pedicle Screw Fixation for Thoracolumbar Burst Fractures. *Orthopedics* **2016**, *39*, e514–e518. [CrossRef]
10. Waqar, M.; Van-Popta, D.; Barone, D.G.; Bhojak, M.; Pillay, R.; Sarsam, Z. Short versus Long-Segment Posterior Fixation in the Treatment of Thoracolumbar Junction Fractures: A Comparison of Outcomes. *Br. J. Neurosurg.* **2017**, *31*, 54–57. [CrossRef]
11. Thaker, R.A.; Gautam, V.K. Study of Vertebral Body Replacement with Reconstruction Spinal Cages in Dorsolumbar Traumatic and Koch's Spine. *Asian Spine J.* **2014**, *8*, 786–792. [CrossRef]
12. Lindtner, R.A.; Mueller, M.; Schmid, R.; Spicher, A.; Zegg, M.; Kammerlander, C.; Krappinger, D. Monosegmental Anterior Column Reconstruction Using an Expandable Vertebral Body Replacement Device in Combined Posterior–Anterior Stabilization of Thoracolumbar Burst Fractures. *Arch. Orthop. Trauma Surg.* **2018**, *138*, 939–951. [CrossRef]
13. Jordan, Y.; Buchowski, J.M.; Mokkarala, M.; Peters, C.; Bumpass, D.B. Outcomes and Cost-Minimization Analysis of Cement Spacers versus Expandable Cages for Posterior-Only Reconstruction of Metastatic Spine Corpectomies. *Ann. Transl. Med.* **2019**, *7*, 212. [CrossRef]
14. Eleraky, M.; Papanastassiou, I.; Tran, N.D.; Dakwar, E.; Vrionis, F.D. Comparison of Polymethylmethacrylate versus Expandable Cage in Anterior Vertebral Column Reconstruction after Posterior Extracavitary Corpectomy in Lumbar and Thoraco-Lumbar Metastatic Spine Tumors. *Eur. Spine J.* **2011**, *20*, 1363–1370. [CrossRef]
15. Akamaru, T.; Kawahara, N.; Sakamoto, J.; Yoshida, A.; Murakami, H.; Hato, T.; Awamori, S.; Oda, J.; Tomita, K. The Transmission of Stress to Grafted Bone inside a Titanium Mesh Cage Used in Anterior Column Reconstruction after Total Spondylectomy: A Finite-Element Analysis. *Spine (Phila Pa 1976)* **2005**, *30*, 2783–2787. [CrossRef] [PubMed]
16. Shin, G.; Mirka, G.A.; Loboa, E.G. Viscoelastic Responses of the Lumbar Spine during Prolonged Stooping. *Proc. Hum. Factors Ergon. Soc. Annu. Meet.* **2016**, *49*, 1269–1273. [CrossRef]
17. Wilcox, R.K.; Allen, D.J.; Hall, R.M.; Limb, D.; Barton, D.C.; Dickson, R.A. A Dynamic Investigation of the Burst Fracture Process Using a Combined Experimental and Finite Element Approach. *Eur. Spine J.* **2004**, *13*, 481–488. [CrossRef] [PubMed]
18. Imai, K. Computed Tomography-Based Finite Element Analysis to Assess Fracture Risk and Osteoporosis Treatment. *World J. Exp. Med.* **2015**, *5*, 182. [CrossRef]
19. Sin, D.A.; Heo, D.H. Comparative Finite Element Analysis of Lumbar Cortical Screws and Pedicle Screws in Transforaminal and Posterior Lumbar Interbody Fusion. *Neurospine* **2019**, *16*, 298. [CrossRef] [PubMed]
20. Rodriguez, A.G.; Rodriguez-Soto, A.E.; Burghardt, A.J.; Berven, S.; Majumdar, S.; Lotz, J.C. Morphology of the Human Vertebral Endplate. *J. Orthop. Res.* **2012**, *30*, 280. [CrossRef]
21. Yeni, Y.N.; Dix, M.R.; Xiao, A.; Oravec, D.J.; Flynn, M.J. Measuring the Thickness of Vertebral Endplate and Shell Using Digital Tomosynthesis. *Bone* **2022**, *157*, 116341. [CrossRef]
22. Palepu, V.; Rayaprolu, S.D.; Nagaraja, S. Differences in Trabecular Bone, Cortical Shell, and Endplate Microstructure across the Lumbar Spine. *Int. J. Spine Surg.* **2019**, *13*, 361–370. [CrossRef] [PubMed]
23. Wong, C.-E.; Hu, H.-T.; Hsieh, M.-P.; Huang, K.-Y. Optimization of Three-Level Cervical Hybrid Surgery to Prevent Adjacent Segment Disease: A Finite Element Study. *Front. Bioeng. Biotechnol.* **2020**, *8*, 154. [CrossRef]
24. Wong, C.-E.; Hu, H.-T.; Tsai, C.-H.; Li, J.-L.; Hsieh, C.-C.; Huang, K.-Y. Comparison of Posterior Fixation Strategies for Thoracolumbar Burst Fracture: A Finite Element Study. *J. Biomech. Eng.* **2021**, *143*, 071007. [CrossRef] [PubMed]
25. Polikeit, A.; Ferguson, S.J.; Nolte, L.P.; Orr, T.E. Factors Influencing Stresses in the Lumbar Spine after the Insertion of Intervertebral Cages: Finite Element Analysis. *Eur. Spine J.* **2003**, *12*, 413–420. [CrossRef] [PubMed]
26. Kumaresan, S.; Yoganandan, N.; Pintar, F.A. Finite Element Analysis of the Cervical Spine: A Material Property Sensitivity Study. *Clin. Biomech.* **1999**, *14*, 41–53. [CrossRef]
27. Goel, V.K.; Park, H.; Kong, W. Investigation of Vibration Characteristics of the Ligamentous Lumbar Spine Using the Finite Element Approach. *J. Biomech. Eng.* **1994**, *116*, 377–383. [CrossRef]
28. Hsieh, Y.Y.; Kuo, Y.J.; Chen, C.H.; Wu, L.C.; Chiang, C.J.; Lin, C.L. Biomechanical Assessment of Vertebroplasty Combined with Cement-Augmented Screw Fixation for Lumbar Burst Fractures: A Finite Element Analysis. *Appl. Sci.* **2020**, *10*, 2133. [CrossRef]
29. Yamamoto, I.; Panjabi, M.M.; Crisco, T.; Oxland, T. Three-Dimensional Movements of the Whole Lumbar Spine and Lumbosacral Joint. *Spine (Phila Pa 1976)* **1989**, *14*, 1256–1260. [CrossRef]
30. Lan, C.-C.; Kuo, C.-S.; Chen, C.-H.; Hu, H.-T. Finite Element Analysis of Biomechanical Behavior of Whole Thoraco-Lumbar Spine with Ligamentous Effect. *Chang. J. Med.* **2013**, *11*, 26–41.
31. Chin, K.R.; Newcomb, A.G.U.; Reis, M.T.; Reyes, P.M.; Hickam, G.A.; Gabriel, J.; Pencle, F.J.R.; Sung, R.D.; Crawford, N.R. Biomechanics of Posterior Instrumentation in L1-L3 Lateral Interbody Fusion: Pedicle Screw Rod Construct vs. Transfacet Pedicle Screws. *Clin. Biomech.* **2016**, *31*, 59–64. [CrossRef]

32. Rustenburg, C.M.E.; Faraj, S.S.A.; Holewijn, R.M.; Kingma, I.; van Royen, B.J.; Stadhouder, A.; Emanuel, K.S. The Biomechanical Effect of Single-Level Laminectomy and Posterior Instrumentation on Spinal Stability in Degenerative Lumbar Scoliosis: A Human Cadaveric Study. *Neurosurg. Focus* **2019**, *46*, E15. [CrossRef] [PubMed]
33. Obid, P.; Danyali, R.; Kueny, R.; Huber, G.; Reichl, M.; Richter, A.; Niemeyer, T.; Morlock, M.; Püschel, K.; Übeyli, H. Hybrid Instrumentation in Lumbar Spinal Fusion. *Glob. Spine J.* **2017**, *7*, 47–53. [CrossRef] [PubMed]
34. Cunningham, B.W.; Kotani, Y.; McNulty, P.S.; Cappuccino, A.; McAfee, P.C. The Effect of Spinal Destabilization and Instrumentation on Lumbar Intradiscal Pressure: An in Vitro Biomechanical Analysis. *Spine (Phila Pa 1976)* **1997**, *22*, 2655–2663. [CrossRef]
35. Brinckmann, P.; Grootenboer, H. Change of Disc Height, Radial Disc Bulge, and Intradiscal Pressure from Discectomy. An in Vitro Investigation on Human Lumbar Discs. *Spine (Phila Pa 1976)* **1991**, *16*, 641–646. [CrossRef]
36. Wilke, H.J.; Wolf, S.; Claes, L.E.; Arand, M.; Wiesend, A. Influence of Varying Muscle Forces on Lumbar Intradiscal Pressure: An in Vitro Study. *J. Biomech.* **1996**, *29*, 549–555. [CrossRef]
37. Buttermann, G.R.; Beaubien, B.P. In Vitro Disc Pressure Profiles below Scoliosis Fusion Constructs. *Spine (Phila Pa 1976)* **2008**, *33*, 2134–2142. [CrossRef] [PubMed]
38. Zhang, Q.; Chon, T.E.; Zhang, Y.; Baker, J.S.; Gu, Y. Finite Element Analysis of the Lumbar Spine in Adolescent Idiopathic Scoliosis Subjected to Different Loads. *Comput. Biol. Med.* **2021**, *136*, 104745. [CrossRef]
39. Reid, J.J.; Johnson, J.S.; Wang, J.C. Challenges to Bone Formation in Spinal Fusion. *J. Biomech.* **2011**, *44*, 213–220. [CrossRef] [PubMed]
40. Heggeness, M.H.; Esses, S.I. Classification of Pseudarthroses of the Lumbar Spine. *Spine (Phila Pa 1976)* **1991**, *16*, S449–S454. [CrossRef]
41. Scholz, M.; Kandziora, F.; Tschauder, T.; Kremer, M.; Pingel, A. Prospective Randomized Controlled Comparison of Posterior vs. Posterior-Anterior Stabilization of Thoracolumbar Incomplete Cranial Burst Fractures in Neurological Intact Patients: The RASPUTHINE Pilot Study. *Eur. Spine J.* **2018**, *27*, 3016–3024. [CrossRef]
42. Lau, D.; Funao, H.; Clark, A.J.; Nicholls, F.; Smith, J.; Bess, S.; Shaffrey, C.; Schwab, F.J.; Lafage, V.; Deviren, V.; et al. The Clinical Correlation of the Hart-ISSG Proximal Junctional Kyphosis Severity Scale With Health-Related Quality-of-Life Outcomes and Need for Revision Surgery. *Spine (Phila Pa 1976)* **2016**, *41*, 213–223. [CrossRef]
43. Reames, D.L.; Kasliwal, M.K.; Smith, J.S.; Hamilton, D.K.; Arlet, V.; Shaffrey, C.I. Time to Development, Clinical and Radiographic Characteristics, and Management of Proximal Junctional Kyphosis Following Adult Thoracolumbar Instrumented Fusion for Spinal Deformity. *J. Spinal Disord. Tech.* **2015**, *28*, E106–E114. [CrossRef]
44. Tezeren, G.; Kuru, I. Posterior Fixation of Thoracolumbar Burst Fracture: Short-Segment Pedicle Fixation versus Long-Segment Instrumentation. *J. Spinal Disord. Tech.* **2005**, *18*, 485–488. [CrossRef] [PubMed]
45. Doblaré, M.; García, J.M.; Gómez, M.J. Modelling Bone Tissue Fracture and Healing: A Review. *Eng. Fract. Mech.* **2004**, *71*, 1809–1840. [CrossRef]
46. Pattin, C.A.; Caler, W.E.; Carter, D.R. Cyclic Mechanical Property Degradation during Fatigue Loading of Cortical Bone. *J. Biomech.* **1996**, *29*, 69–79. [CrossRef]
47. Ponnappan, R.K.; Serhan, H.; Zarda, B.; Patel, R.; Albert, T.; Vaccaro, A.R. Biomechanical Evaluation and Comparison of Polyetheretherketone Rod System to Traditional Titanium Rod Fixation. *Spine J.* **2009**, *9*, 263–267. [CrossRef]
48. Machino, M.; Yukawa, Y.; Ito, K.; Nakashima, H.; Kato, F. Posterior/Anterior Combined Surgery for Thoracolumbar Burst Fractures—Posterior Instrumentation with Pedicle Screws and Laminar Hooks, Anterior Decompression and Strut Grafting. *Spinal Cord.* **2011**, *49*, 573–579. [CrossRef]
49. Bianchi, D.; Falcinelli, C.; Molinari, L.; Gizzi, A.; di Martino, A. Osteolytic vs. Osteoblastic Metastatic Lesion: Computational Modeling of the Mechanical Behavior in the Human Vertebra after Screws Fixation Procedure. *J. Clin. Med.* **2022**, *11*, 2850. [CrossRef]
50. Rivera, A.F.; de Castro Magalhães, F.; Moreno, A.; Rubio, J.C. Assessment of the Highest Stress Concentration Area Generated on the Mandibular Structure Using Meshless Finite Elements Analysis. *Bioengineering* **2020**, *7*, 142. [CrossRef]
51. Knapp, A.; Williams, L.N. Predicting the Effect of Localized ACL Damage on Neighbor Ligament Mechanics via Finite Element Modeling. *Bioengineering* **2022**, *9*, 54. [CrossRef]
52. Molinari, L.; Falcinelli, C.; Gizzi, A.; di Martino, A. Effect of Pedicle Screw Angles on the Fracture Risk of the Human Vertebra: A Patient-Specific Computational Model. *J. Mech. Behav. Biomed. Mater.* **2021**, *116*, 104359. [CrossRef] [PubMed]

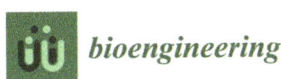

Review

Recent Advances in Coupled MBS and FEM Models of the Spine—A Review

Kati Nispel [1,2,*], Tanja Lerchl [1,2], Veit Senner [1] and Jan S. Kirschke [2]

1. Associate Professorship of Sport Equipment and Sport Materials, School of Engineering and Design, Technical University of Munich, 85748 Garching, Germany
2. Department of Diagnostic and Interventional Neuroradiology, School of Medicine, Klinikum Rechts Der Isar, Technical University of Munich, 81675 Munich, Germany
* Correspondence: kati.nispel@tum.de; Tel.: +49-89-289-15365

Abstract: How back pain is related to intervertebral disc degeneration, spinal loading or sports-related overuse remains an unanswered question of biomechanics. Coupled MBS and FEM simulations can provide a holistic view of the spine by considering both the overall kinematics and kinetics of the spine and the inner stress distribution of flexible components. We reviewed studies that included MBS and FEM co-simulations of the spine. Thereby, we classified the studies into unidirectional and bidirectional co-simulation, according to their data exchange methods. Several studies have demonstrated that using unidirectional co-simulation models provides useful insights into spinal biomechanics, although synchronizing the two distinct models remains a key challenge, often requiring extensive manual intervention. The use of a bidirectional co-simulation features an iterative, automated process with a constant data exchange between integrated subsystems. It reduces manual corrections of vertebra positions or reaction forces and enables detailed modeling of dynamic load cases. Bidirectional co-simulations are thus a promising new research approach for improved spine modeling, as a main challenge in spinal biomechanics is the nonlinear deformation of the intervertebral discs. Future studies will likely include the automated implementation of patient-specific bidirectional co-simulation models using hyper- or poroelastic intervertebral disc FEM models and muscle forces examined by an optimization algorithm in MBS. Applications range from clinical diagnosis to biomechanical analysis of overload situations in sports and injury prediction.

Keywords: multibody simulation; finite element method; co-simulation; spine; spinal loading; sports; biomechanics; degeneration; intervertebral disc; coupled

---

1. Introduction

When humans evolved to adopt an upright position, the spine became a central structure of the human biomechanical system. As such, it can be a source of pain that can significantly impact a person's quality of life. Intervertebral disc (IVD) degeneration and herniation are possible causes of back pain. Research has shown that both aging [1] and overload [2,3], often experienced by ambitious athletes, can contribute to the degeneration process. However, the relationship between abnormal loading and degeneration is not fully understood. In addition, IVD changes that are visible in magnetic resonance imaging (MRI) have not proven to be clear evidence of back pain [4]. To better understand the mechanisms underlying back pain and identify potential solutions, it is important to study the spine and its related structures in a holistic manner, considering the interactions of motion or posture, pain, and IVD biomechanics. However, the difficulty of directly observing these structures in vivo makes this task challenging. Numerical simulations can be useful in modeling and analyzing the mechanics of the spine, to identify factors that contribute to spinal health problems and potential interventions.

Multibody simulation (MBS) is widely used to gain insights into the healthy and pathological biomechanics of the spine from a macroscopic perspective. MBS models

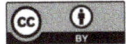

Citation: Nispel, K.; Lerchl, T.; Senner, V.; Kirschke, J.S. Recent Advances in Coupled MBS and FEM Models of the Spine—A Review. *Bioengineering* **2023**, *10*, 315. https://doi.org/10.3390/bioengineering10030315

Academic Editors: Christina Zong-Hao Ma, Zhengrong Li, Chen He, Aurélien Courvoisier and Elena A. Jones

Received: 31 December 2022
Revised: 13 February 2023
Accepted: 22 February 2023
Published: 1 March 2023

Copyright: © 2023 by the authors. Licensee MDPI, Basel, Switzerland. This article is an open access article distributed under the terms and conditions of the Creative Commons Attribution (CC BY) license (https://creativecommons.org/licenses/by/4.0/).

study joint reaction forces, muscle forces and muscle activation patterns in combination with respective movements or positions. There are several such models that include intervertebral joints with three rotational [5–19] or six translational [20–22] degrees of freedom (DoFs) while neglecting passive structures, such as ligaments and facet joints. Using force elements as additions to joints allows individual stiffness definitions for all given DoFs [15–20]. For all models, including rotational joints in at least one dimension, the position of joints is a central issue, as it defines the centers of rotation and therefore, directly influences joint kinematics. The fixed centers of rotation in these studies were set either in the center of the IVD [6,12,17], or according to Pearcy and Bogduk [23], in the posterior half of the upper endplate of the inferior vertebra of each motion segment [9,15,16,24].

Finite element method (FEM) spine models aim to simulate deforming bodies in a detailed manner to reveal their inner stresses. Models may include the whole spine, a segment or only an IVD. Most models contain manually created geometries for IVDs and vertebrae [25], but recent approaches use automated segmentation algorithms to derive patient-specific geometries [26,27]. For IVDs, the current gold standard is a biphasic, poroelastic and nonlinear model including an anulus fibrosus (AF) and a nucleus pulposus (NP) component. While bone is usually modeled with linear material properties [28], or as a rigid body [29], material properties for the IVD commonly include hyperelastic material models, such as the Neo-Hooke and Mooney–Rivlin models [30]. As IVD degeneration is believed to affect IVD biomechanics [31,32], several approaches also deal with degeneration-dependent material properties [33,34]. A key evaluation criterion of FEM spine models is their ability to describe arbitrary material behavior of the IVD while numerically reporting all its biomechanical functions, such as load transfer and bulging events [35].

In summary, MBS models are suitable for investigations of the overall kinematics and kinetics of the trunk, or even the full body. However, detailed information on flexible body deformation and internal stress cannot be provided. Complex, heterogeneous structures, such as the IVD, or even entire functional spinal units (FSU) combining all stabilizing structures (IVD, ligaments, facet joints), are reduced to a resultant mechanical response to external deformation, often in reference to an approximated center of rotation. In contrast, FEM models are beneficial for simulating detailed structures and analyzing inner stresses and deformations. However, detailed FEM meshes may cause large computational costs, and thus, models often include simplifications. Additionally, defining realistic boundary conditions (BC) for FEM models remains a main challenge due to the lack of possibilities for in vivo measurements. Until now, no satisfactory, broad investigations are available containing this data [22].

Coupling MBS and FEM takes advantage of the strengths of each method and offers great potential to analyze the deformations and stresses of IVDs while considering the overall kinematics and kinetics of the trunk. How coupling is implemented can be subdivided into two approaches: One is to calculate acting forces or present deformations completely before starting the other simulation (unidirectional data flow). The second approach considers acting forces or displacements anew in every increment of an ongoing simulation, generating a constant, bidirectional data flow. Unidirectional coupling commonly includes an inverse dynamic MBS simulation with resulting forces and moments, which are subsequently used as loading and BCs in an FEM model [36–43]. Less common approaches use FEM model displacements and stresses to define properties of force elements, occasionally called bushing components, in MBS simulations [44]. Few approaches apply order-reduction techniques to the FEM model before integrating it into an MBS model [45], which reduces computational costs in linear models, but does not support parameter variation after the reduction is carried out. In general, unidirectional coupling is suitable for linearly deforming FEM bodies because the positions of the body's particles do not change substantially, providing the possibility of directly applying the calculated forces of the MBS simulation subsequently to the respective locations in the FEM bodies. Bidirectional coupling is preferential whenever large deformations are present [46,47]. In that case, the deformations of the flexible bodies have a direct impact on multibody kinematics, hindering the option of consecutive simulations.

Hence, by using co-simulation, we can examine the pathological spine in a holistic way to analyze the interactions of various factors, such as motion, posture, back pain and the biomechanics of the IVD. In this work, we review advances in coupled MBS and FEM simulations of the spine. Specifically, we excluded reduced order models and instead focused on the type of data exchange, whether unidirectional or bidirectional, as this is essential for the simulation of large deformations and constant interactions of different components in the spine.

2. Methods

Coupling MBS and FEM models has become a common practice in spine modeling during the last decade. However, no terminology has been established yet to differentiate between what are here called unidirectional and bidirectional co-simulation. To achieve comprehensive coverage of studies using co-simulation, the following keywords were searched in several combinations in different databases: coupled, spine, multibody, MBS, FEM, hybrid, finite element, co-simulation, combined. Resulting articles were manually reviewed and included only if they: (i) contained a type of coupling between MBS and FEM and (ii) were published after 2009 or included models that were still used in studies published after 2009.

3. Unidirectional Co-Simulation of the Spine

We first reviewed MBS and FEM models of the spine using unidirectional coupling, which was characterized by the execution of one simulation and the integration of the results into another simulation. Considering the order of execution, three distinct methods of coupling were identified: MBS execution and transfer of data to an FEM simulation; FEM and transfer of data to MBS; and a threefold data transfer from FEM to MBS and to FEM again. Figure 1 visualizes the representative simulation models with the different coupling methods.

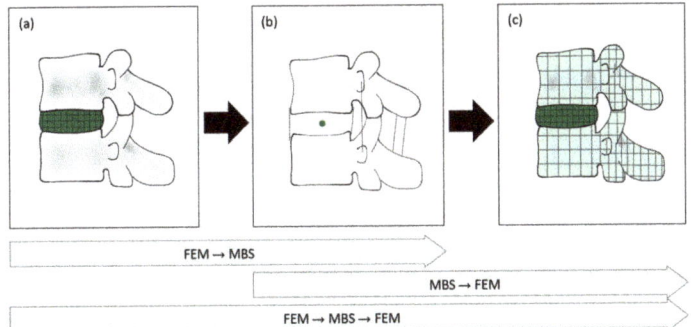

Figure 1. Schematic overview of unidirectional coupling methods. Arrows on the bottom indicate the respective coupling methods. (**a**) Representative FEM model of a FSU containing a detailed IVD, as found in Karajan et al. [44]. Resulting FEM displacements were converted to MBS bushing element parameters. (**b**) Typical MBS model with a joint representing the IVD. Results from the simulation, such as muscle forces or time-dependent displacements of vertebrae or joints, were subsequently included in an FEM simulation. (**c**) Representative FEM model of a FSU or a larger section of the spine. With the BCs defined according to the results of (**b**), these models were often used to calculate IDPs, stress distributions in the IVDs and load-sharing mechanisms.

3.1. MBS → FEM

A unidirectional data transfer from MBS to FEM was the most common approach in unidirectional coupling. Muscle forces, reaction forces or displacements were calculated by an MBS simulation and integrated as boundary conditions (BC) in a subsequent FEM simulation.

Esat et al. [37,38] established a unidirectional MBS and FEM co-simulation of the cervical spine to calculate intradiscal pressure and AF stresses at large impact accelerations. Geometries for rigid MBS bodies were inspired by human anatomy but not specifically derived from medical images. Bodies were created in computer-aided design (CAD) software and imported in Nastran (MSC Software, Garching, Germany) before ligaments and facet joint contacts were integrated. IVD joints were modeled with nonlinear viscoelastic bushing components. One hundred and forty muscles with their respective time-dependent forces were transcribed using a dynamic calculation framework (Virtual Muscle 3.1.5 [48]). The FEM model was then implemented with independent dimensions and locations of IVDs, which were derived from the general quantitative anatomy of the spine in the software Marc/Mentat (MSC Software, Garching, Germany). NP and AF were defined using linear material parameters. Two impact loadings, namely, 15 g frontal and 8.5 g rear-end impacts, were implemented at the neck of the MBS model. The resulting loads—two sagittal forces and one sagittal moment—at the interface points for each IVD, were measured in the MBS model and implemented as time-dependent force BCs in the subsequently set-up FEM model to predict von Mises stresses in the AF and the intradiscal pressure in the NP.

Du et al. [49] investigated the impact of ejection out of, e.g., a plane on the IVDs using unidirectional co-simulation. The MBS model included the entire human body seated in a chair and consisted of 16 rigid elements, with the spine divided only into the neck, upper body and lower body. Joint properties were taken from the literature. The joint between the upper and lower torso was replaced by a spring with a stiffness level of 900 N/mm. Loading was applied through an accelerative load peak of 15 g. The nonlinear FEM model of the thoracolumbar–pelvis complex (T9-S1) included the following material properties: vertebrae and pelvis as isotropic homogeneous elastic material, IVD divided into NP and AF, with the NP containing brick elements of an incompressible, hyperelastic Mooney–Rivlin material model and the AF containing hyperelastic ground substance and 3D cable elements as fibers with nonlinear stress–strain behavior, along with seven ligaments as tension-only cable elements. Attachment points and cross-sectional areas of the ligaments were obtained from Agur et al. [50]. The model was validated statically and quasi-dynamically. The MBS model was used to calculate the translation and rotation of freely chosen reference points (RP), namely, the hip joint and a point at the center of the superior endplate at T9, which were subsequently implemented as time-dependent BCs in the FEM model. For both models, Hypermesh (Altair Engineering Corp., Troy, MI, USA) was used.

Henao et al. [51] simulated surgery procedures to predict potential spinal cord damage. To do so, they implemented a complete, patient-specific FEM spine model that included the spinal cord. A previously developed MBS model of the spine [52] contained 6-DoF springs as IVD and ligament representatives. It was used to calculate the displacements of respective vertebrae, which were then incorporated as BC in the FEM model. No information was given on the stiffness parameters of the spine and how the authors ensured consistency with the FEM IVD model. The study was rated useful for surgery planning, as spinal cord injuries could be predicted by the model. Individualized parameters, especially in the area of the IVD, would likely improve prediction quality.

Honegger et al. [53] investigated the IVD stresses during the sit-to-stand (STS) transfer of lower-limb amputees using a unidirectional co-simulation. The lower-body MBS model was built in OpenSim and included 294 Hill-type muscles and five lumbar vertebrae, which were complemented with three DoF bushing elements containing stiffness values found in the literature [20]. Simulating the STS motion in the MBS model resulted in the lumbar pelvic rhythm, namely, the respective time-dependent joint angles of the lumbar spine and the muscle forces. In a lumbar FEM model taken from Campbell et al. [54], these values were introduced as time-dependent inputs, together with joint contact forces and moments. Results included, among others, the time-dependent AF stresses, facet joint loads and

IDPs during the STS. Comparing the IDPs calculated based on the MBS joint force and the IDPs found in the FEM model showed greater agreement between MBS values and in vivo data [55]. The authors stated that personalized data would possibly improve the muscle force and joint-load estimations from the MBS model, and thus have an impact on the FEM model and final simulation results.

A research group bulit around Shirazi-Adl and Arjmand has been developing numerical models of the spine since 1985 [56] and has started to advance, in parallel, two distinct model versions, which have been known by various names throughout the years. For overview reasons, the two models are herein marked as "I" and "II".

(I) The first model included an initial, detailed FEM representation of the spine.

(II) The second model was based on the detailed model but consisted of rigid bodies and interconnecting beam elements. It is later referred to as the musculoskeletal (MS) model.

Version II was not solved with a classic MBS solver, but included clear characteristics of an MBS model, such as the involvement of mainly rigid bodies and their interconnections by joint-like components. While version II could not represent detailed deformations, it was able to perform large numbers of nonlinear analyses [57]. The researchers refined these models into a passive, osteoligamentous (I) and an active, muscular part (II) and considered their respective roles in a coupled, biomechanical system [57–59]. They implemented their passive FEM model in Abaqus (Dassault Systèmes, Paris, France), consisting of single rigid vertebrae (L1–L5) and one rigid body combining T1–T12. The IVDs were created by extruding the endplate geometries and were infused with rebar elements as AF fibers. The active model was based on a Fortran code. For the coupling process, virtual springs were attached to each vertebra in the passive model (I) to allow the transmission of shear forces and axial, lateral and sagittal moments. Hence, the load sharing between the passive structures and the muscles could be controlled.

In 2002, Shirazi-Adl et al. [60] incorporated a novel, kinematic-based Matlab (the Mathorks Inc., Natick, Massachusetts, USA) algorithm into the simplified model (II) to interactively calculate optimized solutions for muscle- and passive reaction forces. Refer to [61] for a detailed data flow chart. Note, optimization algorithms are commonly used in MBS models for muscle force estimations as well. Beam joints in the active model (II) represented the overall nonlinear stiffness levels of the spinal segments—namely, IVDs, facets and ligaments—with a nonlinear load–displacement curve, which was defined in an iterative process towards yielding the best agreement with the detailed FEM results (I) [57] and was direction-dependent [60]. Ten muscles, five global and five local, were included with six distinct fascicles [62]. The detailed FEM model (I) was based on CT images and consisted of 6 vertebrae (L1-S1) as rigid bodies, five IVDs divided ino AF and NP, 10 contact facet surfaces and 9 sets of ligaments [40]. Fourteen AF lamellae were considered with rebar fibers and a linear elastic ground substance, along with an incompressible NP. Satisfactory agreement considering predicted rotations under flexion, extension and torque loading validated the two respective models against each other [60]. Given IVD cross sectional areas, values in the FEM model (I) were 17% smaller than the ones in the MS model (II) [36].

Azari et al. [36] modified the models by applying the idea of a follower load (FL), which is a method for including simplified muscle forces in passive FEM models (I) to achieve more realistic load conditions [40]. The FL's line of action was aligned with the lumbar spine's curvature, passing the endplates and vertebrae at the approximate center. The FEM model was based on the detailed, passive FEM model (I), but included only the L4–L5 segment. The MS model (II) was adopted mainly unchanged from earlier work by the research group [56,57,60–62]. To estimate stresses and strains in IVDs; ligaments and facets; and load sharing among these structures under realistic loading conditions, Azari et al. applied gravity loads and muscle forces from an MS trunk model (II) to the passive FEM model (I) in several static positions. Twelve static positions were simulated based on the availability of the results of Wilke et al. [55] and the kinematic data gathered by

Arjmand et al. [62]. A resultant force including all gravity loads and muscle forces with upper insertions at and above L4 was calculated using the MS muscle force predictions. After the passive FEM model was rotated manually per IVD to fit the kinematic position of the twelve respective MS models, the research group tried two approaches: directly applying muscle forces estimated by the MS model in the center of the L4 body, and determining a substituting FL by trial and error to yield a similar IDP as derived by the previous approach. The FL was applied as a unilateral, pre-compressed spring between the L4 and L5 centroid.

To analyze scoliotic spine loads and their growth patterns, Kamal et al. [39] established a combined MS and FEM simulation based on subject-specific upright positional data. An MS model data of the bony spine components, including the pelvis, hip and ribcage, was derived from subject-specific CT images using mimics and was subsequently aligned into an estimated upright position with the aid of optical imaging tools. IVD centroids were considered the centers of rotation (CoRs) for the modeled spine section T12–L1 and set up with three nonlinear rotational stiffness values according to Hajihosseinali et al. [17]. Simulations were run statically with all rigid bodies fully constrained. Muscle attachment points for more than 160 muscles were calculated using Matlab. A static optimization algorithm then computed muscle forces and reaction moments, namely, individual forces F_m and reaction moment M_{CoR}, for each muscle. Reaction forces were considered as the sum of gravitational forces and muscle forces. The resulting forces and moments in a static equilibrium condition calculated in the MS model were applied to the vertebral growth plate FEM bodies as distributed pressures and shear stresses. Note, IVDs were solely considered as joints, and the biomechanical focus lay on the growth plates. FEM simulations were carried out with Abaqus (Dassault Systèmes, Paris, France). The resulting stresses in the growth plates were comparable with results from the literature and may be helpful in predicting growth patterns in scoliotic spines.

Further studies included a hybrid model applying muscle forces calculated in the beam-joint-based MS model (II) to the updated, passive T12-S1 FEM model (I) [40]. The MS model consisted of 56 muscles and was solved with an optimization algorithm minimizing the sum of the cubed muscle stresses. The outcome served as a basis for evaluating the loads on the beam joints. Simulations included eight static tasks for which the muscle forces were estimated by connector elements between muscle insertion points in the MS model. Together with the pelvic rotations gathered from in vivo experiments, these forces were substituted into the FEM model. Final deformed positions for the eight tasks were found to vary between the MS and FEM model, and the authors subsequently applied an iterative process, in which the compression-dependent stiffness properties of the MS beam-joints were adapted and resulting forces were again prescribed into the FEM model until the solution was convergent. The hybrid nature of the approach was thus the adaption of the beam-joint parameters based on a passive FEM model deformed position, which was defined actively by MS results. Kinematics of the MS and FEM models differed by less than 1 mm in the final state.

In order to develop a self-defined gold standard of spine modeling, Rajaee et al. [63] further developed the hybrid MS and FEM model introduced by Khoddam-Khorasani et al. [40] towards a coupled model, which enhances the hybrid model by incorporating the musculature of the MS model (II) in the FEM model (I). The manual approach of iteratively updating the nonlinear beam-joint stiffness was thus avoided. The resulting model hence consists of the rigid vertebrae defined earlier in the passive FEM model (I), the detailed geometries of the IVDs and all muscles and ligaments defined in the MS model. In the resulting FEM model, muscle forces are predicted by a procedure similar to the optimization procedure described above [60], and due to the novel method, depend on detailed IVD FEM model deformations. Static positions were simulated to evaluate the performance of the model compared to earlier versions and in vivo data. Stress distributions in IVDs were not available in the study, but compression forces and muscles forces could be compared between different model versions.

To sum up, multiple simulation approaches have been executed using MBS simulation results in FEM models. Transferred data included reaction forces, muscle forces or displacements of vertebrae on different spine levels. The vast majority of MBS studies rely on experimental data to define joint properties of the IVDs. However, one study investigated the potential of FEM simulations to define MBS model properties.

3.2. FEM → MBS

Karajan et al. [44] investigated the possibility of representing IVD behavior in MBS bushing components by polynomial functions previously derived from detailed FEM simulations. In their approach, one FSU was simplified with three cylinders. The IVD model was constructed based on earlier work combining porous and polyconvex material to account for the complex behavior of the IVD [35]. The conversion of the FEM displacements into the three-DoF MBS bushing-element parameters, namely, rotation and translation in the sagittal plane, was realized as follows: From the center of gravity in the IVD, where the bushing component was located, lever arms to the nodes on the top surface of the IVD aid in yielding nodal displacements of surface nodes. Nodal deformations were then summarized in a Cardan rotation tensor. The FEM simulation with the nodal displacements as input yielded a surface-traction vector derived from the reaction stresses of the IVD, which was homogenized by summarizing the stress distribution to one single value for the force and moment acting on the surface. With the resulting force and moment, the load–displacement behavior of the IVD at the center of gravity was computed. However, as their work focused on the coupling scheme, IVD responses were investigated solely for the elastic part of an MBS bushing component, and nonlinear deformations were not considered. Karajan et al. stated that the advantage of the method was the significantly shorter computation times compared to other approaches. The co-simulation aspect here consists of the modification of the bushing component definitions in the MBS analysis based on the FEM simulation results. The authors stated that the developed model yields the same elastic response of the IVD as that expected by the full biphasic FEM model in each time step.

The resulting MBS model with adapted stiffness parameters could potentially be further used to provide information for a detailed FEM simulation, calculating stresses and deformations. This step has been realized by some research groups. Studies are reviewed in the following.

3.3. FEM → MBS → FEM

To investigate the effects of muscle damage as seen in lumbar interbody fusion surgery, Kumaran et al. [64] used multiple data exchanges between an OpenSim MBS and an Abaqus FEM model. Firstly, an existing FEM model of the thoracolumbar spine [65] was loaded with 4 Nm at T1 to gain ranges of motion (ROMs). These were then transferred to an OpenSim MBS model [8] to calculate muscle forces, which were subsequently applied to the lumbar part of the previously mentioned FEM spine model as connector forces. The research group noted that a limiting factor of their model was that these muscle forces did not produce the motion of the vertebrae, but the simulation was implemented with a given displacement to synchronize both models. Thus, the correct interaction of forces and displacement was likely not given.

In 2021, Meszaros et al. presented a study in which they adapted an established neuro-musculoskeletal spine model [22] to match with an FEM model of the spine [66] considering mechanical behavior. They used the Visible Human Male (VHM) of the Visible Human Project (VHP) [67] as an MBS basis model. From the patient-specific FEM model, they derived muscle attachment points (a) and patient-specific bone geometries (b), which were then subsequently morphed into the VHM MBS framework. The MBS framework was further individualized by generic structures (c), namely, joints, muscles, ligaments and IVDs, which were firstly customized in the neuro-musculoskeletal model and then prescribed to it. Next, soft-tissue characteristics of IVDs and ligaments within the VHM framework were adapted based on IVD responses in the FEM model, ligament stiffnesses derived from the FEM model and soft-tissue models in the neuro-musculoskeletal model. Scaling and simulating the resulting MBS VHM model led to time-dependent forces of muscles, tendons and ligaments ($F_{MTU(t)}$). These forces were finally inserted into the FEM VHM model together with the adapted bone geometries (b). The result of Meszaros et al.'s work was therefore an Abaqus FEM model with time-dependent forces $F_{MTU(t)}$ derived from an MBS model. The model allowed for investigations of spinal motion and tissue mechanics on a mechanical level.

Load sharing in the lumbosacral spine was explored by Liu et al. [42] in 2018 using a unidirectional MBS and FEM co-simulation. The MBS model was set up in Anybody (AnyBody Technology A/S, Aalborg, Denmark) with three DoF IVD joints at the centers of the instantaneous axes of rotation, respectively. Stiffness curves were predicted previously by FEM models of FSUs—they were devoid of ligaments and facet joints and loaded with flexion and extension moments. The model included 188 muscles of three different types: straight, via-point and nonlinear. Seven ligaments with fourth-order polynomial force-deformation relationships with respect to the spinal level [68] were added. The FEM model was implemented in Hypermesh and Abaqus based on the MBS model geometry. Endplates were meshed with shell elements, extruded to form brick elements as far as the adjacent vertebrae and divided into NP and AF. While bones and endplates were modeled with linear material parameters, hyperelastic Mooney–Rivlin models were used for the NP and AF ground substance, and nonlinear AF fiber parameters included increasing stiffness towards the outer lamellae [56,69]. Ligament locations and parameters were copied exactly from the MBS model. Moreover, the model included frictionless facet joint contacts. A static equilibrium was calculated in the MBS model following the concept of a spinal rhythm, in which the single FSUs were flexed proportionally and loaded by gravity. The reaction moment, ligament forces and muscle forces were applied to the T12–L1 joint of the FEM model. Results showed a different deformed state of the FEM model afterwards, which Liu et al. explained with the inability of the joint models in the MBS to allow deformations, which was in turn represented in the FEM model. To synchronize the models, Liu et al. translated vertebra L1 along the reaction force F_R line of action until it reached to MBS-predicted position. The novel reaction force R_F obtained was iteratively compared with the initial reaction force F_R while adjusting the translation, until the difference was smaller than a predefined tolerance. In a follow-up work, Liu and El-Rich used the same model, reduced to one functional spinal unit (L4–L5), to investigate the influences of the NP position on the IDP, spinal loads and load sharing during 60° forward flexion. Based on in vivo data, three posterior shifts of the NP were realized by the models: 0, 1.5 and 2.7 mm. Muscles and ligaments forces, and joint forces and moments at L3–L4 were calculated by the MBS model and prescribed to the FEM model. IDP and spinal loads calculated by the FEM model show that the IDP and compressive forces within an FSU were distinctly influenced by the posterior shifts of the NP, and the CoRs calculated by their MBS and FEM model differ. Liu and El-Rich believe the kinetic results predicted by the MBS model to have been affected by single IVD rotating joints and suggest implementing an iterative process combining MBS and FEM models to account for compressive and shear stiffness. [42]

Refer to Table 1 for an overview of the reviewed unidirectional co-simulation studies. Author groups with more than one study mentioned in this review were included in the table only with their most recent studies for clarity reasons.

Independent of the data transfer being solely from MBS to FEM, from FEM to MBS or both, unidirectional co-simulation was often limited by linear deformations and manual adaption processes to synchronize both models [36,40,42]. To overcome these limitations in the field, a few recent studies implemented bidirectional co-simulations of the spine.

Table 1. Recent simulation studies using unidirectional co-simulation to investigate the spine with information on the execution order, transferred data, the software structure and the source of the model geometry.

	MBS Solver [1]	FEM Solver	Execution Order	Transferred Data	Software Structure	Model Geometry
Esat et al., 2005, 2009 [37,38]	visualNastran 4D from MSC Software	Marc/Mentat from MSC Software.	MBS → FEM	Two time-dependent sagittal forces and one sagittal moment at each IVD → BC	Distinct software, manual transfer	Literature
Du et al., 2014 [49]	Hypermesh	Hypermesh (Altair Engineering)	MBS → FEM	Time-dependent translation & rotation at hip joint & T9 endplate → BC	Distinct software, manual transfer	Literature
Henao et al., 2016 [51]	ADAMS [52]	RADIOSSTM (Altair Engineering)	MBS → FEM	Displacement of vertebrae	Distinct software, manual transfer	Patient-specific/Literature
Honegger et al., 2021 [53]	OpenSim	Abaqus	MBS → FEM	Time-dependent joint angles and muscle forces	Distinct software, manual transfer	Preexisting FEM model fitted to patient-specific geometry
Kamal et al., 2019 [39]	Matlab	Abaqus	MBS → FEM	Resulting muscle forces and reaction moments as distributed pressure and shear stress	Distinct software, manual transfer	CT-based
Azari et al., 2018, Khoddam-Khorasani et al., 2018, Rajaee et al., 2021 [36,40,63]	Abaqus/Matlab	Abaqus/In-house	MBS → FEM	Mostly static muscle forces and moments	Distinct software/One software incorporating muscles and detailed passive elements	CT-based
Karajan et al., 2013 [44]	Not mentioned	Not mentioned	FEM → MBS	IVD displacement → bushing component definition	Distinct software, manual transfer	Simplified as cylinders
Kumaran et al., 2021 [64]	OpenSim	Abaqus	FEM → MBS → FEM	FEM → MBS: ROM MBS → FEM: Muscle forces	Distinct software, manual transfer	Literature
Liu et al., 2018,2020 [41,42]	Anybody	Abaqus/Hypermesh	FEM → MBS → FEM	FEM → MBS: Joint stiffness curves of IVDs MBS → FEM: Reaction moment, ligament and muscle forces at T12-L1 joint	Distinct software, manual transfer by trial-and-error	Default Anybody data/Literature
Meszaros et al., 2021 [43]	VHM	Abaqus	FEM → MBS → FEM	FEM → MBS: IVD response as mechanical parameters MBS → FEM: Time-dependent muscle, tendon & ligament forces	Distinct software, manual transfer	VHM for MBS, patient-specific & VHM-based FEM (morphed)

[1] In this definition, we also include models with clear characteristics of MBS models, such as the involvement of mainly rigid bodies and their interconnections by joint-like components.

4. Bidirectional Co-Simulation of the Spine

Bidirectional co-simulation models benefit from an iterative data exchange that requires less manual intervention and more accurately accounts for large deformations of, e.g., IVDs. Approaches using this type of coupling are listed below, again focusing on how data are exchanged between MBS and FEM models.

Monteiro et al. [46] realized a bidirectional data flow to explore intersomatic fusion biomechanics. In their study, the MBS framework included specific reference points, for which the kinematic data, namely, displacements and rotations, were calculated. The results were transferred as initial data to the FEM simulation, which calculated the reaction forces and moments. Those were transmitted back to the MBS software and served as new starting points for another forward dynamic iteration. The process was managed by a co-simulation module, which used a gluing algorithm (an algorithm for bidirectional coupling of numerical models) to communicate between the MBS and FEM model of a C5-C6 or C6-C7 segment. This gluing algorithm was an adaptation of an algorithm developed in 2001 by Tseng et. al. [70], which in turn was based on the coordinate split (CS) technique by Yen et al. [71]. Wang et al. [72] complemented the gluing algorithm with an interfacing communication platform to make it suitable for practical applications. This approach made the single submodels black boxes, which could be coupled with one of three distinct algorithms distinguished by the data provided by the MBS system. Monteiro et al. applied the algorithm in which the MBS system (coordinator) provided kinematic data, as it was more convenient in the case of a forward dynamic analysis with given displacements. The general environment was developed in Abaqus and Apollo, a multibody system dynamics (MSD) simulator based on the Adams–Moulton method. The MBS algorithm was implemented in Fortran code. The co-simulation module core was incorporated into the Apollo code, and the co-simulation partner was Abaqus. The geometry of the IVD was derived from images and divided into NP and AF based on ratios from the literature. Material parameters were chosen as viscoelastic and quasi-incompressible with a hydrostatic NP and a fiber-drawn AF [37]. IVDs non-adjacent to the fused vertebrae were modeled as bushing components for efficacy reasons. Seven ligaments were introduced as viscoelastic, nonlinear elements. For the linkage of the MBS and FEM system, Monteiro et al. implemented so-called co-simulation elements as RPs. The possibility of more than one RP per linkage was mentioned as an option to consider more complex deformations. In his work, however, one master RP and one slave RP were introduced, either to the center of the top side of the IVD (slave) or to the center of the bottom side of the IVD (master). Refer to Figure 2a for a graphical representation of these RPs. The master RP belonged to the constrained master body, while the slave RP drove the deformation of the model. The information flux therefore consisted of the three basic stations: First, the kinematic data of the RPs were analyzed and stored. Second, the FEA was launched by taking into account the kinematic data of the RPs. Third, the kinetic results of step two were processed by the coordinator software. The validation of the model with a sagittal moment of 1.5 Nm applied to the head showed realistic results, confirming the compatibility of the MBS software with the FEM analysis considering the modeling of the spine.

Another coupling method was implemented by Dicko et al. [73] in combination with a composite lumbar spine model. The algorithm worked by dividing the lumbar spine model into particles with either rigid- or flexible-body characteristics. The vertebrae were represented by rigid bodies, each comprising a rigid coordinate system. The IVDs were represented as a discretized, meshed FEM body containing both rigid and flexible particles: Endplate particles were modeled as rigid-body particles; thus, they remained the same distance from each other over time. The remaining part of the IVD consisted of flexible particles, each experiencing an independent deformation (Figure 2b). The advantage of this approach was the reduction of unknowns, as FEM nodes could be attached to rigid-body particles using Lagrange multipliers. The movement of these attached nodes was then fully prescribed by the rigid body movement of the vertebrae, resulting in a reduction in the size of the equation system. A multimapping step reunited all particles before FEM parameters such as inertia and material properties were applied. The authors state that the model delivers accurate results without penalizing precision. The method was inspired by Stavness et al., who already implemented it in their software, ArtiSynth (Vancouver, BC, Canada) [74]. The software defines deformable bodies by representing their nodes as three DoF particles. Together with the other type of dynamic components—six-DoF rigid bodies—the model can be formulated as an ordinary differential Equation (ODE) and solved by a semi-implicit integrator. While particle-based approaches such as ArtiSynth are particularly well-suited for coupled biomechanical simulations, FEM models are approximated by a lumped mass matrix and a linear co-rotation, and other rotation effects are neglected. Linear FEM representations might not be able to adequately represent large deformations, as undergone by the IVD.

In 2021, Remus et al. [47] published a passive spine model created with ArtiSynth combining rigid vertebral bodies and deformable IVDs as FEM bodies. In Remus' work, data were segmented from the VHM [67] and smoothed. Auxiliary vertebral bodies were additionally derived and acted as interfaces to the IVDs. Vertebral bodies and endplates were not differentiated. Facet joints were modeled in the shape of cylindrical rigid bodies. As FEM components, the IVDs were modeled with a Yeoh material model for the NP and a Mooney–Rivlin material model for the four lamellae of the AF, which was composed with multi-point springs linking the external nodes of the lamellae. Ligaments were modeled as multi-point springs or axial springs. The researchers validated their model in a quasi-static framework with multiple load cases and respective kinematics of in vitro literature data and numerical data. They calculated intradiscal pressure by using the negative mean of normal stresses of all FEM nodes in the NP. Values showed high alignment with in vitro literature data of IVDs at all vertebrae levels. Still, no muscular components were integrated into the model. In subsequent studies, the model was used to study the impact of degenerative changes of the IVD on the axis of rotation by altering its mechanical properties [75] and the effects of a simplified intra-abdominal pressure [76] with integrated muscles as active components. Both studies showed reasonable results, as the authors stated.

Refer to Table 2 for an overview of the reviewed bidirectional co-simulation studies. In summary, two main approaches have been used to couple MBS and FEM spine models bidirectionally: a gluing algorithm providing constant data exchange at certain RPs, managed by a co-simulation engine, and a particle-based approach dividing the model into rigid and flexible particles and solving the resulting ODE with a semi-implicit integrator.

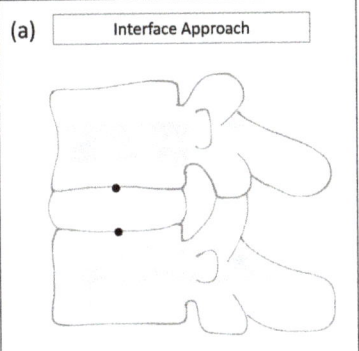 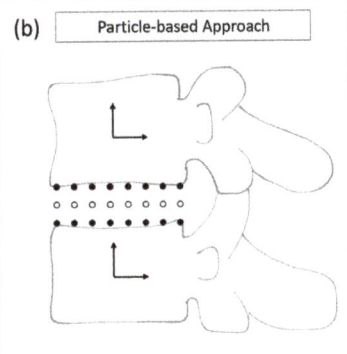

Figure 2. Graphical representation of bidirectional coupling methods found in the literature. (**a**) Coupling algorithm implemented by Monteiro et al. [46]. Two RPs, pictured as black dots, served as an interface between the flexible IVD and the rigid vertebrae. (**b**) Coupling method realized by Dicko et al. [73], which was inspired by an algorithm of Stavness et al. [74]. The model was divided into two types of particles. Rigid particles are illustrated as black dots and flexible particles as circles.

Table 2. Simulation studies using bidirectional co-simulation to investigate the spine with information on the execution order, transferred data, the software structure and the source of the model geometry.

	MBS Solver	FEM Solver	Execution Order	Transferred Data	Software Structure	Model Geometry
Monteiro et al., 2011 [46]	Abaqus	Apollo (Fortran)	constant	Displacements in MBS ↔ reaction forces and moments in FEM	Single software	Literature
Dicko et al., 2015 [73]	Not mentioned	Not mentioned	constant	Integrated approach based on particles	Single software	Literature
Remus et al., 2021 [47]	ArtiSynth	ArtiSynth	constant	Integrated approach based on particles	Single software	Literature (VHM)

5. Limitations and Challenges

Most co-simulation models of the spine use a unidirectional coupling approach, transferring data singularly from one simulation to the other by applying both simulation methods consecutively. MBS spine models can profit by defining joint stiffness parameters based on FEM simulations of the IVD. FEM models of the spine or spinal components can be improved when muscle or ligament forces and moments are implemented as BCs. However, when providing a time-dependent input, the time-dependency is influenced by the deformation properties of a material or component. Equal mechanics cannot be expected when comparing FEM and MBS IVD representations due to their different modeling approaches. The input accomplished by the results of the MBS initially carried out is therefore only partly suitable for being incorporated in a subsequent FEM simulation. This limitation is demonstrated in the effort that has been put into synchronizing the respective models of the unidirectional co-simulations. The manual adaption steps that become necessary may provoke inaccuracies and take much time. Kumaran et al. [64], for example, identified an issue with the interaction of forces and displacement in their simulation and stated that the muscle forces did not produce the desired motion of the vertebrae. They then implemented the simulation with a given displacement rather than a correct interaction of forces and displacement. The same synchronization difficulties were experienced by Khoddam-Khorasani et al. [40] and Liu et al. [41], who both mentioned the need for a manual, iterative process to achieve convergence between the FEM and MBS model or to account for factors such as compressive and shear stiffness. As in Liu et al. [41], the concept of a FL is frequently used to apply summarized loads in the direction of the spinal curvature to provide realistic loading conditions. However, it neither accounts for time-dependent changes in loads, nor dissolves the need of trial and error procedures [36]. In sum, unidirectional co-simulation is often associated with lower accuracy and convergence issues.

To overcome these limitations, a few recent studies have implemented bidirectional co-simulations of the spine. By updating the deformation values of the IVDs and the resulting positions of the vertebrae in every increment, updated reaction moments and forces of muscles, tendons and ligaments can be considered. Of the research groups using bidirectional co-simulation models, all authors found that their models were able to deliver accurate results [46,47,73]. However, two main methods were identified to bidirectionally couple the MBS and FEM solver. Monteiro et al. used an interface approach consisting of two linking RPs, at which the kinematic and kinetic data were exchanged constantly. Although this constant exchange of data solves many of the problems encountered in unidirectional co-simulation, a limiting factor could have been that only one reference node represented the interface between the vertebra and its endplate in this study. The pressure distribution on the IVD thus needed to be derived from one single node, which may have resulted in lowered accuracy. As already reported by Monteiro et al., the implementation of multiple RPs per linkage would be a reasonable adaption to account for more complex deformations.

The particle-based approach divides the whole model into two types of particles, rigid and flexible ones [47,73,74]. Thus, the interface between the flexible FEM and the rigid MBS bodies consists of more than one RP. A mapping step combines the distinct particle sets into one model consisting of a single ODE, which is solved by an integrator. A limiting factor in this approach is the use of a lumped mass matrix and linear co-rotation definitions (neglecting other rotation effects) for the FEM component, which has been associated with less adequate representation of large deformations, as they appear in the IVD. [77]

Despite these limitations, bidirectional co-simulation models of the spine can provide a holistic understanding of the spine because they consider both the overall kinematics with the muscular and gravitational forces and moments, and the detailed mechanics of the IVDs with their deformations and stress distributions.

6. Conclusions and Future Directions

FEM is broadly used in detailed analyses of internal stresses in deforming bodies but lacks computational efficiency. MBS is more efficient, but can only achieve a certain degree of detail when it comes to deformations of model components. A combination of both methods, not only in a unidirectional way, but in a bidirectional manner of data exchange, can provide both accuracy and efficiency.

Future studies will likely include widespread use of bidirectional co-simulation models to understand and predict the behavior of the spine. Including automated segmentation algorithms such as the one implemented by Sekuboyina et al. [26] could accelerate two things: individual, more adequate diagnoses due to patient-specific geometries, and clinical investigations containing large cohorts. Those detailed, personalized simulations of large cohorts could be used to better understand the underlying mechanisms of pathological changes and the biomechanics of overload situations in ambitious athletes, or to predict injuries before they occur.

Author Contributions: Conceptualization, K.N. and J.S.K.; writing—original draft preparation, K.N.; writing—review and editing, T.L., V.S. and J.S.K.; supervision, J.S.K.; project administration, J.S.K.; funding acquisition, J.S.K. All authors have read and agreed to the published version of the manuscript.

Funding: This research was funded by the European Research Council (ERC) under the European Union's Horizon 2020 research and innovation program, Grant No.: 101045128—iBack-epic—ERC-2021-COG.

Institutional Review Board Statement: Not applicable.

Informed Consent Statement: Not applicable.

Data Availability Statement: Not applicable.

Acknowledgments: We thank Andreas Zwölfer for the constructive and helpful exchange.

Conflicts of Interest: J.S.K. is a Co-Founder of Bonescreen GmbH. All other authors declare that the research was conducted in the absence of any commercial or financial relationships that could be construed as a potential conflict of interest.

Abbreviations

The following abbreviations are used in this manuscript:

IVD	Intervertebral Disc
MBS	Multibody Simulation
FEM	Finite Element Method
MRI	Magnetic resonance imaging
DoF	Degrees of Freedom
BC	Boundary Conditions
FSU	Functional Spine Unit
ROM	Range of Motion

CAD	Computer-aided Design
STS	Sit-to-Stand
CoR	Center of Rotation
RP	Reference Point
ODE	Ordinary Differential Equation
VHM	Visible Human Male
CS	Coordinate Split
MSD	Multibody System Dynamics

References

1. Twomey, L.; Taylor, J. Age changes in lumbar intervertebral discs. *Acta Orthop. Scand.* **1985**, *56*, 496–499. [CrossRef] [PubMed]
2. Ball, J.R.; Harris, C.B.; Lee, J.; Vives, M.J. Lumbar Spine Injuries in Sports: Review of the Literature and Current Treatment Recommendations. *Sport. Med.-Open* **2019**, *5*, 26. [CrossRef] [PubMed]
3. Stokes, I.A.; Iatridis, J.C. Mechanical conditions that accelerate intervertebral disc degeneration: overload versus immobilization. *Spine* **2004**, *29*, 2724–2732. [CrossRef] [PubMed]
4. Videman, T.; Battié, M.C.; Gibbons, L.E.; Maravilla, K.; Manninen, H.; Kaprio, J. Associations between back pain history and lumbar MRI findings. *Spine* **2003**, *28*, 582–588. [CrossRef] [PubMed]
5. Actis, J.A.; Honegger, J.D.; Gates, D.H.; Petrella, A.J.; Nolasco, L.A.; Silverman, A.K. Validation of lumbar spine loading from a musculoskeletal model including the lower limbs and lumbar spine. *J. Biomech.* **2018**, *68*, 107–114. [CrossRef]
6. Bassani, T.; Casaroli, G.; Galbusera, F. Dependence of lumbar loads on spinopelvic sagittal alignment: An evaluation based on musculoskeletal modeling. *PLoS ONE* **2019**, *14*, e0207997. [CrossRef]
7. Beaucage-Gauvreau, E.; Robertson, W.S.P.; Brandon, S.C.E.; Fraser, R.; Freeman, B.J.C.; Graham, R.B.; Thewlis, D.; Jones, C.F. Validation of an OpenSim full-body model with detailed lumbar spine for estimating lower lumbar spine loads during symmetric and asymmetric lifting tasks. *Comput. Methods Biomech. Biomed. Eng.* **2019**, *22*, 451–464. [CrossRef]
8. Bruno, A.G.; Bouxsein, M.L.; Anderson, D.E. Development and Validation of a Musculoskeletal Model of the Fully Articulated Thoracolumbar Spine and Rib Cage. *J. Biomech. Eng.* **2015**, *137*, 081003. [CrossRef]
9. Christophy, M.; Faruk Senan, N.A.; Lotz, J.C.; O'Reilly, O.M. A musculoskeletal model for the lumbar spine. *Biomech. Model. Mechanobiol.* **2012**, *11*, 19–34. [CrossRef]
10. Dao, T.T.; Pouletaut, P.; Charleux, F.; Lazàry, A.; Eltes, P.; Varga, P.P.; Ho Ba Tho, M.C. Multimodal medical imaging (CT and dynamic MRI) data and computer-graphics multi-physical model for the estimation of patient specific lumbar spine muscle forces. *Data Knowl. Eng.* **2015**, *96-97*, 3–18. [CrossRef]
11. de Zee, M.; Hansen, L.; Wong, C.; Rasmussen, J.; Simonsen, E.B. A generic detailed rigid-body lumbar spine model. *J. Biomech.* **2007**, *40*, 1219–1227. [CrossRef] [PubMed]
12. Fasser, M.R.; Jokeit, M.; Kalthoff, M.; Gomez Romero, D.A.; Trache, T.; Snedeker, J.G.; Farshad, M.; Widmer, J. Subject-Specific Alignment and Mass Distribution in Musculoskeletal Models of the Lumbar Spine. *Front. Bioeng. Biotechnol.* **2021**, *9*, 721042. [CrossRef] [PubMed]
13. Kim, H.K.; Zhang, Y. Estimation of lumbar spinal loading and trunk muscle forces during asymmetric lifting tasks: application of whole-body musculoskeletal modelling in OpenSim. *Ergonomics* **2017**, *60*, 563–576. [CrossRef] [PubMed]
14. Raabe, M.E.; Chaudhari, A.M.W. An investigation of jogging biomechanics using the full-body lumbar spine model: Model development and validation. *J. Biomech.* **2016**, *49*, 1238–1243. [CrossRef] [PubMed]
15. Bayoglu, R.; Galibarov, P.E.; Verdonschot, N.; Koopman, B.; Homminga, J. Twente Spine Model: A thorough investigation of the spinal loads in a complete and coherent musculoskeletal model of the human spine. *Med. Eng. Phys.* **2019**, *68*, 35–45. [CrossRef]
16. Favier, C.D.; Finnegan, M.E.; Quest, R.A.; Honeyfield, L.; McGregor, A.H.; Phillips, A.T.M. An open-source musculoskeletal model of the lumbar spine and lower limbs: a validation for movements of the lumbar spine. *Comput. Methods Biomech. Biomed. Eng.* **2021**, *24*, 1310–1325. [CrossRef]
17. Hajihosseinali, M.; Arjmand, N.; Shirazi-Adl, A.; Farahmand, F.; Ghiasi, M.S. A novel stability and kinematics-driven trunk biomechanical model to estimate muscle and spinal forces. *Med. Eng. Phys.* **2014**, *36*, 1296–1304. [CrossRef]
18. Han, K.S.; Rohlmann, A.; Yang, S.J.; Kim, B.S.; Lim, T.H. Spinal muscles can create compressive follower loads in the lumbar spine in a neutral standing posture. *Med. Eng. Phys.* **2011**, *33*, 472–478. [CrossRef]
19. Petit, Y.; Aubin, C.E.; Labelle, H. Patient-specific mechanical properties of a flexible multi-body model of the scoliotic spine. *Med. Biol. Eng. Comput.* **2004**, *42*, 55–60. [CrossRef]
20. Senteler, M.; Weisse, B.; Rothenfluh, D.A.; Snedeker, J.G. Intervertebral reaction force prediction using an enhanced assembly of OpenSim models. *Comput. Methods Biomech. Biomed. Eng.* **2016**, *19*, 538–548. [CrossRef]
21. Ignasiak, D.; Dendorfer, S.; Ferguson, S.J. Thoracolumbar spine model with articulated ribcage for the prediction of dynamic spinal loading. *J. Biomech.* **2016**, *49*, 959–966. [CrossRef] [PubMed]
22. Rupp, T.K.; Ehlers, W.; Karajan, N.; Günther, M.; Schmitt, S. A forward dynamics simulation of human lumbar spine flexion predicting the load sharing of intervertebral discs, ligaments, and muscles. *Biomech. Model. Mechanobiol.* **2015**, *14*, 1081–1105. [CrossRef] [PubMed]
23. Pearcy, M.J.; Bogduk, N. Instantaneous axes of rotation of the lumbar intervertebral joints. *Spine* **1988**, *13*, 1033–1041. [CrossRef] [PubMed]

24. Han, K.S.; Zander, T.; Taylor, W.R.; Rohlmann, A. An enhanced and validated generic thoraco-lumbar spine model for prediction of muscle forces. *Med. Eng. Phys.* **2012**, *34*, 709–716. [CrossRef] [PubMed]
25. Peloquin, J.M.; Yoder, J.H.; Jacobs, N.T.; Moon, S.M.; Wright, A.C.; Vresilovic, E.J.; Elliott, D.M. Human L3L4 intervertebral disc mean 3D shape, modes of variation, and their relationship to degeneration. *J. Biomech.* **2014**, *47*, 2452–2459. [CrossRef] [PubMed]
26. Sekuboyina, A.; Rempfler, M.; Valentinitsch, A.; Menze, B.H.; Kirschke, J.S. Labeling Vertebrae with Two-dimensional Reformations of Multidetector CT Images: An Adversarial Approach for Incorporating Prior Knowledge of Spine Anatomy. *Radiol. Artif. Intell.* **2020**, *2*, e190074. [CrossRef] [PubMed]
27. Lavecchia, C.E.; Espino, D.M.; Moerman, K.M.; Tse, K.M.; Robinson, D.; Lee, P.V.S.; Shepherd, D.E.T. Lumbar model generator: a tool for the automated generation of a parametric scalable model of the lumbar spine. *J. R. Soc. Interface* **2018**, *15*, 20170829. [CrossRef]
28. Schmidt, H.; Heuer, F.; Drumm, J.; Klezl, Z.; Claes, L.; Wilke, H.J. Application of a calibration method provides more realistic results for a finite element model of a lumbar spinal segment. *Clin. Biomech.* **2007**, *22*, 377–384. [CrossRef]
29. Dauvilliers, F.; Bendjellal, F.; Weiss, M.; Lavaste, F.; Tarriere, C. Development of a Finite Element Model of the Neck. In Proceedings of the 38th Stapp Car Crash Conference, Fort Lauderdale, FL, USA, 31 October–4 November 1994. [CrossRef]
30. Chetoui, M.A.; Boiron, O.; Ghiss, M.; Dogui, A.; Deplano, V. Assessment of intervertebral disc degeneration-related properties using finite element models based on H-weighted MRI data. *Biomech. Model. Mechanobiol.* **2019**, *18*, 17–28. [CrossRef]
31. Sen, S.; Jacobs, N.T.; Boxberger, J.I.; Elliott, D.M. Human annulus fibrosus dynamic tensile modulus increases with degeneration. *Mech. Mater.* **2012**, *44*, 93–98. [CrossRef]
32. Iatridis, J.C.; Setton, L.A.; Foster, R.J.; Rawlins, B.A.; Weidenbaum, M.; Mow, V. Degeneration affects the anisotropic and nonlinear behaviors of human anulus fibrosus in compression. *J. Biomech.* **1998**, *31*, 535–544. [CrossRef] [PubMed]
33. Massey, C.J.; van Donkelaar, C.C.; Vresilovic, E.; Zavaliangos, A.; Marcolongo, M. Effects of aging and degeneration on the human intervertebral disc during the diurnal cycle: A finite element study. *J. Orthop. Res.* **2012**, *30*, 122–128. [CrossRef] [PubMed]
34. Wu, Y.G.; Wang, Y.H.; Wu, J.H.; Guan, J.J.; Mao, N.F.; Lu, C.W.; Lv, R.X.; Ding, M.C.; Shi, Z.C.; Cai, B. Study of Double-level Degeneration of Lower Lumbar Spines by Finite Element Model. *World Neurosurg.* **2016**, *86*, 294–299. [CrossRef] [PubMed]
35. Ehlers, W.; Karajan, N.; Markert, B. An extended biphasic model for charged hydrated tissues with application to the intervertebral disc. *Biomech. Model. Mechanobiol.* **2009**, *8*, 233–251. [CrossRef]
36. Azari, F.; Arjmand, N.; Shirazi-Adl, A.; Rahimi-Moghaddam, T. A combined passive and active musculoskeletal model study to estimate L4-L5 load sharing. *J. Biomech.* **2018**, *70*, 157–165. [CrossRef]
37. Esat, V.; Acar, M. Viscoelastic finite element analysis of the cervical intervertebral discs in conjunction with a multi-body dynamic model of the human head and neck. *Proc. Inst. Mech. Eng. Part-J. Eng. Med.* **2009**, *223*, 249–262. [CrossRef] [PubMed]
38. Esat, V.; van Lopik, D.W.; Acar, M. Combined multi-body dynamic and Fe models of human head and neck. In *IUTAM Symposium on Impact Biomechanics: From Fundamental Insights to Applications*; Springer: Dordrecht, The Netherlands, 2005; Volume 124, pp. 91–100.
39. Kamal, Z.; Rouhi, G.; Arjmand, N.; Adeeb, S. A stability-based model of a growing spine with adolescent idiopathic scoliosis: A combination of musculoskeletal and finite element approaches. *Med. Eng. Phys.* **2019**, *64*, 46–55. [CrossRef]
40. Khoddam-Khorasani, P.; Arjmand, N.; Shirazi-Adl, A. Trunk Hybrid Passive–Active Musculoskeletal Modeling to Determine the Detailed T12–S1 Response Under In Vivo Loads. *Ann. Biomed. Eng.* **2018**, *46*, 1830–1843. [CrossRef]
41. Liu, T.; El-Rich, M. Effects of nucleus pulposus location on spinal loads and joint centers of rotation and reaction during forward flexion: A combined finite element and Musculoskeletal study. *J. Biomech.* **2020**, *104*, 109740. [CrossRef]
42. Liu, T.; Khalaf, K.; Naserkhaki, S.; El-Rich, M. Load-sharing in the lumbosacral spine in neutral standing & flexed postures - A combined finite element and inverse static study. *J. Biomech.* **2018**, *70*, 43–50. [CrossRef]
43. Meszaros, L.; Hammer, M.; Riede, J.; Pivonka, P.; Little, J.; Schmitt, S. Simulating subject-specific spine mechanics: An integrated finite element and neuro-musculoskeletal modelling framework. In Proceedings of the XXVIII Congress of the International Society of Biomechanics, Stockholm, Sweden, 25–29 July 2021.
44. Karajan, N.; Rohrle, O.; Ehlers, W.; Schmitt, S. Linking continuous and discrete intervertebral disc models through homogenisation. *Biomech. Model. Mechanobiol.* **2013**, *12*, 453–466. [CrossRef] [PubMed]
45. Knapik, G.G.; Mendel, E.; Marras, W.S. Use of a personalized hybrid biomechanical model to assess change in lumbar spine function with a TDR compared to an intact spine. *Eur. Spine J.* **2012**, *21* (Suppl. S5), S641–S652. [CrossRef] [PubMed]
46. Monteiro, N.M.B.; da Silva, M.P.T.; Folgado, J.; Melancia, J.P.L. Structural analysis of the intervertebral discs adjacent to an interbody fusion using multibody dynamics and finite element cosimulation. *Multibody Syst. Dyn.* **2011**, *25*, 245–270. [CrossRef]
47. Remus, R.; Lipphaus, A.; Neumann, M.; Bender, B. Calibration and validation of a novel hybrid model of the lumbosacral spine in ArtiSynth-The passive structures. *PLoS ONE* **2021**, *16*, e0250456. [CrossRef]
48. Cheng, E.J.; Brown, I.E.; Loeb, G.E. Virtual muscle: a computational approach to understanding the effects of muscle properties on motor control. *J. Neurosci. Methods* **2000**, *101*, 117–130. [CrossRef]
49. Du, C.F.; Mo, Z.J.; Tian, S.; Wang, L.Z.; Fan, J.; Liu, S.Y.; Fan, Y.B. Biomechanical investigation of thoracolumbar spine in different postures during ejection using a combined finite element and multi-body approach. *Int. J. Numer. Methods Biomed. Eng.* **2014**, *30*, 1121–1131. [CrossRef]
50. Agur, A.M.R.; Dalley, A.F. *Grant Atlas of Anatomy*, 10th ed.; Williams and Wilkins: Baltimore, MD, USA, 2009.
51. Henao, J.; Aubin, C.E.; Labelle, H.; Arnoux, P.J. Patient-specific finite element model of the spine and spinal cord to assess the neurological impact of scoliosis correction: preliminary application on two cases with and without intraoperative neurological complications. *Comput. Methods Biomech. Biomed. Eng.* **2016**, *19*, 901–910. [CrossRef]

52. Aubin, C.E.; Labelle, H.; Chevrefils, C.; Desroches, G.; Clin, J.; Boivin, A. Preoperative planning simulator for spinal deformity surgeries. *Spine* **2008**, *33*, 2143–2152. [CrossRef]
53. Honegger, J.D.; Actis, J.A.; Gates, D.H.; Silverman, A.K.; Munson, A.H.; Petrella, A.J. Development of a multiscale model of the human lumbar spine for investigation of tissue loads in people with and without a transtibial amputation during sit-to-stand. *Biomech. Model. Mechanobiol.* **2021**, *20*, 339–358. [CrossRef]
54. Campbell, J.Q.; Coombs, D.J.; Rao, M.; Rullkoetter, P.J.; Petrella, A.J. Automated finite element meshing of the lumbar spine: Verification and validation with 18 specimen-specific models. *J. Biomech.* **2016**, *49*, 2669–2676. [CrossRef]
55. Wilke, H.J.; Neef, P.; Caimi, M.; Hoogland, T.; Claes, L.E. New in vivo measurements of pressures in the intervertebral disc in daily life. *Spine* **1999**, *24*, 755–762. [CrossRef] [PubMed]
56. Shirazi-Adl, A.; Ahmed, A.M.; Shrivastava, S.C. Mechanical Response of a Lumbar Motion Segment in Axial Torque Alone and Combined with Compression. *Spine* **1986**, *11*, 914–927. [CrossRef]
57. Shirazi-Adl, A.; Parnianpour, M. Nonlinear response analysis of the human ligamentous lumbar spine in compression. On mechanisms affecting the postural stability. *Spine* **1993**, *18*, 147–158. [CrossRef] [PubMed]
58. Kiefer, A.; Shirazi-Adl, A.; Parnianpour, M. Synergy of the human spine in neutral postures. *Eur. Spine J.* **1998**, *7*, 471–479. [CrossRef]
59. Kiefer, A.; Shirazi-Adl, A.; Parnianpour, M. Stability of the human spine in neutral postures. *Eur. Spine J.* **1997**, *6*, 45–53. [CrossRef]
60. Shirazi-Adl, A.; Sadouk, S.; Parnianpour, M.; Pop, D.; El-Rich, M. Muscle force evaluation and the role of posture in human lumbar spine under compression. *Eur. Spine J.* **2002**, *11*, 519–526. [CrossRef]
61. Arjmand, N.; Shirazi-Adl, A. Biomechanics of Changes in Lumbar Posture in Static Lifting. *Spine* **2005**, *30*, 2648. [CrossRef]
62. Arjmand, N.; Gagnon, D.; Plamondon, A.; Shirazi-Adl, A.; Larivière, C. Comparison of trunk muscle forces and spinal loads estimated by two biomechanical models. *Clin. Biomech.* **2009**, *24*, 533–541. [CrossRef]
63. Rajaee, M.A.; Arjmand, N.; Shirazi-Adl, A. A novel coupled musculoskeletal finite element model of the spine - Critical evaluation of trunk models in some tasks. *J. Biomech.* **2021**, *119*, 110331. [CrossRef] [PubMed]
64. Kumaran, Y.; Shah, A.; Katragadda, A.; Padgaonkar, A.; Zavatsky, J.; McGuire, R.; Serhan, H.; Elgafy, H.; Goel, V.K. Iatrogenic muscle damage in transforaminal lumbar interbody fusion and adjacent segment degeneration: a comparative finite element analysis of open and minimally invasive surgeries. *Eur. Spine J.* **2021**, *30*, 2622–2630. [CrossRef] [PubMed]
65. Shah, A.; Kumaran, Y.; Zavatsky, J.; McGuire, R.; Serhan, H. Development of a Novel Finite Element Model of a Thoracolumbar Spine with Ribcage and Muscle Forces to Simulate Scenarios Closer to in Vivo. In Proceedings of the ORS 2020 Annual Meeting, Phoenix, AZ, USA, 8–11 February 2020.
66. Little, J.P.; Adam, C.J. Geometric sensitivity of patient-specific finite element models of the spine to variability in user-selected anatomical landmarks. *Comput. Methods Biomech. Biomed. Eng.* **2013**, *18*, 676–688. [CrossRef] [PubMed]
67. Ackerman, M.J. The Visible Human Project: a resource for education. *Acad Med.* **1999**, *74*, 667–670. [CrossRef] [PubMed]
68. Rohlmann, A.; Bauer, L.; Zander, T.; Bergmann, G.; Wilke, H.J. Determination of trunk muscle forces for flexion and extension by using a validated finite element model of the lumbar spine and measured in vivo data. *J. Biomech.* **2006**, *39*, 981–989. [CrossRef] [PubMed]
69. Schmidt, H.; Heuer, F.; Simon, U.; Kettler, A.; Rohlmann, A.; Claes, L.; Wilke, H.J. Application of a new calibration method for a three-dimensional finite element model of a human lumbar annulus fibrosus. *Clin. Biomech.* **2006**, *21*, 337–344. [CrossRef] [PubMed]
70. Tseng, F.C.; Hulbert, G.M. A gluing algorithm for network-distributed multibody dynamics simulation. *Multibody Syst. Dyn.* **2001**, *6*, 377–396. [CrossRef]
71. Yen, J.; Petzold, L.R. An efficient Newton-type iteration for the numerical solution of highly oscillatory constrained multibody dynamic systems. *Siam J. Sci. Comput.* **1998**, *19*, 1513–1534. [CrossRef]
72. Wang, J.Z.; Ma, Z.D.; Hulbert, G.M. A gluing algorithm for distributed simulation of multibody systems. *Nonlinear Dyn.* **2003**, *34*, 159–188. [CrossRef]
73. Dicko, A.H.; Tong-Yette, N.; Gilles, B.; Faure, F.; Palombi, O. Construction and validation of a hybrid lumbar spine model for the fast evaluation of intradiscal pressure and mobility. *Int. Sci. Index Med. Health Sci.* **2015**, *9*, 134–145.
74. Stavness, I.; Lloyd, J.E.; Payan, Y.; Fels, S. Coupled hard-soft tissue simulation with contact and constraints applied to jaw-tongue-hyoid dynamics. *Int. J. Numer. Methods Biomed. Eng.* **2011**, *27*, 367–390. [CrossRef]
75. Remus, R.; Uttich, E.; Bender, B. Sensitivity of biomechanical responses in path optimized follower loads considering the lumbosacral load sharing. In Proceedings of the XXVIII Congress of the International Society of Biomechanics, Stockholm, Sweden, 25–29 July 2021.
76. Remus, R.; Lipphaus, A.; Hoffmann, M.; Neumann, M.; Bender, B. An inverse dynamic active hybrid model to predict effects of the intra-abdominal pressure on the lumbar spine. In Proceedings of the 27th Congress of the European Society of Biomechanics, Porto, Portugal, 26–29 June 2022.
77. Mueller, M.; Gross, M. Interactive Virtual Materials. In Proceedings of the Graphics Interface 2004 Conference, London, ON, Canada, 17–19 May 2004.

Disclaimer/Publisher's Note: The statements, opinions and data contained in all publications are solely those of the individual author(s) and contributor(s) and not of MDPI and/or the editor(s). MDPI and/or the editor(s) disclaim responsibility for any injury to people or property resulting from any ideas, methods, instructions or products referred to in the content.

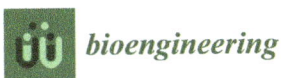

Article

How do Paraspinal Muscles Contract during the Schroth Exercise Treatment in Patients with Adolescent Idiopathic Scoliosis (AIS)?

Chen He [1], Jian-Tao Yang [1,*], Qian Zheng [2], Zhao Mei [3] and Christina Zong-Hao Ma [4]

1. Institute of Rehabilitation Engineering and Technology, University of Shanghai for Science and Technology, Shanghai 200093, China; hechen@usst.edu.cn
2. Department of Rehabilitation Medicine, Tongji Hospital, Tongji Medical College, Huazhong University of Science and Technology, Wuhan 430030, China; qianzhengtongji@163.com
3. Department of Technology, Shanghai Huazhu Medical Institution, Shanghai 201204, China; meizhao2003@163.com
4. Department of Biomedical Engineering, The Hong Kong Polytechnic University, Hong Kong SAR 999077, China; czh.ma@polyu.edu.hk
* Correspondence: jtyang123@outlook.com; Tel.: +86-5527-0127

Abstract: The Schroth exercise can train the paraspinal muscles of patients with adolescent idiopathic scoliosis (AIS), however, muscle performance during the training remains unknown. This study applied surface electromyography (sEMG) to investigate the paraspinal muscle activities before, during and after Schroth exercise in nine AIS patients. This study found that after the Schroth exercise, the paraspinal muscle symmetry index (PMSI) was significantly reduced (PMSI = 1.3), while symmetry exercise significantly lowered the PMSI (PMSI = 0.93 and 0.75), and asymmetric exercise significantly increased the PMSI (PMSI = 2.56 and 1.52) compared to relax standing (PMSI = 1.36) in participants ($p < 0.05$). Among the four exercises, the PMSI of on all fours (exercise 1) and kneeling on one side (exercise 3) was the most and the least close to 1, respectively. The highest root mean square (RMS) of sEMG at the concave and convex side was observed in squatting on the bar (exercise 2) and sitting with side bending (exercise 4), respectively. This study observed that the asymmetric and symmetric exercise induced more sEMG activity on the convex and concave side, respectively, and weight bearing exercise activated more paraspinal muscle contractions on both sides of the scoliotic curve in the included AIS patients. A larger patient sample size needs to be investigated in the future to validate the current observations.

Keywords: adolescent idiopathic scoliosis (AIS); surface electromyography (sEMG); paraspinal muscle; Schroth exercise; paraspinal muscle symmetry index (PMSI)

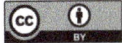

1. Introduction

Scoliosis is a three-dimensional deformity of the lateral curvature and rotated vertebrae, among which adolescent idiopathic scoliosis (AIS) is the most commonly diagnosed. The prevalence of AIS is reported as high as 1.02–2.4% among primary and secondary school students [1,2]. The deformed spine in patients with AIS leads to asymmetric paraspinal muscles that show higher electromyographic (EMG) activity on the convex side than that of the concave side of the scoliotic curve [3–5]. This asymmetry could be due to a lower proportion of oxidative slow-twitch (type 1) fibers on the concave side, which induced a decrease in tonic activity and the ability to sustain contractions, resulting in sustained postural deficits [5,6]. The imbalance and asymmetry in the paraspinal muscles have been suggested to be related to the development and progression of spinal deformity [4] and decreased quality of life in AIS patients [7], which warrants further efforts to identify and validate the appropriate treatment.

Treatment of the musculature is one of the main objectives in AIS, as the effect of the correction in posture needs to be maintained by the musculature. Different treatment exercises have been proposed, and the muscle responses to these exercises have been investigated in a number of previous studies. Schmid et al. (2010) assessed the surface electromyography (sEMG) activity of paraspinal muscles during four back strengthening exercises on patients with AIS, and found that the asymmetric exercises of the front press at the lumbar level and the roman chair and bent-over barbell row at the thoracic level were superior in increasing sEMG amplitudes in the concave side [8]. Chwala et al. (2014) compared sEMG activity symmetry during two symmetric and four asymmetric exercises in girls with AIS, and found that most cases generated an increase in the predominance of sEMG activity at the convex side during symmetric and asymmetric exercises than in the resting position [9]. Strasse et al. (2018) validated the application of sEMG in monitoring the neuromuscular activity after an exercise treatment lasting for 12 weeks. They found improved balance in the recruitment of motor units for the production of muscle strength after exercise, especially at the right side of the spine [10]. Tsai et al. (2010) investigated the difference in bilateral paraspinal muscle activities during resistance isokinetic exercises in people with and without scoliosis [11]. They found that the paraspinal muscle tended to shift sEMG activities from the convex to the concave side, and the lumbar paraspinal muscle supplied the major action in healthy subjects, while thoracic paraspinal muscle compensated to supply actions in patients with a larger scoliosis curve. As a result, they recommended more midback protection during exercises on patients with AIS.

The Schroth exercise is a common approach for paraspinal muscle training for patients with AIS in clinical practice. It was developed by Katharina Schroth in 1920 [12]. The scoliosis-specific exercise is specifically designed to train patients to bring their asymmetric posture into alignment and restore a correct upright position. The repetitive training of the skeletomuscular system could reinforce the effect, so that patients could consciously maintain the corrected posture in daily living activities [13]. The Schroth method also provides sensorimotor and breathing exercises aimed at the recalibration of static/dynamic postural control, spinal stability, and breathing patterns [14]. It has been reported that the Schroth exercise slows curve progression [15], reduces curve severity [16] and reduces scoliosis related pain (>50% intensity and frequency) [17]. Furthermore, the Schroth exercise was also reported to improve the performance capacity of the paraspinal muscles, such as strengthening the musculature, better exploiting muscle activity [12], improving erector spinae activation strategies [6], and correcting the postural defects [18]. These benefits may be presented by a more symmetric sEMG activity on the concave and convex side of the paraspinal muscles.

However, to the best of the authors' knowledge, few previous studies have investigated the sEMG activity while performing the Schroth exercise in patients with AIS. Therefore, this study aimed to address this issue and applied sEMG innovatively to investigate the paraspinal muscles activity before, during and after the Schroth exercise in AIS patients. The muscle performance in the Schroth exercise, as revealed via sEMG signal, will provide evidence and contribute to the individualized and case-specific training of the Schroth exercise for patients with AIS in future clinical practice.

2. Materials and Methods

2.1. Participants

Patients with AIS were recruited through the outpatient clinic specializing in the treatment of scoliosis. The inclusion criteria were: (1) diagnosed as AIS; (2) 10–18 years old with Risser sign ranged from 0 to 5; (3) Cobb angle between 20°~50°; and (4) experienced in the Schroth exercise (i.e., received the Schroth exercise training for at least three times previously) to control and ensure a good exercise performance among the participants. A sample size of 21 subjects was calculated (assuming that the effect size (d) = 0.5; statistical power $(1 - \beta)$ = 0.8; level of significance (α) = 0.05 used for 2-tailed T-test). Patients with severe back pain, spinal surgery history and other neurological symptoms were excluded from this study. All participants gave their written informed consent to participate in the study.

2.2. Assessment Procedure

A Noraxon EMG assessment system with wireless electromyography sensors (Noraxon Inc., Scottsdale, AZ, USA) was used for data collection. The sampling rate of the EMG Sensor System was 1500 Hz with ±24,000 µV EMG input range. The baseline noise was less than 1 µV. The selectable low-pass cut-off and high-pass cut-off were at 500/1000/1500 Hz and 5/10/20 Hz, respectively. The CMRR of EMG preamplifier was more than 100 dB.

2.2.1. Before Exercise

Each participant was instructed to stand in a relaxed position. Surface electrodes were placed on the skin surface of superficial erector spinae muscles, 3-cm from the midline and parallel to the spinous processes of the apical vertebra. The level of the apical vertebra was determined on the radiographs by an experienced clinician. Then, the sEMG signals were recorded for 20 s during the relaxed standing position. The test was repeated three times, with at least 3 min of rest in between to minimize the effect of fatigue in participants.

2.2.2. During Exercise

A physiotherapist specializing in the Schroth exercise instructed participants in performing the exercises. The sEMG data was collected in four different exercise positions, which were performed in a randomized order (Figure 1). Exercise 1 (E1) and exercise 2 (E2) were symmetric exercises, and exercise 3 (E3) and exercise 4 (E4) were asymmetric exercises. It is routine practice that each exercise is repeated three to five times in the clinic as specified in Lehnert-Schroth (2007) [12]. Thus, each test was repeated three times, aiming to minimize the influence of a daily training schedule and reflect the muscle performance in a real clinical situation. Furthermore, rest for at least 3 min in between was allowed to minimize the effects of fatigue in participants. Details of each exercise position are provided below.

E1 (on the fours): The participant kneeled down with the knees apart at shoulder width and kept the thighs in a vertical position. The arms were extended vertically under the shoulders to support the body, with the fingers pointing straight ahead [12]. The participant kept a steady breath and sustained this position for 20 s, during which the sEMG signal was recorded. Each participant repeated this procedure three times to acquire an average sEMG value.

E2 (squatting on the bar): The participant put the feet on the second bar, and the hands apart on bar at shoulder level in a squatting position. The participant would then guide the hip below the rib hump to move laterally, backwards, and downward [12]. Then the participant sustained the downward position for 20 s, during which the sEMG signal was recorded. Each participant repeated this procedure three times to acquire an average sEMG value.

E3 (kneeling on one side): The participant kneeled down with the trunk leaning over to the convex side, then stretched out the leg on the concave side, rotated outwards and placed it laterally to form the leg and the upper body as a line. The participant kept the pelvis upright and hands on the hips. The participant kept a steady breath and sustained this position for 20 s, during which the sEMG signal was recorded. Each participant repeated this procedure three times to acquire an average sEMG value.

E4 (sitting with side bending): The participant sat with the buttock on the heel and kept the pelvis upright, then leaned the trunk over to the convex side and put the hand on the convex side on a block to support the oblique body. Then, the participant sustained this position for 20 s, during which the sEMG signal was recorded. Each participant repeated this procedure three times to acquire an average sEMG value.

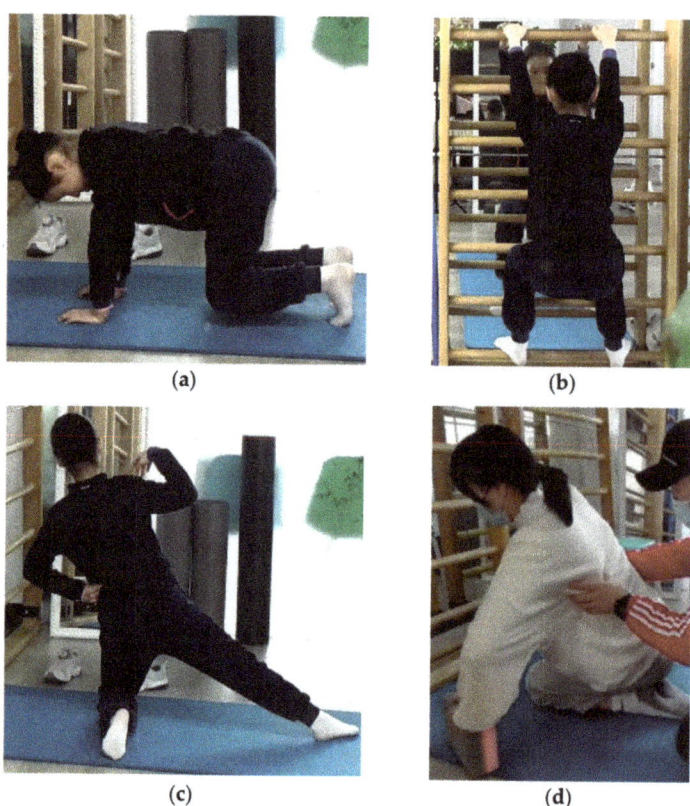

Figure 1. Four different Schroth exercise positions: (**a**) E1—on the fours, (**b**) E2—squatting on the bar, (**c**) E3—kneeling on one side, (**d**) E4—sitting with side bending.

2.2.3. After Exercise

The participant was instructed to stand in the relaxed standing position. The same procedure of sEMG activity measurement as the pre-exercise was taken again, to record the sEMG signals after exercise.

2.3. Data and Statistical Analysis

The obtained sEMG signals were amplified and sampled at 1500 Hz using myoMUSCLE™ software (Noraxon Inc., Scottsdale, AZ, USA). The raw data was band-passed filtered (Butterworth with a cut-off frequency of 20–500 Hz). The sEMG signal of each exercise was divided into three sequences. Each sequence was normalized for time. The root mean square (RMS) quantifying the sEMG amplitude of the averaged sEMG signal was calculated. The paraspinal muscle symmetry index (PMSI) was calculated as $RMS_{convex}/RMS_{concave}$. The PMSI of being close to 1 (e.g., PMSI = 1) referred to the high symmetry of the paraspinal muscle. The PMSI < 1 referred to a greater $RMS_{concave}$ than RMS_{convex}, and PMSI > 1 referred to a greater RMS_{convex} than $RMS_{concave}$ of the scoliotic curve.

The statistical package SPSS, version 22 (SPSS Inc, Chicago, IL, USA), was used for all statistical analyses. One-way repeated ANOVA was used to compare the PMSI before, during and after exercise, and examine for the existence of significant difference. A post hoc adjusted for multiple comparisons with the Bonferroni method was used if significant differences among overall PMSIs were found. Two-way repeated ANOVA and the Bonferroni correction for multiple comparisons was adopted to analyze the RMS of sEMG on the concave and convex side before, during and after exercise, and examine for the existence of significant difference. The level of significance was set at 0.05.

3. Results

3.1. Participants

A total of nine patients with AIS participated in this study. Their demographic data are shown in Table 1.

Table 1. Demographic data ($n = 9$).

Demographic Data	Description
Age	15.2 ± 3.3 years
Gender	9 females
Body Mass Index (BMI)	18.56 ± 1.66
Cobb Angle	$31.56° \pm 8.29°$
Curve Type	C curve
Apex	T7~L2
Risser Sign	0~5

3.2. The PMSI and RMS of sEMG Activity of Paraspinal Muscles

The PMSI and RMS values of sEMG activity of paraspinal muscles are shown in Table 2. The PMSI of pre-exercise and post-exercise in the relaxed standing position was over 1, which meant the sEMG activity of the paraspinal muscle on the concave side was lower than that of the convex side. The PMSI significantly reduced from 1.36 to 1.30 after exercise ($p < 0.05$), indicating the sEMG activity symmetry of the paraspinal muscle between the convex and concave side was improved.

Table 2. Paraspinal muscle symmetry index (PMSI) before, during and after Schroth Exercise ($n = 9$).

	$RMS_{concave}$ (μV)	RMS_{convex} (μV)	PMSI	p Values
Pre-exercise	17.28 ± 6.18	23.51 ± 6.55	1.36 ± 0.19 *	<0.01
E 1	44.08 ± 14.58	41.15 ± 20.49	0.93 ± 0.35	0.08
E 2	81.79 ± 24.01	61.20 ± 44.59	0.75 ± 0.16	0.06
E 3	21.30 ± 15.72	54.47 ± 5.37	2.56 ± 0.60 *	<0.01
E 4	45.13 ± 21.19	68.77 ± 16.51	1.52 ± 0.09 *	<0.01
Post-exercise	19.60 ± 6.17	25.39 ± 5.34	1.30 ± 0.12 *	0.03

* The $RMS_{concave}$ and the RMS_{convex} were significantly different ($p < 0.05$).

3.2.1. The PMSI before, during and after the Schroth Exercise

The PMSI values before, during and after the Schroth exercise are shown in Figure 2. The PMSI during E1 reduced significantly to 0.93 from 1.36 ($p < 0.05$) in the relaxed standing position. It suggested that the sEMG activity of paraspinal muscle at the concave side increased and reached a similar level to that of the convex side, which improved the symmetry of the paraspinal muscles. The PMSI during E1 was closest to 1 among the four exercises, with no significant difference between the $RMS_{concave}$ and the RMS_{convex}; thus, it may be regarded as the exercise with the highest symmetry of the sEMG activity among the four exercises. The PMSI during E2 was reduced to 0.75 from 1.36 ($p < 0.05$) in the relaxed standing position. This suggests that the sEMG activity of paraspinal muscle on the concave side increased and reached to the level closer to the convex side, which improved the symmetry of the paraspinal muscle. The $RMS_{concave}$ and the RMS_{convex} during E2 did not show significant difference.

The PMSI during E3 increased significantly to 2.56 from 1.36 ($p < 0.05$) in the relaxed standing position. This suggested that the sEMG activity of paraspinal muscle at both sides increased but the convex side increased more, which reduced the symmetry of the paraspinal muscle. The PMSI during E3 was the least close to 1 among the four exercises, with the sEMG activity of convex side being significantly higher than that of the concave side ($p < 0.05$). Therefore, it may be regarded as the exercise with the lowest symmetry among the four exercises. The PMSI during E4 increased significantly to 1.52 from 1.36 ($p < 0.05$) in the relaxed standing position. This suggests that the sEMG activity of the paraspinal muscle on both sides increased but the convex side increased more, which reduced the symmetry of the paraspinal muscle.

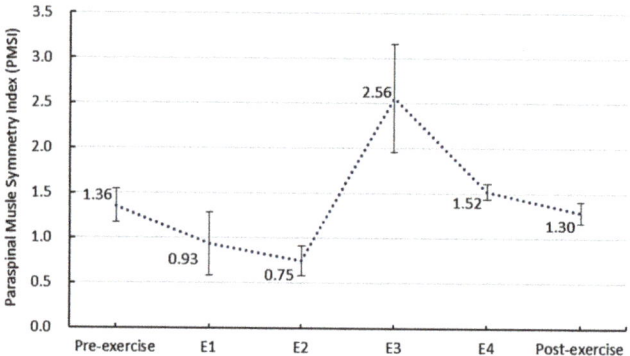

Figure 2. The PMSI before, during and after the Schroth exercise ($n = 9$).

3.2.2. The RMS of sEMG Activity before, during and after the Schroth Exercise

The RMS of sEMG before, during, and after the Schroth exercise is shown in Figure 3. The sEMG activity of paraspinal muscle was higher in all Schroth exercises than that in the relaxed standing position before exercise. The $RMS_{concave}$ significantly increased after exercise (23.51 μV vs. 25.39 μV, $p < 0.05$), while the RMS_{convex} did not significantly change after exercise (17.28 μV vs. 19.60 μV, $p > 0.05$), which indicates that the exercise induced more sEMG activity of paraspinal muscle change on the concave side of the scoliotic curve.

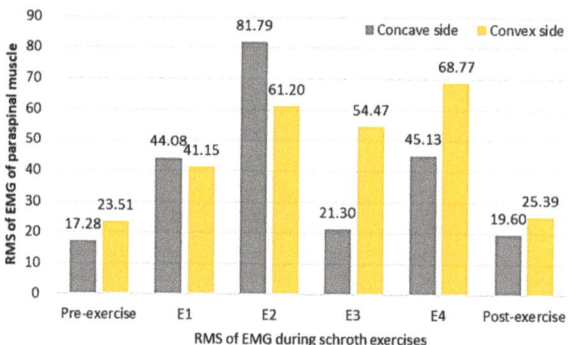

Figure 3. The RMS of sEMG before, during, and after the Schroth exercise ($n = 9$).

The highest $RMS_{concave}$ (81.79 μV) was observed in E2, which was a symmetric exercise against gravity and induced muscle contraction on both sides. The highest RMS_{convex} (68.77 μV) was observed in E4, which was an asymmetric exercise, with side bending to the convex side and stretching of the concave side. Upon comparing the magnitude of sEMG activity of paraspinal muscles, this study observed that E4 > E3 ($p < 0.05$) and E2 > E1 ($p < 0.05$) in both the convex and concave side of the scoliotic curve.

4. Discussion

This study innovatively applied the sEMG to investigate paraspinal muscle activities before, during and after the Schroth exercise in patients with AIS. The findings of this study will provide evidence and support the individualized and case-specific prescription of the Schroth exercise in future clinical practice, which could improve the effectiveness of treatment and improve the quality of life of patients with AIS.

The sEMG activity of the paraspinal muscle on the concave side was found to be lower than that of the convex side during the relaxed standing position in AIS patients. This could be explained by the prolonged stretching of the paraspinal muscles due to deformed vertebrae in AIS patients, which resulted in the asymmetry of muscle fiber types, lengths and locations at bilateral sides [5,19]. The indicated functional imbalance of the paraspinal muscles in AIS suggests that clinicians should prescribe specific exercise to improve muscle balance on both sides according to individual conditions.

This study found that the PMSI of AIS reduced by 4.6% after the Schroth exercise. A previous study also reported the reduced PMSI by 12.0% in the thoracic region and by 7.9% in the lumbar region after the Schroth exercise [6]. Since only patients with single lumbar scoliosis were recruited in the current study, the influence of curve location on the symmetry of paraspinal muscles could be investigated in future studies.

During symmetric exercises, the sEMG activity of the paraspinal muscle was symmetric, while during the relaxed standing position was asymmetric. Chwala et al. [9] also reported higher PMSI during symmetric exercise in comparison with the resting recordings. The possible reason could be that symmetric exercise tried to isolate the muscle contraction between the concave and convex side, and focused more on the atrophied concave side to improve the symmetry of paraspinal muscles [18]. For E1 (on the fours), the sEMG activity on the concave side increased more than the convex side and reached a symmetric sEMG activity on both sides. E1 may be regarded as a symmetric exercise with reduced longitudinal gravity on the spine, which would simultaneously correct the sagittal lordosis and coronal scoliosis of spinal deformity [20]. The symmetric sEMG activity of paraspinal muscles during E1 may be related to both the self-correction of the patients and the spontaneous correction by the postural change. This can also explain the highest $RMS_{concave}$ in E2 (squatting on the bar), which is a symmetric exercise that was against gravity and induced higher muscle contraction on both sides.

During asymmetric exercises, the sEMG activity of paraspinal muscle on the concave side was lower than that of the convex side. The paraspinal muscle fiber was reported to be weaker on the concave side and stretched on the convex side in the scoliotic spine [21]. The convex side was usually used as the dominant side for daily activities. During asymmetric exercise, side bending created an imbalance load on the spine, requiring greater paraspinal muscle contraction to maintain stability. As a result, an increase in the predominance of the sEMG activity on the convex side was instigated. It could be a sign of an adaptive response to the greater use of the muscles on the convex side in patients with AIS. The highest RMS_{convex} was observed in E4 (sitting with side bending), which agreed with Chwala et al.'s study [9] who observed the highest sEMG activity of the convex side of paraspinal muscles in an asymmetric exercise, which involved actively stretching the concave side. They also reported that asymmetric exercises demonstrated larger differences in sEMG activity of the paraspinal muscles in comparison with symmetric exercises.

When considering individual patients, two out of nine patients demonstrated lower sEMG activity at the concave side during symmetric exercise, which was opposite to the other subjects. This might be because each patient had different motor habits and variable attempts when performing exercises. The same exercise could result in diverse performance quality and repeatability of the corrective patterns in practice [9]. Therefore, individualized exercise should be recommended based on the specific muscle response and performance quality of patients. This study validated the feasibility of applying sEMG to evaluate the muscle performance during the Schroth exercise, which will provide evidence and contribute to the case-specific training for patients with AIS in clinical practice. It may also be helpful to adopt some ultrasound imaging technologies [22] to study the internal paraspinal muscle contraction pattern during the exercise in AIS patients in the future.

This study has several limitations. This study only involved nine patients with lumbar scoliosis. A larger sample size with diverse types of scoliosis curve needs to be investigated. Unfortunately, due to the COVID-19 pandemic in China, it is extremely difficult to recruit more AIS patients for this study at this time and in the near future. The current study may serve as pilot investigation providing the theoretical foundation and research direction for future studies to further validate the current observations and deepen the knowledge in this field with larger samples. This study has focused on the immediate effect of the exercise on the paraspinal muscles, but lengthier studies will be necessary to confirm the long-term effects of the Schroth exercise on the performance of the paraspinal muscles. It would also be interesting to investigate whether any difference existed in paraspinal muscle activity during the Schroth exercise between adolescents with and without scoliosis. However, due to the limited number of available children/adolescent participants, it has been difficult to recruit the healthy adolescents without scoliosis to perform the Schroth exercise as a control group, especially under the current pandemic situation. Future studies could recruit some healthy children/adolescents without scoliosis to study the difference in paraspinal muscle activity during the Schroth Exercise.

5. Conclusions

This study observed that the sEMG activity of paraspinal muscle was higher during Schroth exercise than in that of a relaxed standing position in nine patients with AIS. The asymmetric exercise induced more sEMG activity at the convex side, while symmetric exercise induced more sEMG activity at the concave side. Weight bearing exercise tended to activate more muscle contractions on both sides of the scoliotic curve in the included AIS patients. Patients in a larger sample size will need to be investigated in the future to validate the current observations.

Author Contributions: Conceptualization, C.H., J.-T.Y., Q.Z., Z.M., C.Z.-H.M.; methodology, C.H., J.-T.Y., Q.Z., Z.M., C.Z.-H.M.; software, C.H., J.-T.Y., Q.Z., Z.M., C.Z.-H.M.; validation, C.H., J.-T.Y., Q.Z., Z.M., C.Z.-H.M.; formal analysis, C.H., J.-T.Y., Q.Z., Z.M., C.Z.-H.M.; investigation, C.H., J.-T.Y., Q.Z., Z.M., C.Z.-H.M.; resources, C.H., J.-T.Y., Q.Z., Z.M., C.Z.-H.M.; data curation, C.H., J.-T.Y., Q.Z., Z.M., C.Z.-H.M.; writing—original draft preparation, C.H., J.-T.Y., Q.Z., Z.M., C.Z.-H.M.; writing—review and editing, C.H., J.-T.Y., Q.Z., Z.M., C.Z.-H.M.; visualization, C.H., J.-T.Y., Q.Z., Z.M., C.Z.-H.M.; supervision, C.H., J.-T.Y., Q.Z., Z.M., C.Z.-H.M.; project administration, C.H., J.-T.Y., Q.Z., Z.M., C.Z.-H.M.; funding acquisition, C.H., J.-T.Y., Q.Z., Z.M., C.Z.-H.M. All authors have read and agreed to the published version of the manuscript.

Funding: This research was funded by Shanghai Youth Science and Technology Talent Yangfan Program, grant number 20YF1433600.

Institutional Review Board Statement: The study was conducted in accordance with the Declaration of Helsinki, and approved by Medical Ethics Committee of Tongji Medical College, Huazhong University of Science and Technology (protocol code: [2020] (S173); date of approval: 8 July 2020).

Informed Consent Statement: Written informed consent was obtained from all subjects involved in the study.

Data Availability Statement: Data are presented in the article. Initial instrumental output data are available upon request from corresponding author.

Acknowledgments: The authors would like to acknowledge Guoqing Liu for his support in subject recruitment and Yanping Zhang for his clinical suggestions.

Conflicts of Interest: The authors declare no conflict of interest.

References

1. Zhang, H.; Guo, C.; Tang, M.; Liu, S.; Li, J.; Guo, Q.; Chen, L.; Zhu, Y.; Zhao, S. Prevalence of scoliosis among primary and middle school students in Mainland China: A systematic review and meta-analysis. *Spine* **2015**, *40*, 41–49. [CrossRef] [PubMed]
2. Zheng, Y.; Dang, Y.; Wu, X.; Yang, Y.; Reinhardt, J.D.; He, C.; Wong, M. Epidemiological study of adolescent idiopathic scoliosis in Eastern China. *J. Rehabil. Med.* **2017**, *49*, 512–519. [CrossRef] [PubMed]

3. Avikainen, V.J.; Rezasoltani, A.; Kauhanen, H.A. Asymmetry of paraspinal EMG-time characteristics in idiopathic scoliosis. *J. Spinal Disord.* **1999**, *12*, 61–67. [CrossRef] [PubMed]
4. Cheung, J.; Veldhuizen, A.G.; Halbertsma, J.; Maurits, N.M.; Sluiter, W.J.; Cool, J.C.; Horn, J.V. The Relation Between Electromyography and Growth Velocity of the Spine in the Evaluation of Curve Progression in Idiopathic Scoliosis. *Spine* **2004**, *29*, 1011–1016. [CrossRef] [PubMed]
5. Mannion, A.; Meier, M.; Grob, D.; Muntener, M. Paraspinal muscle fibre type alterations associated with scoliosis: An old problem revisited with new evidence. *Eur. Spine J.* **1998**, *7*, 289–293. [CrossRef] [PubMed]
6. Weiss, H.R. Imbalance of electromyographic activity and physical rehabilitation of patients with idiopathic scoliosis. *Eur. Spine J.* **1993**, *1*, 240–243. [CrossRef] [PubMed]
7. Tang, Y.; Yang, S.; Chen, C.; Luo, K.; Chen, Y.; Wang, D.; Tan, J.; Dai, Q.; Zhang, C.; Wu, W. Assessment of the association between paraspinal muscle degeneration and quality of life in patients with degenerative lumbar scoliosis. *Exp. Ther. Med.* **2020**, *20*, 505–511. [CrossRef] [PubMed]
8. Schmid, A.B.; Dyer, L.; Böni, T.; Held, U.; Brunner, F. Paraspinal muscle activity during symmetrical and asymmetrical weight training in idiopathic scoliosis. *J. Sport Rehabil.* **2010**, *19*, 315–327. [CrossRef] [PubMed]
9. Chwala, W.; Koziana, A.; Kasperczyk, T.; Walaszek, R.; Plaszewski, M. Electromyographic assessment of functional symmetry of paraspinal muscles during static exercises in adolescents with idiopathic scoliosis. *Biomed Res. Int.* **2014**, *2014*, 573276. [CrossRef] [PubMed]
10. Strasse, W.; Stadnik, A.; Beraldo, L.M.; Oliveira, K.D. Analysis of the electromyography and symmetrography technologies in the treatment of scoliosis. In Proceedings of the Global Medical Engineering Physics Exchanges/Pan American Health Care Exchanges, Porto, Portugal, 19–24 March 2018; pp. 1–5.
11. Tsai, Y.-T.; Leong, C.-P.; Huang, Y.-C.; Kuo, S.-H.; Wang, H.-C.; Yeh, H.-C.; Lau, Y.-C. The electromyographic responses of paraspinal muscles during isokinetic exercise in adolescents with idiopathic scoliosis with a Cobb's angle less than fifty degrees. *Chang. Gung Med. J.* **2010**, *33*, 540–550. [PubMed]
12. Lehnert-Schroth, C. *Three-Dimensional Treatment for Scoliosis: A Physiotherapeutic Method for Deformities of the Spine*; The Martindale Press: Palo Alto, CA, USA, 2007.
13. Schreiber, S.; Parent, E.C.; Hedden, D.M.; Moreau, M.; Hill, D.; Lou, E. Effect of Schroth exercises on curve characteristics and clinical outcomes in adolescent idiopathic scoliosis: Protocol for a multicentre randomised controlled trial. *J. Physiother.* **2017**, *60*, 234. [CrossRef] [PubMed]
14. Schreiber, S. Schroth Exercises for Adolescent Idiopathic Scoliosis—Reliability, A Randomized Controlled Trial and Clinical Significance. Ph.D. Thesis, University of Alberta, Edmonton, AB, Canada, 2015.
15. Weiss, H.; Weiss, G.; Petermann, F. Incidence of curvature progression in idiopathic scoliosis patients treated with scoliosis in-patient rehabilitation (SIR): An age- and sex-matched cotrolled study. *Pediatr. Rehabil.* **2003**, *6*, 23–30. [CrossRef] [PubMed]
16. Negrini, S.; Fusco, C.; Minozzi, S.; Atanasio, S.; Zaina, F.; Romano, M. Exercises reduce the progression rate of adolescent idiopathic scoliosis: Results of a comprehensive systematic review of the literature. *Disabil. Rehabil.* **2008**, *30*, 772–785. [CrossRef] [PubMed]
17. Weiss, H.-R. Scoliosis-related pain in adults: Treatment influences. *Eur. J. Phys. Med. Rehabil.* **1993**, *3*, 91–94.
18. Otman, S.; Kose, N.; Yakut, Y. The efficacy of Schroth's 3-dimensional exercise therapy in the treatment of AIS in Turkey. *Saudi Med. J.* **2005**, *26*, 1429–1435. [PubMed]
19. Bylund, P.; Jansson, E.; Dahlberg, E.; Eriksson, E. Muscle fiber types in thoracic erector spinae muscles. Fiber types in idiopathic and other forms of scoliosis. *Clin. Orthop. Relat. Res.* **1987**, *214*, 222–228. [CrossRef]
20. He, C.; To, K.T.; Chan, C.K.; Wong, M.S. Significance of recumbent curvature in prediction of in-orthosis correction for adolescent idiopathic scoliosis. *Prosthet. Orthot. Int.* **2019**, *43*, 163–169. [CrossRef] [PubMed]
21. Mattei, T.A. Do not miss it: Paraspinal muscle atrophy in the concave side of the curve in patients with adult degenerative scoliosis. *Spine J.* **2013**, *13*, 987–988. [CrossRef] [PubMed]
22. Ma, Z.H.; Ren, L.J.; Cheng, L.K.; Zheng, Y.P. Mapping of Back Muscle Stiffness along Spine during Standing and Lying in Young Adults: A Pilot Study on Spinal Stiffness Quantification with Ultrasound Imaging. *Sensors* **2020**, *20*, 7317. [CrossRef] [PubMed]

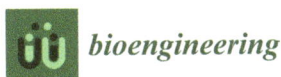

Article

How Does the Use of an Intraoral Scanner Affect Muscle Fatigue? A Preliminary In Vivo Study

KeunBaDa Son [1], Ji-Min Lee [1,2], Young-Tak Son [1,2], Jin-Wook Kim [3,*], Myoung-Uk Jin [4,*] and Kyu-Bok Lee [1,5,*]

1. Advanced Dental Device Development Institute (A3DI), Kyungpook National University, Daegu 41940, Korea; oceanson@knu.ac.kr (K.S.); wlals9408@naver.com (J.-M.L.); dudxkr741@naver.com (Y.-T.S.)
2. Department of Dental Science, Graduate School, Kyungpook National University, Daegu 41940, Korea
3. Department of Conservative Dentistry, School of Dentistry, Kyungpook National University, Daegu 41940, Korea
4. Department of Oral & Maxillofacial Surgery, School of Dentistry, Kyungpook National University, Daegu 41940, Korea
5. Department of Prosthodontics, School of Dentistry, Kyungpook National University, Daegu 41940, Korea
* Correspondence: vocaleo@naver.com (J.-W.K.); musljin@knu.ac.kr (M.-U.J.); kblee@knu.ac.kr (K.-B.L.); Tel.: +82-32-600-7551 (J.-W.K.); +82-32-600-7601 (M.-U.J.); +82-32-660-6825 (K.-B.L.)

Citation: Son, K.; Lee, J.-M.; Son, Y.-T.; Kim, J.-W.; Jin, M.-U.; Lee, K.-B. How Does the Use of an Intraoral Scanner Affect Muscle Fatigue? A Preliminary In Vivo Study. *Bioengineering* 2022, 9, 358. https://doi.org/10.3390/bioengineering9080358

Academic Editors: Christina Zong-Hao Ma, Zhengrong Li and Chen He

Received: 8 July 2022
Accepted: 29 July 2022
Published: 1 August 2022

Publisher's Note: MDPI stays neutral with regard to jurisdictional claims in published maps and institutional affiliations.

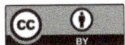

Copyright: © 2022 by the authors. Licensee MDPI, Basel, Switzerland. This article is an open access article distributed under the terms and conditions of the Creative Commons Attribution (CC BY) license (https://creativecommons.org/licenses/by/4.0/).

Abstract: The purpose of this study was to evaluate muscle activation and fatigue in the operator during tooth preparation and intraoral scanning by simulating these tasks in two types of dental unit chair systems (UCS). Six participants were recruited, and the above tasks were simulated. Electrodes were placed on the skin over five types of muscles (arm, neck, and shoulder muscles), and the maximal voluntary contraction (*MVC*) was measured. Electromyography (EMG) was assessed during the simulation, and EMG values were normalized using *MVC*. The root mean square (RMS) EMG (%*MVC*) and muscle fatigue (%) were calculated. Owing to a lack of normal distribution of the data, Mann–Whitney U test and Kruskal–Wallis H test were performed for statistical comparison, and Bonferroni adjustment was performed for multiple comparisons (α = 0.05). There was no significant difference in *RMS EMG* between the two types of dental UCS (intraoral scanning, $p = 0.237$; tooth preparation, $p = 0.543$). Moreover, the *RMS EMG* and muscle fatigue were not significantly different between the two tasks ($p > 0.05$). There was significant muscle fatigue after the intraoral scanner use was simulated thrice ($p < 0.001$). It is necessary to refrain from performing continuous intraoral scanning and tooth preparation and to take appropriate rest to reduce the incidence of musculoskeletal disorders in dentists in clinical settings.

Keywords: dentistry; dental unit chair systems; muscle fatigue; muscle activation; in vivo study

1. Introduction

In dental clinical practice, the use of a dental unit chair system (UCS) is essential for patient diagnosis and treatment [1,2]. Dentists spend most of their work time in the dental UCS for patient care [3]. The dental UCS consists of an operating light and a patient seat, foot controller, water fountain and cuspidor, monitor, bracket table, and dentist's chair [4]. In addition, the dental UCS has been developed to facilitate the use of various dental medical devices and treatment tools [5,6].

Musculoskeletal disorders (MSDs) frequently occur among dental practitioners [7]. It is very difficult for a dentist to adopt an optimal working position because of the limited working space and long duration of treatment [8]. In addition, a high degree of concentration is required by the dentist during treatment resulting in a static posture being maintained for a long time [9]. In the process of maintaining a static posture, the parts of the dentist's body most affected are the back, shoulders, and neck [10,11].

Electromyography (EMG) is a method for measuring electrical signals generated in the skeletal muscles to quantitatively evaluate the magnitude of muscle fatigue or exerted strength [9–12]. Since EMG evaluation can diagnose the functional abnormalities of muscles, it is widely used in various fields, such as medical research, rehabilitation medicine, sports science, and design engineering [9–12]. Muscle fatigue refers to a temporary decrease in the ability of a muscle or muscle group to generate force or perform physical activity and is an essential factor affecting working efficiency [10–12]. Therefore, muscle fatigue is highly correlated with muscle EMG activity and the root mean square (RMS) of EMG [10,11].

Several muscle groups, including the arms, neck, shoulders, and back, are activated during dental work. The arm muscles, flexor digitorum superficialis (FDS), and extensor digitorum communis (EDC) are activated during bending of the wrist and application of force for gripping dental instruments [13]. The sternocleidomastoid muscle (SCM) is involved when turning the head, and the splenius capitis (SC) is involved when bending the head to observe the patient's mouth [9,10,12–15]. The trapezius descendens (T), which is used to raise the shoulder, has also been frequently used for assessment of EMG in dentists [9,10,12–15]. Therefore, it is important to reduce or prevent MSDs in the aforementioned muscles. There are several examples of application of ergonomics in dentistry, including in the patient chair, operator chair, operating light, hand instrumentation, and cabinetry.

Recently, as the application of dental computer-aided design and computer-aided manufacturing (CAD/CAM) has rapidly increased. The use of intraoral scanners has also increased [16]. Although manufacturers have reduced the weight and size of intraoral scanners for usability, these scanners are still one of the heaviest medical devices used directly in the oral cavity [17]. The weight of the intraoral scanner suggested by the manufacturer generally ranges from 113 g to 585 g; the scan time is more than five minutes per complete arch and the device is used repeatedly [17,18]. Although studies have reported the evaluation of EMG when a dentist performs tooth preparation using a high-speed handpiece [9,11], there have been no reports on the effect of intraoral scanner use on the dentist's MSDs.

There is a need for further research on muscle activity and fatigue considering MSDs in various dental practices. Therefore, the purpose of this study was to evaluate muscle activation and fatigue in the operator during tooth preparation and intraoral scanning by simulating these two tasks in the two types of dental UCS. The null hypothesis of this study was that there is no significant difference in muscle activity and fatigue between the two types of dental UCS and the two types of tasks (tooth preparation and intraoral scanning). Additionally, we hypothesized that there is no difference in muscle activity and fatigue caused by repeated use of the intraoral scanner.

2. Materials and Methods

2.1. Participants

This clinical trial was approved by the Clinical Trial Ethics Committee of Kyungpook National University Dental Hospital (IRB No. KNUDH-2021-04-04-00). Right-handed participants with no history of MSDs were recruited. The study inclusion criteria specified that individuals with right-handedness or who presented with musculoskeletal disorders were excluded. The study exclusion criteria specified that individuals with musculoskeletal disorders, sensory or mental abnormalities, debilitating medical conditions, and/or who were pregnant, or lactating were not eligible for assessment in this study. For blinding, all participants did not know the purpose of the present study, and the experiment was performed only according to the instructions of one investigator. The sample size was calculated as at least four participants per group based on the results of a previous study [10] (G*Power version 3.1.9.2; Heinrich-Heine-Universität Düsseldorf, Düsseldorf, Germany) (actual power = 99.11%; power = 95%; $\alpha = 0.05$); the present study included six participants per group. The mean age of the participants was 31.5 ± 3.9 years. The participants had a mean height of 170 ± 6.2 cm, mean weight of 66.3 ± 10 kg, and a dental clinical experience of 3.6 ± 1.1 years. The six participants consisted of two women and four men.

2.2. Data Collection: Ag/AgCl Electrode Placement on Sampled Muscles

The present study refers to the location for evaluation of MSDs that develop during dental treatment in the dental UCS as observed in previous studies [6–11]. The muscles to be assessed for surface EMG, EDC, and FDS were the arm muscles; neck muscles (SCM and SC); and shoulder muscle (T) (Figure 1). For the arm muscles, a pair of 20 mm diameter silver or silver chloride solid adhesive pre-gelled electrodes (Covidien, Mansfield, MA, USA) were attached only to the right hand to perform the task (Figure 1). For the other muscles, the electrodes were symmetrically attached to the left and right sides (Figure 1). Before attaching the electrode, the attachment site was made free of excess hair and thoroughly washed with a 70% isopropyl alcohol swab. According to the guidelines of the surface electromyography for the non-invasive assessment of muscles (SENIAM) protocol for each muscle location, two electrodes were attached to the movement point of each muscle in the direction of the muscle fiber [19]. The center distance between the two electrodes was 20 mm, and the ground electrode was attached to the sphenoid process of the left ulna (Figure 1) [19].

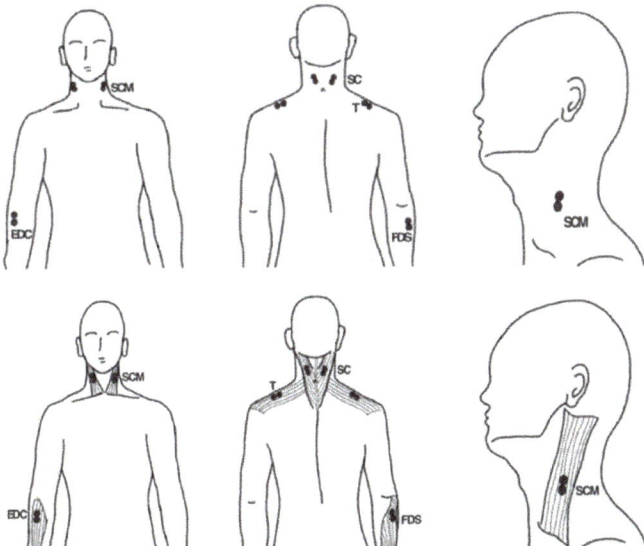

Figure 1. Schematic of the electrode attachment position for electromyography. EDC, extensor digitorum communis; FDS, flexor digitorum superficialis; SCM, sternocleidomastoid muscle; SC, splenius capitis; T, trapezius descendens.

For the EDC, the electrodes were attached to the quarter point between the lateral epicondyle of the humerus and the styloid process of the ulna (Figure 1) [20,21]. For the FDS, the electrodes were attached to the quarter of the medial border of the medial epicondyle of the humerus and the coronoid process of the ulna (Figure 1) [20]. For the SCM, the electrodes were attached at the third point between the mastoid process and the sternal notch toward the sternal portion of the muscle [20]. For the SC, the electrodes were attached to the midpoint between the mastoid process and vertebra C7. For the T, the electrodes were attached to the midpoint between the acromion and vertebra C7 (Figure 1) [20].

After electrode placement, the electrode was connected to an EMG measuring system (WEMG-8; LAXTHA, Daejeon, Korea). In the measurement system, each channel was amplified to 244 µV through the EMG preamplifier, and the analog and digital signals were converted to a 10-bit resolution through the AD converter. The sample was collected at a sampling rate of 1024 Hz. Real-time EMG measurement software (TeleScan ver 3.29; LAXTHA, Daejeon, Korea) was used to collect real-time EMG data.

2.3. Data Collection: Maximal Voluntary Contraction (MVC) Measurement

To normalize the EMG data, *MVC* was measured according to the guidelines of the SENIAM protocol [11,21]. All *MVC* measurements were performed while sitting on a dentist's chair and supporting the lower back on the backrest. When measuring the *MVC* of the arm muscles, the forearm was supported on a desk and the elbow was bent at 90°. The EDC was measured by providing the maximum resistance force when opening the back of the hand and fingers, and the FDS measured the force to maximally close the fingers and palms using a grip force meter. The SCM was measured while providing the maximum resistance to the left and right rotations of the head with both arms lowered. The shoulder muscle (T) was measured by providing the maximum resistance force when trying to lift the shoulder upward. Each muscle was assessed three times at 5 s intervals, and the highest value was defined as the *MVC*.

2.4. Data Collection: Muscle Activation Measurement

After taking a break for 30 min after the *MVC* measurement, dental work simulations were performed on a dental mannequin (Simple Manikin III, NISSIN, Kyoto, Japan) installed in the dental UCS, and muscle activity was recorded in eight EMG channels. The participants performed simulations for intraoral scanning and tooth preparation tasks for two days at intervals of one week to prevent fatigue accumulation between tasks, and the work order was randomly selected by listing all orders (Figure 2).

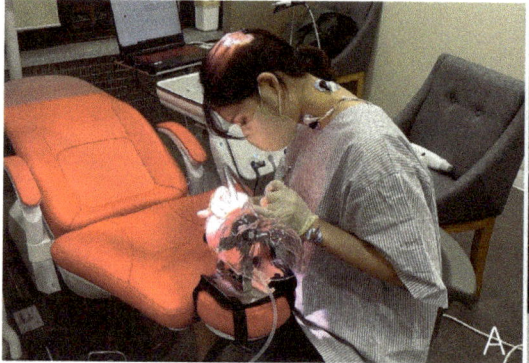
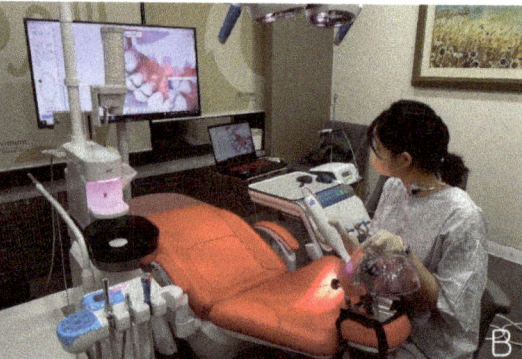

Figure 2. Electromyography measurements during dental simulations. (**A**) Tooth preparation simulation; (**B**) Intraoral scanning simulation.

The digital integrated dental UCS (MEGAGEN, Daegu, Korea) used an intraoral scanner (i500; MEDIT, Seoul, Korea) and monitored the dental UCS, and the conventional dental UCS (Maxpert; SHINHUNG, Seoul, Korea) showed the scanning process on a separate monitor, other than that of the dental UCS, connected to an intraoral scanner. The participants performed all work procedures after adjusting the dentist's chair and the patient's chair to fit their posture and body.

The intraoral scanning task was performed by consecutively scanning the maxillary and mandibular models for dental education (D85DP-500B.1; Nissin Dental, Kyoto, Japan) three times using an intraoral scanner (i500; MEDIT, Seoul, Korea; Figure 2). The scanning strategy was to scan the complete arch in the order of occlusal, buccal, and lingual, and all participants performed a scan so that there were no empty spaces in any of the teeth (Figure 2). The weight of an intraoral scanner used in the present study was 280 g.

The tooth preparation task was performed by preparing the maxillary right first molar (D85DP-500B.1; Nissin Dental, Kyoto, Japan) for a single ceramic crown and chamfer margin using a high-speed dental handpiece (TG-98; W&H, Bürmoos, Austria; Figure 2). Participants performed the tooth preparation task without a magnification system (Figure 2).

One investigator (J.M.L.) recorded the muscle activity in real time only when the participant performed any action for the tasks and did not record the muscle activity unless the participant performed the simulation. In addition, all working times were recorded.

2.5. Data Collection: Muscle Activation Analysis

Muscle activation and muscle fatigue were calculated from the data measured using *EMG* measurement software (TeleScan ver 3.29; LAXTHA, Daejeon, Korea). *EMG* data from dental work were normalized and expressed as percentages, and the activation of each muscle was calculated as follows [9,12] (1):

$$RMS\ EMG(\%MVC) = \frac{Muscle\ activation\ during\ tasks\ (\mu V)}{MVC} \times 100 \quad (1)$$

RMS EMG (%*MVC*) indicates muscle activation that occurs during dental work compared to MVC. As the *RMS EMG* (%*MVC*) increased, the risk of MSDs increased, and the ergonomic risk level according to the activation level of each muscle was evaluated according to previous literature: *MVC* in the range of 0–10% means "low risk"; 11–20% means "moderate risk," and more than 21% means "high risk" [9,12,13].

Muscle fatigue can be identified by increasing and decreasing median edge frequency (*MEF*) values, and as *MEF* decreases, muscle fatigue increases [22–25]. The *MEF* value can be obtained in the frequency range of 1–400 Hz after applying the fast Fourier transform, which transforms the *EMG* signal that changes with time into a frequency. Among the total working time, *MEF* in the first 60 s and next 60 s were calculated, and muscle fatigue was calculated according to the following formula [23,24] (2):

$$Muscle\ fatigue(\%) = \frac{MEF\ in\ the\ second\ 60\ s - MEF\ in\ the\ first\ 60\ s}{MEF\ in\ the\ first\ 60\ s} \times 100 \quad (2)$$

When *MEF* in the first 60 s of dental work was compared with *MEF* in the next 60 s, a negative value was obtained when the value of *MEF* in the second 60 s was low, indicating the increase in muscle fatigue [23,24].

2.6. Statistical Analysis

IBM SPSS statistical Statistics for Windows, version 25 (IBM Corp., Armonk, NY, USA) was used to analyze all data (α = 0.05). First, the distribution of the data was investigated using the Shapiro–Wilk test; the data were not normally distributed. Therefore, Mann–Whitney U test was performed to compare the two types of dental UCS in EMG and muscle fatigue and to compare dental tasks (intraoral scanning and tooth preparation simulation). A Kruskal–Wallis H test was performed to compare the differences in EMG and muscle fatigue according to the muscles. The Bonferroni adjustment was performed for multiple comparisons.

3. Results

The mean working time was 444.7 $\pm$ 195.2 s for the tooth preparation task and 509.6 $\pm$ 142.6 s for the intraoral scanning task (1st: 571.5 $\pm$ 169.0 s, second: 496.3 $\pm$ 145.2 s, third: 461.0 $\pm$ 113.6 s). The time for the intraoral scanning task showed a significant decrease during the three repetitions ($p < 0.001$).

In both types of dental UCS, the *RMS EMG* of the tooth preparation task was higher than that of intraoral scanning, but there was no statistically significant difference ($p = 0.147$; Table 1). In addition, there was no significant difference between the muscle fatigue for the two types of simulations measured in the two types of dental UCS ($p = 0.435$; Table 2).

Table 1. Comparison of mean RMS EMG (%MVC) according to muscle type and dental unit chair system.

Muscle Type	Intraoral Scanning Task			Tooth Preparation Task		
	Dental Unit Chair System		p *	Dental Unit Chair System		p *
	Integrated	Conventional		Integrated	Conventional	
Extensor digitorum communis	13.6 ± 4.0 [ac]	11.7 ± 2.5 [a]	0.368	16.4 ± 4.8 [ab]	17.9 ± 6.9 [ab]	0.668
Flexor digitorum superficialis	10.5 ± 5.5 [ab]	5.5 ± 3.2 [a]	0.209	15.4 ± 8.0 [ab]	12.7 ± 4.3 [ab]	0.487
Left sternocleidomastoid muscle	8.5 ± 6.2 [ab]	6.0 ± 3.2 [a]	0.409	9.4 ± 5.2 [a]	9.3 ± 6.9 [a]	0.967
Right sternocleidomastoid muscle	4.6 ± 2.5 [b]	5.3 ± 1.3 [a]	0.551	5.5 ± 3.9 [a]	7.7 ± 6.2 [a]	0.490
Left splenius capitis	9.4 ± 4.8 [ab]	12.0 ± 4.9 [a]	0.397	11.8 ± 4.6 [ab]	12.8 ± 4.5 [ab]	0.712
Right splenius capitis	10.2 ± 4.0 [ab]	7.1 ± 3.8 [a]	0.207	8.8 ± 4.1 [a]	7.7 ± 4.5 [a]	0.675
Left trapezius descendens	17.0 ± 4.4 [ac]	11.1 ± 5.6 [a]	0.077	14.2 ± 6.5 [ab]	10.6 ± 4.3 [ab]	0.298
Right trapezius descendens	19.5 ± 5.7 [c]	20.7 ± 7.7 [b]	0.755	20.3 ± 8.8 [b]	16.1 ± 9.4 [ab]	0.451
Mean	11.7 ± 6.3	10.1 ± 6.3		12.7 ± 7.1	11.8 ± 6.7	
p **	<0.001	<0.001		0.003	0.042	
p ***		0.237			0.543	
p ****			0.147			

Significance was determined by the Mann–Whitney U test (*, comparison according to unit chair system in each muscle; ***, comparison of unit chair systems in overall mean; and ****, comparison of two simulations), $p < 0.05$. **, Significance determined by Kruskal–Wallis H test (comparison of each muscle), $p < 0.05$. RMS, root mean square; EMG, Electromyography.

Table 2. Comparison of mean muscle fatigue (%) according to muscle type and dental unit chair system.

Muscle Type	Intraoral Scanning Task			Tooth Preparation Task		
	Dental Unit Chair System		p *	Dental Unit Chair System		p *
	Integrated	Conventional		Integrated	Conventional	
Extensor digitorum communis	−6.7 ± 3.4	−9.6 ± 9.0	0.488	−2.8 ± 5.1	−7.2 ± 14.8	0.513
Flexor digitorum superficialis	−4.4 ± 6.6	−1.2 ± 10.7	0.554	−4.2 ± 9.4	−9.4 ± 13.3	0.455
Left sternocleidomastoid muscle	−17.8 ± 7.2	−0.9 ± 18.0	0.058	−17.0 ± 19.0	−3.9 ± 6.2	0.142
Right sternocleidomastoid muscle	−8.0 ± 11.9	3.4 ± 12.1	0.126	15.3 ± 42.4	5.7 ± 16.3	0.623
Left splenius capitis	8.7 ± 9.9	−2.9 ± 4.2	0.033	2.9 ± 11.1	−11.2 ± 10.4	0.047
Right splenius capitis	−7.2 ± 9.7	0.6 ± 5.8	0.127	3.2 ± 8.4	3.5 ± 11.7	0.960
Left trapezius descendens	3.2 ± 11.1	−3.4 ± 3.4	0.190	3.2 ± 16.7	1.7 ± 5.7	0.847
Right trapezius descendens	−0.3 ± 5.0	1.9 ± 4.3	0.407	3.4 ± 7.8	−3.4 ± 10.8	0.240
Mean	−4.0 ± 11.0	−1.5 ± 9.7		0.5 ± 19.3	−3.0 ± 12.3	
p **	0.148	0.417		0.219	0.141	
p ***		0.228			0.287	
p ****			0.435			

Significance was determined by the Mann–Whitney U test (*, comparison according to unit chair system in each muscle; ***, comparison of unit chair systems in overall mean; and ****, comparison of two simulations), $p < 0.05$. **, Significance determined by Kruskal–Wallis H test (comparison of each muscle), $p < 0.05$.

The intraoral scanning task and tooth preparation task showed a low risk level only in the SCM and a moderate risk level in other muscles (Table 1). During the intraoral scanning task, the digital integrated dental UCS showed significantly higher RMS EMG in the EDC and T ($p < 0.001$), while the conventional dental UCS showed significantly higher RMS EMG in the right T ($p < 0.001$; Table 1). During the tooth preparation task, both types of dental UCS showed significantly higher RMS EMG in the EDC, FDS, left SC, and T ($p < 0.05$;

Table 1). There was also no significant difference between the *RMS EMG* with the two dental UCS (intraoral scanning task, $p = 0.237$; tooth preparation task, $p = 0.543$; Table 1).

In digital integrated dental UCS, there was no significant difference in muscle fatigue according to muscle in the intraoral scanning task ($p = 0.138$) and tooth preparation task ($p = 0.219$; Table 2). Similarly, in conventional dental UCS, there was no significant difference in muscle fatigue according to the muscle in the intraoral scanning task ($p = 0.417$) and tooth preparation task ($p = 0.141$; Table 2).

When comparing the two tasks (intraoral scanning and tooth preparation), there was a significant difference in the *RMS EMG* of EDC ($p = 0.033$), and there was no significant difference in the *RMS EMG* and muscle fatigue between the two tasks in other muscles ($p > 0.05$). Both tasks showed moderate risk levels of *RMS EMG* in the T and EDC (Figure 3), and high muscle fatigue in the EDC and FDS (Figure 4).

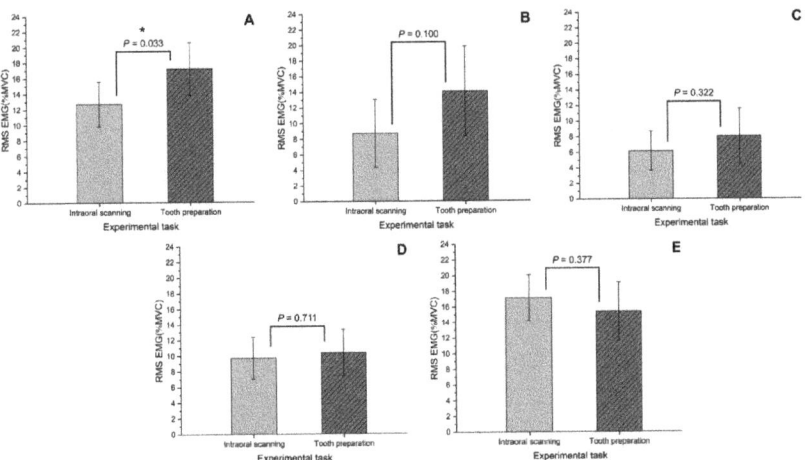

Figure 3. Comparison of *RMS EMG* (%MVC) according to the experimental task. (**A**) extensor digitorum communis; (**B**) flexor digitorum superficialis; (**C**) sternocleidomastoid muscle; (**D**) splenius capitis; (**E**) trapezius descendens.

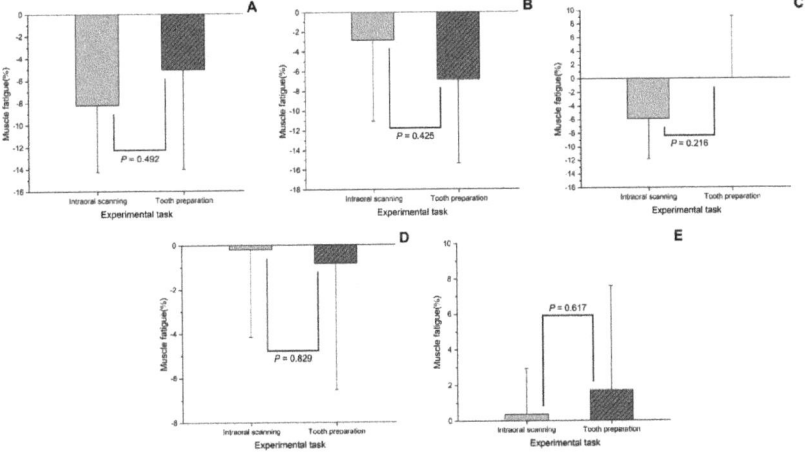

Figure 4. Comparison of muscle fatigue (%) according to the experimental task. (**A**) extensor digitorum communis; (**B**) flexor digitorum superficialis; (**C**) sternocleidomastoid muscle; (**D**) splenius capitis; (**E**) trapezius descendens.

Repeated use of the intraoral scanner three times did not show a significant change in RMS EMG ($p = 0.639$; Table 3) but showed a significant difference in muscle fatigue ($p < 0.001$; Table 4). In the FDS and SCM, using the intraoral scanner three times increased the muscle fatigue significantly (FDS, $p = 0.043$; SCM, $p = 0.027$; Table 4).

Table 3. Comparison of mean RMS EMG (%MVC) in the first, second, and third repetitions of the intraoral scanning task.

Muscle Type	Trial No.			p **	p ***
	1	2	3		
Extensor digitorumcommunis	11.9 ± 2.4 [a]	11.7 ± 3.1 [ab]	13.2 ± 3.3 [ab]	0.656	
Flexor digitorumsuperficialis	5.6 ± 2.7 [b]	6.5 ± 3.0 [b]	6.9 ± 3.2 [b]	0.765	
sternocleidomastoid muscle	5.9 ± 1.0 [b]	5.7 ± 2.8 [b]	7.7 ± 3.8 [b]	0.434	0.639
splenius capitis	10.8 ± 4.7 [ab]	8.9 ± 3.2 [b]	8.9 ± 4.0 [b]	0.661	
trapezius descendens	15.5 ± 4.7 [a]	15.9 ± 5.5 [a]	18.1 ± 5.4 [a]	0.653	
p *	<0.001	<0.001	<0.001		

The same superscript lowercase letters (column) are not significantly different according to the Mann–Whitney U-test and Bonferroni correction method. Significance was determined by the Kruskal–Wallis H test (*, comparison of each muscle; **, comparison of task repetitions in each muscle; and ***, comparison of task repetitions overall); $p < 0.05$. RMS, root mean square; EMG, Electromyography.

Table 4. Comparison of intraoral scanning task mean muscle fatigue (%) in the first, second, and third repetitions.

Muscle Type	Trial No.			p **	p ***
	1	2	3		
Extensor digitorumcommunis	−5.3 ± 8.8	−10.4 ± 10.7 [a]	−11 ± 7.1	0.509	
Flexor digitorumsuperficialis	1.9 ± 17.2 [A]	0.9 ± 8.1 [abA]	−16.8 ± 12.2 [B]	0.043	
sternocleidomastoid muscle	−2.3 ± 9.3 [A]	2.1 ± 6.7 [bA]	−10.5 ± 5.2 [B]	0.027	<0.001
splenius capitis	−1.7 ± 6.9	0.1 ± 3.5 [ab]	−3.8 ± 3.5	0.406	
trapezius descendens	−0.4 ± 6.5	−0.5 ± 4.6 [ab]	−4.6 ± 5.4	0.351	
p *	0.814	0.041	0.066		

The same superscript lowercase letters (column) and same superscript uppercase letters (row) are not significantly different according to the Mann–Whitney U-test and Bonferroni correction method. Significance was determined by the Kruskal–Wallis H test (*, comparison of each muscle; **, comparison of task repetitions in each muscle; and ***, comparison of task repetitions overall); $p < 0.05$.

4. Discussion

The purpose of the present preliminary in vivo study was to evaluate muscle activation and fatigue in dentists during tooth preparation and intraoral scanning by performing simulations of the same with two types of dental UCS. The null hypothesis of our study was partially rejected ($p > 0.05$). There was no significant difference between muscle activity and fatigue with the two types of dental UCS (RMS EMG: $p = 0.237$ and $p = 0.543$; muscle fatigue: $p = 0.228$ and $p = 0.287$; Tables 1 and 2), and there was no significant difference between muscle activity and fatigue with the two types of simulations (RMS EMG: $p = 0.147$; muscle fatigue: $p = 0.435$; Tables 1 and 2). Repetitive learning of the intraoral scanner had no effect on muscle activity ($p = 0.639$; Table 3) but had a significant effect on muscle fatigue ($p < 0.001$; Table 4).

The learning effect (reduction in working time) according to repeated learning with the intraoral scanner has been confirmed in previous studies [26–28]. Similarly, in the present study, a significant decrease in the working time was observed with repetition of the intraoral scanning task ($p < 0.001$). In the previous study, the mean time of full-arch scanning using the intraoral scanner was reported to be 1255 s [29], but in the present study, the mean time was 509.6 s. This difference in scan time is due to rapid advances in intraoral scanners and the shift toward digital workflows. Although the task time was shortened, muscle activation was confirmed to be the same during the three repetitions due to the quantitative amount of the same task ($p = 0.639$; Table 3). However, contrary to the results of muscle activation, muscle fatigue showed significant accumulation after three repetitions ($p < 0.001$; Table 4); in particular, significant accumulation of muscle fatigue was confirmed in the arm (FDS: $p = 0.043$) and neck muscles (SCM: $p = 0.027$) after three repetitions (Table 4).

The weight of the intraoral scanner has been found to range from 113 g to 585 g [17]. In addition, because the manufacturing process of dental prostheses is being digitalized, the use of intraoral scanners is increasing. Therefore, considering the weight and increasing use of the intraoral scanner, it becomes necessary to evaluate muscle activation and fatigue. To the best of our knowledge, the present study is the first to evaluate this. The weight of an intraoral scanner used in the present study was 280 g. Our results suggest that continuous and repetitive intraoral scanning tasks should be avoided, and sufficient rest is important after an intraoral scanning task. In a previous study, a difference in muscle activation was observed with the type of muscle involved in performing the task [8–10]. Contrary to these results, a previous study reported that there were no significant differences in elbow or shoulder pain in 110 participants using either a light wide-handle curette or a narrow-handled heavy curette for scaling in 16 weeks [30].

In the present study, the intraoral scanning task and the tooth preparation task both showed a low risk level only in the SCM and a moderate risk level in the other muscles (Table 1). In the present study, high muscle activation was observed in the shoulder muscle (T) during the intraoral scanning task and in the two arm muscles (EDC and FDS) and in the shoulder muscle (T) in the tooth preparation task (Table 1). A previous study reported that a force of 0.9 N or more is applied to the teeth during tooth preparation for a desired shape [28]. Therefore, it can be inferred that the high activation of the arm muscles (EDC and FDS) during the tooth preparation task in the present study was because of gripping the dental ultra-fast handpiece and pressing it against the teeth (Figure 3). In addition, because the intraoral scanner is heavier than the high-speed dental handpiece [17], it can be inferred that the shoulder muscle (T) showed relatively high muscle activation during the intraoral scanning task compared to that during the tooth preparation task (Figure 3).

A previous study reported a difference in the neck muscle activation depending on the posture of the dentist when observing the oral cavity [8]. The posture for observing the oral cavity was corrected through the use of magnification lenses, and this lowered the activation of the neck muscles [8]. A previous study reported that the use of an ergonomic saddle and a dental magnifying glass improved working posture [31]. In a previous study, it was reported that the vision of an operator may accompany changes in the head and neck posture, which may affect the EMG [32]. In the present study, it was observed that activation of the neck muscle (SCM) increased during the intraoral scanning task compared with that during the tooth preparation task (Figure 3). This is because the intraoral scanning task is performed while observing a separate monitor while the scan is in progress, and the tooth preparation task is performed by bending the neck to observe the oral cavity (Figure 2). Muscle fatigue occurred regardless of the muscle type in both the intraoral scanning and tooth preparation tasks (Table 2). Therefore, it is important to note that activation of the neck muscles can be increased during the tooth preparation task [8], and sufficient rest is required after the task.

According to previous studies, various designs for dental UCS have been considered to help dentists provide treatment in the dental clinical environment [1–3]. In the present study, the design of the dental UCS had no effect on muscle activation and fatigue ($p > 0.05$; Tables 1 and 2). Therefore, before performing each task, the participants adjusted the dentist's chair and the patient's chair according to their needs. Since both types of dental UCS used in the present study were adjusted for body type and convenience, it is presumed that the difference in dental UCS did not affect muscle activation and fatigue.

The present preliminary in vivo study has several limitations. First, the following variables were not considered during the simulation: postures, other than sitting, for treatment; various types of teeth involved in tooth preparation tasks; and types of high-speed dental handpieces and intraoral scanners. The mannequin used in the present study was difficult to reflect the patient's oral environment. In actual clinical practice, the oral cavity does not remain fixed even if the patient cooperates. Moreover, the muscle tone associated with the presence of temporomandibular joint disorder can affect the degree of opening of the mouth, which can affect the dentist's posture. This is a preliminary in vivo study, which has limitations in experimental configuration, and the findings should be further verified through additional studies. Second, although the sample size was determined by referring to a previous study [10], the present study included a small number of participants (six participants). In the present study, various factors were controlled for, and only participants who had a high willingness to participate, were very cooperative, and had a high understanding of its purpose were included. In addition, it is difficult for participants recruited in the present study to represent the results of various age and sex groups [33]. With increasing age, musculoskeletal disorders may increase, which may affect muscle fatigue and activation during certain activities. Finally, factors that may affect fatigue and muscle activation during work activities were not considered: subjective working positions, vision, practitioner parafunctions and bad habits, type of services performed, daily working hours, individual physical activity, degree of experience in the use of specific dental equipment. Conversely, a long-term clinical trial should be conducted by increasing the number of participants.

5. Conclusions

The difference between the two types of dental UCS did not affect muscle activation or fatigue. In addition, similar muscle activation and fatigue were observed during intraoral scanning and tooth preparation. However, in the present in vivo study, a moderate risk level of muscle activation was confirmed in the arm muscle (EDC) and shoulder muscle (T), and successive and repeated use of the intraoral scanner may have caused an increase in the muscle fatigue. Therefore, to reduce the occurrence of MSDs in dentists, it is recommended to take appropriate rest after performing continuous intraoral scanning and tooth preparation tasks. In addition, further studies are needed considering the number of participants and factors affecting fatigue and muscle activation during work activities.

Author Contributions: K.S. contributed to the conception and design, analysis, and writing of the original draft; Y.-T.S. contributed to data acquisition and interpretation; J.-M.L. contributed to data acquisition and interpretation; J.-W.K., M.-U.J. and K.-B.L. contributed to supervision and project administration. All authors have read and agreed to the published version of the manuscript.

Funding: This research was financially supported by the Ministry of Trade, Industry, and Energy (MOTIE) and the Korea Institute for the Advancement of Technology (KIAT) through the National Innovation Cluster R&D program (P0016241_User-friendly chair unit development for digital information provision).

Institutional Review Board Statement: The study protocol was approved by the Kyungpook National University Dental Hospital Institutional Review Board (approval number: KNUDH-2021-04-04-00). All methods were carried out in accordance with relevant guidelines and regulations. The informed consent was obtained from all subjects.

Informed Consent Statement: Informed consent was obtained from all subjects involved in the study. Written informed consent has been obtained from the patients to publish this paper.

Data Availability Statement: The datasets used and/or analyzed during the current study are available from the corresponding author on reasonable request.

Acknowledgments: The authors thank the researchers at the Advanced Dental Device Development Institute, Kyungpook National University, for their time and contribution to the study. This research was financially supported by the Ministry of Trade, Industry, and Energy (MOTIE) and the Korea Institute for the Advancement of Technology (KIAT) through the National Innovation Cluster R&D program (P0016241_User-friendly chair unit development for digital information provision).

Conflicts of Interest: The authors declare no conflict of interest.

References

1. Haddad, O.; Sanjari, M.A.; Amirfazli, A.; Narimani, R.; Parnianpour, M. Trapezius muscle activity in using ordinary and ergonomically designed dentistry chairs. *Int. J. Occup. Environ. Med.* **2012**, *3*, 76–83. [PubMed]
2. Lakshmi, K.; Madankumar, P.D. Development of modified dental chair to accomodate both wheelchair bound patients and general population. *Disabil. Rehabil. Assist. Technol.* **2020**, *15*, 467–470. [CrossRef] [PubMed]
3. Choi, J.O.; Lee, Y.H.; Nam, S.H. Factors affecting surface management of dental unit chair. *Biomed. Res.* **2018**, *29*, 15.
4. Tiwari, A.; Shyagali, T.; Kohli, S.; Joshi, R.; Gupta, A.; Tiwari, R. Effect of dental chair light on enamel bonding of orthodontic brackets using light cure based adhesive system: An in-vitro study. *Acta Inform. Med.* **2016**, *24*, 317. [CrossRef]
5. Rafeemanesh, E.; Jafari, Z.; Kashani, F.O.; Rahimpour, F. A study on job postures and musculoskeletal illnesses in dentists. *Int. J. Occup. Med. Environ. Health* **2013**, *26*, 615–620. [CrossRef] [PubMed]
6. Dong, H.; Loomer, P.; Barr, A.; LaRoche, C.; Young, E.; Rempel, D. The effect of tool handle shape on hand muscle load and pinch force in a simulated dental scaling task. *Appl. Ergon.* **2007**, *38*, 525–531. [CrossRef]
7. Gandavadi, A.; Ramsay, J.R.E.; Burke, F.J.T. Assessment of dental student posture in two seating conditions using RULA methodology–a pilot study. *Br. Dent. J.* **2007**, *203*, 601–605. [CrossRef]
8. García-Vidal, J.A.; López-Nicolás, M.; Sánchez-Sobrado, A.C.; Escolar-Reina, M.P.; Medina-Mirapeix, F.; Bernabeu-Mora, R. The combination of different ergonomic supports during dental procedures reduces the muscle activity of the neck and shoulder. *J. Clin. Med.* **2019**, *8*, 1230. [CrossRef]
9. Petrović, V.; Pejčić, N.; Bulat, P.; Djurić-Jovičić, M.; Miljković, N.; Marković, D. Evaluation of ergonomic risks during dental work. *Balk J. Dent. Med.* **2016**, *20*, 33–39. [CrossRef]
10. Ng, A.; Hayes, M.J.; Polster, A. Musculoskeletal disorders and working posture among dental and oral health students. *Healthcare* **2016**, *4*, 13.
11. Pejčić, N.; Petrović, V.; Đurić-Jovičić, M.; Medojević, N.; Nikodijević-Latinović, A. Analysis and prevention of ergonomic risk factors among dental students. *Eur. J. Dent. Educ.* **2021**, *25*, 460–479. [CrossRef] [PubMed]
12. Pejčić, N.; Đurić-Jovičić, M.; Miljković, N.; Popović, D.B.; Petrović, V. Posture in dentists: Sitting vs. standing positions during dentistry work: An EMG study. *Srp. Arh. Celok. Lek.* **2016**, *144*, 181–187. [CrossRef] [PubMed]
13. Astrand, P.; Rodahl, K. *Textbook of Work Physiology: Physiological Basis of Exercise*; McGraw-Hill: New York, NY, USA, 1986; pp. 115–122.
14. Alexopoulos, E.C.; Stathi, I.C.; Charizani, F. Prevalence of musculoskeletal disorders in dentists. *BMC Musculoskelet. Disord.* **2004**, *5*, 16. [CrossRef] [PubMed]
15. Milerad, E.; Ekenvall, L. Symptoms of the neck and upper extremities in dentists. *Scand. J. Work Environ. Health* **1990**, *16*, 129–134. [CrossRef] [PubMed]
16. Son, K.; Son, Y.T.; Lee, J.M.; Lee, K.B. Marginal and internal fit and intaglio surface trueness of interim crowns fabricated from tooth preparation of four finish line locations. *Sci. Rep.* **2021**, *11*, 13947. [CrossRef] [PubMed]
17. Róth, I.; Czigola, A.; Fehér, D.; Vitai, V.; Joós-Kovács, G.L.; Hermann, P.; Vecsei, B. Digital intraoral scanner devices: A validation study based on common evaluation criteria. *BMC Oral Health* **2022**, *22*, 140. [CrossRef]
18. Park, H.R.; Park, J.M.; Chun, Y.S.; Lee, K.N.; Kim, M. Changes in views on digital intraoral scanners among dental hygienists after training in digital impression taking. *BMC Oral Health* **2015**, *15*, 151. [CrossRef]
19. Hermens, H.J.; Freriks, B.; Disselhorst-Klug, C.; Rau, G. Development of recommendations for SEMG sensors and sensor placement procedures. *J. Electromyogr. Kinesiol.* **2000**, *10*, 361–374. [CrossRef]
20. Díez, J.A.; Catalán, J.M.; Lledo, L.D.; Badesa, F.J.; Garcia-Aracil, N. Multimodal robotic system for upper-limb rehabilitation in physical environment. *Adv. Mech. Eng.* **2016**, *8*, 1687814016670282. [CrossRef]
21. Roman-Liu, D.; Bartuzi, P. The influence of wrist posture on the time and frequency EMG signal measures of forearm muscles. *Gait Posture* **2013**, *37*, 340–344. [CrossRef]
22. Almosnino, S.; Pelland, L.; Pedlow, S.V.; Stevenson, J.M. Between-day reliability of electromechanical delay of selected neck muscles during performance of maximal isometric efforts. *BMC Sports Sci. Med. Rehabil.* **2009**, *1*, 22. [CrossRef] [PubMed]
23. Balasubramanian, V.; Dutt, A.; Rai, S. Analysis of muscle fatigue in helicopter pilots. *Appl. Ergon.* **2011**, *42*, 913–918. [CrossRef]
24. Balasubramanian, V.; Adalarasu, K.; Regulapati, R. Comparing dynamic and stationary standing postures in an assembly task. *Int. J. Ind. Ergon.* **2009**, *39*, 649–654. [CrossRef]
25. Alhaag, M.H.; Ramadan, M.Z.; Al-harkan, I.M.; Alessa, F.M.; Alkhalefah, H.; Abidi, M.H.; Sayed, A.E. Determining the fatigue associated with different task complexity during maintenance operations in males using electromyography features. *Int. J. Ind. Ergon.* **2022**, *88*, 103273. [CrossRef]

26. Al Hamad, K.Q. Learning curve of intraoral scanning by prosthodontic residents. *J. Prosthet. Dent.* **2020**, *123*, 277–283. [CrossRef] [PubMed]
27. Zarauz, C.; Sailer, I.; Pitta, J.; Robles-Medina, M.; Hussein, A.A.; Pradíes, G. Influence of age and scanning system on the learning curve of experienced and novel intraoral scanner operators: A multi-centric clinical trial. *J. Dent.* **2021**, *115*, 103860. [CrossRef]
28. Kim, D.Y.; Son, K.; Lee, K.B. Evaluation of High-Speed Handpiece Cutting Efficiency According to Bur Eccentricity: An In Vitro Study. *Appl. Sci.* **2019**, *9*, 3395. [CrossRef]
29. Patzelt, S.B.; Lamprinos, C.; Stampf, S.; Att, W. The time efficiency of intraoral scanners: An in vitro comparative study. *J. Am. Dent. Assoc.* **2014**, *145*, 542–551. [CrossRef]
30. Mulimani, P.; Hoe, V.C.; Hayes, M.J.; Idiculla, J.J.; Abas, A.B.; Karanth, L. Ergonomic interventions for preventing musculoskeletal disorders in dental care practitioners. *Cochrane Database Syst. Rev.* **2018**, *10*, CD011261. [CrossRef] [PubMed]
31. Plessas, A.; Bernardes Delgado, M. The role of ergonomic saddle seats and magnification loupes in the prevention of musculoskeletal disorders. A systematic review. *Int. J. Dent. Hyg.* **2018**, *16*, 430–440. [CrossRef]
32. Ciavarella, D.; Palazzo, A.; De Lillo, A.; Russo, L.L.; Paduano, S.; Laino, L.; Muzio, L.L. Influence of vision on masticatory muscles function: Surface electromyographic evaluation. *Ann. Stomatol.* **2014**, *5*, 61. [CrossRef]
33. Rickert, C.; Fels, U.; Gosheger, G.; Kalisch, T.; Liem, D.; Klingebiel, S.; Schorn, D. Prevalence of Musculoskeletal Diseases of the Upper Extremity Among Dental Professionals in Germany. *Risk Manag. Healthc. Policy* **2021**, *14*, 3755. [CrossRef] [PubMed]

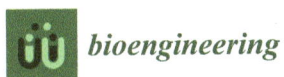

Communication

Electromyography–Force Relation and Muscle Fiber Conduction Velocity Affected by Spinal Cord Injury

Le Li [1,†], Huijing Hu [1,†], Bo Yao [2], Chengjun Huang [3], Zhiyuan Lu [4], Cliff S. Klein [5] and Ping Zhou [4,*]

1. Institute of Medical Research, Northwestern Polytechnical University, Xi'an 710072, China
2. Institute of Biomedical Engineering, Chinese Academy of Medical Sciences & Peking Medical College, Beijing 100006, China
3. Department of Neuroscience, Baylor College of Medicine, Houston, TX 77030, USA
4. School of Rehabilitation Science and Engineering, University of Health and Rehabilitation Sciences, Qingdao 266072, China
5. Rehabilitation Research Institute, Guangdong Work Injury Rehabilitation Center, Guangzhou 510440, China
* Correspondence: ping.zhou@uor.edu.cn
† These authors contributed equally to this work.

Abstract: A surface electromyography (EMG) analysis was performed in this study to examine central neural and peripheral muscle changes after a spinal cord injury (SCI). A linear electrode array was used to record surface EMG signals from the biceps brachii (BB) in 15 SCI subjects and 14 matched healthy control subjects as they performed elbow flexor isometric contractions from 10% to 80% maximum voluntary contraction. Muscle fiber conduction velocity (MFCV) and BB EMG–force relation were examined. MFCV was found to be significantly slower in the SCI group than the control group, evident at all force levels. The BB EMG–force relation was well fit by quadratic functions in both groups. All healthy control EMG–force relations were best fit with positive quadratic coefficients. In contrast, the EMG–force relation in eight SCI subjects was best fit with negative quadratic coefficients, suggesting impaired EMG modulation at high forces. The alterations in MFCV and EMG–force relation after SCI suggest complex neuromuscular changes after SCI, including alterations in central neural drive and muscle properties.

Keywords: spinal cord injury (SCI); muscle fiber conduction velocity (MFCV); surface electromyography (EMG); EMG–force relation

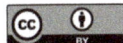

1. Introduction

Spinal cord injuries (SCIs) can cause motor dysfunction including loss of maximal strength and impaired force control that is partially explained by altered muscle activation [1]. In patients with incomplete SCIs, there is a reduction in nervous system activation of skeletal muscle below the lesion. Hence, some motor units (motor neurons) of a muscle may not be recruited despite maximal effort, due to denervation or loss of central neural activation, whereas others may discharge at lower than normal rates [2,3]. Recording of muscle activity by electromyography (EMG) has proved to be useful for evaluating central and peripheral determinants of motor dysfunction [4,5]. In contrast to clinical measures of motor function, EMG is sensitive enough to detect muscle activity after SCI in the absence of palpable muscle contraction and joint movement [6]. Abnormal EMG findings from impaired muscles after SCI include long-lasting involuntary motor activation [7,8], loss of functioning motor units [9–15], impaired motor unit voluntary control [16–18], and muscle fiber denervation and reinnervation [3,19,20]. EMG has demonstrated to be a valuable tool for assessment of paralyzed muscle changes in persons with SCI.

The relation between surface EMG amplitude and voluntary isometric muscle force has been explored in people with motor disorders such as stroke [21–24]. Alterations in EMG–force relation compared with matched healthy control subjects have been observed, that may be related to altered motor control and motor unit properties. In contrast with stroke, few have examined the EMG–force relation after SCI. Thomas and colleagues reported linear (or curvilinear) EMG–force relations in the triceps brachii of persons with chronic SCI that were similar to healthy controls [25].

The EMG–force relation has mainly been examined with conventional single channel surface electrodes. High density surface EMG (HD-sEMG) arrays provide advantages over conventional single channel EMG [26]. For example, Jordanic et al. compared the performance of HD-sEMG and single channel EMG in the upper limb of SCI subjects and found that spatial activation of motor units was dependent on the contraction intensities and the type of exercise, and the related spatial features can improve the identification of specific co-activation patterns during motor performance [27]. Among various HD-sEMG array designs, a one-dimensional linear electrode array is convenient to use [28]. The linear electrode array can simultaneously measure EMG from different locations of the muscle fibers and thus may detect activity in severely paralyzed muscles that may be undetected using conventional single channel EMG. Linear electrode arrays have other useful applications including estimation of locations of innervation zones (IZ) and muscle fiber conduction velocity (MFCV) [29–32].

In this study, we completed an analysis of surface EMG from linear electrode array attached on the biceps brachii (BB) muscle in persons with SCI and a matched group of healthy controls. The purpose of the study was to characterize the BB MFCV and EMG–force relationship, and whether they are affected by SCI.

2. Materials and Methods

2.1. Subjects

The participants of this study included 15 SCI survivors (3 female and 12 male, 44.6 ± 16.1 years,) with injury duration 1–36 years, injury level from C2–C8 and American Spinal Injury Association (ASIA) impairment scale A to D. More information on injury level and ASIA impairment scale can be found in [33]. All SCI survivors were recruited from the outpatient clinic of TIRR Memorial Hermann Hospital (Houston, TX, USA). Their clinical characteristics are summarized in Table 1. In addition, 14 able-bodied subjects (3 female and 11 male, 39.7 ± 12.4 years) with no known history of neuromuscular disorder were recruited as the control group. There was no age difference between the two groups ($p = 0.37$). This study was approved by the Institutional Review Board of the University of Texas Health Science Center at Houston and TIRR Memorial Hermann Hospital and performed in accordance with the Declaration of Helsinki. All subjects gave written consents (or had a witnessed verbal consent if unable to write) before participating in the experiment.

Table 1. SCI subject information.

Subject No	Age (years)	Gender	Years Past Injury	Neurological Level	ASIA Impairment Scale
1	38	Female	10	C6	B
2	47	Male	10	C5	C
3	50	Male	26	C5	D
4	23	Male	9	C3	A
5	39	Male	3	C6	D
6	62	Female	11	C8	D
7	65	Male	2	C2	C
8	32	Male	1	C8	C
9	59	Male	8	C5	D
10	50	Female	30	C5	C
11	25	Male	2.5	C4	D
12	54	Male	36	C4	C
13	19	Male	4	C2	D
14	36	Male	4	C5	C
15	71	Male	3	C4	C

2.2. Experiment

The participants were seated in a chair which is adjustable for comfortable height and were instructed to hold the arm position with the elbow in 90° of flexion and the shoulder in 45° of abduction during the data collection (Figure 1A). A Velcro strap was used to restrain the shoulder and trunk from moving during the experiment. The wrist and forearm were immobilized in a handmade fiberglass cast and placed on a fixed platform. The wrist joint was restricted inside a ring interface, which was mounted to the platform. The ring interface was connected to a load cell (ATI, Apex, NC, USA). Force signals were recorded with a sampling frequency of 2 kHz and digitized by a BNC-2090A data acquisition board (National Instruments, Austin, TX, USA). The fiberglass cast helped to fix the upper limb well and minimize the movement and variation between subjects.

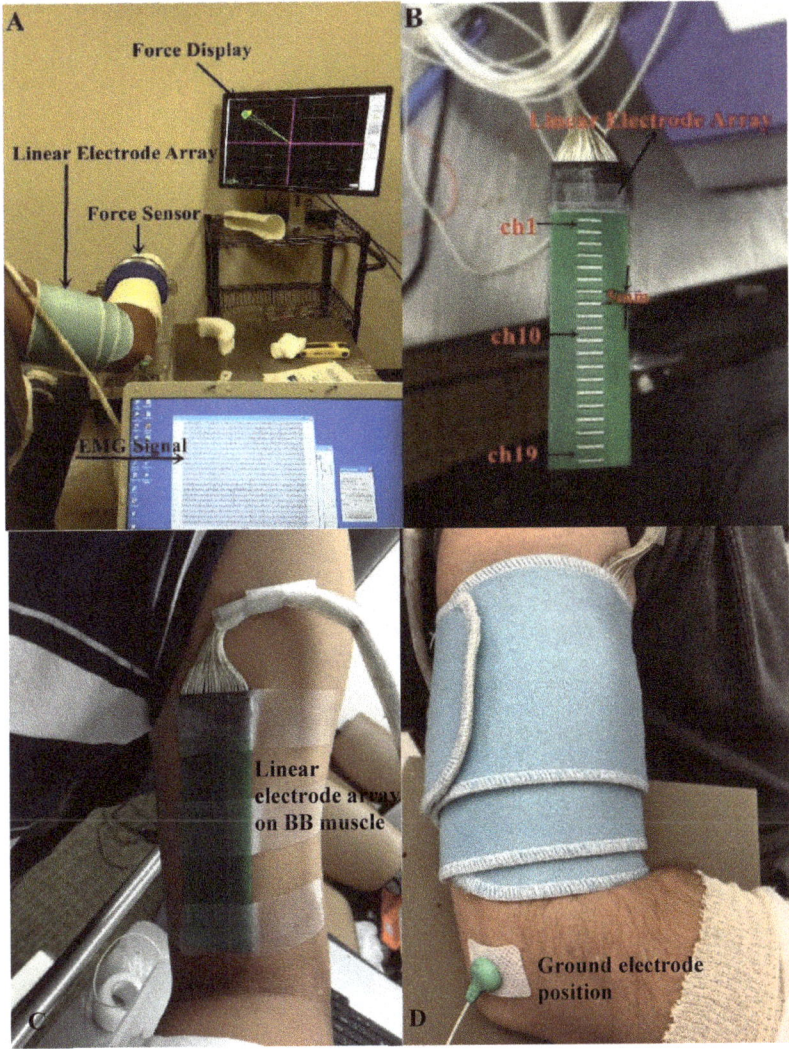

Figure 1. Experimental setup. (**A**) Force display and EMG recording; (**B**) The linear electrode array used for surface EMG recording; (**C**) The placement of the linear electrode array on BB muscle belly; (**D**) The fixation of the linear electrode array.

The maximum voluntary contraction (MVC) of the weaker side of the SCI subjects (determined by self-report and clinical assessment) and the non-dominant side of the control subjects was determined. Each subject conducted three MVC trials of the BB muscle. The largest one was defined as the MVC value. The target force of 10–80% MVC (in 10% MVC increment) was marked as a circle with a line connecting the circle and the center of the computer screen (representing the rest state) (Figure 1A). For each desired force level, there was a computer-generated cursor tracking the force in real time. The subject was asked to move the cursor to follow the force line. When the target circle was reached (indicated by color change in the cursor), the subject was instructed to keep the cursor as stable as possible inside the target circle. In the case of having difficulty in reaching the target (especially for the high force level tasks), the subject was verbally encouraged to control the cursor as close as possible to the target. The whole process (moving the cursor to the target and holding the cursor) lasted for at least 10 s. Each subject was allowed to perform practice trials to become familiar with the contraction task before data recording. The sequence of different muscle contraction levels was randomized. Each muscle contraction level was repeated twice. The subjects were explicitly instructed not to change or move trunk position during task performance. To avoid mental or muscle fatigue, subjects were allowed to have at least 2 min break between trials.

Surface EMG was captured from the BB muscle by a linear electrode array designed and manufactured in our lab. The array has 20 silver bars, with each bar being 10 mm in length and 1 mm in width. The inter-bar distance is 5 mm (Figure 1B). Skin preparation was performed with sandpaper, alcohol pads, and conductive gel. The array was positioned over the midline of the BB muscle longitudinally from the bicipital groove to the biceps tendon insertion (Figure 1C). Such placement ensured that the electrode array covered the major portion of the muscle. In addition, self-adhesive cuff was used to wrap the linear electrode array and secure a good attachment on the skin surface of the BB muscle during the experiment (Figure 1D). The reference electrode was attached on the lateral condyle of the subject's tested arm. Surface EMG signals were recorded via the Porti EMG acquisition system (TMS International, Oldenzaal, The Netherlands). The sampling frequency was 2 kHz per channel. There is a 1st order low pass filter before the ADC with a -3 dB point at 4.8 kHz. The ADC of the Porti has a digital sinc3 filter with a cutoff frequency of $0.27\times$ sample frequency.

2.3. Data Analysis

2.3.1. Data Preprocessing

Surface EMG and force data were processed offline in MATLAB (MathWorks, Natick, MA, USA). A 6th order Butterworth (10–500 Hz) was applied to the EMG signals. The power line interference in the EMG signal was eliminated using a spectrum interpolation algorithm [34]. Force signals were manually inspected to select a relatively stable 5 s segment. Surface EMG and force signals within the epochs were extracted for further analysis.

2.3.2. Calculation of MFCV

Prior to the analysis of MFCV, EMG signals were differentiated between consecutive channels to generate 19 channels of bipolar signals. The IZ was determined by either visual inspection or analysis of the bipolar signals. The IZ was estimated to be the channel with the lowest amplitude, or between the channels that demonstrated reverse signal polarity and a clear pattern of bidirectional signal propagation from the IZ channel to the tendons [35]. The MFCV was determined based on detection of the temporal delay between adjacent single differential channels. Specifically, MFCV was defined and computed as d/τ, where d is the inter-electrode distance between the channels and τ is the time delay between two channels (calculated from cross-correlation analysis). Channels containing IZ or adjacent to IZ were excluded for MFCV estimation. The MFCV calculated at each contraction level was averaged over all contraction levels for further comparison between groups.

2.3.3. EMG–Force Relation

The force signal from individual trials was averaged over the selected epoch. The corresponding surface EMG amplitude was obtained by calculation of the root mean square (RMS) value from each channel. Channels close to the proximal and distal tendons were excluded from analysis. The channel producing the maximal RMS values (by evaluating the eight target force contractions and the MVC) was used for estimation of the EMG–force relation. Next, the RMS values from the selected channel were averaged across the 2 trials for each force level. The force was also averaged across the trials. The RMS and force values were then normalized to the MVC values for determination of the EMG–force relation.

The EMG–force relation was estimated in each SCI and control subject. Given that curvilinear EMG–force relation has been widely reported for large muscles such as BB [36,37], we applied quadratic fitting to describe the BB EMG–force relation. The quadratic equation was expressed as: $y = ax^2 + bx + c$, where x represents force and y represents EMG amplitude. The coefficient of determination (R^2) for quadratic fitting was calculated for each subject.

2.4. Statistical Analysis

Descriptive statistics were performed. A normal distribution of MVC and MFCV values was confirmed by the Kolmogorov–Smirnov test. The independent t test was applied to compare the difference of MVC between the SCI and healthy control groups. A linear-mixed effects model was applied to analyze the main effects of group (SCI and Control), force (8 levels from 10% to 80% MVC) and the interaction of the two main effects on MFCV. The coefficient of determination of the quadratic fitting of the EMG–force relation was calculated for both control and SCI groups. Statistical analysis was conducted using SPSS (SPSS Inc., Chicago, IL, USA) with a significance level of $p < 0.05$. All values in the text are presented as mean ± SD.

3. Results

The SCI participants were significantly weaker compared to the controls (SCI MVC: 98.5 ± 69.9 N, range: 11.9–307.6 N; control MVC: 212.7 ± 111.3 N, range: 70.6–314.9 N, $p = 0.005$). Examination of differences of average MFCV value revealed a significantly slower value in the SCI group compared with the healthy control group (SCI: 3.97 ± 0.55 m/s, control: 4.62 ± 0.86 m/s, $p = 0.025$, Figure 2A). The results showed a significant main effect of group (presence of SCI) ($\beta = -0.87$, SE = 0.29, t = -2.97, $p = 0.005$), while the main effect of contraction level ($\beta = -0.04$, SE = 0.02, t = -1.67, $p = 0.096$) and interaction of the two main effects ($\beta = 0.002$, SE = -0.004, t = 1.79, $p = 0.075$) were not significant. Although a trend of increasing MFCV with muscle contraction level was observed in some subjects (Figure 2B), linear-mixed effects model analysis indicated that MFCV was not significantly related to the different target forces.

Normalized EMG–force relations in all the tested healthy control subjects and the averaged relation are shown in Figure 3A. For all 14 healthy control subjects, the EMG–force relation was well fit by a quadratic function ($R^2 = 0.96$, range: 0.89–0.99). All the control subjects had a positive quadratic coefficient (i.e., a > 0), suggesting that EMG tended to increase relatively more than force during the stronger target contractions. In contrast, a more diverse EMG–force relation was observed in the SCI subjects, although data for the group was also well fit by a quadratic function ($R^2 = 0.87$, range: 0.50–0.99). Two different quadratic patterns were observed after SCI. Among the 15 tested SCI subjects, seven had a positive quadratic coefficient (i.e., a > 0, Figure 3B), consistent with the responses in the controls. The other eight SCI subjects had a negative quadratic coefficient (i.e., a < 0, Figure 3C), suggesting that EMG tended to increase relatively less than force during the stronger target contractions. The two SCI sub-groups with negative and positive quadratic coefficients did not have significant differences in age, years post injury, ASIA scale, neurological level, and MVC force ($p > 0.05$).

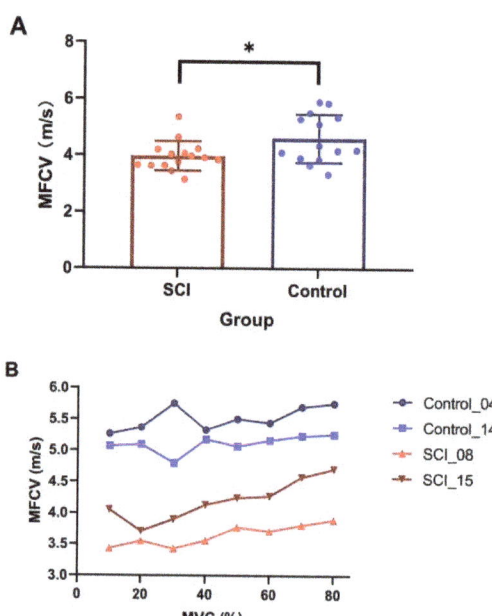

Figure 2. Comparison of MFCV between SCI and control subjects. (**A**) Mean and individual MFCVs in each group (* $p < 0.05$, error bar represents standard deviation); (**B**) MFCV at the different target forces in two subjects from SCI and control groups, respectively.

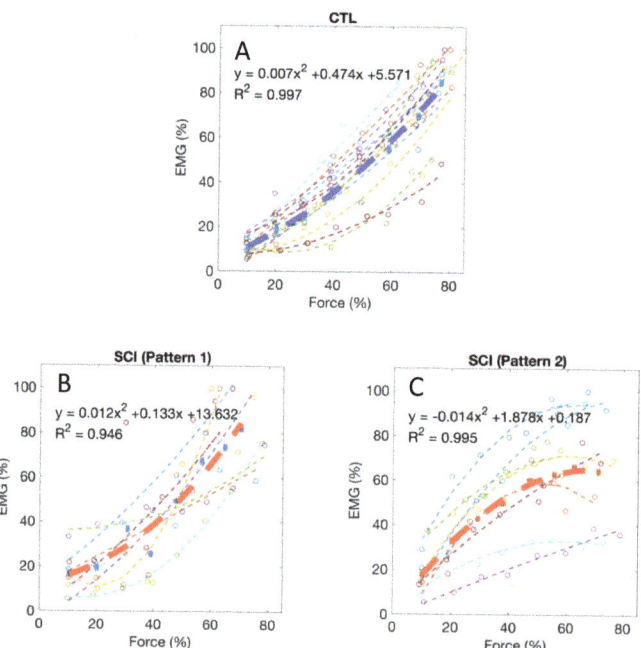

Figure 3. (**A**) Normalized EMG–force relations from all healthy control subjects and the averaged relation (the thick line); (**B**,**C**) Two typical patterns of EMG–force relations from all the tested SCI subjects and the averaged relations (the thick lines).

4. Discussion

A linear electrode array was applied in this study to examine the BB partially paralyzed by cervical SCI. The average MVC of the examined muscles was approximately 50% of healthy control subjects, and this weakness likely reflects both central neural (i.e., paralysis) and peripheral muscular changes. In the subacute or chronic stage after SCI, muscles innervated by spinal segments at and caudal to the SCI are prone to atrophy from both denervation and disuse [38]. A decrease in the number of motor units or axons following spinal motor neuron death could occur [9–15]. There were only a few motor units that remained under voluntary control since the injury interrupted many of the descending inputs to the motor neuron pool [39]. The disturbances of motor neuron control and contractile properties persist in chronic SCI survivors, and represent an important source of muscular weakness and increased fatigability [40]. These neurophysiological changes were also reflected in the current linear electrode array EMG analysis of the SCI subjects, focused on the MFCV and the EMG–force relation.

MFCV, which is directly related to membrane excitability, can reflect the dynamic changes and redistribution of ions during voluntary muscle contraction [41]. MFCVs calculated in the BB muscles were reported to range from 3.4 ± 0.2 to 5.0 ± 0.6 m/s in healthy subjects [28,42]. Our results from healthy control subjects (4.62 ± 0.86 m/s) are in similar range with the previous findings. Changes in MFCV have been reported after neuromuscular disorders. For example, BB MFCV during isometric contractions were found to be significantly slower in patients with Duchenne muscular dystrophy compared to healthy controls [43]. MFCV was also shown to be significantly slower in paretic muscles of stroke survivors [29]. In this study, BB MFCV was significantly slower after SCI compared to control subjects. This could be due to muscle fiber atrophy or degeneration of large motor units after SCI. Given that the BB has motor unit recruitment range up to 80% MVC, a clear correlation was expected between muscle force and MFCV to be revealed in current study. However, our results indicated no significant correlation between the averaged MFCV and muscle contraction level for both groups. For the SCI group, this is likely due to complex neuromuscular changes that may compromise the relationship between MFCV and muscle force. Admittedly, our results from healthy control subjects are somewhat different from most of the previous literatures [44–46], although a similar finding was also reported in a recent study that BB MFCV of healthy control subjects increased only slightly but non-significantly with force [47]. According to size principle, later recruited motor units are supposed to have larger muscle fiber diameters and thus higher MFCV. Although some of the healthy control subjects showed an increase trend of MFCV with muscle contraction level, group analysis did not reveal a significant relation. There might be multiple factors that likely compromise the MFCV of the healthy control subjects in this study, which were also suggested in previous studies. For example, Masuda et al. (1996) [48] examined MFCVs from vastus lateralis, tabialis anterior, and BB muscles of seven healthy subjects. Although increased MFCV was observed with increasing force of the vastus lateralis muscle, the results from BB muscle showed that the MFCV reduced rapidly with time before the muscle contraction force reached the designed target levels of 70% or 90% MVC. MFCV at these larger force levels was smaller than that at 50% MVC and then consequently MFCV in the BB showed no dependent on the contraction levels. These results suggest that although MFCV basically increases with muscle contraction force but this relation can become unclear when MFCV decreases rapidly with time. Other factors may also contribute to compromising the relation such as variability in interference surface EMG, variability between different sessions (especially at higher contraction force), muscle temperature variability (which may also affect MFCV) [49], and muscle fatigue. Although muscle fatigue was a controlled factor during experiment and subjects were allowed sufficient rest, it would be difficult to completely avoid its effect on MFCV, especially at high force levels when large and fast-fatigable motor units are recruited [50].

The EMG–force relation was also examined in this study, which can provide additional insights pertaining to neuromuscular changes in pathological conditions. Application of a linear electrode array can characterize the EMG–force relation unconfounded by muscle IZ effects on the EMG signal. This is important because surface EMG parameters can be significantly affected by IZs, and the uncertainty of electrode locations (with respect to the IZ) might compromise the signal interpretation [51,52]. Both linear and nonlinear EMG–force relations were reported in the literature [36,37]. For small muscles such as the first dorsal interosseous (FDI) whose force generation is dominated by motor unit rate coding, a linear EMG–force relation is often observed. For large muscles such as BB, motor unit recruitment takes an important role in muscle force generation, and the progressively recruited motor units have larger action potentials, increase EMG more than force despite the effect of action potential amplitude cancellation, thus resulting in a nonlinear EMG–force relation. In this study, we observed that for all healthy control subjects, the quadratic term coefficient of the EMG–force relation fitting was positive, suggesting that EMG increased faster than force, which is consistent with previous reports [36].

An interesting finding is that for the SCI group, diverse EMG–force relations were observed. In about half of the SCI subjects, a negative quadratic term coefficient of the EMG–force relation fitting was revealed, indicating that EMG tended to increase slower than force. There are various factors that may contribute to this EMG–force relation change after SCI. Previously, the effects of different motor unit property changes on the EMG–force relation were systematically investigated by simulating activities of motor neuron pool, surface EMG and force of the FDI muscle [53]. For example, it was found that reductions in motor unit firing rate would tend to increase the slope of EMG–force relation, which was experimentally confirmed in stroke subjects [21–23]. Jahanmiri-Nezhad et al. found a trend of decreased slope of the EMG–force relation in the FDI muscle of patients with amyotrophic lateral sclerosis compared with healthy control subjects, which could be related to selective degeneration of motor units with high threshold or a change in motor unit contractile properties [54]. In the current study of the SCI BB, the unusual negative quadratic term coefficients could be caused by motor unit property changes after SCI, such as the loss of large motor units, and altered motor unit recruitment as well as firing behavior. For example, Johanson et al. found two of the four SCI subjects had significantly reduced motor neuron recruitment and high firing rates, likely a compensatory effect of dramatic motor neuron loss after SCI, while the other two subjects with stronger elbow extension had relatively normal recruitment and firing rates [55]. It is worth noting that there are various interactive factors that can influence the EMG–force relation in different ways. Those positive quadratic term coefficients of the fitting in SCI subjects consistent with the healthy control group might be viewed as a collective effect of various factors, which can drive the EMG–force relation in opposite directions.

There are several limitations in the present study. We solely applied global surface EMG parameters and it might be difficult to differentiate or quantify various motor unit properties that may contribute to the changes in surface EMG. Surface EMG decomposition is required to perform analysis at the motor unit level. Given that it is more ideal to perform surface EMG decomposition using 2-dimensional electrode arrays which provide EMG recordings not only parallel to but also perpendicular to muscle fibers, surface EMG decomposition was not attempted in this study. Motor unit number, size, and control property changes after SCI can readily be examined through 2-dimensional high density surface EMG recording and decomposition in future studies [56,57]. Considering that surface electrode only records superficial regions of a muscle, intramuscular recording with needle or fine wire electrodes is necessary in order to capture activity of deeper motor units in the muscle. As computational modeling provides a useful approach in neuromuscular performance investigations [53,58], a delicate simulation analysis incorporating experimental motor unit behaviors can help understand the global surface EMG parameter alterations after SCI. The current study focused on MFCV and the relation of EMG amplitude and muscle force for a relatively steady segment of signals, while there are more advanced or complex signal processing methods which can be applied in data analysis. For example, wavelet transform is promising to explore time and frequency dependence of the examined parameters [59]. In this study, EMG was not recorded from synergistic and antagonistic muscles, although a previous SCI study found that BB coactivation did not have a major effect on the triceps brachii EMG–force relation [25]. Simultaneous recording from synergistic and antagonistic muscles is suggested in the future study, which can assess the potential effects of the "sharing load" strategy, especially during strong contractions. In addition, the shoulder and trunk position may influence EMG signal measurement [60], and this should be considered in data analysis and interpretation. Finally, this study is limited by a relatively small subject number for performing meaningful sub-group analysis.

In summary, this study presents findings from a linear electrode array surface EMG examination of the BB in chronic cervical SCI subjects. The results demonstrated significantly slower MFCV in SCI subjects compared with healthy controls. The EMG–force relation was also altered in a subset of the SCI participants. Using quadratic fitting of the EMG–force relation, approximately half of the SCI participants demonstrated a negative quadratic term coefficient, possibly reflecting impaired motor unit control at high forces. In contrast, positive quadratic coefficients were observed for all healthy control subjects. These findings suggest both central neural and peripheral muscular changes in the BB after SCI.

Author Contributions: Conceptualization, C.S.K. and P.Z.; methodology, L.L., H.H. and P.Z.; software, B.Y., C.H. and Z.L.; validation, B.Y., C.H. and Z.L.; formal analysis, L.L. and H.H; investigation, L.L., H.H., B.Y., C.H. and Z.L.; resources, P.Z.; data curation, L.L., H.H. and B.Y.; writing—original draft preparation, L.L. and H.H; writing—revision, review and editing, C.S.K. and P.Z.; visualization, L.L., H.H. and C.S.K.; supervision, P.Z.; project administration, L.L. and P.Z. All authors have read and agreed to the published version of the manuscript.

Funding: This work was supported by Shandong Provincial Natural Science Foundation (ZR2020KF012), National Natural Science Foundation of China (32071316, 32211530049, 82102179), the Fundamental Research Funds for the Central Universities (G2021KY05101, W016204, G2022WD01006), the Key Research and Development Project of Shaanxi province (2022SF-117), and the Natural Science Foundation of Shaanxi province (2022-JM482).

Institutional Review Board Statement: The study was conducted in accordance with the Declaration of Helsinki, and approved by the Committee of Protection of Human Subjects of University of Texas Health Science Center at Houston and TIRR Memorial Hermann Hospital (Approval Code: HSC-MS-14-1031, Approval Date: 18 August 2015).

Informed Consent Statement: Informed consent was obtained from all subjects involved in the study.

Data Availability Statement: The data that support the findings of this study are available from the corresponding author upon reasonable request.

Acknowledgments: We acknowledge the help of Henry Shin, Xiaoyan Li, Argyrios Stampas, and Zichong Luo during performance of this study.

Conflicts of Interest: The authors declare no conflict of interest. The funders had no role in the design of the study; in the collection, analyses, or interpretation of data; in the writing of the manuscript; or in the decision to publish the results.

References

1. Sherwood, A.M.; McKay, W.B.; Dimitrijević, M.R. Motor control after spinal cord injury: Assessment using surface EMG. *Muscle Nerve* **1996**, *19*, 966–979. [CrossRef]
2. Thomas, C.K.; Zaidner, E.Y.; Calancie, B.; Broton, J.G.; Bigland-Ritchie, B.R. Muscle weakness, paralysis, and atrophy after human cervical spinal cord injury. *Exp. Neurol.* **1997**, *148*, 414–423. [CrossRef]
3. Thomas, C.K.; Bakels, R.; Klein, C.S.; Zijdewind, I. Human spinal cord injury: Motor unit properties and behavior. *Acta Physiol.* **2014**, *210*, 5–19.
4. Calancie, B.; Molano, M.R.; Broton, J.G.; Bean, J.A.; Alexeeva, N. Relationship between EMG and muscle force after spinal cord injury. *J. Spinal Cord Med.* **2001**, *24*, 19–25. [CrossRef]
5. de Vargas Ferreira, V.M.; Varoto, R.; Cacho, Ê.W.A.; Cliquet, A., Jr. Relationship between function, strength and electromyography of upper extremities of persons with tetraplegia. *Spinal Cord* **2012**, *50*, 28–32. [CrossRef]
6. Calancie, B.; Molano, M.D.R.; Broton, J.G. Neural plasticity as revealed by the natural progression of movement expression-both voluntary and involuntary—In humans after spinal cord injury. *Prog. Brain Res.* **2000**, *128*, 71–88.

7. McKay, W.B.; Ovechkin, A.V.; Vitaz, T.W.; de Paleville, D.G.T.; Harkema, S.J. Long-lasting involuntary motor activity after spinal cord injury. *Spinal Cord* **2011**, *49*, 87–93. [CrossRef]
8. Zijdewind, I.; Thomas, C.K. Spontaneous motor unit behavior in human thenar muscles after spinal cord injury. *Muscle Nerve* **2001**, *24*, 952–962. [CrossRef]
9. Xiong, G.X.; Zhang, J.W.; Hong, Y.; Guan, Y.; Guan, H. Motor unit number estimation of the tibialis anterior muscle in spinal cord injury. *Spinal Cord* **2008**, *46*, 696–702. [CrossRef]
10. Li, X.; Jahanmiri-Nezhad, F.; Rymer, W.Z.; Zhou, P. An examination of the motor unit number index (MUNIX) in muscles paralyzed by spinal cord injury. *IEEE Trans. Inf. Technol. Biomed.* **2012**, *16*, 1143–1149.
11. Li, L.; Li, X.; Liu, J.; Zhou, P. Alterations in multidimensional motor unit number index of hand muscles after incomplete cervical spinal cord injury. *Front. Hum. Neurosci.* **2015**, *9*, 238. [CrossRef]
12. Zong, Y.; Lu, Z.; Chen, M.; Li, X.; Stampas, A.; Deng, L.; Zhou, P. CMAP scan examination of the first dorsal interosseous muscle after spinal cord injury. *IEEE Trans. Neural Syst. Rehabil. Eng.* **2021**, *29*, 1199–1205. [CrossRef]
13. Lu, Z.; Chen, M.; Zong, Y.; Li, X.; Zhou, P. A Novel Analysis of CMAP Scans from Perspective of Information Theory: CMAP Distribution Index (CDIX). *IEEE Trans. Biomed. Eng.* **2022**. ahead of print. [CrossRef]
14. Li, J.; Zhu, Y.; Li, Y.; He, S.; Wang, D. Motor unit number index detects the effectiveness of surgical treatment in improving distal motor neuron loss in patients with incomplete cervical spinal cord injury. *BMC Musculoskelet. Disord.* **2020**, *21*, 549. [CrossRef]
15. Witt, A.; Fuglsang-Frederiksen, A.; Finnerup, N.B.; Kasch, H.; Tankisi, H. Detecting peripheral motor nervous system involvement in chronic spinal cord injury using two novel methods: MScanFit MUNE and muscle velocity recovery cycles. *Clin. Neurophysiol.* **2020**, *131*, 2383–2392. [CrossRef]
16. Smith, H.C.; Davey, N.J.; Savic, G.; Maskill, D.W.; Ellaway, P.H.; Frankel, H.L. Motor unit discharge characteristics during voluntary contraction in patients with incomplete spinal cord injury. *Exp. Physiol.* **1999**, *84*, 1151–1160. [CrossRef]
17. Zijdewind, I.; Thomas, C.K. Motor unit firing during and after voluntary contractions of human thenar muscles weakened by spinal cord injury. *J. Neurophysiol.* **2003**, *89*, 2065–2071. [CrossRef]
18. Thomas, C.K.; Broton, J.G.; Calancie, B. Motor unit forces and recruitment patterns after cervical spinal cord injury. *Muscle Nerve* **1997**, *20*, 212–220. [CrossRef]
19. Riley, D.A.; Burns, A.S.; Carrion-Jones, M.; Dillingham, T.R. Electrophysiological dysfunction in the peripheral nervous system following spinal cord injury. *PM&R* **2011**, *3*, 419–425.
20. Zhang, X.; Li, X.; Tang, X.; Chen, X.; Chen, X.; Zhou, P. Spatial filtering for enhanced high-density surface electromyographic examination of neuromuscular changes and its application to spinal cord injury. *J. Neuroeng. Rehabil.* **2020**, *17*, 160. [CrossRef]
21. Zhou, P.; Li, X.; Rymer, W.Z. EMG-force relations during isometric contractions of the first dorsal interosseous muscle after stroke. *Top. Stroke Rehabil.* **2013**, *20*, 537–544. [CrossRef]
22. Suresh, N.L.; Concepcion, N.S.; Madoff, J.; Rymer, W.Z. Anomalous EMG-force relations during low-force isometric tasks in hemiparetic stroke survivors. *Exp. Brain Res.* **2015**, *233*, 15–25. [CrossRef]
23. Bhadane, M.; Liu, J.; Rymer, W.Z.; Zhou, P.; Li, S. Re-evaluation of EMG-torque relation in chronic stroke using linear electrode array EMG recordings. *Sci. Rep.* **2016**, *6*, 28957. [CrossRef]
24. Zhang, X.; Wang, D.; Yu, Z.; Chen, X.; Li, S.; Zhou, P. EMG-torque relation in chronic stroke: A novel EMG complexity representation with a linear electrode array. *IEEE J. Biomed. Health Inform.* **2017**, *21*, 1562–1572. [CrossRef]
25. Thomas, C.K.; Tucker, M.E.; Bigland-Ritchie, B. Voluntary muscle weakness and co-activation after chronic cervical spinal cord injury. *J. Neurotrauma* **1998**, *15*, 149–161. [CrossRef]
26. Drost, G.; Stegeman, D.F.; van Engelen, B.G.; Zwarts, M.J. Clinical applications of high-density surface EMG: A systematic review. *J. Electromyogr. Kinesiol.* **2006**, *16*, 586–602. [CrossRef]
27. Jordanic, M.; Rojas-Martínez, M.; Mañanas, M.A.; Alonso, J.F. Spatial distribution of HD-EMG improves identification of task and force in patients with incomplete spinal cord injury. *J. Neuroeng. Rehabil.* **2016**, *13*, 41. [CrossRef]
28. Merletti, R.; Farina, D.; Gazzoni, M. The linear electrode array: A useful tool with many applications. *J. Electromyogr. Kinesiol.* **2003**, *13*, 37–47. [CrossRef]
29. Yao, B.; Zhang, X.; Li, S.; Li, X.; Chen, X.; Klein, C.S.; Zhou, P. Analysis of linear electrode array EMG for assessment of hemiparetic biceps brachii muscles. *Front. Hum. Neurosci.* **2015**, *9*, 569. [CrossRef]
30. Conrad, M.O.; Qiu, D.; Hoffmann, G.; Zhou, P.; Kamper, D.G. Analysis of muscle fiber conduction velocity during finger flexion and extension after stroke. *Top. Stroke Rehabil.* **2017**, *24*, 262–268. [CrossRef]
31. Jahanmiri-Nezhad, F.; Li, X.; Barkhaus, P.E.; Rymer, W.Z.; Zhou, P. A clinically applicable approach for detecting spontaneous action potential spikes in amyotrophic lateral sclerosis with a linear electrode array. *J. Clin. Neurophysiol.* **2014**, *31*, 35–40. [CrossRef] [PubMed]
32. Li, X.; Lu, Z.; Wang, I.; Li, L.; Stampas, A.; Zhou, P. Assessing redistribution of muscle innervation zones after spinal cord injuries. *J. Electromyogr. Kinesiol.* **2021**, *59*, 102550. [CrossRef] [PubMed]
33. Burns, S.; Biering-Sørensen, F.; Donovan, W.; Graves, D.; Jha, A.; Johansen, M.; Jones, L.; Krassioukov, A.; Kirshblum, S.; Mulcahey, M.J.; et al. International Standards for Neurological Classification of Spinal Cord Injury, Revised 2011. *Top. Spinal Cord Inj. Rehabil.* **2012**, *18*, 85–99. [CrossRef] [PubMed]
34. Mewett, D.T.; Reynolds, K.J.; Nazeran, H. Reducing power line interference in digitised electromyogram recordings by spectrum interpolation. *Med. Biol. Eng. Comput.* **2004**, *42*, 24–31. [CrossRef]

35. Beck, T.W.; Housh, T.J.; Cramer, J.T.; Mielke, M.; Hendrix, R. The influence of electrode shift over the innervation zone and normalization on the electromyographic amplitude and mean power frequency versus isometric torque relationships for the vastus medialis muscle. *J. Neurosci. Methods* **2008**, *169*, 100–108. [CrossRef] [PubMed]
36. Woods, J.J.; Bigland-Ritchie, B. Linear and non-linear surface EMG/force relationships in human muscles. An anatomical/functional argument for the existence of both. *Am. J. Phys. Med.* **1983**, *62*, 287–299. [PubMed]
37. Zhou, P.; Rymer, W.Z. Factors governing the form of the relation between muscle force and the EMG: A simulation study. *J. Neurophysiol.* **2004**, *92*, 2878–2886. [CrossRef]
38. Biering-Sørensen, B.; Kristensen, I.B.; Kjaer, M.; Biering-Sørensen, F. Muscle after spinal cord injury. *Muscle Nerve* **2009**, *40*, 499–519. [CrossRef] [PubMed]
39. Thomas, C.K.; del Valle, A. The role of motor unit rate modulation versus recruitment in repeated submaximal voluntary contractions performed by control and spinal cord injured subjects. *J. Electromyogr. Kinesiol.* **2001**, *11*, 217–229. [CrossRef]
40. Klein, C.S.; Häger-Ross, C.K.; Thomas, C.K. Fatigue properties of human thenar motor units paralysed by chronic spinal cord injury. *J. Physiol.* **2006**, *573 Pt 1*, 161–171. [CrossRef] [PubMed]
41. McGill, K.C.; Lateva, Z.C. History dependence of human muscle-fiber conduction velocity during voluntary isometric contractions. *J. Appl. Physiol.* **2011**, *111*, 630–641. [CrossRef]
42. Nishihara, K.; Chiba, Y.; Moriyama, H.; Hosoda, M.; Suzuki, Y.; Gomi, T. Noninvasive estimation of muscle fiber conduction velocity distribution using an electromyographic processing technique. *Med. Sci. Monit.* **2009**, *15*, 113–120.
43. Martinez, A.C.; Terradas, J.M.L. Conduction velocity along muscle fibers in situ in Duchenne muscular dystrophy. *Arch. Phys. Med. Rehabil.* **1990**, *71*, 558–561.
44. Rainoldi, A.; Galardi, G.; Maderna, L.; Comi, G.; Lo Conte, L.; Merletti, R. Repeatability of surface EMG variables during voluntary isometric contractions of the biceps brachii muscle. *J. Electromyogr. Kinesiol.* **1999**, *9*, 105–119. [CrossRef] [PubMed]
45. Sadoyama, T.; Masuda, T. Changes of the average muscle fiber conduction velocity during a varying force contraction. *Electroencephalogr. Clin. Neurophysiol.* **1987**, *67*, 495–497. [CrossRef] [PubMed]
46. Andreassen, S.; Arendt-Nielsen, L. Muscle fibre conduction velocity in motor units of the human anterior tibial muscle: A new size principle parameter. *J. Physiol.* **1987**, *1391*, 561–571. [CrossRef]
47. Klaver-Krol, E.G.; Hermens, H.J.; Vermeulen, R.C.; Klaver, M.M.; Luyten, H.; Henriquez, N.R.; Zwarts, M.J. Chronic fatigue syndrome: Abnormally fast muscle fiber conduction in the membranes of motor units at low static force load. *Clin. Neurophysiol.* **2021**, *132*, 967–974. [CrossRef]
48. Masuda, T.; Sadoyama, T.; Shiraishi, M. Dependence of average muscle fiber conduction velocity on voluntary contraction force. *J. Electromyogr. Kinesiol.* **1996**, *6*, 267–276. [CrossRef]
49. Troni, W.; DeMattei, M.; Contegiacomo, V. The effect of temperature on conduction velocity in human muscle fibers. *J. Electromyogr. Kinesiol.* **1997**, *1*, 281–287. [CrossRef]
50. Arendt-Nielsen, L.; Mills, K.R.; Forster, A. Changes in muscle fiber conduction velocity, mean power frequency, and mean EMG voltage during prolonged submaximal contractions. *Muscle Nerve* **1989**, *12*, 493–497. [CrossRef]
51. Beck, T.W.; Housh, T.J.; Cramer, J.T.; Weir, J.P. The effect of the estimated innervation zone on EMG amplitude and center frequency. *Med. Sci. Sport. Exerc.* **2007**, *39*, 1282–1290. [CrossRef]
52. Huang, C.; Klein, C.S.; Meng, Z.; Zhang, Y.; Li, S.; Zhou, P. Innervation zone distribution of the biceps brachii muscle examined using voluntary and electrically-evoked high-density surface EMG. *J. Neuroeng. Rehabil.* **2019**, *16*, 73. [CrossRef]
53. Zhou, P.; Suresh, N.L.; Rymer, W.Z. Model based sensitivity analysis of EMG-force relation with respect to motor unit properties: Applications to muscle paresis in stroke. *Ann. Biomed. Eng.* **2007**, *35*, 1521–1531. [CrossRef]
54. Jahanmiri-Nezhad, F.; Hu, X.; Suresh, N.L.; Rymer, W.Z.; Zhou, P. EMG-force relation in the first dorsal interosseous muscle of patients with amyotrophic lateral sclerosis. *NeuroRehabilitation* **2014**, *35*, 307–314. [CrossRef]
55. Johanson, M.E.; Lateva, Z.C.; Jaramillo, J.; Kiratli, B.J.; McGill, K.C. Triceps Brachii in incomplete tetraplegia: EMG and dynamometer evaluation of residual motor resources and capacity for strengthening. *Top. Spinal Cord Inj. Rehabil.* **2013**, *19*, 300–310. [CrossRef]
56. Chen, M.; Zhou, P. A Novel Framework Based on FastICA for High Density Surface EMG Decomposition. *IEEE Trans. Neural Syst. Rehabil. Eng.* **2016**, *24*, 117–127. [CrossRef]
57. Chen, M.; Zhang, X.; Chen, X.; Zhou, P. Automatic Implementation of Progressive FastICA Peel-Off for High Density Surface EMG Decomposition. *IEEE Trans. Neural Syst. Rehabil. Eng.* **2018**, *26*, 144–152. [CrossRef]
58. Sybilski, K.; Mazurkiewicz, L.; Jurkokc, J.; Michnik, R.; Malachowski, J. Evaluation of the effect of muscle forces implementation on the behavior of a dummy during a head-on collision. *Acta Bioeng. Biomech.* **2021**, *23*, 4. [CrossRef]
59. von Tscharner, V.; Barandun, M. Wavelet based correlation and coherence analysis reveals frequency dependent motor unit conduction velocity of the abductor pollicis brevis muscle. *J. Electromyogr. Kinesiol.* **2010**, *20*, 1088–1096. [CrossRef]
60. Dejneka, A.; Malachowski, J.; Mazurkiewicz, L. Identification of muscle movements and activity by experimental methods for selected cases—Stage. *Acta Bioeng. Biomech.* **2022**, *24*. [CrossRef]

Disclaimer/Publisher's Note: The statements, opinions and data contained in all publications are solely those of the individual author(s) and contributor(s) and not of MDPI and/or the editor(s). MDPI and/or the editor(s) disclaim responsibility for any injury to people or property resulting from any ideas, methods, instructions or products referred to in the content.

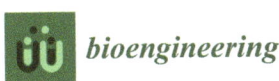

Article

Leveraging Multivariable Linear Regression Analysis to Identify Patients with Anterior Cruciate Ligament Deficiency Using a Composite Index of the Knee Flexion and Muscle Force

Haoran Li [1], Hongshi Huang [2], Shuang Ren [2,*] and Qiguo Rong [1,*]

1. Department of Mechanics and Engineering Science, College of Engineering, Peking University, Beijing 100871, China
2. Department of Sports Medicine, Peking University Third Hospital, Institute of Sports Medicine of Peking University, Beijing 100871, China
* Correspondence: xixishuang123@126.com (S.R.); qrong@pku.edu.cn (Q.R.)

Abstract: Patients with anterior cruciate ligament (ACL) deficiency (ACLD) tend to have altered lower extremity kinematics and dynamics. Clinical diagnosis of ACLD requires more objective and convenient evaluation criteria. Twenty-five patients with ACLD before ACL reconstruction and nine healthy volunteers were recruited. Five experimental jogging data sets of each participant were collected and calculated using a musculoskeletal model. The resulting knee flexion and muscle force data were analyzed using a t-test for characteristic points, which were the time points in the gait cycle when the most significant difference between the two groups was observed. The data of the characteristic points were processed with principal component analysis to generate a composite index for multivariable linear regression. The accuracy rate of the regression model in diagnosing patients with ACLD was 81.4%. This study demonstrates that the multivariable linear regression model and composite index can be used to diagnose patients with ACLD. The composite index and characteristic points can be clinically objective and can be used to extract effective information quickly and conveniently.

Keywords: composite index; characteristic points; multivariable linear regression; anterior cruciate ligament deficiency

1. Introduction

Anterior cruciate ligament (ACL) deficiency (ACLD) is a common injury in people who play sports. The ACL plays an important role in maintaining the stability of the knee joint. However, because of the complexity of the knee joint and ACL, it is difficult to conduct kinematic and dynamic research on patients with ACLD. Studies have focused on building a mechanical model of ACL in vitro [1,2]. Since the establishment of a muscle model by Zajac et al. [3], musculoskeletal models have improved [4,5]. With the help of musculoskeletal models, many studies have investigated the kinematics and dynamics in ACLD-affected knees. Some studies have shown that patients with ACLD adopted quadricep avoidance [6,7] and a stiffening strategy [8], resulting in reductions in the knee flexion moment and peak knee flexion angle. ACLD affects a patient's gait patterns and further kinematics and dynamics [9]. Ren et al. [10] and Yin et al. [11], respectively, studied the kinematics and dynamics in patients with ACLD. Shelburne et al. [7] considered the role of muscles, explaining that in patients with ACLD, quadricep avoidance occurred to restore anterior tibial translation. Furthermore, increasing hamstring force was also sufficient, implying muscle compensation in the knee instability. Even after ACL reconstruction, patients still have a high risk of osteoarthritis [12,13] because of the loss of normal muscle compensation in patients with ACL reconstruction [14,15].

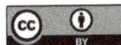

Citation: Li, H.; Huang, H.; Ren, S.; Rong, Q. Leveraging Multivariable Linear Regression Analysis to Identify Patients with Anterior Cruciate Ligament Deficiency Using a Composite Index of the Knee Flexion and Muscle Force. *Bioengineering* 2023, 10, 284. https://doi.org/10.3390/bioengineering10030284

Academic Editors: Christina Zong-Hao Ma, Zhengrong Li, Chen He and Aurélien Courvoisier

Received: 9 January 2023
Revised: 10 February 2023
Accepted: 17 February 2023
Published: 22 February 2023

Copyright: © 2023 by the authors. Licensee MDPI, Basel, Switzerland. This article is an open access article distributed under the terms and conditions of the Creative Commons Attribution (CC BY) license (https://creativecommons.org/licenses/by/4.0/).

The clinical diagnosis of ACLD is complicated and expensive, and the diagnosis process requires the subjective judgment of clinicians. For auxiliary diagnosis, many studies have used statistics to study the gait of ACLD. Christian et al. [16] trained the gait trajectory points of patients with ACLD using support vector machines (SVMs) to extract trajectory features. Berruto et al. [17] counted the fluctuation range of the acceleration of the patient's legs with one ACL reconstruction in a pivot-shift test and demonstrated a significant difference between the ACLD-affected and contralateral sides. Zeng et al. [18] used kinematic data extracted by a motion capture system as features for neural network training. Kokkotics et al. [19] used different machine learning methods to identify patients with ACLD and ACL reconstruction from kinematics and dynamics data. However, only a few studies have used kinematics and dynamics data to diagnose patients with ACLD. There are even fewer studies that can be directly reproduced and can rapidly diagnose patients.

The feature choice is the most important variable, regardless of the statistical method. Reinbolt et al. [20] performed t-tests on the entire gait cycle and selected the peak points of the statistics as features to predict outcomes of rectus femoris transfer surgeries. Principal component analysis (PCA) has been widely used for dimensionality reduction and feature extraction [21]. Armstrong et al. [22] used PCA to extract the feature points of kinematics and reconstruct the kinematics process. Based on multiple parameters extracted from gait data, some indexes were developed to identify walking patterns of normal [23] and abnormal [24–27] gait. Schutte et al. [26] proposed a normalcy index to reflect gait deviations from the mean of normal gait. Liu et al. [28] assessed the abnormal gait in patients with ACLD using the normalcy index calculated by PCA based on kinematics and dynamics data. Similarly, Rozumalski et al. [29] combined a single muscle strength score using PCA to describe the overall lower body joint strength. Hicks et al. [30] used this score as a variable for multivariable regression to study crouch gait. Their regression model had 71% classification accuracy when the parameters were analyzed in detail. However, few studies have combined kinematics and muscle forces to extract features.

This study was performed to identify patients with ACLD using multivariable linear regression through a composite index that combined kinematics and muscle forces.

2. Materials and Methods

2.1. Participants

Twenty-five patients with unilateral chronic ACLD (the contralateral side was intact) were recruited before ACL reconstruction (ACLD group). Their knees had been injured 6 months to 4 years before testing. Most injuries occurred during basketball. Exclusion criteria were that the patient had no prior ACL and concomitant meniscal and ligament rupture and no history of musculoskeletal disease of the hip or ankle. Their physical activity levels were assessed by the Tegner score, which is a reliable and valid tool for assessing the activity level of patients with ACLD [31]. Average activity level of all patients was normal before knee injuries (score range 3.0–6.0). A control group comprising nine healthy volunteers with no history of musculoskeletal injury or surgery in the lower extremities was selected (Control group). All participants were young males to rule out biomechanical differences between sexes [32]. Ethical approval was obtained from the university's ethics committee, and written informed consent was obtained from all participants. The morphological data are shown in Table 1, and the participants' characteristics of the groups were not significantly different.

Table 1. Characteristics of the participants in each group.

Parameters	Control	ACLD
Age (years)	29.22 ± 5.61	27.20 ± 4.19
Height (cm)	173.67 ± 1.95	178.36 ± 7.23
Weight (kg)	74.06 ± 4.73	82.04 ± 11.55
BMI (kg/m^2)	24.56 ± 1.62	25.75 ± 2.93
Pace (m/s)	2.32 ± 0.17	2.36 ± 0.25
Time since injury (months)	/	11.10 ± 6.87
Tegner score	/	4.16 ± 1.72

Data are presented as mean ± standard deviation. ACLD, anterior cruciate ligament deficiency; BMI, body mass index.

2.2. Data Collection and Modeling Analysis

From January 2014 to December 2016, the experimental 3D data were collected while the patients were jogging using an optical motion capture system (Vicon MX; Oxford Metrics, Yarnton, Oxfordshire, UK). The marker trajectory data were filtered at 12 Hz, and the force data were filtered at 100 Hz using a low-pass Butterworth filter. To track the segmental motion during jogging, all participants had a set of markers attached to their anatomical lower limbs at specific locations based on the plug-in-gait model. The participants were asked to run along a 10-m path at a self-selected speed, and the kinematic data were recorded by eight cameras. No participants reported pain during jogging. Ground reaction forces were collected using two embedded force plates at a sampling rate of 1000 Hz (AMTI, Advanced Mechanical Technology Inc., Watertown, MA, USA). Each participant stepped on the force plates at their self-selected speed. For each participant, five successful jogging trials were recorded, and these results were imported into multi-body dynamics software, AnyBody Modeling System version 6.0.5 (AnyBody Technology, Aalborg, Denmark), to estimate the kinetics of the knee joint.

A lower extremity model [33] implemented in the AnyBody Modeling System was used for the analysis. The model comprised 12 body segments, and 11 joints were used to connect the segments. Six joint degrees of freedom were considered for each leg, with a spherical joint with three degrees of freedom for the hip joint and a universal joint with two degrees of freedom for the ankle joint. The knee joint was modeled as a hinge joint with one degree of freedom because of the soft tissue artifact error [34]. Based on the morphological parameters measured from each subject, each model was scaled with a mass-fat scaling algorithm to perform the subject-specific jogging simulation. The min/max recruitment principle solver based on the optimization of the objective function [35,36], which has good numerical convergence and physiological representation, was used to predict the muscle force during the inverse dynamics analysis. The objective function is generally formulated as follows [5]:

$$Minimize\ max\left(\frac{f_i^{(M)}}{N_i}\right) \quad (1)$$

Subject to

$$\mathbf{Cf} = \mathbf{d},\ 0 \leq f_i^{(M)} \leq N_i,\ i \in \left\{1,\cdots,n^{(M)}\right\} \quad (2)$$

where $n^{(M)}$ is the number of muscles, $f_i^{(M)}$ is the respective muscle force, and N_i is the strength of the muscle. f contains all unknown forces in the optimization problem. C is the coefficient-matrix for the unknown forces. d contains all known applied loads and inertia forces. Muscle parameters were obtained from a comprehensive musculoskeletal geometry dataset [37]. Some studies have validated the ability of computational muscle forces [38,39].

2.3. Muscle Data Processing

According to the characteristics of the model and anatomy related to the knee muscles, force data were output from 13 muscles: rectus femoris (RF), popliteus (POP), vastus (VAS), gastrocnemius lateralis (GL), gastrocnemius medialis (GM), soleus medialis (SOLm), soleus lateralis (SOLl), semitendinosus (ST), semimembranosus (SM), proximal sartorius (SAp), distal sartorius (SAd), biceps femoris long head (BFlh), and biceps femoris short head (BFsh). For each participant, separate simulations were performed based on the data from five different jogging trials. The average values of the five calculations were used to perform dynamics analysis using MATLAB version 2019b (MathWorks, Natick, MA, USA).

The acquired muscle force data was processed in a dimensionless manner, and the nondimensionalization of the force data was divided by the subject's gravity (mass × 9.8) [40]. To investigate one gait cycle, the kinematics and dynamics data were interpolated to a 0%–100% gait cycle. Additionally, to more intuitively study the patterns of knee flexion and muscle strength, all flexion and muscle data were normalized to their maximal muscle force within that cycle, leading to a normalized amplitude between 0 and 1 [41].

2.4. Extracting Features

In this study, PCA was adopted as a statistical method for data dimensionality reduction. The main algorithm of PCA is to map the original n-dimensional data to a new k-dimensional feature that retains the largest variance. Thus, the other parts where the variance is close to zero can be ignored and the loss of information is guaranteed to be small. The flow of PCA is as follows:

1. Collect an m × n matrix G, where m is the sample size and n is the n-dimensional variable.
2. Subtract the respective mean from each variable.
3. Compute the covariance matrix of the de-averaged matrix.
4. Calculate the eigenvalues and eigenvectors of the covariance matrix by singular value decomposition.
5. Sort the eigenvalues from large to small, and select the largest k eigenvalues among them. In this study, the ratio of selected eigenvalues to the sum of all eigenvalues was used to assess the information content. Arrange the eigenvectors in the same order as the eigenvalues to form a matrix of principal component coefficients (PCcoeff).
6. Transform the data into a new space, i.e., the new data samples = G × PCcoeff. The first k columns are the required features.

Therefore, data are reduced to k dimensions. If a new sample (1 × n) needs to be predicted, perform the same de-average operation first (the centered sample = the new sample—the variable mean of G from Step 2). Then, the centered sample × PCcoeff produces the predicted value of the sample after the same processing, and the first k columns can be selected as the features of the new sample.

Inspired by the NI index [28] and the strength score [29,30], the first three features used in the calculation are the average force of each muscle during the stance/swing phase of each participant and the value of each person's knee flexion during the swing phase. The specific process was to first obtain the average value of the stance/swing phase of 13 muscle forces and then perform PCA on the average muscle force to obtain a column variable. PCA was also used to process the knee flexion data in the swing phase to obtain a column variable. Only one column variable for each feature after PCA was used because the information content was sufficiently large. For the data of knee flexion in the stance phase and other columns after PCA, their regression parameters in the following multivariable regression were not significant and did not affect the final accuracy.

2.5. Composite Index

In addition to the above features, a composite index containing the data of the knee flexion and muscle forces' characteristic points, which were the time points in the gait cycle when the most significant difference was observed between the two groups, was used in this study. Comparing the ACLD and Control groups based on knee flexion and muscle force data for all participants, t-tests were performed at each point during a 0–100% gait cycle. The data of the characteristic points ($p < 0.05$ and p values were minimal) were finally filtered out as a matrix to calculate the composite index. The selection method of the characteristic points is shown in Figure 1 (using the rectus femoris as an example), and the filtered characteristic points are shown in Figure 2. The muscle force/knee flexion at these characteristic points were filtered out to form a matrix, where the rows of the matrix were the number of participants and the columns of the matrix were the number of characteristic points. Finally, PCA was used to process this matrix to select the representative columns as features.

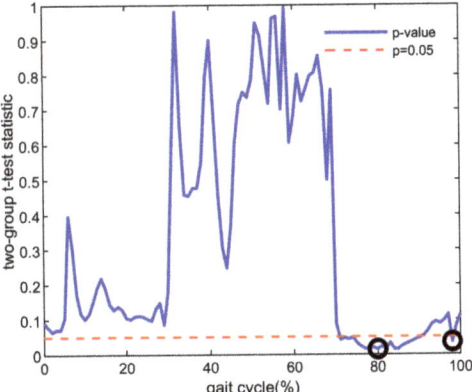

Figure 1. Example of p values between the ACLD and Control groups (taking the muscle force of rectus femoris as an example). The red dotted line means that the p value equals 0.05. The black circle is the selected characteristic point used to calculate the composite index, which is the minimum value in the range of significant differences ($p < 0.05$). ACLD, anterior cruciate ligament deficiency.

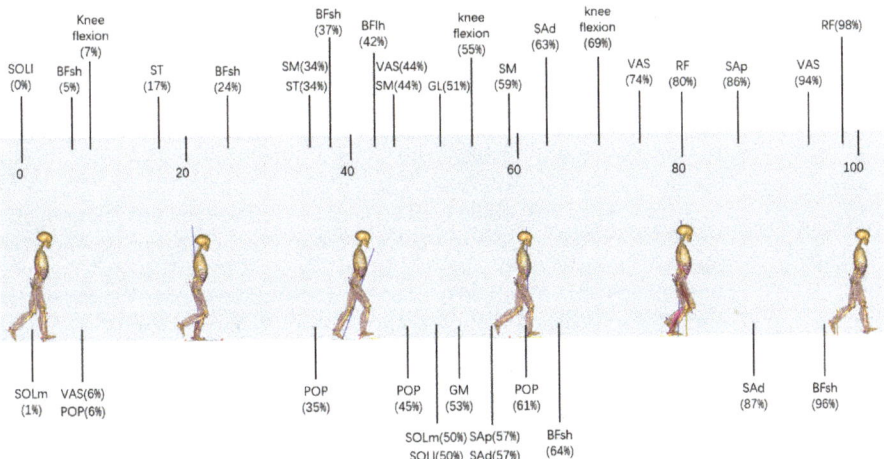

Figure 2. The filtered characteristic points, which were the time points in the gait cycle when the most significant difference ($p < 0.05$ and p values were minimal) occurred between the ACLD and Control groups according to the two-sample t-test method. Characteristic points are shown at their corresponding points during the 0–100% gait cycle. ACLD, anterior cruciate ligament deficiency.

2.6. Statistical Analysis

Using the above variables and samples, we built a multivariable linear regression model. The general form of this model is:

$$Y_{diagnosis} = \beta_0 + \beta_1 X_1 + \beta_2 X_2 + \cdots + \beta_q X_q \tag{3}$$

The outcome variable $Y_{diagnosis}$ was a diagnosis of whether the participant was a patient with ACLD, such that positive values correspond with patients with ACLD and negative values correspond to the Control group. In the data used for training, the ACLD group had $Y_{diagnosis} = 1$ and the Control group had $Y_{diagnosis} = -1$. X_i are the predictive features in the data obtained above and β_i are the linear weighting coefficients for the predictive features. The formulation and prediction of the model were conducted in MATLAB.

3. Results

For these 43 samples (the affected legs of the 25 patients in the ACLD group and both legs of the 9 participants in the Control group), the number of variables selected will affect the final accuracy. The final prediction accuracy changes with feature selection changes are shown in Table 2, where 5-fold cross-validation was used to estimate the predictive ability of the regression model. The second column showed whether only the composite index was used as features. If not, the first column showed the first three features (knee flexion and mean values of muscle force during the stance/swing phase) + the number of features retained in the composite index. If yes, the first column showed only the number of features retained in the composite index. The composite index produced eight features when 90% of the PCA information content was preserved. Therefore, when just using the composite index as features and considering all eight features produced by the composite index, the maximum accuracy achieved was 81.4%. The last column showed the p values in the t-test for the coefficients of the features of the composite index during regression. The smaller the p value, the more significant the corresponding feature. $p < 0.001$ indicated very significant findings and was replaced by 0.001 in Table 2. When using the first 3 features + the composite index, the accuracy gradually increased as the features produced by the composite index increased. When the features produced by the composite index were more than three, the accuracy remained the same and the p value of the newly introduced features increased and was not significant. When the features produced by the composite index were equal to five, the p value of the last feature was 0.999, indicating that the newly introduced feature had no new information. For a comprehensive comparison, the optimal condition was to select six features (the first three features + three composite index features), and the accuracy rate after 5-fold cross-validation was 81.4%. For comparison and validation, under the condition of using only three composite index features, the accuracy was 79.1%.

The classification ability evaluation of the optimal condition is shown in Table 3. The actual results of classification and the accuracy, precision, recall, specificity, and F1-score were used to evaluate the classification ability of the regression model under the optimal condition. Most of the actual results were correctly classified. All evaluation criteria were above 80%, which proved the good performance of the regression model.

Finally, multivariable linear regression was performed on all samples, and the resulting model is shown in Table 4. In Table 4, the coefficients of the average muscle force during the swing phase, Composite Index 1, and Composite Index 2 were negative and their absolute values were the largest among all coefficients. The p value of Composite Index 1 was less than 0.001, the p value of Composite Index 2 was 0.006, and the p value of Composite Index 3 was 0.208. The overall p value of the regression model was less than 0.001.

Table 2. Accuracy changes as the number of features change.

Number of Features	Use of the Composite Index Only	Accuracy	p Value for the t-Test of Regression Coefficients for the Composite Index
3 + 1	No	67.4%	0.001
3 + 2	No	74.4%	0.001 0.001
3 + 3	No	81.4%	0.001 0.006 0.208
3 + 4	No	81.4%	0.001 0.008 0.209 0.686
3 + 5	No	81.4%	0.001 0.009 0.225 0.692 0.999
0 + 1	Yes	72.1%	0.001
0 + 3	Yes	79.1%	0.001 0.001 0.75
0 + 8	Yes	81.4%	0.001 0.001 0.74 0.66 0.45 0.01 0.3 0.48

If the composite index is used as features only, the first column shows 0 + the number of features retained in the composite index. If not, the first column shows three features (knee flexion and mean values of muscle force during the stance/swing phase) + the number of features retained in the composite index. $p < 0.001$ indicates very significant results and is replaced by 0.001 in the last column.

Table 3. Evaluation criteria for the classification ability.

TP	FP	FN	TN	Accuracy	Precision	Recall	Specificity	F1-Score
20	3	5	15	81.4%	87.0%	80.0%	83.3%	83.3%

TP = true positive, samples are classified as positive (ACLD group) and the judgment is correct. FN = false negative, samples are classified as negative (Control group) and the judgment is wrong. FP = false positive, samples are classified as positive and the judgment is wrong. TN = true negative, samples are classified as negative and the judgment is correct. Accuracy = (TP + TN)/(TP + TN + FP + FN). Precision = TP/(TP + FP). Recall = TP/(TP + FN). F1-score represents the harmonic mean of precision and recall. ACLD, anterior cruciate ligament deficiency.

Table 4. Multivariable linear regression model of all samples.

Features	Coefficient	Standard Error of the Coefficients	p Value [a]
Constant	0.1628	0.1113	0.152
Mean muscle force during the stance phase	0.2384	0.1850	0.205
Average muscle force during the swing phase	−2.5339	0.1968	0.206
Knee flexion during the swing phase	0.7346	0.5518	0.191
Composite Index 1	−2.3055	0.5040	<0.001
Composite Index 2	−1.5697	0.5468	0.006
Composite Index 3	1.2417	0.9698	0.208
RMSE		0.73	
R-squared		0.542	
p value [b]		<0.001	

[a] p value for the t-test of each regression coefficient. [b] p value for the F-test on the model. Composite index 1–3 represent the first three features of the composite index, respectively. RMSE, root mean squared error.

4. Discussion

The multivariable linear regression model using the composite index was able to predict, with 81.4% accuracy, whether participants had ACLD. Under the optimal condition (Table 3), data were well classified, and the evaluation criteria were greater than 80%. Among them, the value of precision was high (87.0%), meaning that the correct proportion of the samples classified as the ACLD group was high. Our model was very capable in diagnosing patients with ACLD. The F1-score was high (83.3%), indicating that our model was effective.

As shown in Table 2, when the composite index was used as features only, the best accuracy of 81.4% was achieved by retaining all eight variables. With only one variable of the composite index, there was still 72.1% accuracy. After importing the first three features and retaining three features of the composite index, the best accuracy of 81.4% was achieved. Therefore, this composite index characterized the information of kinematics and dynamics. Using only the three features of the composite index can also achieve an accuracy of 79.1%. Based on the optimal condition of six features, when more composite index features were imported, the accuracy remained unchanged and the p value of the coefficient continued to increase closer to 1, indicating that the introduction of more features was no longer significant. Therefore, the composite index contained more information in the model. Most information in knee flexion and muscle force can be covered in the composite index.

Interpretation of the model must be taken with caution (Table 4). The R-squared value of the regression was 0.542, which indicated that the model was able to explain 54.2% of the variance in the diagnosis of patients with ACLD [30]. For all samples, the optimal features used for regression were significant at the $p = 0.21$ level by the t-test. For the F-test on the model, $p < 0.001$ indicated that the fitting process of the model was very significant. The root mean squared error, which estimated the standard deviation of the error distribution, was equal to 0.73, indicating that the model fit well. As shown in Table 4, there was a significant ($p < 0.001$) negative relationship between Composite Index 1 and the diagnostic outcome, with an expected 2.3055 decline in the final outcome for each one-point increase in the first variable of the composite index. Additionally, there was also a significant ($p < 0.05$) negative relationship between Composite Index 2 and the outcome, indicating that the composite index, especially the first two variables, played the most important role in the regression model.

The composite index was determined by the data of the characteristic points in muscle force and knee flexion (Figure 2). Each muscle selected was associated with the knee joint, which aids in understanding gait pathology and planning treatment using gait analysis and biomechanical models [20,30]. As shown in Figure 2, most of the characteristic points in thigh muscles were concentrated at the terminal of the stance phase, which also corresponded to the previous studies, especially decreased quadriceps [6,7] and increased hamstring [7,42,43]. Alternatively, although tibialis triceps were active during the mid-stance phase, they had more of an impact on ankle dorsiflexion during this period and thus were not significantly different in patients with ACLD [44]. In this study, the muscle force and knee flexion were normalized. Therefore, in further research or clinical diagnosis and treatment, even if the muscle force or knee flexion is obtained in different principles, the characteristic points in Figure 2 can still be directly selected.

With further validation, the regression model can be used to aid clinical practice [30]. Table 5 describes the characteristics of two hypothetical subjects from the ACLD and Control groups. These two subjects have feature values close to the mean of their respective groups. Their expected final outcomes are 0.6164 and −0.4672, respectively, which can be clearly classified into the ACLD group and Control group. Of all the features, the expected improvements in Composite Index 1 and Composite Index 2 have the most impact on the final outcomes. Notably, the subject values of the ACLD group are all less than 0, while the subject values of the Control group are all greater than 0. With t-tests between the two groups on the composite index, we were able to obtain $p < 0.001$ for the first variable of the composite index and $p < 0.05$ for the second variable, verifying the validity of the composite index in the regression model and demonstrating that using only the composite index is also a successful evaluation index, similar to the normalcy index [28] and strength score [29,30].

Some limitations of this study should be noted. First, some patients with ACLD also had meniscus injuries. One study [45] has shown that about 40% to 80% of patients with ACLD have a concurrent meniscal injury. Grouping the data more deeply will help improve our accuracy. Second, data quality can be further improved. The compensatory patterns in the knee joint change depending on the time after ACLD. Limited by clinical data, the period of patients' injuries in this study was not concentrated. Unconcentrated data may affect the accuracy of the final results. Third, electromyography (EMG) data can be introduced. EMG can assist in validating the muscle forces obtained from the calculations [46]. In addition, EMG data can be directly involved in the calculation to obtain a composite index. Fourth, the results of the composite index need further validation for the assessment of walking.

Table 5. Characteristics of two hypothetical subjects from the ACLD and Control groups.

Features	ACLD Group		Control Group	
	Subject Value	Expected Improvement	Subject Value	Expected Improvement
Constant	1	0.1628	1	0.1628
Mean muscle force during the stance phase	−0.1757	−0.0419	0.2440	0.0582
Average muscle force during the swing phase	−0.0063	0.0160	0.0088	−0.0223
Knee flexion during the swing phase	−0.0051	−0.0037	0.0071	0.0052
Composite Index 1	−0.1490	0.3435	0.2069	−0.4771
Composite Index 2	−0.0937	0.1470	0.1301	−0.2042
Composite Index 3	−0.0059	−0.0073	0.0082	0.0102
Expected outcome		0.6164		−0.4672

Composite Index 1–3 are respectively the first three features of the composite index. ACLD, anterior cruciate ligament deficiency.

5. Conclusions

We built a multivariable linear regression model to diagnose patients with ACLD using a composite index that combined knee flexion and muscle forces. This statistical model and composite index can aid clinical diagnosis. The composite index and characteristic points can help avoid complex subjective diagnosis in clinical practice and can be used to extract effective information more quickly and conveniently for diagnosis.

Author Contributions: Conceptualization, Q.R.; methodology, H.L.; software, H.L.; validation, Q.R., H.H. and S.R.; formal analysis, H.L.; investigation, H.L.; resources, H.H. and S.R.; data curation, H.H. and S.R.; writing—original draft preparation, H.L.; writing—review and editing, Q.R. and H.L.; visualization, S.R.; supervision, Q.R.; project administration, Q.R.; funding acquisition, Q.R. All authors have read and agreed to the published version of the manuscript.

Funding: This research was funded by the Natural Science Foundation of China (Grant No: 11872074, 82202821, 31900943), Beijing Municipal Natural Science Foundation (Grant No: L222138), Peking University Third Hospital (Grant No: BYSYZHKC2022119, BYSY2022058, BYSYZD2021012).

Institutional Review Board Statement: The study was conducted in accordance with the Declaration of Helsinki and was approved by the Ethics Committee of Peking University Third Hospital (IRB00006761-2012010).

Informed Consent Statement: Informed consent was obtained from all subjects involved in the study.

Data Availability Statement: Not applicable.

Conflicts of Interest: The authors declare no conflict of interest.

References

1. Kanamori, A.; Zeminski, J.; Rudy, T.W.; Li, G.; Fu, F.H.; Woo, S.L.-Y. The effect of axial tibial torque on the function of the anterior cruciate ligament: A biomechanical study of a simulated pivot shift test. *Arthrosc. J. Arthrosc. Relat. Surg.* **2002**, *18*, 394–398. [CrossRef] [PubMed]
2. Sakane, M.; Woo, S.L.-Y.; Hildebrand, K.A.; Fox, R.J. The contribution of the anterior cruciate ligament to knee joint kinematics: Evaluation of its in situ forces using a robot/universal force-moment sensor test system. *J. Orthop. Sci.* **1996**, *1*, 335–347. [CrossRef]
3. Zajac, F.E. Muscle and tendon: Properties, models, scaling, and application to biomechanics and motor control. *Crit. Rev. Biomed. Eng.* **1989**, *17*, 359–411.
4. Delp, S.L.; Anderson, F.C.; Arnold, A.S.; Loan, P.; Habib, A.; John, C.T.; Guendelman, E.; Thelen, D.G. OpenSim: Open-Source Software to Create and Analyze Dynamic Simulations of Movement. *IEEE Trans. Biomed. Eng.* **2007**, *54*, 1940–1950. [CrossRef]
5. Damsgaard, M.; Rasmussen, J.; Christensen, S.T.; Surma, E.; de Zee, M. Analysis of musculoskeletal systems in the AnyBody Modeling System. *Simul. Model. Pract. Theory* **2006**, *14*, 1100–1111. [CrossRef]

6. Berchuck, M.; Andriacchi, T.P.; Bach, B.R.; Reider, B. Gait adaptations by patients who have a deficient anterior cruciate ligament. *JBJS* **1990**, *72*, 871–877. [CrossRef]
7. Shelburne, K.B.; Torry, M.R.; Pandy, M.G. Effect of Muscle Compensation on Knee Instability during ACL-Deficient Gait. *Med. Sci. Sports Exerc.* **2005**, *37*, 642–648. [CrossRef]
8. Hurd, W.J.; Snyder-Mackler, L. Knee instability after acute ACL rupture affects movement patterns during the mid-stance phase of gait. *J. Orthop. Res.* **2007**, *25*, 1369–1377. [CrossRef]
9. Zhang, Y.; Huang, W.-H.; Yao, Z.; Ma, L.; Lin, Z.; Wang, S.; Huang, H. Anterior Cruciate Ligament Injuries Alter the Kinematics of Knees with or without Meniscal Deficiency. *Am. J. Sports Med.* **2016**, *44*, 3132–3139. [CrossRef]
10. Ren, S.; Yu, Y.; Shi, H.; Miao, X.; Jiang, Y.; Liang, Z.; Hu, X.; Huang, H.; Ao, Y. Three dimensional knee kinematics and kinetics in ACL-deficient patients with and without medial meniscus posterior horn tear during level walking. *Gait Posture* **2018**, *66*, 26–31. [CrossRef]
11. Yin, W.; Ren, S.; Huang, H.; Yu, Y.; Liang, Z.; Ao, Y.; Rong, Q. Dynamical Characteristics of Anterior Cruciate Ligament Deficiency Combined Meniscus Injury Knees. In *Advanced Computational Methods in Life System Modeling and Simulation*; Springer: Singapore, 2017; pp. 132–139.
12. Barenius, B.; Ponzer, S.; Shalabi, A.; Bujak, R.; Norlén, L.; Eriksson, K. Increased Risk of Osteoarthritis After Anterior Cruciate Ligament Reconstruction: A 14-year follow-up study of a randomized controlled trial. *Am. J. Sports Med.* **2014**, *42*, 1049–1057. [CrossRef]
13. Wellsandt, E.; Gardinier, E.S.; Manal, K.; Axe, M.J.; Buchanan, T.S.; Snyder-Mackler, L. Decreased Knee Joint Loading Associated with Early Knee Osteoarthritis After Anterior Cruciate Ligament Injury. *Am. J. Sports Med.* **2016**, *44*, 143–151. [CrossRef] [PubMed]
14. Makihara, Y.; Nishino, A.; Fukubayashi, T.; Kanamori, A. Decrease of knee flexion torque in patients with ACL reconstruction: Combined analysis of the architecture and function of the knee flexor muscles. *Knee Surg. Sports Traumatol. Arthrosc.* **2006**, *14*, 310–317. [CrossRef] [PubMed]
15. Smeets, A.; Willems, M.; Gilson, L.; Verschueren, S.; Staes, F.; Vandenneucker, H.; Claes, S.; Vanrenterghem, J. Neuromuscular and biomechanical landing alterations persist in athletes returning to sport after anterior cruciate ligament reconstruction. *Knee* **2021**, *33*, 305–317. [CrossRef]
16. Christian, J.; Kröll, J.; Strutzenberger, G.; Alexander, N.; Ofner, M.; Schwameder, H. Computer aided analysis of gait patterns in patients with acute anterior cruciate ligament injury. *Clin. Biomech.* **2016**, *33*, 55–60. [CrossRef]
17. Berruto, M.; Uboldi, F.; Gala, L.; Marelli, B.; Albisetti, W. Is triaxial accelerometer reliable in the evaluation and grading of knee pivot-shift phenomenon? *Knee Surg. Sports Traumatol. Arthrosc.* **2013**, *21*, 981–985. [CrossRef]
18. Zeng, W.; Ismail, S.A.; Pappas, E. Classification of gait patterns in patients with unilateral anterior cruciate ligament deficiency based on phase space reconstruction, Euclidean distance and neural networks. *Soft Comput.* **2020**, *24*, 1851–1868. [CrossRef]
19. Kokkotis, C.; Moustakidis, S.; Tsatalas, T.; Ntakolia, C.; Chalatsis, G.; Konstadakos, S.; Hantes, M.E.; Giakas, G.; Tsaopoulos, D. Leveraging explainable machine learning to identify gait biomechanical parameters associated with anterior cruciate ligament injury. *Sci. Rep.* **2022**, *12*, 6647. [CrossRef]
20. Reinbolt, J.A.; Fox, M.D.; Schwartz, M.H.; Delp, S.L. Predicting outcomes of rectus femoris transfer surgery. *Gait Posture* **2009**, *30*, 100–105. [CrossRef]
21. Deluzio, K.; Astephen, J. Biomechanical features of gait waveform data associated with knee osteoarthritis: An application of principal component analysis. *Gait Posture* **2007**, *25*, 86–93. [CrossRef]
22. Armstrong, D.P.; Pretty, S.P.; Weaver, T.B.; Fischer, S.L.; Laing, A.C. Application of Principal Component Analysis to Forward Reactive Stepping: Whole-body Movement Strategy Differs as a Function of Age and Sex. *Gait Posture* **2021**, *89*, 38–44. [CrossRef]
23. Tingley, M.; Wilson, C.; Biden, E.; Knight, W. An index to quantify normality of gait in young children. *Gait Posture* **2002**, *16*, 149–158. [CrossRef]
24. Leporace, G.; Batista, L.A.; Muniz, A.M.; Zeitoune, G.; Luciano, T.; Metsavaht, L.; Nadal, J. Classification of gait kinematics of anterior cruciate ligament reconstructed subjects using principal component analysis and regressions modelling. In Proceedings of the 2012 Annual International Conference of the IEEE Engineering in Medicine and Biology Society, San Diego, CA, USA, 28 August–1 September 2012; pp. 6514–6517. [CrossRef]
25. Romei, M.; Galli, M.; Motta, F.; Schwartz, M.; Crivellini, M. Use of the normalcy index for the evaluation of gait pathology. *Gait Posture* **2004**, *19*, 85–90. [CrossRef]
26. Schutte, L.M.; Narayanan, U.; Stout, J.L.; Selber, P.; Gage, J.R.; Schwartz, M.H. An index for quantifying deviations from normal gait. *Gait Posture* **2000**, *11*, 25–31. [CrossRef]
27. Shin, K.-Y.; Rim, Y.H.; Kim, Y.S.; Kim, H.S.; Han, J.W.; Choi, C.H.; Lee, K.S.; Mun, J.H. A joint normalcy index to evaluate patients with gait pathologies in the functional aspects of joint mobility. *J. Mech. Sci. Technol.* **2010**, *24*, 1901–1909. [CrossRef]
28. Liu, X.; Huang, H.; Ren, S.; Rong, Q.; Ao, Y. Use of the normalcy index for the assessment of abnormal gait in the anterior cruciate ligament deficiency combined with meniscus injury. *Comput. Methods Biomech. Biomed. Eng.* **2020**, *23*, 1102–1108. [CrossRef]
29. Rozumalski, A.; Schwartz, M.H. Crouch gait patterns defined using k-means cluster analysis are related to underlying clinical pathology. *Gait Posture* **2009**, *30*, 155–160. [CrossRef]
30. Hicks, J.L.; Delp, S.L.; Schwartz, M.H. Can biomechanical variables predict improvement in crouch gait? *Gait Posture* **2011**, *34*, 197–201. [CrossRef]

31. Huang, H.; Zhang, D.; Jiang, Y.; Yang, J.; Feng, T.; Gong, X.; Wang, J.; Ao, Y. Translation, validation and cross-cultural adaptation of a simplified-Chinese version of the Tegner Activity Score in Chinese patients with anterior cruciate ligament injury. *PLoS ONE* **2016**, *11*, e0155463. [CrossRef]
32. Théoret, D.; Lamontagne, M. Study on three-dimensional kinematics and electromyography of ACL deficient knee participants wearing a functional knee brace during running. *Knee Surg. Sports Traumatol. Arthrosc.* **2006**, *14*, 555–563. [CrossRef]
33. Horsman, M.K.; Koopman, H.; van der Helm, F.; Prosé, L.P.; Veeger, H. Morphological muscle and joint parameters for musculoskeletal modelling of the lower extremity. *Clin. Biomech.* **2007**, *22*, 239–247. [CrossRef]
34. Andersen, M.S.; Benoit, D.L.; Damsgaard, M.; Ramsey, D.K.; Rasmussen, J. Do kinematic models reduce the effects of soft tissue artefacts in skin marker-based motion analysis? An in vivo study of knee kinematics. *J. Biomech.* **2010**, *43*, 268–273. [CrossRef]
35. Marra, M.A.; Vanheule, V.; Fluit, R.; Koopman, B.H.F.J.M.; Rasmussen, J.; Verdonschot, N.; Andersen, M.S. A Subject-Specific Musculoskeletal Modeling Framework to Predict In Vivo Mechanics of Total Knee Arthroplasty. *J. Biomech. Eng.* **2015**, *137*, 020904. [CrossRef]
36. Crowninshield, R. Use of optimization techniques to predict muscle forces. *J. Biomech.* **1979**, *12*, 627. [CrossRef]
37. Carbone, V.; Fluit, R.; Pellikaan, P.; van der Krogt, M.M.; Janssen, D.; Damsgaard, M.; Vigneron, L.; Feilkas, T.; Koopman, H.F.J.M.; Verdonschot, N. TLEM 2.0—A comprehensive musculoskeletal geometry dataset for subject-specific modeling of lower extremity. *J. Biomech.* **2015**, *48*, 734–741. [CrossRef]
38. Carbone, V.; van der Krogt, M.M.; Koopman, H.F.; Verdonschot, N. Sensitivity of subject-specific models to Hill muscle–tendon model parameters in simulations of gait. *J. Biomech.* **2016**, *49*, 1953–1960. [CrossRef] [PubMed]
39. Trinler, U.; Schwameder, H.; Baker, R.; Alexander, N. Muscle force estimation in clinical gait analysis using AnyBody and OpenSim. *J. Biomech.* **2019**, *86*, 55–63. [CrossRef]
40. Andriacchi, T.P.; Dyrby, C.O. Interactions between kinematics and loading during walking for the normal and ACL deficient knee. *J. Biomech.* **2005**, *38*, 293–298. [CrossRef]
41. Hug, F.; Vogel, C.; Tucker, K.; Dorel, S.; Deschamps, T.; Le Carpentier, É.; Lacourpaille, L. Individuals have unique muscle activation signatures as revealed during gait and pedaling. *J. Appl. Physiol.* **2019**, *127*, 1165–1174. [CrossRef] [PubMed]
42. Liu, W.; Maitland, M.E. The effect of hamstring muscle compensation for anterior laxity in the ACL-deficient knee during gait. *J. Biomech.* **2000**, *33*, 871–879. [CrossRef]
43. Catalfamo, P.F.; Aguiar, G.; Curi, J.; Braidot, A. Anterior Cruciate Ligament Injury: Compensation during Gait using Hamstring Muscle Activity. *Open Biomed. Eng. J.* **2010**, *4*, 99–106. [CrossRef]
44. Lenhart, R.L.; Francis, C.A.; Lenz, A.L.; Thelen, D.G. Empirical evaluation of gastrocnemius and soleus function during walking. *J. Biomech.* **2014**, *47*, 2969–2974. [CrossRef] [PubMed]
45. Granan, L.-P.; Inacio, M.C.; Maletis, G.B.; Funahashi, T.T.; Engebretsen, L. Sport-Specific Injury Pattern Recorded During Anterior Cruciate Ligament Reconstruction. *Am. J. Sports Med.* **2013**, *41*, 2814–2818. [CrossRef] [PubMed]
46. Lenhart, R.L.; Thelen, D.G.; Wille, C.M.; Chumanov, E.S.; Heiderscheit, B.C. Increasing Running Step Rate Reduces Patellofemoral Joint Forces. *Med. Sci. Sports Exerc.* **2014**, *46*, 557–564. [CrossRef] [PubMed]

Disclaimer/Publisher's Note: The statements, opinions and data contained in all publications are solely those of the individual author(s) and contributor(s) and not of MDPI and/or the editor(s). MDPI and/or the editor(s) disclaim responsibility for any injury to people or property resulting from any ideas, methods, instructions or products referred to in the content.

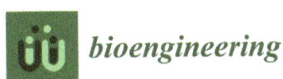

Article

Simultaneous Estimation of the Vertical Stiffness in the Knee and Hip for Healthy Human Subjects during Walking

Huan Zhao [1], Junyi Cao [1,*] and Wei-Hsin Liao [2]

[1] Key Laboratory of Education Ministry for Modern Design and Rotor Bearing System, Xi'an Jiaotong University, 28 Xianning West Road, Xi'an 710049, China
[2] Department of Mechanical and Automation Engineering, The Chinese University of Hong Kong, Shatin, N.T., Hong Kong 999077, China
* Correspondence: caojy@mail.xjtu.edu.cn

Abstract: The stiffness of lower limb joints is a critical characteristic of walking. To investigate the potential of establishing a simple and universal model to describe the characteristics related to vertical vibration during human walking, vertical stiffness is introduced at the knee and hip. A multi-mass-spring model of the human body is established in the vertical direction. In the Fourier form, results of experiments on 14 healthy adults show that the vertical displacements of joints are a function of the leg length and walking cadence, while the ground reaction force is a function of the body weight and walking cadence. The obtained universal equations of vertical displacement and ground reaction force are employed as the input parameters to the proposed multi-mass-spring model. Thus, the vertical stiffness in the knee and hip can then be estimated simultaneously by the subject's weight, leg length, and walking cadence. The variation of vertical stiffness shows different time-varying trends in different gait phases across the entire gait cycle. Finally, the proposed model for vertical stiffness estimation is validated by the vertical oscillation of the pelvis. The average error across three gait cycles for all subjects is 20.48%, with a standard deviation of 5.44%. These results display that the vertical stiffness of knee and hip across the entire gait cycle can be directly estimated by individual parameters that are easy to measure. It provides a different view of human walking analysis and may be applied in future pathological gait recognition, bipedal robots, and lower limb exoskeletons.

Keywords: ground reaction force; knee and hip; lower limb; normal walking

1. Introduction

Walking is one of the most common daily activities of humans, and a large number of engineered locomotion systems are designed to emulate human walking, such as bipedal walkers [1,2], biologically inspired prosthetic limbs [3], and lower limb exoskeletons [4,5]. Research in these fields requires knowledge of the stiffness of lower limbs [6–8] since lower limbs act as supports and actuators in walking [9,10]. As stiffness is a multifactorial expression of the musculoskeletal system [11–14], stiffness in the lower limbs has been studied a lot [15–17]. There are several types of 'stiffness' such as leg stiffness, joint stiffness, and vertical stiffness [18,19]. Leg stiffness is the quotient of ground reaction force (GRF) and the change in leg length. The joint stiffness is the torsional stiffness, which is calculated as the quotient of the moment and joint angle for passive walking. Furthermore, the instantaneous slope of the joint's torque-angle profile is described and defined as quasi-stiffness [20,21]. In addition, joint stiffness at the ankle, knee, and hip is typically defined as the ratio of the change in muscle moment to joint angular displacement [22,23]. Vertical stiffness is generally used to describe the linear movements that occur in the vertical direction, such as hopping and jumping [24]. It was defined as the quotient of vertical ground reaction force (VGRF) and the center of mass displacement [25].

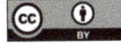

At times, vertical stiffness and leg stiffness were used interchangeably for jumping activities, but it is actually vertical stiffness rather than leg stiffness [26]. Moreover, the relationships between the leg stiffness, vertical stiffness, and joint stiffness of the stance phase in running are compared [27]. It also illustrated that joint stiffness was associated with limb stiffness (vertical stiffness and leg stiffness). As for walking, leg stiffness is calculated as the resultant GRF in the direction of the connection between the center of pressure and hip joint center, and symmetry in bilateral leg stiffness and stiffness sharing proved useful for a more complete gait assessment in children with diplegic cerebral palsy [28].

As reviewed in [29], loading, motion, and cycle all influenced the mechanical characteristics components of walking. Walking metrics such as vertical oscillation, cadence, speed, and step length can be employed to estimate the GRF during walking by a deep learning network regression algorithm [30]. To analyze the inner relationship between stiffness and walking characteristics, some dynamic models have been established. A human gait model in two degrees of freedom was developed to calculate the time-varying stiffness of the joint, and the stiffness is found to be affected by gait pattern and cadence [31]. To realize human-like GRF patterns, an actuated dissipative spring-mass model was also proposed by introducing spring-damping units to the optimization-based minimal biped model [32]. Results illustrated that stiffness and objective weight affect the number and size of peaks in the VGRF and stance time. The vertical movement of the center of mass was related to the stabilization strategies of the double support phase and the single support phase, and the difference was also reflected in the GRF [33]. In addition, the alterations of VGRF during walking were also associated with the appearance of neurodegenerative diseases [34,35].

From the above studies, it can be summarized that the vertical characteristic is crucial for assessing the walking ability of humans. However, the vertical characteristic of joints has not been studied since the reported 'vertical stiffness' was at the whole-body level and the joint stiffness was focused on the moment and angle applied to them. In addition, all kinds of the mentioned 'stiffness' were calculated only at the stance phase and based on the measured GRF, displacement, angle, and moment, which are expensive to measure.

Therefore, the objective of this study is twofold: (i) to establish a universal gait dynamic model that can estimate both the immeasurable stiffness and measurable displacement, and (ii) to estimate the vertical stiffness of the knee and hip during walking by the individual parameters. Based on these concepts, the vertical stiffness of lower limb joints is hypothesized to be directly estimated by individual parameters like leg length, body weight, and walking cadence.

2. Materials and Methods

To evaluate the vertical stiffness of lower limb joints continuously and completely, a multi-mass-spring model of the lower limbs is established. Then the vertical displacements of the lower limb during walking are collected and summarized into a uniform equation. Moreover, the vertical stiffness of the hip and knee is derived. The entire process is displayed in Figure 1.

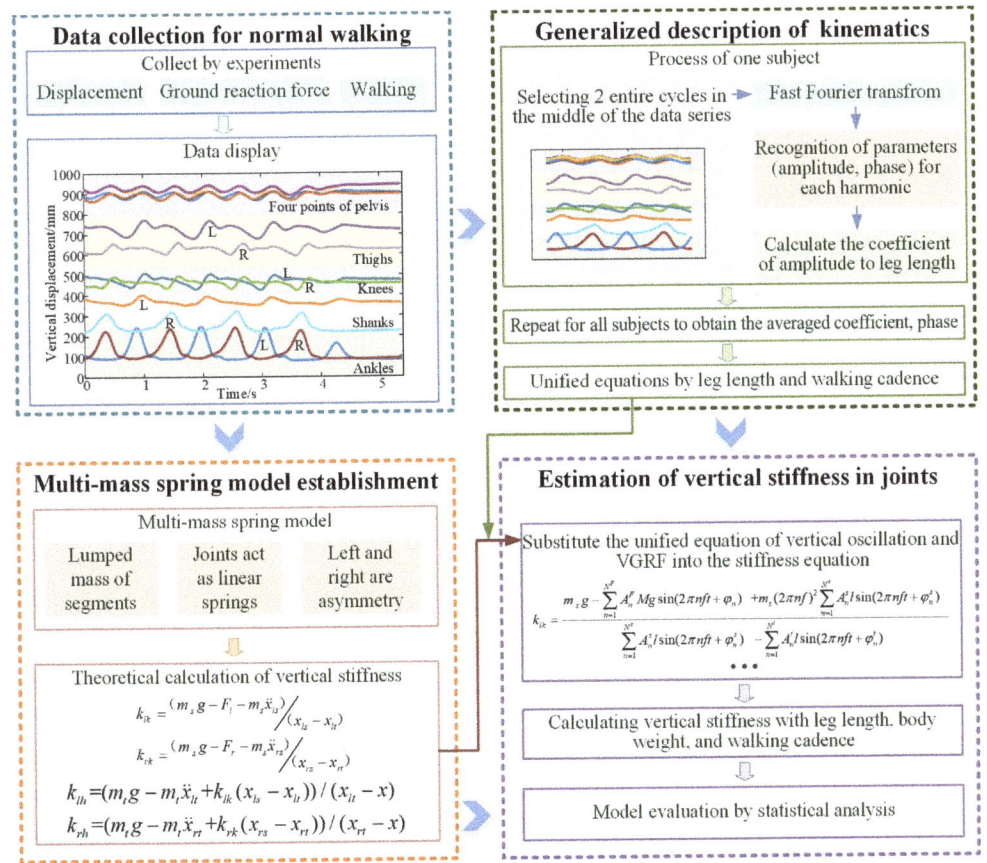

Figure 1. The process of the estimation of vertical stiffness by a dynamic model.

2.1. Subjects

This study was developed according to the Declaration of Helsinki, and all the subjects signed an approved informed consent. Lower limb displacement was measured in 14 young healthy subjects (five females and nine males; age: 25 ± 2 years old; height: 167.9 ± 10.1 cm; and body mass: 58.7 ± 10.3 kg). Subjects were free of any lower-limb musculoskeletal-related injury for at least 3 years before testing.

2.2. Experiments

In a gait laboratory, subjects walked at their preferred speed while wearing 16 retroreflective markers, as shown in Figure 2. The 3D trajectories are collected at 100 Hz by a 12 camera optical capture system (Vicon MX, OML, UK). The GRF was collected at 1000 Hz by three force plates (AMTI, 40060, Advanced Mechanical Technology, Inc., Watertown, MA, USA). Anthropometric parameters including height, mass, and leg length of each subject were measured and recorded. All the subjects were asked to walk barefoot at their preferred walking cadence. The distance of the walking track was about 7 m and had 3 force plates embedded in it. For all subjects, 15 trials of data were recorded for each subject.

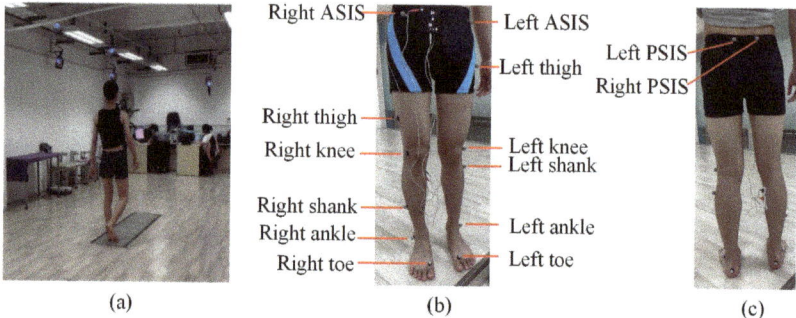

Figure 2. Measurement of lower limb displacement during level ground walking. (**a**) The experimental setup; (**b**) the reflective markers on the front side; and (**c**) the reflective markers on the back side.

2.3. Multi-Mass-Spring Model of the Lower Limbs

A simple model that can characterize the dynamic behaviors of the lower limbs during walking is the foundation for understanding human motion. To describe the kinematics and kinetics in the vertical direction of both the left and right lower limbs, a multi-mass-spring model that includes both the knee and hip joints of the lower limbs is proposed as shown in Figure 3. The trunk and upper limbs are assumed to be concentrated mass points; moreover, the thigh and shank are both characterized as mass points.

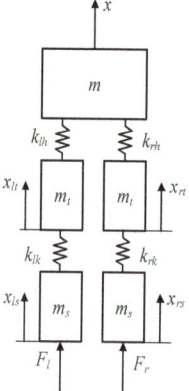

Figure 3. The dynamic model of the human body with ground reaction force.

The analytical formula can then be written as:

$$\begin{bmatrix} m & 0 & 0 & 0 & 0 \\ 0 & m_t & 0 & 0 & 0 \\ 0 & 0 & m_t & 0 & 0 \\ 0 & 0 & 0 & m_s & 0 \\ 0 & 0 & 0 & 0 & m_s \end{bmatrix} \begin{bmatrix} \ddot{x} \\ \ddot{x}_{lt} \\ \ddot{x}_{rt} \\ \ddot{x}_{ls} \\ \ddot{x}_{rs} \end{bmatrix} + \begin{bmatrix} k_{lh}+k_{rh} & -k_{lh} & -k_{rh} & 0 & 0 \\ -k_{lh} & k_{lh}+k_{lk} & 0 & -k_{lk} & 0 \\ -k_{rh} & 0 & k_{rh}+k_{rk} & 0 & -k_{rk} \\ 0 & -k_{lk} & 0 & k_{lk} & 0 \\ 0 & 0 & -k_{rk} & 0 & k_{rk} \end{bmatrix} \begin{bmatrix} x \\ x_{lt} \\ x_{rt} \\ x_{ls} \\ x_{rs} \end{bmatrix} = \begin{bmatrix} mg \\ m_t g \\ m_t g \\ m_s g - F_l \\ m_s g - F_r \end{bmatrix}, \quad (1)$$

where m is the mass of the trunk, upper limbs, and head in total, m_t and m_s are the masses of the thighs and shanks, respectively, based on the relationship of the segment mass to body mass 'M' given by Leva [36], $m^{male} = 0.6028*M$; $m^{female} = 0.5824*M$, $m_t^{male} = 0.1416*M$; $m_t^{female} = 0.1478*M$, the foot is neglected in the model and its mass is included in the shank, $m_s^{male} = 0.057*M$; $m_s^{female} = 0.061*M$; x_{lt} and x_{rt} denote the vertical displacements of the left and right thigh, respectively; x_{ls} and x_{rs} refer to the vertical displacements of the left and right shanks, respectively; F_l and F_r are the left and right GRF in vertical, respectively; k_{lh} and k_{rh} indicate the vertical stiffness of left and right hip, respectively; and k_{lk} and k_{rk} correspond to the vertical stiffness of left and right knee, respectively.

Then the vertical stiffness of the hip and knee are derived as follows:

$$\begin{cases} (k_{lh}+k_{rh})x - k_{lh}x_{lt} - k_{rh}x_{rt} = mg - m\ddot{x} \\ -k_{lh}x + (k_{lh}+k_{lk})x_{lt} - k_{lk}x_{ls} = m_tg - m_t\ddot{x}_{lt} \\ -k_{rh}x + (k_{rh}+k_{rk})x_{rt} - k_{rk}x_{rs} = m_tg - m_t\ddot{x}_{rs} \\ -k_{lk}x_{lt} + k_{lk}x_{ls} = m_sg - F_l - m_s\ddot{x}_{ls} \\ -k_{rk}x_{rt} + k_{rk}x_{rs} = m_sg - F_r - m_s\ddot{x}_{rs} \end{cases} \quad (2)$$

The solution to vertical stiffness in the knee is as follows:

$$\begin{aligned} k_{lk} &= \frac{(m_sg - F_l - m_s\ddot{x}_{lk})}{(x_{lk} - x_{lt})} \\ k_{rk} &= \frac{(m_sg - F_r - m_s\ddot{x}_{rk})}{(x_{rk} - x_{rt})} \end{aligned} \quad (3)$$

Moreover, the pelvis displacement can be derived as:

$$\begin{aligned} & Ax^2 + Bx + C = 0 \\ & A = -2m_tg + 2m_t\ddot{x}_{lt} - k_{lk}(x_{ls}-x_{lt}) - m_tg + m_t\ddot{x}_{rt} - k_{rk}(x_{rs}-x_{rt}) \\ & B = m_tgx_{rt} - m_t\ddot{x}_{lt}x_{rt} + k_{lk}(x_{ls}-x_{lt})x_{rt} + m_tgx_{lt} - m_t\ddot{x}_{rt}x_{lt} \\ & \quad + k_{rk}(x_{rs}-x_{rt})x_{lt} + m_tgx_{lt} - m_t\ddot{x}_{lt}x_{lt} + k_{lk}x_{ls}x_{lt} - k_{lk}x_{lt}^2 \\ & \quad + m_tgx_{rt} - m_t\ddot{x}_{rt}x_{rt} + k_{rk}x_{rs}x_{rt} - k_{rk}x_{rt}^2 + (m_tg - m_t\ddot{x}_{lt})(x_{lt} + x_{rt}) \\ & C = -2x_{lt}x_{rt}m_tg + m_tx_{lt}x_{rt}(\ddot{x}_{lt} + \ddot{x}_{rt}) - k_{lk}x_{lt}x_{rt}x_{ls} + k_{lk}x_{lt}^2x_{rt} \\ & \quad - k_{rk}x_{lt}x_{rt}x_{rs} + k_{lk}x_{lt}x_{rt}^2 - x_{lt}x_{rt}(m_tg - m_t\ddot{x}_{lt}) \\ & x = \frac{-B \pm \sqrt{B^2 - 4AC}}{2A} \end{aligned} \quad (4)$$

The stiffness of the hip can be described as:

$$\begin{aligned} k_{lh} &= (m_tg - m_t\ddot{x}_{lt} + k_{lk}(x_{ls} - x_{lt}))/(x_{lt} - x) \\ k_{rh} &= (m_tg - m_t\ddot{x}_{rt} + k_{rk}(x_{rs} - x_{rt}))/(x_{rt} - x) \end{aligned} \quad (5)$$

therefore, the outputs of the model are hip stiffness, knee stiffness, and the vertical displacement of the pelvis, and they can be calculated from the inputs such as the ground reaction force, mass, and vertical displacement of the thighs and shanks. As for the vertical displacement of both left and right thighs and shanks, they can be represented with anthropometric parameters as conducted in the following section.

2.4. Generalized Description of Kinematics and VGRF

The collected gait signals in Section 2.2 are analyzed with the process shown in Figure 4.

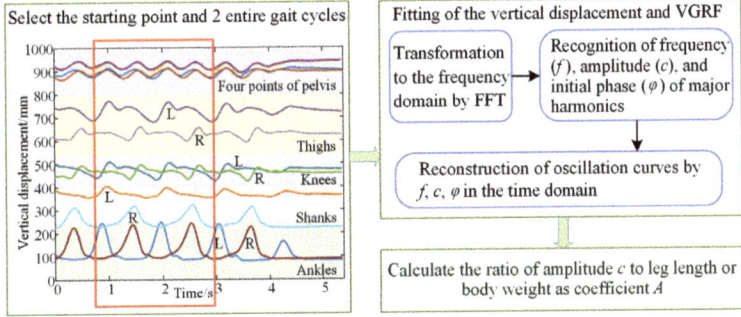

Figure 4. The generalizing process of the lower limb displacement description.

Because the collected gait signals begin and end with standing, the initial and final effects should be eliminated by selecting data points from the median segment. Firstly, the starting point of stable walking and 2 entire gait cycles are selected for analysis. Then the fast Fourier transformation (FFT) is used to transform the signal into the frequency domain since gait is quasiperiodic. The frequency and amplitude of major harmonics are then recognized from the frequency domain, as displayed in Figure 5.

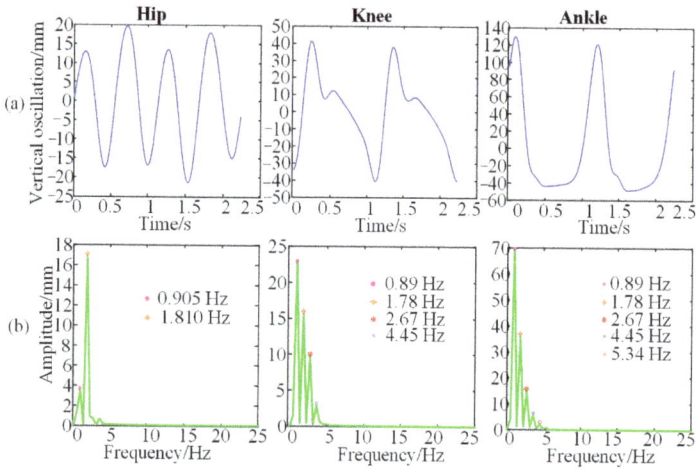

Figure 5. The vertical displacement and the spectrum of the joints for one subject. (**a**) The vertical oscillations of hip, knee, and ankle. (**b**) The spectrums of vertical oscillations of hip, knee, and ankle.

It can be observed in Figure 5b that the vertical oscillation of the hip is mainly accumulated at the first two harmonics, while the vertical oscillation of knee is mainly at the first three harmonics, and the vertical oscillation of ankle is composed mainly of the first four harmonics.. Therefore, the vertical displacement of the hip, knee, and ankle can be represented by the two, three, and four harmonics, respectively. The Fourier series is considered to fit the oscillation trajectory of the lower limb as follows:

$$S_N x = \frac{a_0}{2} + \sum_{n=1}^{N} (a_n \cos 2\pi n x + b_n \sin 2\pi n x), \quad (6)$$

The sine component and the cosine component of the same frequency can be synthesized into a sine component represented as:

$$S_N x = \frac{a_0}{2} + \sum_{n=1}^{N} c_n \sin(2\pi n x + \varphi_n), \quad (7)$$

where $c_n = \sqrt{a_n^2 + b_n^2}$ refers to the amplitude of each harmonic and $\varphi_n = \arctan\left(\frac{a_n}{b_n}\right)$ is the initial phase of the harmonic component in each order; N is the number of the harmonic order. The amplitude is assumed to be proportional to the leg length; therefore, the amplitude of each harmonic in the series is then divided by the leg length of the subject, and thus the ratio of amplitude to leg length is obtained. Then the mean of the ratio and the initial phase of all the subjects are calculated for a general description of lower limb displacements. Finally, the change in vertical displacement can then be derived as:

$$y = \sum_{n=1}^{N} A_n l \sin(2\pi n f t + \varphi_n), \quad (8)$$

where A_n is the coefficient of each harmonic, l is the leg length of the subject, f refers to the real walking cadence, and it is the number of strides in one second; thus, it can also be calculated by the gait cycle time T since $f = \frac{1}{T}$.

The theoretical displacement of one limb can also be derived from the contralateral limb since human walking has the characteristics of symmetry both in space and time. The locomotion of one limb lags a half-gait cycle compared to the contralateral limb. Thus, if a half-gait cycle is introduced to Equation (8), which means t in Equation (8) becomes $(t - \frac{T}{2})$, then the oscillation of the contralateral lower limb joints can be expressed as:

$$y_r = \sum A_i l \sin(2\pi i f t + \varphi_i + (i-1)\pi) + A_j l \sin(2\pi j f t + \varphi_j) \quad i = 1,3,\ldots; j = 2,4,\ldots, \tag{9}$$

where i represents the order of the odd harmonics, and j refers to the order of the even harmonics.

The measured VGRF is also a quasiperiodic signal, as displayed in Figure 4. Similar to the dealing process for kinematic signals, the VGRF can also be represented as:

$$F = \sum_{n=1}^{N} A_n M g \sin(2\pi n f t + \varphi_n), \tag{10}$$

$$F_r = \sum A_i M g \sin(2\pi i f t + \varphi_i + (i-1)\pi) + A_j M g \sin(2\pi j f t + \varphi_j) i = 1,3,\ldots; j = 2,4,\ldots, \tag{11}$$

where F refers to the VGRF of one foot and F_r is the VGRF of the other foot, M is the mass of the body, and $M = m + 2m_t + 2m_s$.

Walking is commonly studied as a repetitively periodic activity using the "gait cycle" [37]. The gait cycle is defined as the duration from the heel strike to the next heel strike of the same limb. It can also be subdivided into the stance phase (accounts for 60% of the gait cycle) and the swing phase (which accounts for 40% of the gait cycle). Moreover, the stance phase and the swing phase can be further subdivided, respectively. These phases can be determined based on the change in VGRF. The details of each gait phase and its corresponding VGRF are shown in Figure 6.

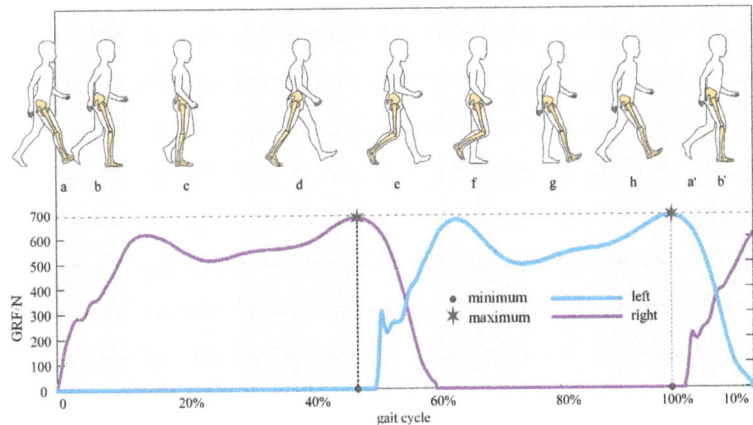

Figure 6. Gait cycles and corresponding ground reaction force. (**a**) Initial contact when heel strike, and it accounts for 2% gait cycle; (**b**) loading response that means foot flatting, and it accounts for 10% gait cycle; (**c**) midstance, and it accounts for 17% gait cycle; (**d**) terminal stance when heeling off, and it accounts for 19% gait cycle; (**e**) pre swing means toe-off, and it accounts for 12% gait cycle; (**f**) initial swing, and it accounts for 13% gait cycle; (**g**) mid swing, and it accounts for 12% gait cycle; and (**h**) terminal swing, and it accounts for 13% gait cycle; (**a′**,**b′**) are phases in the next gait cycle and their determination are the same as (**a**,**b**) respectively.

2.5. Estimation of Vertical Stiffness in Joints

The vertical oscillation of both the left and right thighs and shanks, as well as the VGRF, are represented in Equations (8)–(11) by individual parameters in a universal form. Therefore, by substituting Equations (8)–(11) into Equations (3)–(5), the vertical stiffness of the hip and knee can then be theoretically derived. Here, an equation of vertical stiffness for the left knee is displayed as:

$$k_{lk} = \frac{m_s g - \sum_{n=1}^{N^F} A_n^F M g \sin(2\pi n f t + \varphi_n) + m_s (2\pi n f)^2 \sum_{n=1}^{N^s} A_n^s l \sin(2\pi n f t + \varphi_n^s)}{\sum_{n=1}^{N^s} A_n^s l \sin(2\pi n f t + \varphi_n^s) - \sum_{n=1}^{N^t} A_n^t l \sin(2\pi n f t + \varphi_n^t)}, \quad (12)$$

where the superscript F indicates VGRF, s refers to the shank, and t corresponds to the thigh. Other theoretical equations, like the vertical stiffness of the right knee and hip, are obtained with the same process as Equation (12).

2.6. Statistical Analysis

The distributions of individual parameters such as body weight and height are near normal since they were tested using the Shapiro–Wilk test ($p > 0.05$) [38]. To obtain more accurate descriptions, the coefficient, initial phase, and walking cadence are averaged across the two selected gait cycles for all the subjects. Moreover, the average value and standard deviation of the model errors from all the subjects were calculated to evaluate the dynamic model. All calculations and statistical analyses in this study were carried out using MATLAB (9.6.0.1072779 (R2019a)).

3. Results

3.1. The Empirical Parameters of Unified Representation

As obtained from Section 2.4, all the vertical oscillations of lower limb joints and segments can be obtained with amplitude coefficients and initial phases as represented in Equations (8) and (9). Furthermore, Equations (10) and (11) represent the VGRF with amplitude coefficients, initial phases, walking cadence, and body weight. Their average value across all the subjects is obtained as illustrated in Section 2.5, and they are displayed in Table 1. The vertical displacement of the lower limb can be expressed directly with leg length and walking cadence using these parameters. Moreover, the estimated vertical oscillations were compared to the measured data, as shown in Figure 7. It can be seen that the unified equation with the empirical parameters obtained in Table 1 fits the measured oscillation of the lower limbs well.

Table 1. The parameters of the vertical displacement of the lower limbs.

Parameters	Pelvis	Thigh	Knee	Shank	Ankle	VGRF
A_1	0.007	0.014	0.019	0.022	0.073	0.58
A_2	0.018	0.014	0.017	0.019	0.040	0.08
A_3	0	0.009	0.011	0.016	0.018	0.22
A_4	0	0	0	0.006	0.006	0.03
A_5	0	0	0	0	0	0.07
A_6	0	0	0	0	0	0.03
φ_1	−0.93	−0.59	−0.59	1.08	1.08	2.47
φ_2	−0.49	−1.04	−1.04	0.61	0.61	3.18
φ_3	0	−2.14	−2.14	0.10	0.10	0.98
φ_4	0	0	0	0	0	3.13
φ_5	0	0	0	0	0	−0.42
φ_6	0	0	0	0	0	1.15

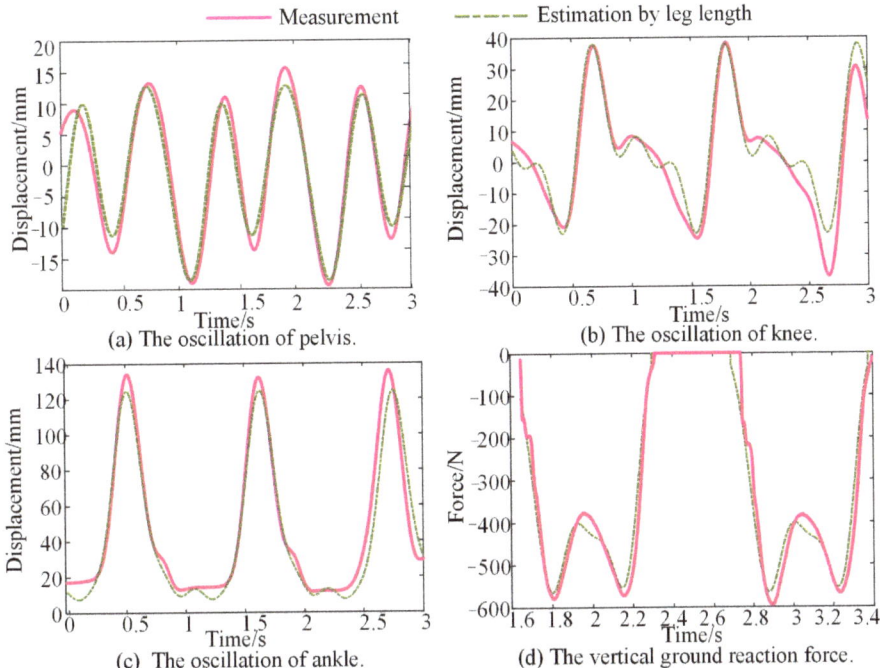

Figure 7. Comparison of vertical displacement between the measurement and the estimation by the individual parameters.

This unification of the quantitative description of human lower limb oscillation during overground walking helps to establish a general representation of the dynamic characteristics such as stiffness.

3.2. The Vertical Stiffness of the Knee

The vertical displacements of the thigh and shank can be represented by the leg length and walking cadence, as illustrated in Equation (12). Figure 8a shows the obtained vertical stiffness of the left knee across several gait cycles after substituting the empirical coefficients and initial phase shown in Table 1 into Equation (12) and then calculating it with MATLAB 2019 a. With the same process, the vertical stiffness of the right knee is calculated and displayed in Figure 8b. In addition, the corresponding ground reaction force is shown in Figure 8c. It can be observed that the vertical stiffness in the knee experienced three changing stages in one stride cycle.

As shown in Figure 8, the vertical stiffness of the knee fluctuated around zero during the first 40% of the gait cycle, from the loading response phase to the terminal stance phase. Moreover, this duration equals the swing duration of the contralateral leg. At the terminal stance phase, the vertical stiffness of the knee appears as the discontinuity point of the first kind, and then it maintains a wide 'U' shape until the mid-swing phase with the duration of 30% of the gait cycle. There is also a discontinuity point of the first kind at the mid-swing phase, and a curve similar to a sinusoid is produced from the mid-swing phase to the loading phase with a duration of 30% of the gait cycle. The duration of the 'U' shape and the sinusoid stiffness curve is the exact stance duration of the contralateral leg. Furthermore, the changing tendencies of the two double support phases differ. When the limb is preparing to swing, there is a discontinuity, and when the limb is preparing for stance, the stiffness variation is continuous. Additionally, the vertical stiffness of the right knee is delaying or ahead of the left knee by half of the gait cycle.

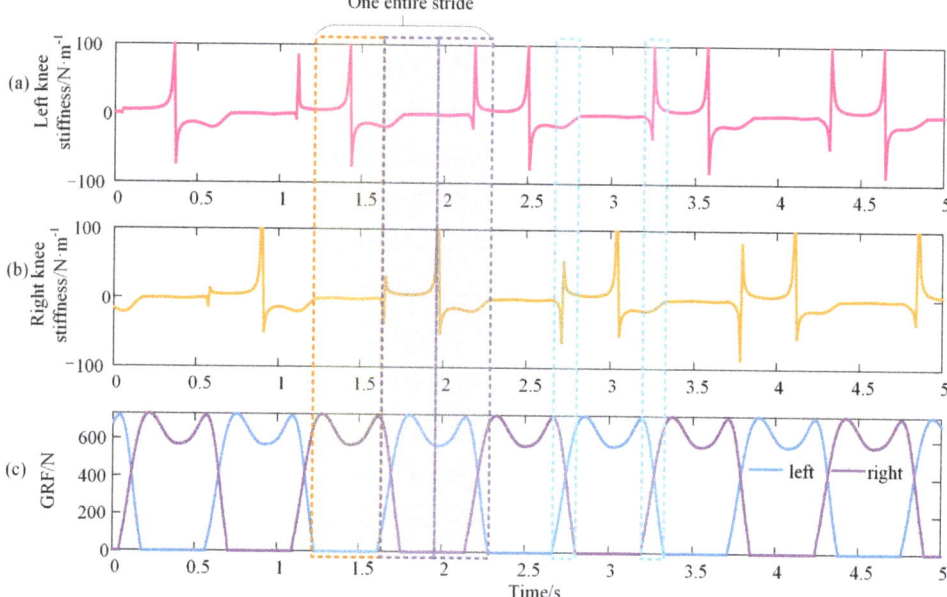

Figure 8. Vertical stiffness of the knee during walking. (**a,b**) denote the left and right knees, respectively, and (**c**) is the corresponding vertical GRF. The yellow rectangle shows the loading response phase to the terminal stance phase of the right leg and the mid-swing phase of the left leg. The purple rectangle represents the terminal stance phase to the loading response phase and is equally separated by the mid-swing phase of the right leg as well as the stance phase of the left leg. The blue rectangles are the double support phase.

3.3. The Vertical Stiffness of the Hip

The empirical coefficients and initial phases of thighs and shanks shown in Table 1 are substituted into Equations (8)–(11) and Equation (4), and these equations are then substituted into Equation (5) to calculate the vertical stiffness of the hip. The obtained vertical stiffness of the left and right hips is shown in Figure 9a,b, respectively. The maximum value of hip stiffness reaches approximately 1×10^6 N/m, and its fluctuation accounts for half of the gait cycle. The stiffness in another half cycle is approaching zero, which seems unchanged. To study the unchanged section, the highly fluctuating section is hidden, as shown in Figure 9c. The theoretical GRF of both lower limbs is shown in Figure 9d to recognize the corresponding gait phase of the two sections.

The vertical stiffness of the hip is extremely high when its corresponding leg goes from the mid-stance phase to the mid-swing phase. From the mid-swing phase to the mid-stance phase, the vertical stiffness of the hip is rather small at about 5 N/m but with a regular shape like 'w'. There is a discontinuity of the first kind at the mid-stance phase and the mid-swing phase. Furthermore, the vertical stiffness between the right and left hips, like the knee, has a time delay for half of the gait cycle. During walking, the vertical stiffness of the knee and hip varies with the gait phase (time).

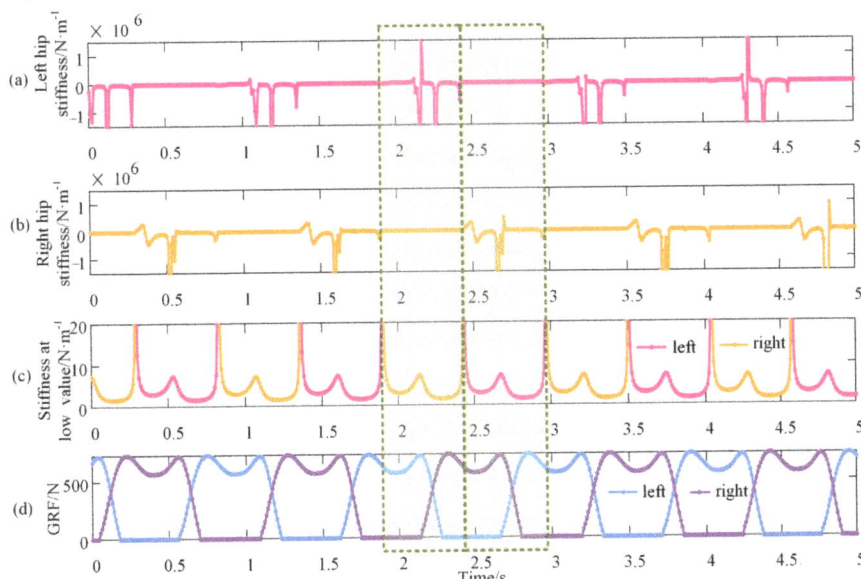

Figure 9. Vertical stiffness of the hip during walking. (**a**,**b**) denote the left and right hip, respectively, and it is evident that the fluctuation is rather high with a magnitude of 10^6; (**c**) shows the hip stiffness at the section of low value; and (**d**) is the vertical GRF of the double lower limbs. The green rectangles stand for half of the gait cycle.

3.4. Validation of the Model

It is reasonable to validate the model by evaluating the pelvis displacement estimated by the model because the vertical stiffness has been difficult, if not impossible, to measure during walking until now. Errors between the model solution and the measured displacement of the pelvis are calculated. The measured displacement was collected in the experiment in Section 2.2. It contains three strides, and each stride has differences in oscillation. Therefore, the variable of time 't' in Equation (8) is set to 3.5 s in order to include three strides. With the empirical coefficients and phases in Table 1, the vertical displacement of the thigh and shank is expressed and substituted into Equation (4). The obtained vertical displacement of the pelvis for one subject is then compared to the measured displacement as presented in Figure 10.

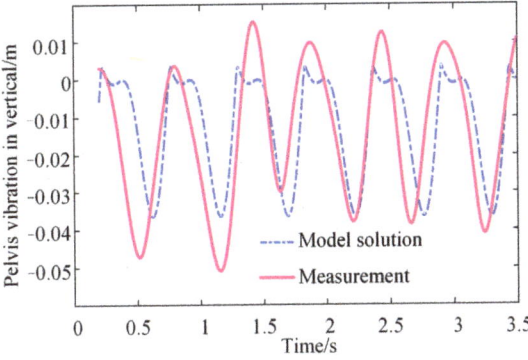

Figure 10. The pelvis trajectory calculated by the model and real measurement.

It can be observed that the model solution of the pelvis displacement is approximately consistent with the measured displacement. This proved that the proposed model could characterize walking characteristics such as vertical stiffness and pelvis oscillation by leg length, body weight, and walking cadence. Moreover, to illustrate the universality and stability of the identification process, the model error is calculated from the solved pelvis displacement and the measured pelvis displacement as follows:

$$E = \frac{1}{t * F_s} \sum_{nt=1}^{t*F_s} \frac{x_{nt}^{measure} - x_{nt}^{solutiom}}{x_{nt}^{measure}}, \quad (13)$$

where t equals 3.5 s as mentioned before, F_s equals the sampling frequency of the motion capture system, which is 100, and subscript nt refers to the number of time points. The errors for all the subjects are shown in Table 2. For different individuals, the errors range from 11.94 to 29.14%, and the mean error is 20.48% while the standard deviation is 5.44%.

Table 2. The error of the estimated pelvis displacement by model.

No	1	2	3	4	5	6	7	8	9	10	11	12	13	14
Errors (%)	29.14	18.87	11.94	23.22	27.95	24.00	16.45	23.49	15.47	27.95	16.48	17.76	18.34	15.62

4. Discussion

The primary aim of this study is to estimate the vertical stiffness of the knee and hip using individual parameters that are easy to measure during walking. To achieve this aim, a multi-mass-spring model was established. Furthermore, the Fourier series was used to fit the vertical displacements of lower limb segments and VGRF required in the established model with individual parameters such as leg length and walking cadence. According to the established model, the vertical stiffness of the knee and hip was estimated by leg length, body weight, and walking cadence across the entire gait cycle. Furthermore, the established lower limb model was validated by its solution of pelvic displacement and real measurement.

Firstly, our results implied that the established multi-spring model is effective at characterizing walking characteristics. There were different dynamic models for stiffness calculation, as shown in Table 3. A typical human gait model using a nonlinear angular spring and dash pot at each point was established to find the optimum joint stiffness of the hip and ankle in the stance phase [31]. It also found that stiffness variation was affected by gait pattern and cadence. An actuated dissipative model combining the optimization-based minimal biped model and the spring-loaded inverted-pendulum model was established for the stance phase, and 2×10^4 N/m (5×10^3 to 1×10^5 N/m) of the leg stiffness achieved the closest GRF profile [32]. This supported our finding that the vertical stiffness of the hip in the stance phase is sometimes varied at a high value level, as displayed in Figure 9. The quasi-stiffness of the knee and ankle was predicted using statistical models based on subject weight and height [18,20]. They provided the foundation for the idea that immeasurable characteristics can be predicted by measurable parameters. A point mass with two massless springs was also established as a dynamic model to calculate the leg stiffness in the stance phase [39] and to predict the trajectory of the center of mass. Compared to these dynamic models for stiffness estimation in the stance phase, the multi-mass spring model established in this study can estimate stiffness across the entire gait cycle, and its solution of pelvis displacement has been validated.

Table 3. The comparison between the typical and proposed dynamic models for stiffness calculation.

Models	Components	Aim Stiffness	Gait Phase	Input Parameters
Two-link conceptual model [31]		Joint stiffness of hip and ankle	Stance	Joint angle and moment
Spring-mass walking model [32]		Leg stiffness	Stance	Leg length and position
Statistic model [18,20]		Quasi-stiffness of knee and hip separately	Stance	Body weight, height, and walking speed
Mass-spring model [39]		Leg stiffness	Stance	Angle and leg length change
Multi-mass spring model Proposed in this paper		Vertical stiffness of knee and hip simultaneous	Entire gait cycle	Body weight, leg length, and walking cadence

Aside from the ability of the proposed model in our study to be consistent across the entire gait cycle, the vertical stiffness of joints in our study was a different concept from traditional joint stiffness. Traditionally, the stiffness of the knee and hip was calculated as the quotient of the moment and joint angle change in the sagittal plane, and the moment was calculated by the trajectory data and the GRF [40]. This joint stiffness illustrated the relationship between the angle and the corresponding moment applied to the joints during walking. While the vertical stiffness of the joints investigated in this study shows a link between vertical oscillation of lower limb segments and VGRF.

During the model solution, the vertical oscillations of lower limb segments and VGR were utilized. The vertical oscillation of lower limb segments was fitted by the Fourier series with leg length and walking cadence, while the VGRF was represented with body weight and walking cadence. The amplitude coefficient and initial phases shown in Table 1 contributed to a universal and mathematical expression. These findings were supported by previous findings. Fourier series, for example, had been used to characterize the pelvic trajectory [41].

Since the vertical stiffness of the knee and hip was obtained solely by individual parameters such as body weight, leg length, and walking cadence, which are all easy and cheap to measure, it implies that VGRF, body weight, and vertical oscillation of body segments have inherent relationships. This is similar to the previous research. The body weight influenced the GRF, and the vertical displacement of the body for a given individual was determined by the effective leg length [32]. Furthermore, it was demonstrated that the VGRF estimated the vertical displacement of the body mass [42].

Moreover, when compared to previous studies, our study illustrates the time-varying process of vertical stiffness corresponding to the gait phase across the entire gait cycle. In vertical, knee stiffness is near zero in the midstance and high in the terminal stance and initial swing. These findings are consistent with previous research, which found that the knee stiffness determined by the slope of the knee moment-angle curve is approximately zero at the start of the stance and increases in the late stance [21]. In addition, it is worthy to note that the vertical stiffness of the knee across the entire cycle is varied in the same order of magnitude while being different for the hip.

The contributions of this study are as follows: (1) the uniform equation to depict the vertical oscillations and VGRF of different people is obtained with individual walking cadences as well as leg length and body weight, respectively; (2) the multi-mass-spring model is established to identify the vertical stiffness of hip and knee simultaneously, and this stiffness can be represented by the body weight, leg length, and walking cadences; and (3) the obtained vertical stiffness is validated by the comparison between the estimated displacement and the measured displacement of the pelvis.

There are also some limitations that need to be considered. The main limitation is the size of the subject. Fourteen subjects walked at their preferred speed, obtaining a homogeneous sample. The analyses could be generalized only to the range of age, height, and walking cadence that the statistical significance supports. Similar estimations could be carried out for other groups, such as older adults and children. Another limitation is that several simplifications were employed. Both the mass and length of the left and right lower limbs were regarded as the same, and the ankle and foot were ignored. A more sophisticated model could be considered to take the asymmetrical factors and eliminated terms into account.

5. Conclusions

In summary, the vertical stiffness of the knee and hip can be simultaneously estimated by a multi-mass-spring model. It has been found that the vertical oscillations of lower limb segments were universally expressed by walking cadence and leg length, while vertical ground reaction force was represented by walking cadence and body weight. Moreover, the vertical stiffness of the knee and hip were finally estimated by the walking cadence, leg length, and body weight. The variation of the estimated vertical stiffness across the entire gait cycle displayed different trends toward different gait phases. Additionally, the proposed model was validated efficiently by the estimated vertical oscillation of the pelvis across three gait cycles for the 14 different subjects. The remarkable results obtained in this study represent a different view for future studies on human walking analysis. In the near future, more sophisticated models that consider ankle and damping will be constructed and extended to more human groups.

Author Contributions: Conceptualization, H.Z. and J.C.; methodology, H.Z.; software, H.Z.; validation, H.Z., J.C. and W.-H.L.; formal analysis, H.Z.; investigation, H.Z.; resources, J.C. and W.-H.L.; data curation, H.Z.; writing—original draft preparation, H.Z.; writing—review and editing, H.Z., J.C. and W.-H.L.; visualization, H.Z.; supervision, J.C. and W.-H.L.; project administration, J.C. and W.-H.L.; funding acquisition, J.C. and W.-H.L. All authors have read and agreed to the published version of the manuscript.

Funding: This work was supported by the National Key Research and Development Program of China [grant number 2021YFE0203400], the Innovation and Technology Commission under the Mainland-Hong Kong Joint Funding Scheme (MHKJFS), and the Hong Kong Special Administrative Region, China [Project No. MHP/043/20].

Institutional Review Board Statement: The study was conducted in accordance with the Declaration of Helsinki and approved by the Institutional Review Board of Xi'an Jiaotong University (protocol code 2020-1330 and date of approval: 26 October 2020).

Informed Consent Statement: Informed consent was obtained from all subjects involved in the study.

Data Availability Statement: The data presented in this study are available on request from the corresponding author.

Acknowledgments: We would like to thank some colleagues for their useful discussion.

Conflicts of Interest: The authors declare no conflict of interest.

References

1. Collins, S.; Ruina, A.; Tedrake, R.; Wisse, M. Efficient Bipedal Robots Based on Passive-Dynamic Walkers. *Science* **2005**, *307*, 1082–1085. [CrossRef]
2. Lin, B.; Zhang, Q.; Fan, F.; Shen, S. Reproducing vertical human walking loads on rigid level surfaces with a damped bipedal inverted pendulum. *Structures* **2021**, *33*, 1789–1801. [CrossRef]
3. Agboola-Dobson, A.; Wei, G.; Ren, L. Biologically inspired design and development of a variable stiffness powered ankle-foot prosthesis. *J. Mech. Robot* **2019**, *11*, 4. [CrossRef]
4. Sanchez-Villamañan, M.D.C.; Gonzalez-Vargas, J.; Torricelli, D.; Moreno, J.C.; Pons, J.L. Compliant lower limb exoskeletons: A comprehensive review on mechanical design principles. *J. Neuroeng. Rehabil* **2019**, *16*, 55. [CrossRef] [PubMed]
5. Saypulaev, M.R.; Zuev, Y.; Saypulaev, G.R. Development of the lower extremity exoskeleton dynamics model using in the task of the patient verticalization. *J. Phys. Conf. Ser.* **2021**, *2096*, 12042. [CrossRef]
6. Zhang, L.; Liu, G.; Han, B.; Wang, Z.; Yan, Y.; Ma, J.; Wei, P. Knee joint biomechanics in physiological conditions and how pathologies can affect it: A systematic review. *Appl. Bionics Biomech.* **2020**, *2020*, 7451683. [CrossRef]
7. Li, T.; Wang, L.; Yi, J.; Li, Q.; Liu, T. Reconstructing walking dynamics from two shank-mounted inertial measurement units. *IEEE/ASME Trans. Mechatron.* **2021**, *26*, 3040–3050. [CrossRef]
8. Jin, D.; Liu, Y.; Ma, X.; Song, Q. Long time prediction of human lower limb movement based on IPSO-BPNN. *J. Phys. Conf. Ser.* **2021**, *1865*, 42099. [CrossRef]
9. Higueras-Ruiz, D.R.; Nishikawa, K.; Feigenbaum, H.; Shafer, M. What is an artificial muscle? A comparison of soft actuators to biological muscles. *Bioinspir. Biomim.* **2021**, *17*, 011001. [CrossRef] [PubMed]
10. Yang, H.; Wu, B.; Li, J.; Bao, Y.; Xu, G. A spring-loaded inverted pendulum model for analysis of human-structure interaction on vibrating surfaces. *J. Sound Vib.* **2022**, *522*, 116727. [CrossRef]
11. Latash, M.L.; Zatsiorsky, V.M. Joint stiffness: Myth or reality. *Hum. Mov. Sci.* **1993**, *12*, 653–692. [CrossRef]
12. Struzik, A.; Karamanidis, K.; Lorimer, A.; Keogh, J.W.; Gajewski, J. Application of leg, vertical, and joint stiffness in running performance: A literature overview. *Appl. Bionics Biomech.* **2021**, *2021*, 9914278. [CrossRef]
13. Wang, K.; Raychoudhury, S.; Hu, D.; Ren, L.; Liu, J.; Xiu, H.; Liang, W.; Li, B.; Wei, G.; Qian, Z. The impact of locomotor speed on the human metatarsophalangeal joint kinematics. *Front. Bioeng. Biotechnol.* **2021**, *9*, 644582. [CrossRef] [PubMed]
14. Santos, T.R.; Araújo, V.L.; Khuu, A.; Lee, S.; Lewis, C.L.; Souza, T.R.; Holt, K.G.; Fonseca, S.T. Effects of sex and walking speed on the dynamic stiffness of lower limb joints. *J. Biomech.* **2021**, *129*, 110803. [CrossRef] [PubMed]
15. van der Kooij, H.; Fricke, S.S.; Veld, R.C.; Prieto, A.V.; Keemink, A.Q.; Schouten, A.C.; van Asseldonk, E.H. A device and method to identify hip, knee and ankle joint impedance during walking. *arXiv* **2021**, arXiv:2112.05564. [CrossRef]
16. Russell, F.; Takeda, Y.; Kormushev, P.; Vaidyanathan, R.; Ellison, P. Stiffness modulation in a humanoid robotic leg and knee. *IEEE Robot. Autom. Lett.* **2021**, *6*, 2563–2570. [CrossRef]
17. Qiu, S.; Guo, W.; Caldwell, D.; Chen, F. Exoskeleton online learning and estimation of human walking intention based on dynamical movement primitives. *IEEE Trans. Cogn. Dev. Syst.* **2021**, *13*, 67–79. [CrossRef]
18. Shamaei, K.; Sawicki, G.; Dollar, A.M. Estimation of quasi-stiffness of the human knee in the stance phase of walking. *PLoS ONE* **2013**, *8*, e59993. [CrossRef]
19. Fajardo, C.D.C.; Cardoso, T.B.; Gontijo, B.A.; de Magalhães, F.A.; de Souza, T.R.; da Fonseca, S.T.; Ocarino, J.D.M.; Resende, R.A. Hip passive stiffness is associated with midfoot passive stiffness. *Braz. J. Phys. Ther.* **2021**, *25*, 530–535. [CrossRef]
20. Shamaei, K.; Sawicki, G.; Dollar, A.M. Estimation of Quasi-Stiffness and propulsive work of the human ankle in the stance phase of walking. *PLoS ONE* **2013**, *8*, e59935. [CrossRef] [PubMed]
21. Rouse, E.J.; Gregg, R.; Hargrove, L.; Sensinger, J.W. The difference between stiffness and quasi-stiffness in the context of biomechanical modeling. *IEEE T. Bio.-Med. Eng.* **2013**, *60*, 562–568. [CrossRef] [PubMed]
22. Davis, R.B.; DeLuca, P.A. Gait characterization via dynamic joint stiffness. *Gait Posture* **1996**, *4*, 224–231. [CrossRef]
23. Dixon, S.J.; Hinman, R.; Creaby, M.; Kemp, G.; Crossley, K.M. Knee joint stiffness during walking in knee osteoarthritis. *Arthrit. Care Res.* **2010**, *62*, 38–44. [CrossRef]
24. Serpell, B.G.; Ball, N.; Scarvell, J.; Smith, P. A review of models of vertical, leg, and knee stiffness in adults for running, jumping or hopping tasks. *J. Sports Sci.* **2012**, *30*, 1347–1363. [CrossRef]
25. Pappas, P.; Paradisis, G.; Vagenas, G. Leg and vertical stiffness (a)symmetry between dominant and non-dominant legs in young male runners. *Hum. Mov. Sci.* **2015**, *40*, 273–283. [CrossRef] [PubMed]
26. Struzik, A.; Winiarski, S.; Zawadzki, J. Inter-Limb Asymmetry of Leg Stiffness in National Second-League Basketball Players during Countermovement Jumps. *Symmetry* **2022**, *14*, 440. [CrossRef]
27. Jin, L.; Hahn, M.E. Relationship between Joint Stiffness, Limb Stiffness and Whole–Body Center of Mass Mechanical Work across Running Speeds. *Biomechanics* **2022**, *2*, 441–452. [CrossRef]
28. Kuo, C.-C.; Huang, H.-P.; Lu, H.-Y.; Chen, T.-Y.; Wang, T.-M.; Lu, T.-W. Effects of Tendon Release Surgery on Inter-Limb Leg Stiffness Control in Children with Spastic Diplegic Cerebral Palsy during Gait. *Appl. Sci.* **2021**, *11*, 4562. [CrossRef]
29. Jamari, J.; Ammarullah, M.; Santoso, G.; Sugiharto, S.; Supriyono, T.; Permana, M.; Winarni, T.; van der Heide, E. Adopted walking condition for computational simulation approach on bearing of hip joint prosthesis: Review over the past 30 years. *Heliyon* **2022**, *8*, e12050. [CrossRef] [PubMed]

30. Davidson, P.; Virekunnas, H.; Sharma, D.; Piche, R.; Cronin, N. Continuous Analysis of Running Mechanics by Means of an Integrated INS/GPS Device. *Sensors* **2019**, *19*, 1480. [CrossRef] [PubMed]
31. Duan, X.H.; Allen, R.; Sun, J.Q. A stiffness-varying model of human gait. *Med. Eng. Phys.* **1997**, *19*, 518–524. [CrossRef] [PubMed]
32. Li, T.; Li, Q.; Liu, T. An actuated dissipative spring-mass walking model: Predicting human-like ground reaction forces and the effects of model parameters. *J. Biomech.* **2019**, *90*, 58–64. [CrossRef]
33. Vielemeyer, J.; Müller, R.; Staufenberg, N.; Renjewski, D.; Abel, R. Ground reaction forces intersect above the center of mass in single support, but not in double support of human walking. *J. Biomech.* **2021**, *120*, 110387. [CrossRef]
34. Zhao, H.; Wang, R.; Lei, Y.; Liao, W.; Cao, H.; Cao, J. Severity level diagnosis of Parkinson's disease by ensemble K-nearest neighbor under imbalanced data. *Expert Syst. Appl.* **2022**, *189*, 116113. [CrossRef]
35. Zhao, H.; Cao, J.; Wang, R.; Lei, Y.; Liao, W.; Cao, H. Accurate identification of Parkinson's disease by distinctive features and ensemble decision trees. *Biomed. Signal Process.* **2021**, *69*, 102860. [CrossRef]
36. de Leva, P. Adjustments to Zatsiorsky-Seluyanov's segment inertia parameters. *J. Biomech.* **1996**, *29*, 1223–1230. [CrossRef]
37. Jamari, J.; Ammarullah, M.; Saad, A.; Syahrom, A.; Uddin, M.; van der Heide, E.; Basri, H. The Effect of Bottom Profile Dimples on the Femoral Head on Wear in Metal-on-Metal Total Hip Arthroplasty. *J. Funct. Biomater.* **2021**, *12*, 38. [CrossRef] [PubMed]
38. Rubio-Peiroten, A.; Garcia-Pinillos, F.; Jaen-Carrillo, D.; Carton-Llorente, A.; Abat, F.; Roche-Seruendo, L. Relationship between Connective Tissue Morphology and Lower-Limb Stiffness in Endurance Runners. A Prospective Study. *Int. J. Environ. Res. Public Health* **2021**, *18*, 8353. [CrossRef] [PubMed]
39. Lipfert, S.W.; Günther, M.; Renjewski, D.; Grimmer, S.; Seyfarth, A. A model-experiment comparison of system dynamics for human walking and running. *J. Theor. Biol.* **2012**, *292*, 11–17. [CrossRef] [PubMed]
40. Gustafson, J.A.; Gorman, S.; Fitzgerald, G.; Farrokhi, S. Alterations in walking knee joint stiffness in individuals with knee osteoarthritis and self-reported knee instability. *Gait Posture* **2016**, *43*, 210–215. [CrossRef] [PubMed]
41. Panero, E.; Anastasio, D.; Massazza, G.; Gastaldi, L. Fourier Analysis of Center of Mass Trajectory in Hemiparetic Gait. In *The International Conference of IFToMM ITALY*; Springer: Berlin/Heidelberg, Germany, 2022; pp. 568–576. [CrossRef]
42. Saini, M.; Kerrigan, D.; Thirunarayan, M.; Duff-Raffaele, M. The vertical displacement of the center of mass during walking: A comparison of four measurement methods. *J. Biomech. Eng.* **1998**, *120*, 133–139. [CrossRef] [PubMed]

Disclaimer/Publisher's Note: The statements, opinions and data contained in all publications are solely those of the individual author(s) and contributor(s) and not of MDPI and/or the editor(s). MDPI and/or the editor(s) disclaim responsibility for any injury to people or property resulting from any ideas, methods, instructions or products referred to in the content.

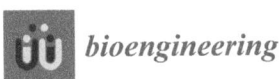

Article

Turmell-Meter: A Device for Estimating the Subtalar and Talocrural Axes of the Human Ankle Joint by Applying the Product of Exponentials Formula

Óscar Agudelo-Varela [1,†], Julio Vargas-Riaño [2,*] and Ángel Valera [2,†]

1. Facultad de Ciencias Básicas e Ingeniería, Universidad de los Llanos, Villavicencio 500002, Colombia; oscar.agudelo@unillanos.edu.co
2. Instituto Universitario de Automática e Informática Industrial (Instituto ai2), Universitat Politècnica de València, 46022 Valencia, Spain; giuprog@isa.upv.es
* Correspondence: julio_h_vargas_r@ieee.org
† These authors contributed equally to this work.

Abstract: The human ankle is a complex joint, most commonly represented as the talocrural and subtalar axes. It is troublesome to take in vivo measurements of the ankle joint. There are no instruments for patients lying on flat surfaces; employed in outdoor or remote sites. We have developed a "Turmell-meter" to address these issues. It started with the study of ankle anatomy and anthropometry. We also use the product of exponentials' formula to visualize the movements. We built a prototype using human proportions and statistics. For pose estimation, we used a trilateration method by applying tetrahedral geometry. We computed the axis direction by fitting circles in 3D, plotting the manifold and chart as an ankle joint model. We presented the results of simulations, a prototype comprising 45 parts, specifically designed draw-wire sensors, and electronics. Finally, we tested the device by capturing positions and fitting them into the bi-axial ankle model as a Riemannian manifold. The Turmell-meter is a hardware platform for human ankle joint axes estimation. The measurement accuracy and precision depend on the sensor quality; we address this issue by designing an electronics capture circuit, measuring the real measurement with a Vernier caliper. Then, we adjust the analog voltages and filter the 10-bit digital value. The Technology Readiness Level is 2. The proposed ankle joint model has the properties of a chart in a geometric manifold, and we provided the details.

Keywords: human ankle model; product of exponentials formula; anthropometry; biomechanics; coordinate measuring machines; kinematics; pose estimation; position measurement; biomedical informatics

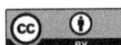

1. Introduction

Taking in vivo measurements in the human ankle joint is troublesome because the ankle is a complex mechanism [1]. Deviations in the axis increase the pronation or supination moments, causing instability and enhancing injuries risk. In this work, we present a device intended for the study of the human ankle joint (HAJ). Modeling and measuring this lower limb joint is essential in physiology, biomechanics, and rehabilitation (also in humanoid robotic limb development).

Our primary aim is to develop a device for the two axes model estimation of the human ankle joint. Secondary objectives are: it must be non-invasive, compact, energy-efficient, and easy to set up and transport. It should also be compatible with laying positions, such as with the foot in the elevated position. To accomplish the objectives, we followed a plan, first by understanding the ankle movements. Then, we used statistics for dimensional determination. We also use a modern approach, such as the Product of Exponential (POE) formula. We then designed the structure based on embedded non-invasive distance sensors.

Our contribution to the ankle joint axis localization is the holistic development of a specific device. Draw-wire sensors measure distance, are composed of a wire wound around a drum, and are attached to a potentiometer and a spring. They are retractile with constant tension. For bias correction and gain calibration, we designed a capture system. We adjust the voltage to avoid the maximal value of the analog-to-digital conversion. We calibrated each sensor through direct measuring with a Vernier caliper. Then, we measured the voltage and adjusted the offset and gain by a calibration program in Processing (Software). Limitation measurements are by 10-bit analog-to-digital converters and digitally filtered in the acquisition board. Technology Readiness Level (TRL) is 2.

We highlight our approach over traditional methods because we apply the POE formula to the ankle kinematic model. Furthermore, we estimate the ankle axis localization by a geometric approach, solved algebraically. We computed it from the pseudo-inverse application. For the talocrural and subtalar axes estimation, we use circle fitting. As an alternative ankle joint representation, we propose a Riemannian chart. We have limited the scope to the human ankle joint (HAJ) model. There are applications in physical therapy and HAJ mobility diagnosis.

The state of the art in the ankle localization is detailed in [1–14].

There are different HAJ models in the literature; we focus on the two-axes approach. The approach is recommended by the International Society of Biomechanics (ISB) [15], anatomy and biomechanics books [3,16–19], and simulation software [20]. We found models of the ankle joints in several articles [14,21–26]. Contributions to the study of the ankle joint axes are in [2,8,9,27]. The most cited research about the subtalar axis are in [5,7,10–13]. A literature review of functional representations is in [4].

Draw-wire sensors (DWS) are distance measurement sensors, who use a wire coiled on a drum attached to a potentiometer and a spiral spring that are retractile at constant tension. Similar robotic applications are in [28–30], also in linear position tracking [31], and easy robot programming [32]. Inertial measurement units (IMU) were post-processed and complemented with other sensors [33–37]. We shall employ our device for the HAJ bi-axial measurements and for other models as well [38]. Biodex^{TM} and Humacnorm^{TM} are manufacturers of general kinetics machines.

We divide the materials and methods section into two subsections: the motion theory and the mechatronics design. In the first section, we study anatomy, statistics, proportions, and anthropometry to understand the functional HAJ movements and standard dimensions. Then we perform the HAJ simulation using the POE formula. Here, we do not include a deep study of infinitesimal kinematics. We intend to design a device for a healthy HAJ with no singularities with a continuous range of movement. We describe the trilateration method to find the platform pose. It is a geometrical method based on tetrahedrons; we avoid numerical solutions that depend on finite derivative terms. The tetrahedron is a well-defined 3D geometrical structure. Solving tetrahedron geometry is the expansion of planar trigonometry. Knowing the sides allows us to find the height of a tetrahedron. We attach the platform to the foot; the sensors are passive elements and do not support or add high tensile forces. We have selected the first seven sensor configurations 3-2-2 (seven sensors) instead of 3-3-3 (nine sensors) or 3-2-1 (five sensors) for hardware limitations, sensor redundancy, and symmetrical design (for both limb use).

The device's mechatronics design and implementation are in the second subsection. We used Draw-wire sensors to measure the tetrahedron sides. These sensors have a constant tension because they comprise a drum attached to a spiral spring. We limit them to the maximal distance, and the precision depends on the potentiometer and electronics signal conditioning with a high common-mode rejection ratio (CMRR). The calibration process deals with accuracy and precision. First, we made rough adjustments to the acquisition system. Second, the software calibration process makes fine adjustments. Our proposed method avoids numerical errors because it uses geometric formulas. We validate the position through sensor redundancy. We conduct calibration and testing in a healthy patient and represent the HAJ movements as a manifold chart. The complementary source code was uploaded to [39].

2. Materials and Methods

This section is grouped in two main subsections, first the motion theory, and second the mechatronic system. For the first part, we show the simulation using anthropometric values and the POE formula. Using the plots, we estimate the DWS maximal length. Next, we present the device's geometrical design and the trilateration method. Finally, we compute the axis position by circle fitting and modeling the ankle joint as a Riemannian manifold chart. In the second subsection, we describe the mechanics design and implementation, we used SolidWorks® (2017–2018 Student Edition, Dassault Systèmes, Vélizy-Villacoublay, France), KiCad©(6.0.4, Jean-Pierre Charras and KiCad developers, CERN, Linux Foundation), and FreeCad© (0.19, Jürgen Riegel, Werner Mayer, Yorik van Havre and others) StepUp tools addon.

2.1. Motion Theory

For the simulation with the POE formula, we adapt the data from [40], proportions from [41,42], and statistics from [43].

2.1.1. References Assignment

Figure 1 presents the reference points and the mean distances taken from [40].

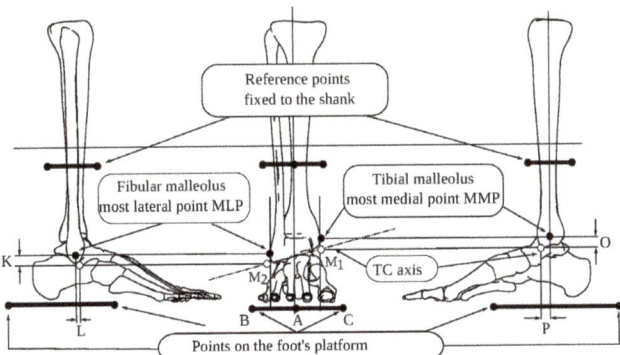

Figure 1. Reference points from anthropometric values K, L, O, and P.

A, B, and C are the triangle's vertices in a platform fixed to the foot, the K, L, and O distances from the most medial and lateral points from the black-filled to the white-filled marker. M_1 and M_2 define the talocrural (TC) axis. We show top-transverse and right-lateral views in Figure 2 with distances Q, W, and w. N_1 and N_2 determine the subtalar (ST) axis.

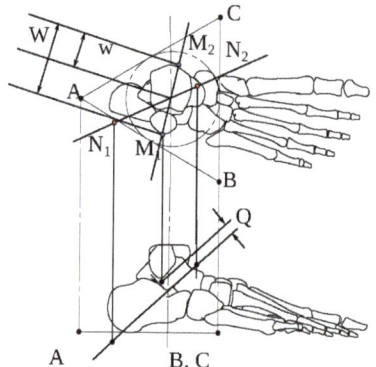

Figure 2. Q, W, and w distances from lateral and transverse views.

Table 1 enumerates the mean values of Figures 1 and 2.

Table 1. Mean values of anthropometric measurements.

Variable	K (cm)	L (cm)	O (cm)	P (cm)	Q (cm)	R = W/w
Mean	1.2 cm	1.1 cm	1.6 cm	1.0 cm	0.5 cm	0.54 cm

In Figure 3, we show the ST and TC axes from several viewpoints. The TC axis refers

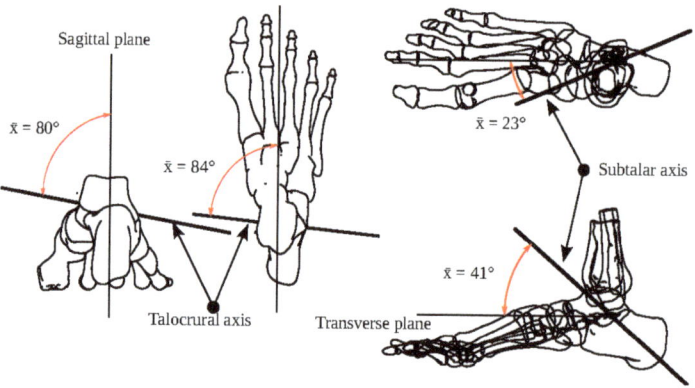

Figure 3. Mean relative position of the ST and TC axis.

2.1.2. Anatomical and Geometrical Correspondence

We define the sagittal (lateral) plane as the X-Z plane (perpendicular to the y-axis). The coronal (frontal) plane is the Y-Z plane (x-axis is normal to it); the transverse (axial) plane is the X-Y plane (perpendicular to the z-axis). Figure 4, left, shows this corresponding references.

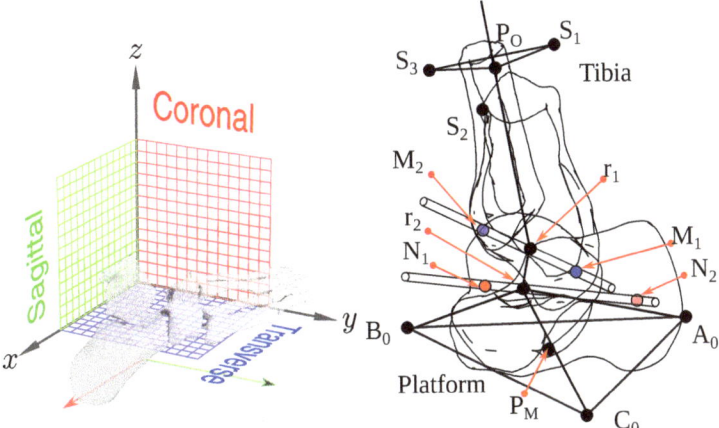

Figure 4. Planes, axes, and points of corresponding references.

With this reference frame, we can define the TC axis orientation from a unitary vector in the z-direction. We first rotate it $-80°$ around the x-axis; then we turn it $-6°$ around the z-axis. A unitary vector in the x-axis direction defines the ST axis, rotating $41°$ about the y-axis, followed by a $23°$ rotation around the z-axis.

We show the fibula, tibia, talus, calcaneus 3D position, reference points, TC, and ST axes in Figure 4, right.

In this image, A_0, B_0, and C_0 are the vertices from the platform fixed to the foot, and P_M is the triangle's center. S_1, S_2, and S_3 are fixed to the shank relative to the origin point P_0. M_1 and M_2 define the TC axis; N_1 and N_2 correspond to the ST axis. We define r_1 and r_2 as the sagittal plane intersection with the TC and ST axes.

2.1.3. Size and Dimensions

This first part help us to determine the HAJ axes direction and orientation for some cases. However, it is difficult to design a device that fits all humans, and we cannot make a device that fits 90 % percentiles; we intend to design a device scalable and adjustable in a defined population group. We also make an effort to design adjustable foot and shank attachments. To do so, we select the device dimensions using the proportions extracted from [41]. The heigh is H, and the proportions we use are: distance from the knee to the foot is 0.285H, the distance from the ankle to the foot is 0.039H and the foot widht is 0.055H and the foot length is 0.152H.

We select the origin of coordinates between the knee and the ankle, d_m is the distance from P_M to P_0. This distance is proportional to the body's height H. To do so, we define d_m as follows:

$$d_m = \|P_0 - P_M\| = \left[\frac{0.285 - 0.039}{2} + 0.039\right] \cdot H = 0.162 \cdot H. \quad (1)$$

For the sake of obtaining the prototype dimensions, we use statistics for a specific population. In [43], the mean height H of an adult male is 175 cm; by substituting this value into the equation, the knee-ankle distance is 28.35 cm. The distance d_{p12} between points r_1 and r_2 about the TC and ST axes on the sagittal plane is:

$$d_{p12} = \|r_1 - r_2\| = Q, \quad (2)$$

the projection of the most medial point (MMP) on the sagittal plane is:

$$P_{MMP} = (x_{MMP}, 0, z_{MMP}), \quad (3)$$

and for the most lateral point is:

$$P_{MLP} = (x_{MLP}, 0, z_{MLP}). \tag{4}$$

The point M_{1p} is the projection of M_1 on the sagittal plane; we calculate it from the P and O values.

$$M_{1p} = (x_{MMP} - P, 0, z_{MMP} - O), \tag{5}$$

also, M_{2p} is M_2; we estimate the projection from L and K through:

$$M_{2p} = (x_{MLP} - L, 0, z_{MLP} - K). \tag{6}$$

Therefore, the segment $\overline{M_2M_1}$ has the sagittal projection $\overline{M_{2p}M_{1p}}$; it has the same proportional relation $R = W/w$ in respect to $\overline{M_{2p}r_1}$, then:

$$\frac{M_2 - M_1}{M_2 - r_1} = \frac{W}{w} = R, \tag{7}$$

solving for r_1 gives the following:

$$r_1 = M_2 - \frac{M_2 - M_1}{R}. \tag{8}$$

By knowing the distance Q projected in the sagittal plane and r_1, the angle 41° we calculate r_2 from:

$$r_2 = Q[\cos(41°), 0, \sin(41°)] + r_1, \tag{9}$$

The distance from the origin P_O to the plantar surface of the foot is d_m, we choose a circumscribed equilateral triangle with vertices A_0, B_0, C_0 as the platform base. The coordinates of A_0 are:

$$A_0 = (r_p, 0, -d_m), \tag{10}$$

for B_0 are:

$$B_0 = (r_p \cos 60°, r_p \sin 60°, -d_m), \tag{11}$$

and for C_0:

$$C_0 = (r_p \cos -60°, r_p \sin -60°, -d_m), \tag{12}$$

where r_p is proportional to H, then:

$$r_p = \tfrac{2}{3} \cdot H. \tag{13}$$

In summary, we estimate P_0, r_1, r_2; and the platform's vertices A_0, B_0, and C_0. They are not arbitrarily selected, on the contrary, we employed anthropometry, statistics, and proportions.

2.1.4. Product of Exponentials Formula

In this section, we employ the PoE formula. We follow the intuitive concept that inter-bone contact surfaces determine HAJ movements. Therefore, we represent these movements as a Special Euclidean group SE(3) in matrix form:

$$\mathfrak{g} = \begin{bmatrix} R & \hat{p}_T \\ 0_{1\times 3} & 1 \end{bmatrix}, \tag{14}$$

where $R_{3\times 3}$ is the rotation matrix and $\hat{p}_T$ is the translation vector.

For the initial point A_0:

$$\mathfrak{g}_A(0) = \begin{bmatrix} I_{3\times 3} & \hat{A}_0 \\ 0_{1\times 3} & 1 \end{bmatrix}, \tag{15}$$

for B_0:
$$g_B(0) = \begin{bmatrix} I_{3\times 3} & \hat{B}_0 \\ 0_{1\times 3} & 1 \end{bmatrix}, \qquad (16)$$

and for C_0
$$g_C(0) = \begin{bmatrix} I_{3\times 3} & \hat{C}_0 \\ 0_{1\times 3} & 1 \end{bmatrix} \qquad (17)$$

We define $\hat{\omega}_1 = (\omega_{x1}, \omega_{y1}, \omega_{z1})$ as a unitary vector for the TC axis direction given by:
$$\hat{\omega}_1 = \frac{M_2 - M_1}{\|M_2 - M_1\|}, \qquad (18)$$

and a directed vector $\hat{r}_1$ from P_O to r_1 is:
$$\hat{r}_1 = r_1 - P_O, \qquad (19)$$

then, an orthogonal vector to $\hat{r}_1$ and $\hat{\omega}_1$ is:
$$\hat{v}_{\theta_1 r_{2z}} = -\hat{\omega}_1 \times \hat{r}_1, \qquad (20)$$

together, $\hat{\omega}_1$ and $\hat{v}_{\theta_1 r_{2z}}$ compound the six-dimensional vector $\hat{\xi}_1$:
$$\hat{\xi}_1 = \begin{pmatrix} \hat{v}_1 \\ \hat{\omega}_1 \end{pmatrix}. \qquad (21)$$

In the same way, there are correspondent vectors for the TC axis:
$$\hat{\omega}_2 = \frac{N_2 - N_1}{\|N_2 - N_1\|}, \qquad (22)$$

$$\hat{r}_2 = r_2 - P_O, \qquad (23)$$

$$\hat{v}_2 = -\hat{\omega}_2 \times \hat{r}_2, \qquad (24)$$

and:
$$\hat{\xi}_2 = \begin{pmatrix} \hat{v}_2 \\ \hat{\omega}_2 \end{pmatrix}. \qquad (25)$$

We compute R for each joint $i = 1, 2$ from the Rodrigues' formula:
$$e^{(\Omega_i \theta_i)} = I_{3\times 3} + \Omega \sin\theta_i + \Omega^2(1 - \cos\theta_i), \qquad (26)$$

where Ω is the skew symmetric matrix:
$$\Omega = \begin{bmatrix} 0 & -\omega_{zi} & \omega_{yi} \\ \omega_{zi} & 0 & -\omega_{xi} \\ -\omega_{yi} & \omega_{xi} & 0 \end{bmatrix}. \qquad (27)$$

The exponential formula is:
$$e^{\hat{\xi}_i \theta_i} = \begin{bmatrix} e^{\Omega_i \theta_i} & \tau_i \\ 0_{1\times 3} & 1 \end{bmatrix}, \qquad (28)$$

and, τ_i is translation vector:
$$\tau_i = \left(I_{3\times 3} - e^{\hat{\omega}_i \theta_i}\right)\hat{\omega}_i \times \hat{v} + \hat{\omega}_i \hat{\omega}_i^T \hat{v}_i \theta_i \qquad (29)$$

Points A, B, and C have invariant relative positions, and there are two rotating joints; the PoE formula for A is:

$$\mathfrak{g}_A = e^{\hat{\xi}_1 \theta_1} e^{\hat{\xi}_2 \theta_2} \mathfrak{g}_A(0) = \begin{bmatrix} R & \hat{p}_A \\ 0 & 1 \end{bmatrix}, \tag{30}$$

where $\hat{p}_A$ is the instantaneous position vector of A, the PoE for B:

$$\mathfrak{g}_B = e^{\hat{\xi}_1 \theta_1} e^{\hat{\xi}_2 \theta_2} \mathfrak{g}_B(0) = \begin{bmatrix} R & \hat{p}_B \\ 0 & 1 \end{bmatrix}, \tag{31}$$

and the PoE for C is:

$$\mathfrak{g}_C = e^{\hat{\xi}_1 \theta_1} e^{\hat{\xi}_2 \theta_2} \mathfrak{g}_C(0) = \begin{bmatrix} R & \hat{p}_C \\ 0 & 1 \end{bmatrix}, \tag{32}$$

θ_1 is the TC rotation angle from the zero position, and θ_2 is the ST rotation from the zero position. For the sake of clarity, we show the section of the ankle with the vectors $\hat{r}_1$, $\hat{\omega}_1$, $\hat{\nu}_1$ and $\hat{r}_2$; also the points A, B, C, and P_O in Figure 5.

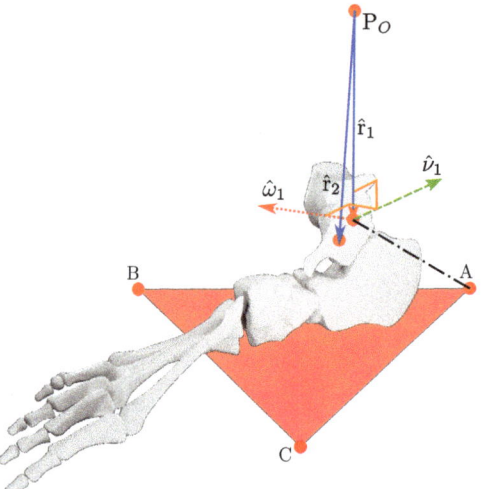

Figure 5. Vectors and points on the sagittal plane.

2.1.5. Forward Kinematics

In this subsection, we show the simulation of the movements of the ankle by using the measurements and the PoE. The code is in SageMath Computer Algebraic System (CAS), which lets us manage symbolic notation, and interactive plotting in a Jupyter notebook. All source was uploaded to Git-Hub [39].

The simulation plot for the platform's central point is in Figure 6a. We show the points P_O, A_0, B_0, C_0, r_1, r_2, and the surfaces representing each group of movements. The forward kinematics with $\theta_{1range} = \theta_{2range} = [-15°, 15°]$ and $\theta_1 = \theta_2 = 10°$ is in Figure 6b. For $\theta_{1range} = \theta_{2range} = [-10°, 10°]$ and $\theta_1 = \theta_2 = 5°$ is in Figure 6c.

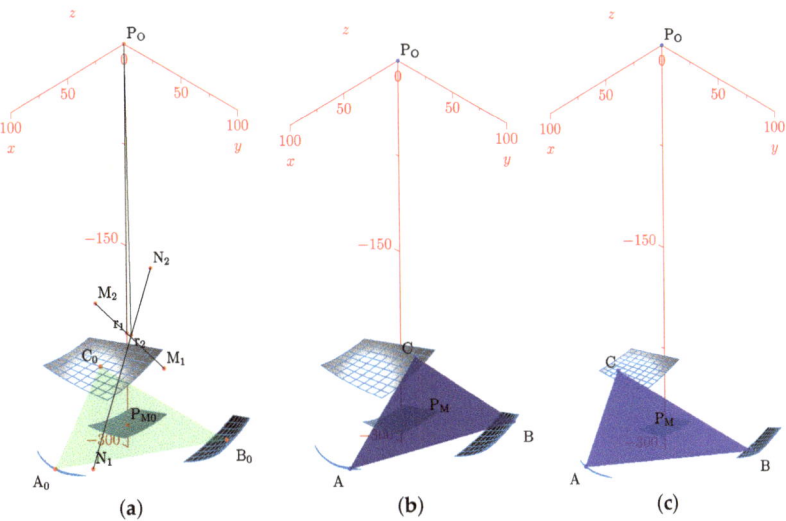

Figure 6. Forward kinematics for (**a**) initial position and (**b**) $\theta_{1range} = \theta_{2range} = [-15°, 15°], \theta_1 = \theta_2 = 10°$ and (**c**) $\theta_{1range} = \theta_{2range} = [-10°, 10°], \theta_1 = \theta_2 = 5°$.

Such a representation lets us compute the ankle joint ROM in all directions. Groups of A, B, C, and PM movements are smooth surfaces or geometric manifolds. They have two DOF, with a limited domain due to the axes ROM.

2.1.6. Geometric Design and Trilateration Method

In the last section, we note that in a healthy ankle, the range of motion from three points in a platform attached to the foot, pertain to a surface without singularities. Moreover, we note that we can trace tetrahedrons from the reference base on the shank to the platform points. Tetrahedrons can be solved by knowing the triangle base, and the sides. We choose the complete tetrahedron with three distance sensors in the point A for symmetry conservation in the case of using the device in the left or right foot. We avoid the use of numerical methods such as the Newton–Raphson (NR), for reducing time of computation. Furthermore, we choose the symmetry and redundancy in the apexes B and C. We realize that by knowing the platform dimensions, two sensors and the apex A coordinates, we can define a plane rotated with respect to the base and solve other tetrahedrons corresponding to the B and C apexes. We also take a holistic approach, we knew that micro-controller systems often have two cores and eight or ten analog to digital converter channels. We used 7 channels, leaving three for temperature, battery level, and voltage input detection.

Finally, based on such considerations, we show a geometric design in the Figure 7a platform center, and in Figure 7b are the vertices.

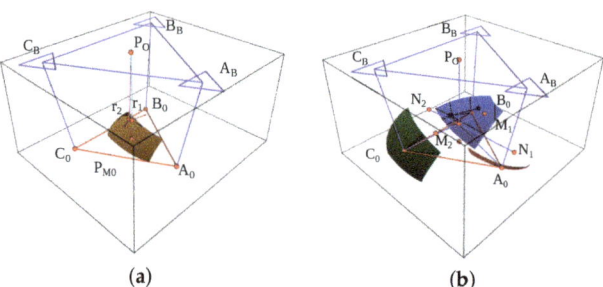

Figure 7. Geometric design: (**a**) is the platform center, base, and r_1, r_2; and (**b**) platform vertices with talocrural and subtalar axis.

By considering the distances between the origin and the vertices, we estimate the DWS maximal length in every module.

$$l_{max} = \max[\|p_A(\theta_1, \theta_2) - A\| + r_m] \qquad (33)$$

Here, l_{max} is the maximal possible length from the triangular inequality, p_A is the positions group in $\mathfrak{g}_A$, r_m is the module's radius, and A_B is the base point.

The main design requirement is the localization of three points attached to the foot. We estimate the actual position employing a DWS array in a tetrahedral structure to find the apex, which is a platform vertex. In Figure 8 we show the design structure.

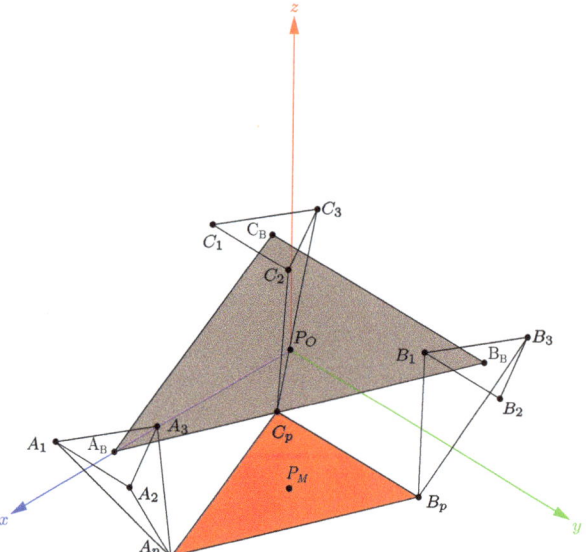

Figure 8. Geometric design of the DWS arrays.

P_O and P_M are the base and platform reference frames. The platform has known dimensions and the number of sensors is seven. First, we compute A_p from three distances: $l_{A1} = \|A_p - A_1\|$, $l_{A2} = \|A_p - A_2\|$, and $l_{A3} = \|A_p - A_3\|$. Then, we compute B_p and B_p apexes after A_p employing two DWS. We summarize the method in a flowchart; Figure 9.

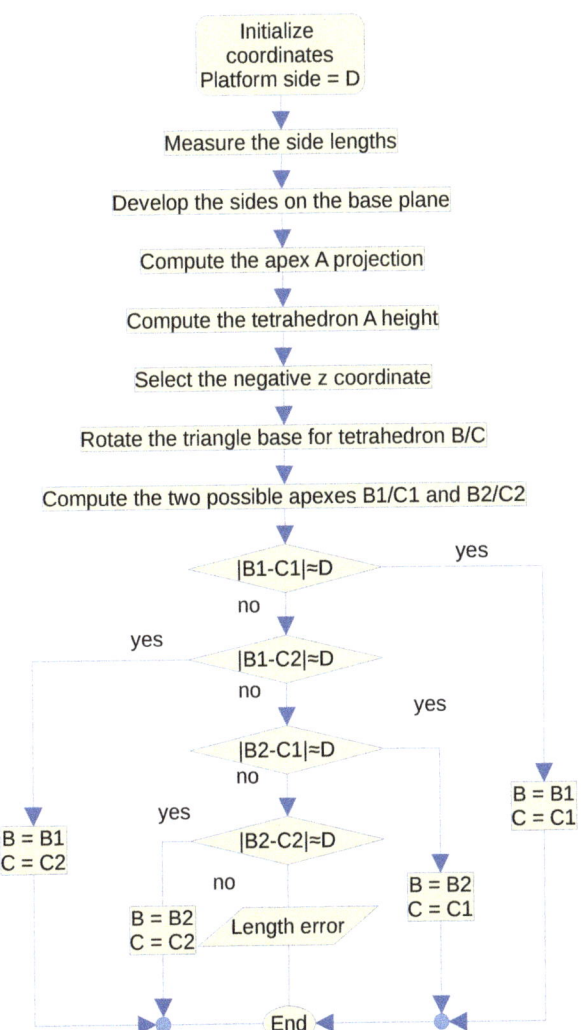

Figure 9. Tetrahedron trilateration flowchart.

2.1.7. Finding the Apex in Tetrahedron A

In this section, we compute the tetrahedron T_A with base $\triangle_A = [A_1, A_2, A_3]$ and apex A_p. Figure 10 shows the method we use.

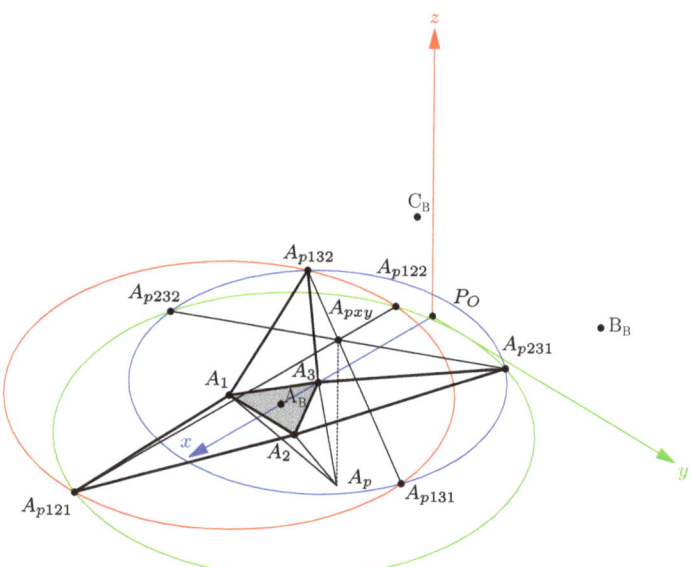

Figure 10. Finding the apex A_p.

In Figure 10 we see that triangles $\triangle_{132} = [A_1, A_3, A_{p132}]$ and $\triangle_{231} = [A_2, A_3, A_{p231}]$ are two sides of the tetrahedron T_A developed on the base plane.

We compute the A_{p132} and A_{p231} orthogonal projection on each adjacent side of the module base triangle $\triangle [A_1, A_2, A_3]$ by tracing a circle centered on A_1 with radius $\|A_p - A_2\|$ and the circle centered on A_3 with radius $\|A_p - A_3\|$; resulting in A_{p132} and A_{p131} intersection points. In addition, the circle centered on A_2 with radius $\|A_p - A_2\|$ intersects the circle centered in A_3 at points A_{p231} and A_{p232}. The segment from A_{p132} to A_{p131} intersects the points defined by A_{p231} and A_{p232} at A_{pxy}. In the case of tetrahedron T_A, we determine $A_{pxy} = (Apx, Apy, 0)$ as A_p projection on the base plane. It is easy to realize that the height of T_A is the absolute value of the A_{pz} coordinate. Then, we can find the distance from A_{pxy} to A_3 as a triangle $\triangle [Apxy, A_3, A_p]$ side; the other is A_{pz}, and the hypotenuse is the distance $l_{A3} = \|A_p - A_3\|$, then, A_{pz} is:

$$A_{pz} = \sqrt{l_{A3}^2 - (A_{pxy} - A_3)^2} \qquad (34)$$

2.1.8. Tetrahedrons B and C Apexes

In this subsection, we show that, by knowing A_p, the point B_p needs two sensors to be found. To determine the result of the tetrahedron T_B, we consider the base of a triangle $\triangle [B_1, B_3, A_p]$ in Figure 11a.

We compute the angle α from the XY plane to a normal vector $\hat{n}_{ApB}$:

$$\hat{n}_{ApB} = \frac{(B_3 - Ap) \times (B_3 - Ap)}{\|(B_3 - Ap) \times (B_3 - Ap)\|}, \qquad (35)$$

and, the angle α is:

$$\alpha = acos(\hat{n}_{ApB} \cdot \hat{n}_z), \qquad (36)$$

where $\hat{n}_z$ is the unitary vector normal to the XY plane.

The tetrahedron sides are the lengths $lB1 = \|Bp - B1\|$, $lB3 = \|Bp - B3\|$, and $d_{ApBp} = \|Bp - Ap\|$. The rotation axis is in the direction $B1 - B3$. The Bpr is Bps rotated α in angle about this axis. In Figure 11b, we show how to find the Bpr apex, similarly to that of a tetrahedron T_A. Finally, when Bpr is found, the contrary rotation about the axis $B_1 - B_3$ gives the Bps.

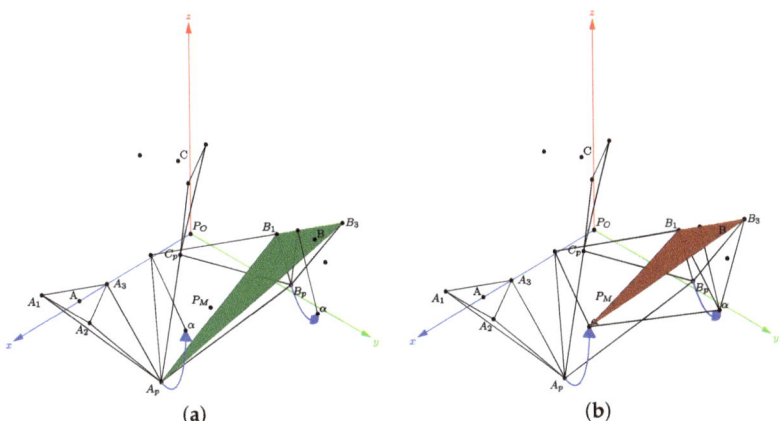

Figure 11. Rotation of α angle about the axis $B_1 - B_3$: (**a**) original tetrahedron, T_B (**b**) rotated tetrahedron.

There are two possible apex values: $Bps1$ over, and $Bps2$ below of the XY plane. We show the Bpr apex below the XY plane in Figure 12.

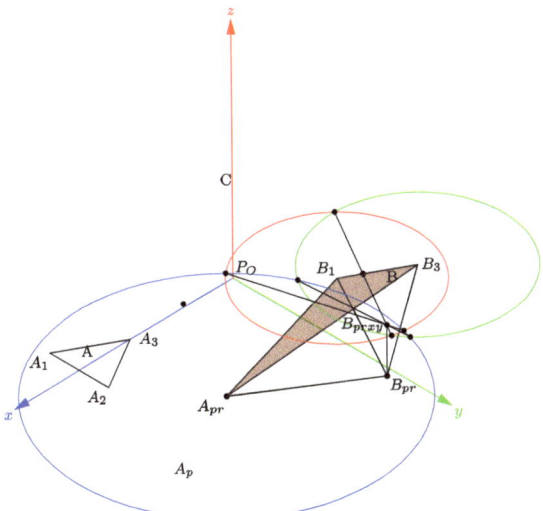

Figure 12. Finding the apex B_{pr}.

We use the same method to solve the T_C apex. For the correct apex selection, the condition when the side of the platform distance d_{CpBp} is:

$$d_{CpBp} = \|Bps - Cps\|. \tag{37}$$

2.1.9. Procedure for Found Platform Positions

We must fix the shank and the foot to the base and platform. Then we mark the MMP and the MLP. To do so, we design a detachable reference point from module A. Initially, we attach the foot and the shank to the device, and then we mark and record the MMP and MLP; Figure 13 shows the detailed view.

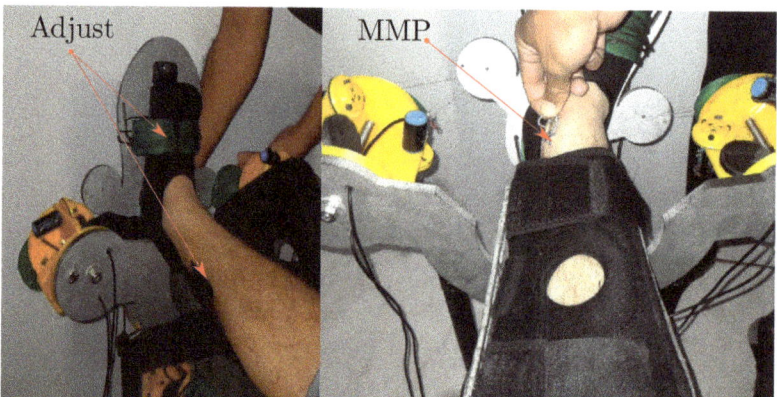

Figure 13. Adjusting the foot, the shank and the Most Medial Point reference.

We compute the platform position from the seven sensor lengths. The main steps for capture data series are:

1. Capture the initial position at horizontal relative position from $dr = IMU2 - IMU1$ readings;
2. Compute jerk $jrk = |dr_i - dr_{i-1}|$;
3. Move the foot continuously until jerk crosses zero again.

First, we capture the sensor lengths by activating a button in the computer software. Every time, we compute the absolute difference from IMU2 to the IMU1 readings. If the differences are constants, then there is no platform and base relative movement. We compute the jerk by relative acceleration differentiation. The data capturing process ends when the acceleration change crosses zero. Jerk changes activate the capture of IMU data.

The symbolic equations to find A_p, B_p, and C_p from the captured data, were found by the SageMath CAS. By using the prototype dimensions and the sensor lengths, we compute the platform's position and orientation. Here, the origin is from the initial DWS lengths l_{Mi0}, where M is the module A, B, or C; and i is the sensor number $i = 1, 2, 3$.

After MLP and MMP registering, we attach the apex of module A to the platform, define the sagittal plane perpendicular to the ABC base plane, and intersect point A. By implementing the trilateration method mentioned before, we compute the points A_0, B_0, and C_0.

Figure 14a illustrate the point positions with the device in the initial portable configuration. The apexes' computation are in Figure 14b–d.

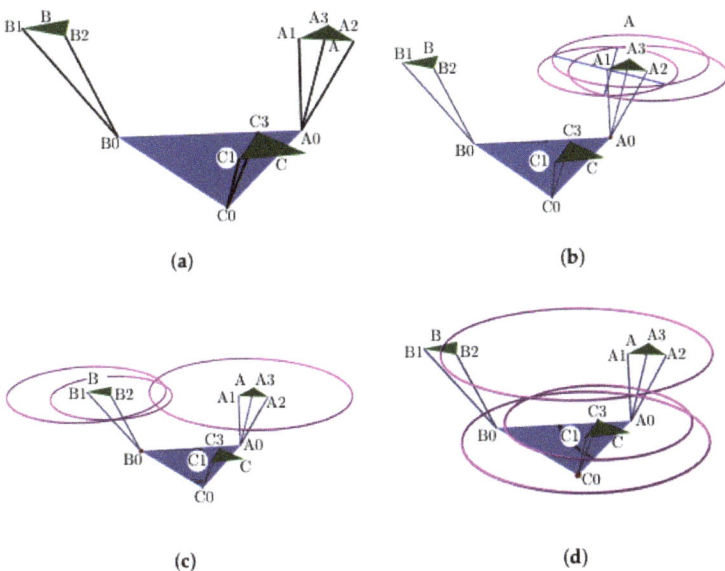

Figure 14. Computed positions from sensor lengths at portable configuration: (**a**) the rest position, (**b**) apex A, (**c**) apex B, and (**d**) apex C.

2.1.10. Computing the Axis Position and Direction

From the anthropometric values [40], we put a mean model in the Turmell-Meter. The TC axis will be defined by M_{1_0} and M_{2_0}. The sagittal plane intersection with the $\overline{M_1 M_2}$ segment is r_1. For example, the TC axis approximation is computed from most lateral point (MLP), the most medial point (MMP) and L, K, P, and O:

$$M_{1_0} = MLP - [L, 0, K], \qquad (38)$$

and:

$$M_{2_0} = MMP - [-P, 0, O], \qquad (39)$$

from these values, we solve for r_1 from the plane $y = 0$ intersection with the line L_{TC}:

$$L_{TC} = V - M1 = \rho \frac{(M_2 - M_1)}{\|M_2 - M_1\|}, \qquad (40)$$

where V is a point pertaining to L_{TC}.

The ST axis sagittal intersection r_2 initial point is:

$$r_2 = r_1 + \tfrac{\sqrt{2}}{2}[Q, 0, Q]. \qquad (41)$$

Here, r_1 and r_2 are reference values computed from the previously mentioned anthropometric mean values. Such initial points are for reference, comparison and validation of the trilateration and regression method. The tracked trajectory data set is processed offline. We use the least squares normal vector to the plane, this direction is similar to the circle approximation. From here, we compute the TC axis first, and then the ST axis. To do so, we compute the TC axis position by employing dorsiflexion and plantarflexion, because the TC axis is the most dominant in such movements. The method used is circle fitting in a plane containing the trajectory points. A further model refinement can be made with optimization, and machine learning methods, such as gradient descent and the symbolic product of exponential formula.

First, we found the TC axis orientation ω_1 by registering several trajectories. For each trajectory, we have a list of data points $P = [x, y, z]$, which pertain to a plane:

$$ax + by + cz + d = 0, \tag{42}$$

where a, b, and c are the components of a direction vector perpendicular to a plane containing the points. Solving out for z, we have the system:

$$\begin{bmatrix} x_0 & y_0 & 1 \\ x_1 & y_1 & 1 \\ \vdots & \vdots & \vdots \\ x_{n-1} & y_{n-1} & 1 \end{bmatrix} \begin{bmatrix} a \\ b \\ d \end{bmatrix} = -c \begin{bmatrix} z_0 \\ z_1 \\ \cdots \\ z_{n-1} \end{bmatrix} \tag{43}$$

which has the form:

$$Ax = B \tag{44}$$

there are more equations than unknowns. From linear algebra and least squares we knew that the pseudo inverse is $A^+ = (A^T A)^{-1} A^T$, then a normal vector is:

$$\begin{bmatrix} a \\ b \\ d \end{bmatrix} = (A^T A)^{-1} A^T B \tag{45}$$

Now, we compute c by replacing a, b, d in the plane equation, and finally we get $\hat{n} = [a, b, c]^T$. We found the angle between the normal plane and the X-Y plane, after knowing the normal vector by applying the Rodrigues' formula, $\hat{v} = \hat{n} \times \hat{k}$, with $\hat{k} = [0, 0, 1]^T$

$$P_r = P\cos(\theta) + (\hat{v} \times P)\sin(\theta) + \hat{v}(\hat{v} \cdot P)(1 - \cos\theta). \tag{46}$$

where $\theta = \arccos\left(\frac{\hat{n} \cdot \hat{k}}{\|\hat{n}\|}\right)$.

After this, we estimate the plane, and rotate all the data points onto the X-Y plane. We search for a circle in the X-Y plane, and rearrange the equation for least squares estimation by using a variable substitution.

$$\begin{array}{rcl} (x - x_c)^2 + (y - y_c)^2 & = & r^2 \\ (2x_c)x + (2y_c)y + (r^2 - x_c^2 - y_c^2) & = & x^2 + y^2 \\ c_0 x + c_1 y + c_2 & = & x^2 + y^2 \end{array} \tag{47}$$

where $c = [c_0, c_1, c_2]^T$ with $c_0 = 2x_c$, $c_1 = 2y_c$, and $c_2 = r^2 - x_c^2 - y_c^2$.

By taking the rotated points, P_r we have a linear system:

$$\begin{bmatrix} x_0 & y_0 & 1 \\ x_1 & y_1 & 1 \\ \vdots & \vdots & \vdots \\ x_{n-1} & y_{n-1} & 1 \end{bmatrix} \begin{bmatrix} c_0 \\ c_1 \\ c_2 \end{bmatrix} = \begin{bmatrix} x_0^2 + y_0^2 \\ x_1^2 + y_1^2 \\ \vdots \\ x_{n-1}^2 + y_{n-1}^2 \end{bmatrix}. \tag{48}$$

that has the form:

$$Ac = b \tag{49}$$

In this system, we have more equations than unknowns, then, we search for the c values that minimize the squared difference $\|b - Ac\|^2$.

$$\arg\min_{c \in \mathbb{R}^3} \|b - Ac\|^2. \tag{50}$$

We found the center point $C_p = [x_c, y_c]$ and radius r by solving:

$$\begin{array}{rcl} 2x_c & = & c_0 \\ 2y_c & = & c_1 \\ r^2 - x_c^2 - y_c^2 & = & c_2 \end{array}. \quad (51)$$

Finally, we apply a rotation to the center in respect to the original plane. This point pertains to the TC axis. For each trajectory A, B, C, we get three planes, and three centers, the TC line direction is parallel to the planes' normal vectors. The information is complete by determining the plane orientation.

The ST axis estimation is similar, but employs trajectories from inversion and eversion movements.

This is a basic estimation; by conducting optimization on the product of the exponential formula, we enhance the accuracy of the axis position estimation.

2.1.11. Ankle Joint Movements as a Manifold

In this subsection, we explain how the centers r_1, r_2 and directions ω_1, ω_2 define a manifold representing the HAJ movements. The circle center points calculated pertain to the TC and ST axes; they are the initial data to fit the product of the exponential formula. In Figure 15a, we show the complete platform's center point manifold. It is topologically similar to a torus.

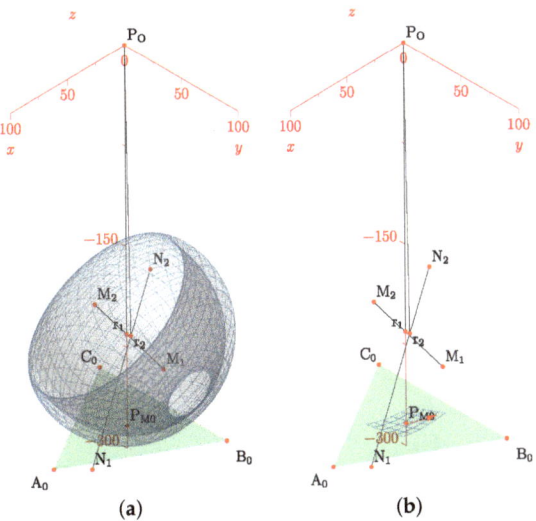

Figure 15. Simulation of the platform central point with variations in the mean statistical values: (a) platform's center point manifold, (b) manifold chart and a geodesic.

A manifold chart represents the range of motion limits, we show an example of the geodesic as a trajectory on the manifold in Figure 15b; this explains how to map ankle coordinates, and a straight trajectory with initial velocity and no external force action. We have the data necessary for the line intersection with the sagittal plane, the center points, and the direction gives a line:

$$\hat{p}_l = \hat{l}_0 + \hat{l}d, \quad (52)$$

where $\hat{p}_l$ is the parametric line, $\hat{l}$ is a parallel vector to it, $\hat{l}_0$ is a known vector in such line, and $d \in \Re$, replacing the parametric equation in the plane equation:

$$(\hat{p}_l - \hat{p}_0) \cdot (\hat{n}_p) = 0, \quad (53)$$

where $\hat{p}_0$ is a known vector in the plane, and $\hat{n}_p$ is the plane's normal vector, solving for d, gives:

$$d = \frac{(\hat{p}_0 - \hat{l}_0) \cdot \hat{n}_p}{\hat{l} \cdot \hat{n}_p}, \tag{54}$$

and replacing in the TC axis line equation:

$$r_1 = c_1 + \omega_1 d, \tag{55}$$

where r_1 is the TC axis intersection with the sagittal plane. The point c_1 is the center, and the axis direction ω_1, both were found by circle fitting. Furthermore, packing in six dimensional Plücker line coordinates, we have:

$$\hat{m}_1 = r_1 \times \omega_1, \tag{56}$$

and the l_1 six dimensional vector is:

$$l_1 = [\omega_{1_x} : \omega_{1_y} : \omega_{1_z} : m_{1_x} : m_{1_y} : m_{1_z}]. \tag{57}$$

We include those data for the PoE formula simulation and the manifold representation.

2.2. Mechatronic System Design

In this section, we design DWS to measure the lengths of the tetrahedron sides; they are arranged as structural parts. Their maximal length estimation is from the forward kinematics simulation. We design the shank attachment from the dimensions, proportions, and statistical data.

2.2.1. Draw-Wire Sensor

We use flat springs. They are not exposed to a high load against gravity, and are in two or three concurrent groups. In Figure 16, we depict the design, composed of three 3D printed parts, potentiometer, flat spring, bolts, and nuts.

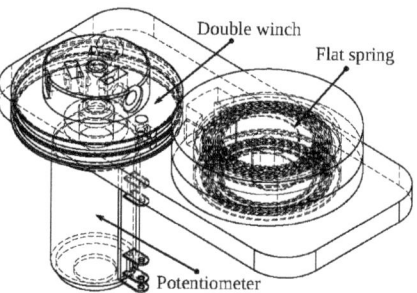

Figure 16. Draw-wire sensor design.

A two-coil winch drives the potentiometer; a flat spring retracts a wire attached to the winch. When we pull the wire, the spring retracts it. The value of each turn is from the nominal value of the potentiometer, $R_n = 2.2$ kΩ, divided into ten turns, that is 220 Ω per turn. The diameter is D = 3.8 cm, the spring could be compressed in four turns. The maximal length is as follows:

$$l_{max} = 4 \cdot D \cdot \pi \tag{58}$$

Which is 47.75 cm approximately, this value is greater than l_{max} for all groups of movements.

2.2.2. Mechanical Parts

The attachment on the calf has a size according to the simulation. We use the mesh model of a leg to guide the shape of the calf support, as in Figure 17a. We also scale and divide this structure into seven parts for 3D printing. An aluminum tube is the support structure, as in Figure 17b, and a neoprene band attaches the shank to the support with Velcro fabric.

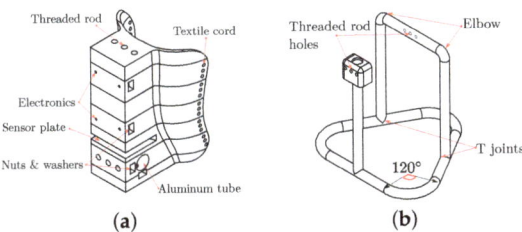

Figure 17. Mechanical attachment: (**a**) calf support and (**b**) aluminum tube structure.

All the DWS modules are in a plate, the A module has three DWS, B and C modules has two DWS, as in Figure 18a. The design of the foot attachment is from standard measurements to adjust the foot's length and width, as in Figure 18b.

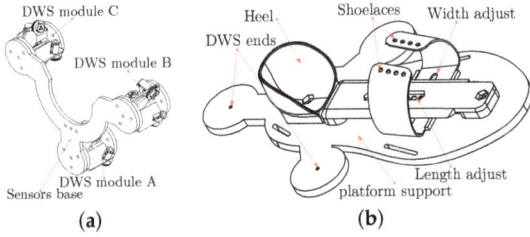

Figure 18. Base and platform: (**a**) DWS modules support (**b**) platform with foot's size adjustment.

2.2.3. Electronics

Two operational amplifiers in instrumentation configuration are the base block of the acquisition system, as Figure 19 shows. We employ the KiCad software for the circuit design.

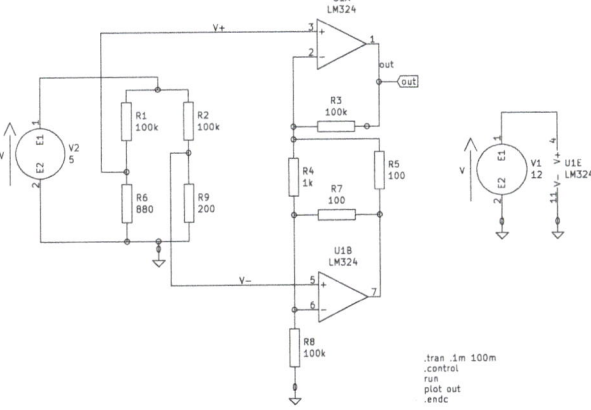

Figure 19. Two Op. Amp. instrumentation amplifier.

The voltage gain in the instrumentation amplifier is:

$$A_v = \frac{v_o}{v_i} = \left[1 = \frac{R_2}{R_1} + \frac{2R_2}{R_1}\right], \quad (59)$$

By selecting $R_2 = 100$ kΩ, $R_1 = 1$ kΩ, and $R_G = 5$ kΩ, the voltage gain is 141. With 34 mV as voltage input, we get:

$$v_o = A_v \cdot v_i = 4.794 \text{ V} \quad (60)$$

The final acquisition circuit has seven instrumentation amplifiers, with bias and gain trimmers for calibration. We design the printed board circuit as an ™Arduino Mega 2560 Shield, and assemble the components to the board by throw-hole soldering. We feed the circuits with a power system with two 18650 Li-Ion batteries in series, a backup pack, a Battery Management System (BMS); a 5V buck and a 12V boost converters. The Figure 20 shows the schematics. Finally, we add connectors for the MPU, OLED, and Bluetooth modules.

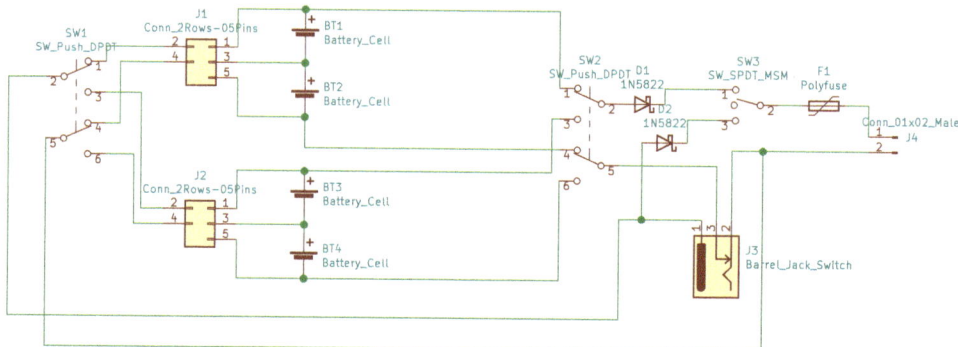

Figure 20. Power system with backup, BMS, boost, and buck converters.

2.2.4. Electronics Casing

We export the KiCad printed circuit design to FreeCAD StepUp to design the case containing all the components, focusing on a compact configuration design. The two main electronic components are the Arduino Mega 2560 and the Orange Pi One single board computer. We place the components, such as the Dual Pole Dual Throw (DPDT) toggle switches, symmetrically on the box sides. Figure 21 shows the main sides and the final assembly of the electronics case.

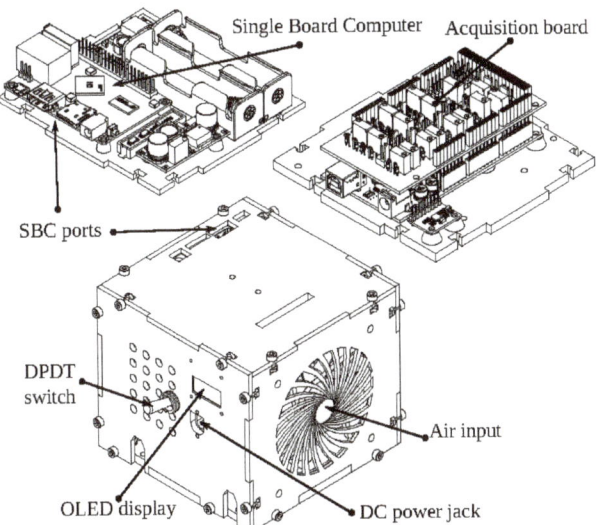

Figure 21. Modular electronics casing.

Each box has attached components to optimize the space. We test every component, and then install the support structure.

2.2.5. Final Mechanical Assembly

The prototype consist of 45 3D printed parts, the union of main components is by an 8 mm steel threaded rod. The sub-assemblies uses M3 bolts and nuts. Figure 22 shows the assembly CAD.

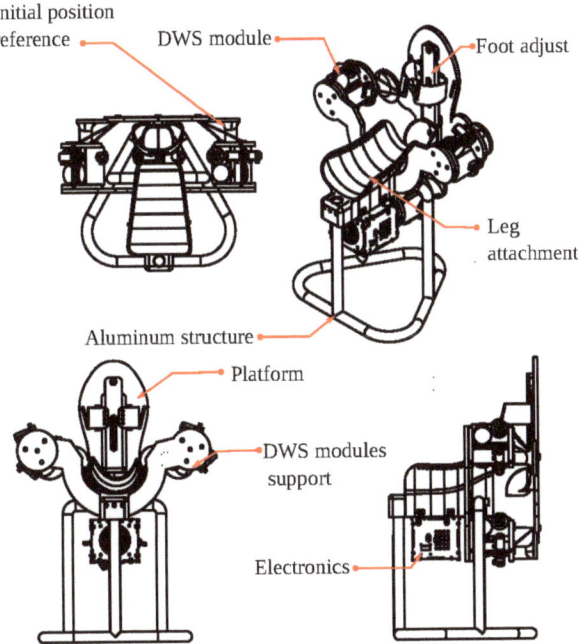

Figure 22. Complete prototype.

2.2.6. Calibration and Validation Software

Calibration is with the Arduino board connected to the PC, running a calibration program in processing. The basic program reads the IMU measurements and captures readings from the draw-wire sensors through the ADC inputs. The raw data are integer values with signs 2 bytes wide, the two 1-byte registers converted to 2-byte integers. An exponentially weighted moving average (EWMA) algorithm filters the raw signals and sends them to the PC via a serial port. The lengths computed are from the initial values plus the scaled sensor inputs with:

$$l_{iMj} = d_{iMj} + \frac{m_{iMj}}{s_{iMj}}, \tag{61}$$

here, l_{iMj} is the length in cm from the i wire to the j module, d_{iMj} is the initial distance, m_{iMj} is the measured digital value, and s_{iM} is the scale factor in digital units per cm.

We present a rendered image with a scaled 175 cm model in Figure 23.

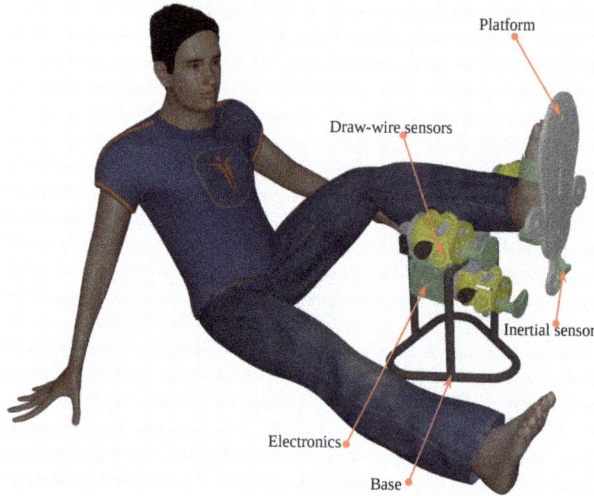

Figure 23. Rendered image with a 175 cm height patient.

3. Results

We organize this section as follows: first, we show the simulation; second, the final prototype; third, the trilateration and axis orientation; and finally, an ankle manifold representation.

3.1. Simulation Results

In this subsection, we use different values from Table 1 to estimate the work-space and range of motion. First, we show the variation of mean value results, and second the platform position simulation by changing the range of movement and angles.

Changing Statistical Mean Values

Figure 24a shows the complete manifold, taking into account the intervals $\theta_1, \theta_2 \in [-180°, 180°]$. It also shows the platform's initial position, the TC axis reference, the initial ST reference, the initial orientation, and a parametric trajectory with equal angle rate variation. In Figure 24b is the attaching point A simulation; Figure 24c,d depicts the simulations of B and C, respectively.

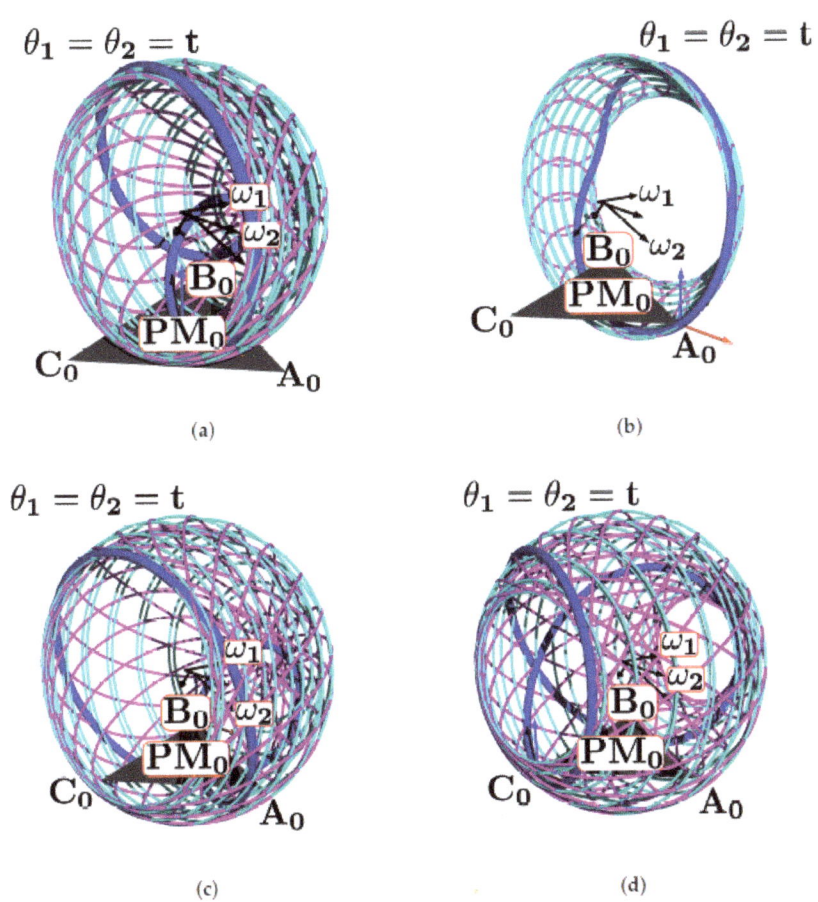

Figure 24. Simulation of all points: (**a**) platform's central point, (**b**) attachment a, (**c**) attachment b, and (**d**) attachment c.

In Figure 25a we show the platform' central point simulation with variations of 10% below the statistical mean values; Figure 25b shows the simulation changing 10% over the statistical mean values; Figure 26a is the attaching point A simulation adding the 10% mean values; and Figure 26b subtracts 10% of the mean values. Figure 27a,b are the results for the platform attaching point B. We show the results for the attaching point C in Figure 28a,b.

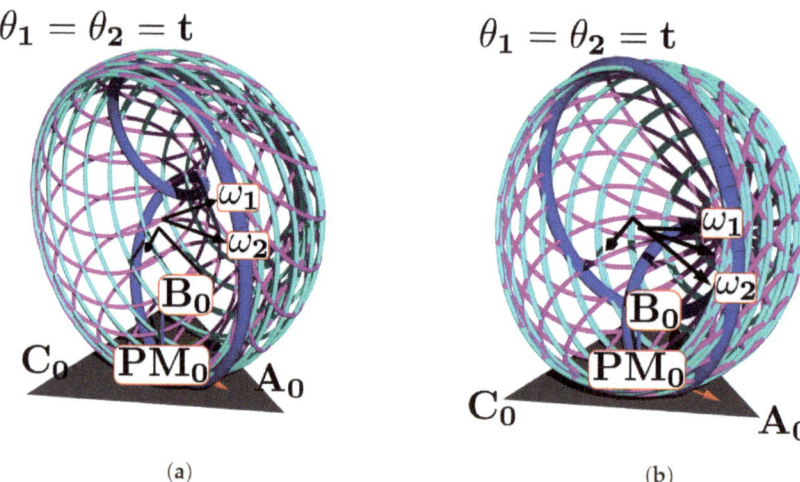

Figure 25. Simulation of the platform central point with variations in the mean statistical values: (**a**) 10% below, and (**b**) 10% over.

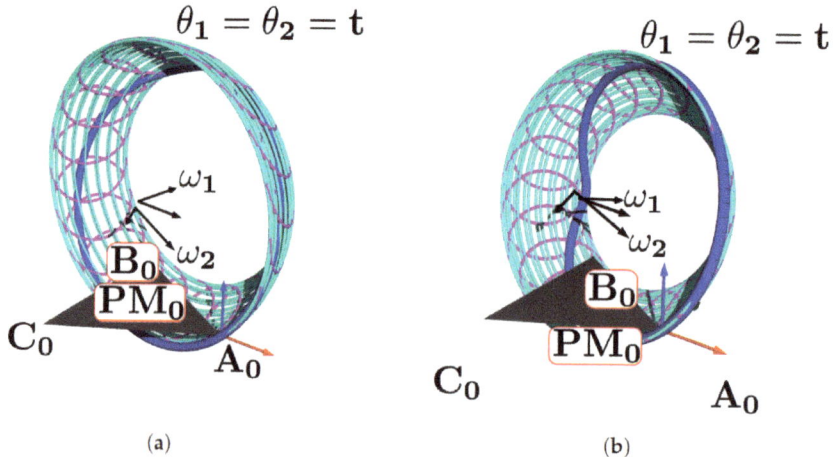

Figure 26. Simulation of the platform's attaching point A: (**a**) mean values plus 10%, (**b**) mean values minus 10%.

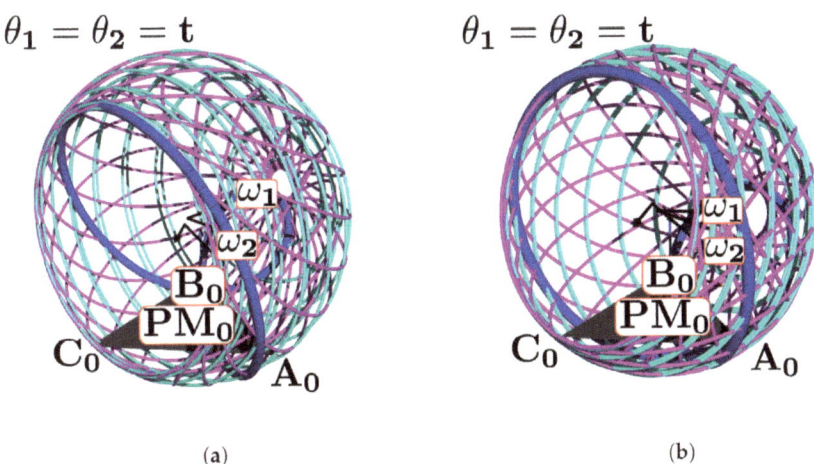

Figure 27. Attaching point B simulation: (**a**) adding 10% to the statistic mean values, (**b**) subtracting 10%.

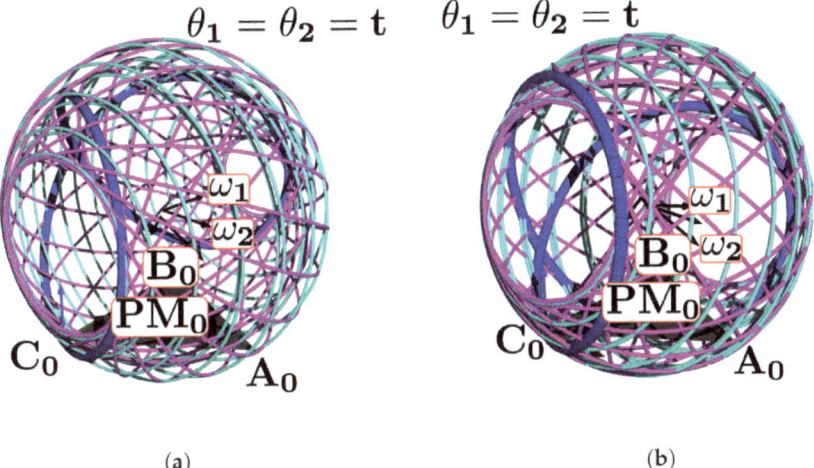

Figure 28. Simulation results for C: (**a**) mean values plus 10%, (**b**) mean values minus 10%.

Finally, by changing the range of maximum and minimum angles, an example of the interactive simulation is in Figure 29a,b. We capture the view of the sliders and also show the simulation rendering result.

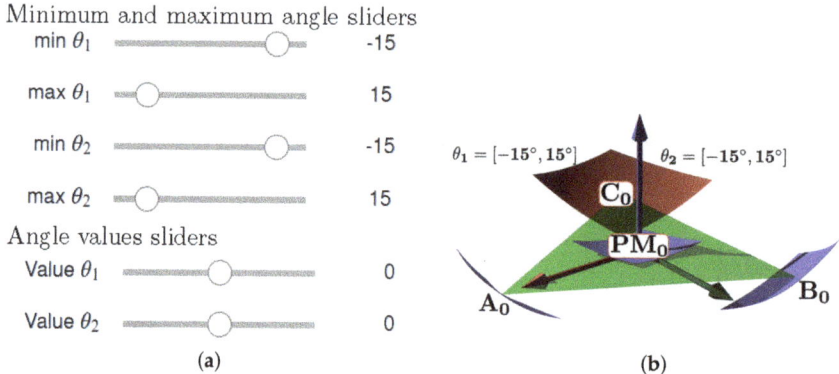

Figure 29. Interactive simulation example: (**a**) sliders, (**b**) rendering.

3.2. Final Prototype

In this section, we describe the results of the TM design, which are the assembled device and calibration. We try several designs and finally the CAD model is in [44]. First, we show images of the connected electronics parts. Second, we assemble the structure and perform calibrations. Third, we probe the device in a healthy patient to validate the prototype adaptability. We print the structural parts using ABS and the draw-wire sensor using PLA; PETG is in the supports and the case.

3.2.1. Printed and Connected Electronics

We place the electronics in each side. In Figure 30, the connections and box sides and charge of the batteries.

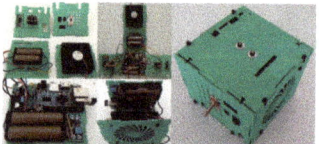

Figure 30. Connections and electronics.

3.2.2. Printed and Assembled Structure

We assemble all structural components carefully, putting them together with stainless-steel threaded rods; then we place the draw-wire sensors, the acquisition board, connections, and final structure for calibration. Figure 31 shows the assembly.

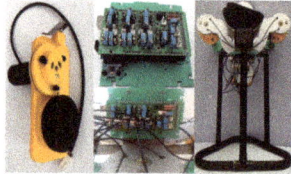

Figure 31. Assembled structure.

3.2.3. Calibration Results

We calibrate the system by using a personal computer. The resulting calibration, and measures of the lengths, are in Figure 32. The lecture is at the initial position, then we compare with the SolidWorks® model measurements and the Vernier caliper real measurements for each DWS. The Table 2 shows the calibration results.

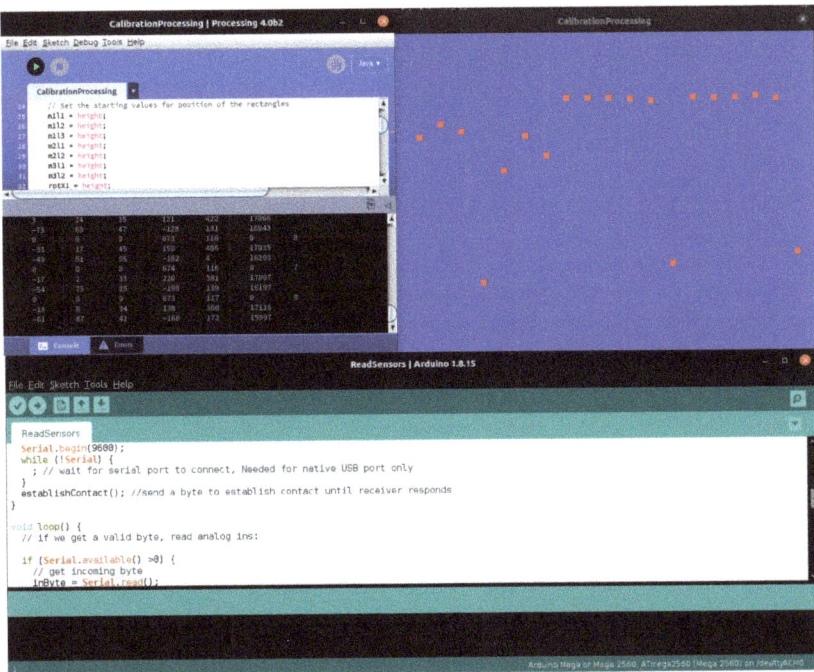

Figure 32. Processing calibration interface.

Table 2. Calibration results with digital measurements and real measurements.

Measurements	l1M1	l2M1	l3M1	l1M2	l2M2	l1M3	l2M3
BCD value	239	330	246	265	177	252	242
Vernier Caliper, cm	8.0 cm	5.3 cm	6.9 cm	13.0 cm	8.4 cm	7.8 cm	11.5 cm

Figure 33a shows the length with a SolidWorks® Measurement tool for module A, sensor 1; the lecture for sensor 2 is in Figure 33b. In Figure 33c, is the sensor 3 length. Table 3 shows the error measured in the real prototype and in SolidWorks®.

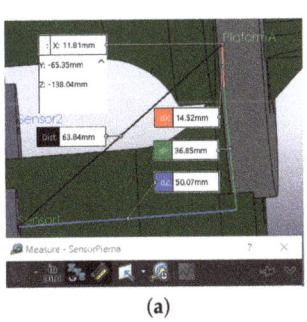
(a)

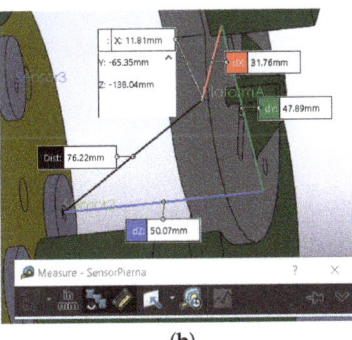
(b)

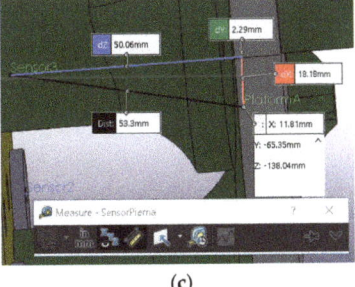
(c)

Figure 33. Measuring in SolidWorks (2017–2018 Student Edition, Dassault Systèmes, Vélizy-Villacoublay, France)®: (**a**) sensor 1, (**b**) sensor 2, (**c**) sensor 3.

Table 3. Error compared with SolidWorks® measurements.

Measurements	l1M1	l2M1	l3M1
Measured distance	7.622 cm	5.33 cm	6.384 cm
Error in cm	0.38 cm	−0.030 cm	0.52 cm

3.3. Trilateration Results

In this section, we use the measurements from the sensors to compute trilateration, then we compare them with the simulation results. The foot and shank fit in the adjustable platform and support structure, respectively, as is shown in the initial procedure in Figure 13. By introducing the DWS lengths to the virtual model, we compute the A, B and C coordinates in four consecutive positions. In the Table 4 are the seven sensors lenghts, and in the Table 5, we show the A, B and C coordinates for the four positions. The resulting figures for the first two positions are in Figure 34a,b, and for the latest two positions in Figure 35a,b. We show the base triangles, the points, the sensors, the platform and the circles on the base.

Table 4. Sensor measurements in four different positions.

Positions	l1M1	l2M1	l3M1	l1M2	l2M2	l1M3	l2M3
Pos1., cm	11.0 cm	12.6 cm	12.5 cm	14.8 cm	10.8 cm	15.2 cm	11.9 cm
Pos2., cm	10.2 cm	11.7 cm	11.6 cm	15.2 cm	11.3 cm	15.5 cm	12.2 cm
Pos3., cm	9.40 cm	10.8 cm	10.8 cm	15.6 cm	11.7 cm	15.8 cm	12.5 cm
Pos4., cm	8.56 cm	9.89 cm	9.95 cm	16.0 cm	12.2 cm	16.0 cm	12.7 cm

Table 5. A, B and C coordinates computed from the four positions.

Positions	A	B	C
Pos1., cm	(−11.7, −1.06, −11.0) cm	(6.11, −9.77, −8.76) cm	(5.54, 8.81, −9.35) cm
Pos2., cm	(−12.1, −0.93, −10.2) cm	(5.62, −9.92, −9.37) cm	(4.83, 9.46, −10.1) cm
Pos3., cm	(−12.4, −0.65, −9.39) cm	(5.27, −9.79, −9.68) cm	(4.94, 9.03, −10.2) cm
Pos4., cm	(−12.7, −0.48, −8.53) cm	(4.68, −10.0, −10.3) cm	(3.54, 10.7, −11.1) cm

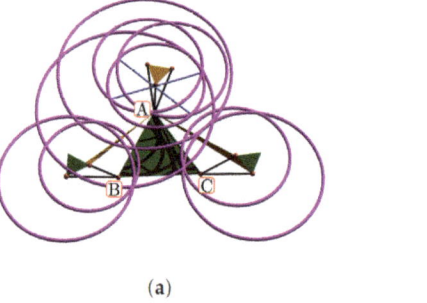
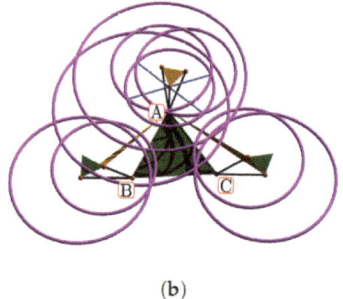

(a)   (b)

Figure 34. First two trilateration results: (**a**) position 1, (**b**) position 2.

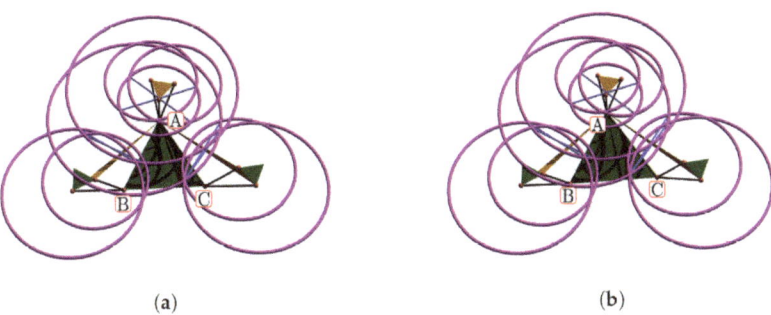

Figure 35. Latest two trilateration results: (**a**) position 3, (**b**) position 4.

3.4. TC Axis Circle Fitting

The results of circle fitting for trajectories A, B, and C are in Table 6, corresponding to ankle joint plantar/dorsiflexion movements. We show the circle fitting for trajectories A, B, C, and PM in the Figure 36a–d.

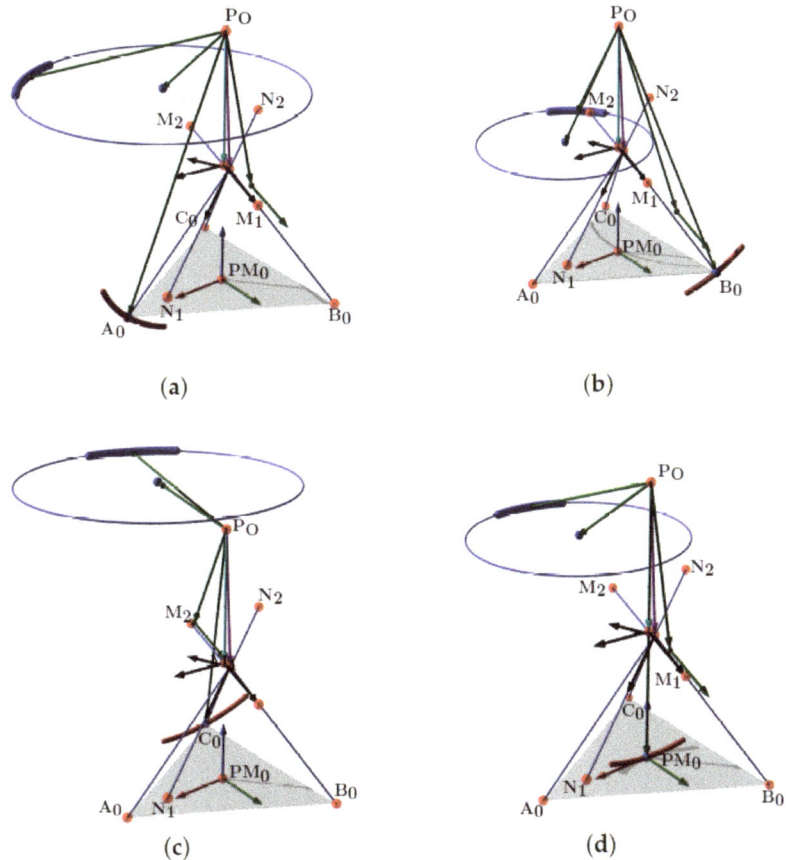

Figure 36. TC axis circle fitting: (**a**) trajectory A, (**b**) trajectory B, (**c**) trajectory C, (**d**) trajectory PM.

Table 6. TC axis circle fitting.

Trajectory	Center	Direction	Radius
A	(0.08649, 2.138, −6.712) cm	(−0.089, −0.95, 0.31)	7.666
B	(0.5713, 5.531, −7.824) cm	(−0.089, −0.95, 0.31)	5.246 cm
C	(−0.2442, −2.669, −5.315) cm	(−0.089, −0.95, 0.31)	7.206 cm
PM	(0.1552, 1.642, −6.683) cm	(−0.089, −0.95, 0.31)	5.375 cm

3.5. ST Axis Circle Fitting

The results of ST circle fitting for trajectories A, B, C, and PM are in Table 7, corresponding to ankle joint inversion movements. We show the circle fitting for trajectories A, B, C, and PM in the Figure 37a–d.

Table 7. ST axis circle fitting.

Trajectory	Center	Direction	Radius
A	(4.444, 1.825, −9.008) cm	(−0.75, −0.28, 0.60)	2.428 cm
B	(1.757, 0.6768, −6.925) cm	(−0.75, −0.28, 0.60)	6.567 cm
C	(0.1578, 0.1819, −5.807) cm	((−0.75, −0.28, 0.60)	6.935 cm
PM	(2.087, 0.8882, −7.281) cm	(−0.75, −0.28, 0.60)	3.875

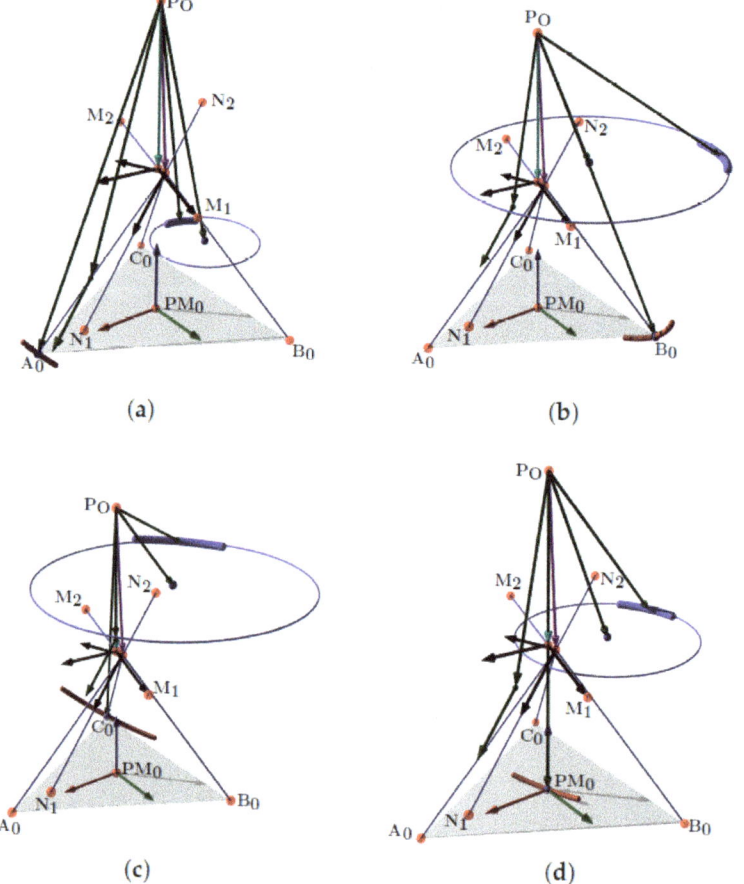

Figure 37. ST axis circle fitting: (**a**) trajectory A, (**b**) trajectory B, (**c**) trajectory C, (**d**) trajectory PM.

3.6. Ankle Manifold Representation

In this section, we show the results in the software SageMath Manifolds. We load the model and visualize it as a manifold, we show the axis and the sagittal plane intersection. With the model parameters loaded, $r_1, r_2, \omega_1, \omega_2$, and the origin established in the center of the base modules. We apply the equation:

$$\hat{r}_1 = \bar{c}_0 + \hat{n}_p \cdot d \qquad (62)$$

where $\bar{c}_0$ is the median center computed from trajectories A, B, and C center fitting, and $\hat{n}_p$ is the median planes' normal vectors containing the circles. Table 8 shows values for the TC axis in the PM chart. In Table 9, we show the Plucker coordinates for the TC and ST axes.

Finally, Figure 38a shows the ankle manifold, and Figure 38b, the chart representing the range of movement and angle coordinates.

Table 8. Axis estimation data.

Axis	Median Center	Median Normal	r	ω
TC	(1.92, 0.783, −7.10) cm	(−0.750, −0.280, 0.600)	(−0.174, 0.000, −5.43) cm	(−0.750, −0.280, 0.600)
ST	(0.121, 1.89, −6.70) cm	(−0.0890, −0.950, 0.310)	(−0.0562, 0.000, −6.08) cm	(−0.0890, −0.950, 0.310)

Table 9. Plucker line coordinates.

Axis	Plucker Line Coordinates
TC	[−0.750 : −0.280 : 0.600: −1.52: 4.17: 0.0487]
ST	[−0.0890: −0.950: 0.310: −5.78: 0.559: 0.0534]

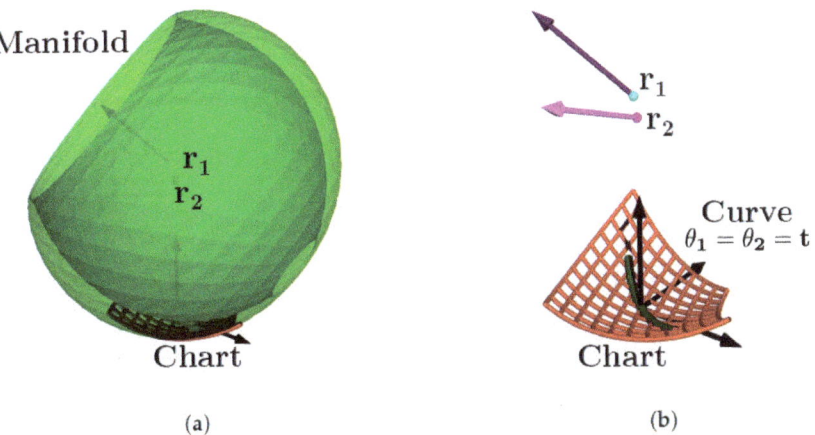

Figure 38. Ankle joint manifold. (**a**) Manifold for PM, (**b**) chart with ankle axis coordinates.

4. Discussion

In this work, we addressed the human ankle joint model from an alternative approach. We used statistical measurements for the development of a new device, specially designed to capture the human ankle joint movements. In animal joints, it is difficult to place encoders and linear sensors to measure the range of movement of complex joints in each internal living tissue reference frame. The product of exponential formulas uses only two frames, and it is useful in this case. Furthermore, in our work, we used a trilateration method for finding the device's platform position, which is an analytic method. Therefore we avoid numerical approximations that can diverge and reduce rounding errors. We proposed the ankle joint model as a Riemannian manifold. We can define a chart as a subset of such a manifold with angle coordinates for measuring the range of movement. Our presented device is lightweight, non-invasive, and can be used in remote places, on beds, or on the floor. By characterizing the ankle parameters, we can conduct symmetry studies by correlating the left and right ankle joints. We can enhance the device configuration in future versions by replacing the draw-wire sensors used from potentiometers to digital encoders connected by a CAN bus, reducing wiring, space, weight, and energy consumption. We will use the model for the synthesis and reconfiguration of an ankle parallel rehabilitation robot, programmed by symmetrical movements at the opposite ankle. By employing the axis location and the screw theory, forces, and torques, we will study the ankle dynamics by using reciprocal screws to the axis location in a re-configurable platform. The robot will be lightweight because of the use of cable-driven actuators, inspired by antagonistic muscles that work with reciprocal inhibition for energy optimization. The robot will reconfigure the structure, considering the ankle joint as a central mast, and referenced it with MMP and MLP markers.

Figure 39 shows a schematic of the re-configurable approach.

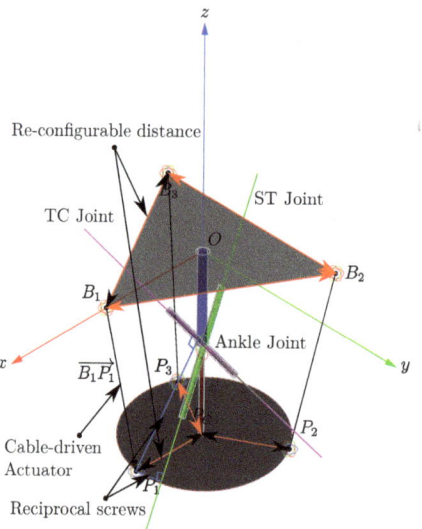

Figure 39. Re-configurable cable-driven robot concept.

Other applications are, for example, by visualizing the platform trajectories one can explain how the calcaneal Achilles insertion is near to the platform's A point. The platform's normal vector changes abruptly near this region, as was depicted in Figures 24b and 26a,b. Furthermore, Riemannian models have different properties. We will explore diagnosis and treatments based on the model and metrics by employing machine learning algorithms. This approach can be applied to other joints in humans and other animals, by designing specialized re-configurable hardware and software. Tracking the parameters in different ages and weight conditions, and comparing the ankle models in healthy and injured people.

5. Conclusions

Computer tomography (CT) and magnetic resonance (MR) images have greater precision and accuracy. Measurements in medical imaging will help us compare the errors (RMS) in the HAJ. In biomechanics, we have not found an ideal model for error comparison. Then, we will compare the error with an accurate measurement. The device has limitations regarding mechanical precision and deformation of its parts. We face up to the error through the electronic design system. The calibration process is imperative for enhancing accuracy.

The calibration process is human-dependent. We read the digital measurement and compare it with caliper measurements directly in the sensor. Then, we register the data in a table to find the equivalence. An electronic board with trimmers avoids saturation, bias, and calibration; a 10 bit ADC and an exponentially weighted moving average (EWMA) filter the noise signals. We have implemented a processing (Software) calibration interface. We avoid adding more specific technical data, such as CMRR, ADC speed, mechanical tolerance, and other issues inherent to the measuring devices.

Digital sensors, communications, and POE function fitting use machine learning techniques.

The ankle is the most commonly injured joint of the lower limb, fundamental to the human body's balance; it is necessary to measure the range of motion by in vivo methods for patients in lying positions in reduced or remote places. The device's development considers ankle anatomy and anthropometry. We propose a Riemannian manifold model based on the device's data readings. Performing simulations enabled us to design the size of the device and the maximal length of the wires. We present a trilateration algorithm, projecting the tetrahedron's sides on the base plane. The sensors are modular and part of the device's lightweight and portable structure. The electronic system is modular, replaced by other single-board computers (SBC) and microcontroller unities. We will also use the TM for ankle characterization and diagnosis for rehabilitation robotics, prosthesis, and orthosis design. The prototype is not a finished product (the TRL is 2). The work's scope is to validate the use of a modern alternative biomechanic representation of the human ankle joint. It is a platform for testing an alternative trilateration method that employs draw-wire sensors (DWS). Such sensors have a constant tension, coiled on a drum attached to a potentiometer, and a flat spiral spring. We also attempted to develop a flexible device design for several foot sizes. We are working on a newer device version with an enhanced attachment system, a more compact design, and digital DWS compatible with a configurable robot. Machine learning and edge computing will assist in disease diagnosis and rehabilitation of patients.

Author Contributions: Conceptualization, J.V.-R., Á.V. and Ó.A.-V.; methodology, Á.V. and Ó.A.-V.; software, J.V.-R.; validation, Á.V. and Ó.A.-V.; formal analysis, J.V.-R.; investigation, J.V.-R.; resources, Á.V. and Ó.A.-V.; data curation, Á.V. and Ó.A.-V.; writing—original draft preparation, J.V.-R.; writing—review and editing, Á.V. and Ó.A.-V.; visualization, J.V.-R.; supervision, Á.V.; project administration, Á.V. ; funding acquisition, J.V.-R., Á.V. and Ó.A.-V. All authors have read and agreed to the published version of the manuscript.

Funding: This research was partially funded by Colciencias-Colfuturo PhD Scholarships Program Educational Credit Forgivable grant number 568, and by Vicerrectorado de Investigación de la Universitat Politècnica de València (PAID-11-21).

Institutional Review Board Statement: Not applicable.

Informed Consent Statement: Informed consent was obtained from all subjects involved in the study.

Data Availability Statement: The code and CAD electronics and mechanical designs are available.

Acknowledgments: The authors thank the Colfuturo Colciencias Collaboration for supporting this work, as well as the Universitat Politècnica de València and the Universidad de los Llanos.

Conflicts of Interest: The authors declare no conflict of interest.

Abbreviations

The following abbreviations are used in this manuscript:

HAJ	Human Ankle Joint
ISB	International Society of Biomechanics
DWS	Draw-Wire Sensors
IMU	Inertial Measurement Units
PoE	Product of Exponentials
DoF	Degrees of Freedom
RoM	Range of Motion
BMS	Battery Management System

References

1. Krähenbühl, N.; Horn-Lang, T.; Hintermann, B.; Knupp, M. The subtalar joint. *EFORT Open Rev.* **2017**, *2*, 309–316. [CrossRef] [PubMed]
2. Nichols, J.A.; Roach, K.E.; Fiorentino, N.M.; Anderson, A.E. Predicting tibiotalar and subtalar joint angles from skin-marker data with dual-fluoroscopy as a reference standard. *Gait Posture* **2016**, *49*, 136–143. [CrossRef] [PubMed]
3. Xie, S.S. Kinematic and Computational Model of Human Ankle. In *Advanced Robotics for Medical Rehabilitation: Current State of the Art and Recent Advances*; Xie, S.S., Ed.; Springer Tracts in Advanced Robotics; Springer International Publishing: Cham, Switzerland, 2016; pp. 185–221. [CrossRef]
4. Jastifer, J.R.; Gustafson, P.A. The subtalar joint: Biomechanics and functional representations in the literature. *Foot* **2014**, *24*, 203–209. [CrossRef]
5. Van Alsenoy, K.; De Schepper, J.; Santos, D.; Vereecke, E.; D'Août, K. The Subtalar Joint Axis Palpation Technique: Part 1—Validating a Clinical Mechanical Model. *J. Am. Podiatr. Med. Assoc.* **2014**, *104*, 238–246. [CrossRef] [PubMed]
6. Van Alsenoy, K.K.; D'Août, K.; Vereecke, E.E.; De Schepper, J.; Santos, D. The Subtalar Joint Axis Palpation Technique: Part 2: Reliability and Validity Results Using Cadaver Feet. *J. Am. Podiatr. Med. Assoc.* **2014**, *104*, 365–374. [CrossRef]
7. De Schepper, J.; Van Alsenoy, K.; Rijckaert, J.; De Mits, S.; Lootens, T.; Roosen, P. Intratest reliability in determining the subtalar joint axis using the palpation technique described by K. Kirby. *J. Am. Podiatr. Med. Assoc.* **2012**, *102*, 122–129.
8. Parr, W.C.H.; Chatterjee, H.J.; Soligo, C. Calculating the axes of rotation for the subtalar and talocrural joints using 3D bone reconstructions. *J. Biomech.* **2012**, *45*, 1103–1107. [CrossRef]
9. Leitch, J.; Stebbins, J.; Zavatsky, A.B. Subject-specific axes of the ankle joint complex. *J. Biomech.* **2010**, *43*, 2923–2928. [CrossRef]
10. Lewis, G.S.; Cohen, T.L.; Seisler, A.R.; Kirby, K.A.; Sheehan, F.T.; Piazza, S.J. In vivo tests of an improved method for functional location of the subtalar joint axis. *J. Biomech.* **2009**, *42*, 146–151. [CrossRef]
11. Lewis, G.S.; Kirby, K.A.; Piazza, S.J. Determination of subtalar joint axis location by restriction of talocrural joint motion. *Gait Posture* **2007**, *25*, 63–69. [CrossRef]
12. Spooner, S.; Kirby, K. The subtalar joint axis locator: A preliminary report. *J. Am. Podiatr. Med. Assoc.* **2006**, *96*, 212–219. [CrossRef] [PubMed]
13. Kirby, K.A. Subtalar Joint Axis Location and Rotational Equilibrium Theory of Foot Function. *J. Am. Podiatr. Med. Assoc.* **2001**, *91*, 465–487. [CrossRef] [PubMed]
14. Dul, J.; Johnson, G.E. A kinematic model of the human ankle. *J. Biomed. Eng.* **1985**, *7*, 137–143. [CrossRef]
15. Wu, G.; Siegler, S.; Allard, P.; Kirtley, C.; Leardini, A.; Rosenbaum, D.; Whittle, M.; D'Lima, D.D.; Cristofolini, L.; Witte, H.; et al. ISB recommendation on definitions of joint coordinate system of various joints for the reporting of human joint motion—Part I: Ankle, hip, and spine. *J. Biomech.* **2002**, *35*, 543–548. [CrossRef]
16. Mann, R.A. Biomechanics of the Ankle. In *Joint Surgery Up to Date*; Hirohata, K., Kurosaka, M., Cooke, T.D.V., Eds.; Springer: Tokyo, Japan, 1989; pp. 73–81. [CrossRef]
17. Winter, D.A. *Biomechanics and Motor Control of Human Movement*; John Wiley & Sons: Hoboken, NJ, USA, 2009.
18. Dawe, E.J.C.; Davis, J. (vi) Anatomy and biomechanics of the foot and ankle. *Orthop. Trauma* **2011**, *25*, 279–286. [CrossRef]
19. Coughlin, M.J.; Saltzman, C.L.; Mann, R.A. *Mann's Surgery of the Foot and Ankle E-Book: Expert Consult-Online*; Elsevier Health Sciences: Amsterdam, The Netherlands, 2013.
20. Delp, S.; Loan, J.; Hoy, M.; Zajac, F.; Topp, E.; Rosen, J. An interactive graphics-based model of the lower extremity to study orthopaedic surgical procedures. *IEEE Trans. Biomed. Eng.* **1990**, *37*, 757–767. [CrossRef]
21. Donatelli, R. Normal Biomechanics of the Foot and Ankle. *J. Orthop. Sport. Phys. Ther.* **1985**, *7*, 91–95. [CrossRef]
22. Bähler, A. The biomechanics of the foot. *Clin. Prosthetics Orthot.* **1986**, *10*, 8–14.
23. Lundberg, A.; K Svensson, O.; Németh, G.; Selvik, G. The axis of rotation of the ankle joint. *J. Bone Jt. Surg. Br. Vol.* **1989**, *71*, 94–99. [CrossRef]
24. Singh, A.K.; Starkweather, K.D.; Hollister, A.M.; Jatana, S.; Lupichuk, A.G. Kinematics of the Ankle: A Hinge Axis Model. *Foot Ankle Int.* **1992**, *13*, 439–446. [CrossRef]
25. Leardini, A.; O'Connor, J.; Catani, F.; Giannini, S. A geometric model of the human ankle joint. *J. Biomech.* **1999**, *32*, 585–591. [CrossRef]
26. Brockett, C.L.; Chapman, G.J. Biomechanics of the ankle. *Orthop. Trauma* **2016**, *30*, 232–238. [CrossRef] [PubMed]
27. Bruening, D.; Richards, J. Skiing-Skating: Optimal ankle axis position for articulated boots. *Sport. Biomech.* **2005**, *4*, 215–225. [CrossRef] [PubMed]

28. Andrade-Cetto, J.; Thomas, F. A Wire-Based Active Tracker. *IEEE Trans. Robot.* **2008**, *24*, 642–651. [CrossRef]
29. Thomas, F.; Ottaviano, E.; Ros, L.; Ceccarelli, M. Coordinate-free formulation of a 3-2-1 wire-based tracking device using Cayley-Menger determinants. In Proceedings of the 2003 IEEE International Conference on Robotics and Automation (Cat. No.03CH37422), Taipei, Taiwan, 14–19 September 2003; Volume 1, pp. 355–361, ISSN: 1050-4729. [CrossRef]
30. Thomas, F.; Ros, L. Revisiting trilateration for robot localization. *IEEE Trans. Robot.* **2005**, *21*, 93–101. [CrossRef]
31. Salleh, S.; Rahmat, M.F.; Othman, S.M.; Abidin, H.Z. Application of draw wire sensor in the tracking control of an electro hydraulic actuator system. *J. Teknol.* **2015**, *73*, 51–57. [CrossRef]
32. Jiafan, Z.; Jinsong, L.; Liwei, Q.; Dandan, Z. Kinematic analysis of a 6-DOF wire-based tracking device and control strategy for its application in robot easy programming. 2009 IEEE International Conference on Robotics and Biomimetics (ROBIO), Guilin, China, 9–23 December 2009; pp. 1591–1596. [CrossRef]
33. Bulling, A.; Blanke, U.; Schiele, B. A Tutorial on Human Activity Recognition Using Body-worn Inertial Sensors. *ACM Comput. Surv.* **2014**, *46*, 1–33. [CrossRef]
34. Chermak, L.; Aouf, N.; Richardson, M.A.; Visentin, G. *Real-Time Smart and Standalone Vision/IMU Navigation Sensor*; Springer Science and Business Media LLC.: Berlin/Heidelberg, Germany, 2016. [CrossRef]
35. Ong, Z.C.; Noroozi, S. *Development of an Economic Wireless Human Motion Analysis Device for Quantitative Assessment of Human Body Joint*; Elsevier BV: Amsterdam, The Netherlands, 2018. [CrossRef]
36. Porciuncula, F.; Roto, A.V.; Kumar, D.; Davis, I.; Roy, S.; Walsh, C.J.; Awad, L.N. Wearable Movement Sensors for Rehabilitation: A Focused Review of Technological and Clinical Advances. *PM&R* **2018**, *10*, S220–S232. [CrossRef]
37. Wahyudi, W.; Listiyana, M.S.; Sudjadi, S.; Ngatelan, N. Tracking Object based on GPS and IMU Sensor. In Proceedings of the 5th International Conference on Information Technology, Computer, and Electrical Engineering (ICITACEE), Semarang, Indonesia, 26–28 September 2018; pp. 214–218. [CrossRef]
38. Gregorio, R.D.; Parenti-Castelli, V.; O Connor, J.J.; Leardini, A. Mathematical models of passive motion at the human ankle joint by equivalent spatial parallel mechanisms. *Med. Biol. Eng. Comput.* **2007**, *45*, 305–313. [CrossRef]
39. Vargas-Riaño, J.H. Turmell-Meter. 2022. Available online: https://github.com/juliohvr/Turmell-Meter (accessed on 29 April 2022).
40. Isman, R.E.; Inman, V.T.; Poor, P.M. Anthropometric studies of the human foot and ankle. *Bull. Prosthet. Res.* **1969**, *11*, 97–129.
41. Drillis, R.; Contini, R.; Bluestein, M. *Body Segment Parameters*; New York University, School of Engineering and Science: New York, NY, USA, 1966.
42. Hebbelinck, M.; Ross, W.D. Kinanthropometry and biomechanics. In *Biomechanics IV*; Springer: Berlin/Heidelberg, Germany, 1974; pp. 535–552.
43. Fryar, C.D.; Carroll, M.D.; Gu, Q.; Afful, J.; Ogden, C.L. *Anthropometric Reference Data for Children and Adults: United States, 2015–2018*; Vital & Health Statistics. Series 3 Analytical and Epidemiological Studies; CDC: Atlanta, GA, USA, 2021; pp. 1–44.
44. Vargas Riaño, J.; Valera, Á.; Agudelo Varela, O. Turmell-Metre|3D CAD Model Library|GrabCAD. Available online: https://grabcad.com/library/turmell-metre-1 (accessed on 29 April 2022).

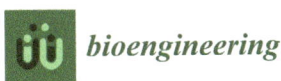

Article

Gait Event Prediction Using Surface Electromyography in Parkinsonian Patients

Stefan Haufe [1,2,3,4,*], Ioannis U. Isaias [5,6], Franziska Pellegrini [3,4] and Chiara Palmisano [5]

1. Uncertainty, Inverse Modeling and Machine Learning Group, Technical University of Berlin, 10587 Berlin, Germany
2. Mathematical Modelling and Data Analysis Department, Physikalisch-Technische Bundesanstalt Braunschweig und Berlin, 10587 Berlin, Germany
3. Berlin Center for Advanced Neuroimaging, Charité–Universitätsmedizin Berlin, 10117 Berlin, Germany
4. Bernstein Center for Computational Neuroscience Berlin, 10115 Berlin, Germany
5. Department of Neurology, University Hospital Würzburg and Julius-Maximilians-Universität Würzburg, 97080 Würzburg, Germany
6. Centro Parkinson, ASST G. Pini-CTO, 20126 Milano, Italy
* Correspondence: haufe@tu-berlin.de

Abstract: Gait disturbances are common manifestations of Parkinson's disease (PD), with unmet therapeutic needs. Inertial measurement units (IMUs) are capable of monitoring gait, but they lack neurophysiological information that may be crucial for studying gait disturbances in these patients. Here, we present a machine learning approach to approximate IMU angular velocity profiles and subsequently gait events using electromyographic (EMG) channels during overground walking in patients with PD. We recorded six parkinsonian patients while they walked for at least three minutes. Patient-agnostic regression models were trained on temporally embedded EMG time series of different combinations of up to five leg muscles bilaterally (i.e., tibialis anterior, soleus, gastrocnemius medialis, gastrocnemius lateralis, and vastus lateralis). Gait events could be detected with high temporal precision (median displacement of <50 ms), low numbers of missed events (<2%), and next to no false-positive event detections (<0.1%). Swing and stance phases could thus be determined with high fidelity (median F1-score of ~0.9). Interestingly, the best performance was obtained using as few as two EMG probes placed on the left and right vastus lateralis. Our results demonstrate the practical utility of the proposed EMG-based system for gait event prediction, which allows the simultaneous acquisition of an electromyographic signal to be performed. This gait analysis approach has the potential to make additional measurement devices such as IMUs and force plates less essential, thereby reducing financial and preparation overheads and discomfort factors in gait studies.

Keywords: electromyography; inertial measurement units; gait-phase prediction; machine learning; Parkinson's disease

Citation: Haufe, S.; Isaias, I.U.; Pellegrini, F.; Palmisano, C. Gait Event Prediction Using Surface Electromyography in Parkinsonian Patients. *Bioengineering* 2023, 10, 212. https://doi.org/10.3390/bioengineering10020212

Academic Editor: Christina Zong-Hao Ma

Received: 3 January 2023
Revised: 31 January 2023
Accepted: 3 February 2023
Published: 6 February 2023

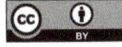

Copyright: © 2023 by the authors. Licensee MDPI, Basel, Switzerland. This article is an open access article distributed under the terms and conditions of the Creative Commons Attribution (CC BY) license (https://creativecommons.org/licenses/by/4.0/).

1. Introduction

Gait and balance disturbances are common and important clinical manifestations of Parkinson's disease (PD), leading to mobility impairment and falls [1]. Current treatments (pharmacological and deep brain stimulation (DBS)) provide only partial benefits in gait derangements in PD, with a wide variability in outcomes [2–5].

Despite detailed testing, specific factors that are critical to predicting locomotor deterioration in PD remain elusive [6–9]. Beside subtle onset and clinical heterogeneity [10], technical limitations have hampered the timely and direct recording of supraspinal locomotor derangements in these patients. Only recently have advances in portable electroencephalography systems [11,12] and new DBS devices capable of on-demand recording using chronically implanted electrodes (e.g., Activa PC+S and Percept PC (Medtronic PLC or AlphaDBS (Newronika Srl)) [13–15] enabled the recording of ongoing brain activity during actual gait in PD to be performed [16–18].

The precise assessment of gait dynamics should account for its context dependency. New study setups employing fully immersive virtual reality (VR) or augmented reality allow gait assessment (with optoelectronic systems, force plates, etc.) to be conducted in environments that deliver patient-specific triggers of gait impairment (e.g., [19]). These setups could facilitate the identification of biomarkers for the fine-tuning of therapy delivery, e.g., adaptive DBS programming and so-called VR Exposure Therapy [20].

An open challenge is the continuous monitoring of gait parameters in laboratory as well as real-world environments. Technically, parameters such as the timings of heel strike and toe-off events, which define swing and stance phases and provide valuable information about cadence patterns, etc., can be assessed with optoelectronic systems and force plates. Both systems, however, are expensive, require qualified personnel, and do not offer monitoring in ecological settings. Video-based analyses of gait have also been proposed [21], although it is unclear whether these could reach the required precision to identify individual events within a gait cycle, especially for clinical applications and in ecological settings. Wearable motion sensors such as inertial measurement units (IMUs) are another viable option to capture gait events in natural environments with high temporal accuracy [22,23]. However, they do not contain further neurophysiological information that may be crucial to understanding and predicting gait derangements [24]. Surface electromyography (EMG) provides the missing link between neural signals and kinematics that makes the comprehensive characterization of pathological gait possible. EMG measurements have been used to predict lower-limb motion in advance [25,26] for real-time control of a prosthesis [27–29] or adaptive DBS devices [16–18,25,26,30,31]. EMG profiles of the gait cycle have also been shown to anticipate specific gait derangements in PD, such as freezing of gait [32], a sudden episodic inability to produce effective stepping despite the intention to walk. The combined use of IMU and EMG signals would make the description of the motor actions and intentions underlying gait kinematic features and alterations possible.

However, some practical limitations should be considered when applying additional sensors on severely ill patients, especially when performing recordings after suspension of medications. For example, in patients with PD, the overnight suspension of dopaminergic drugs is fundamental to evoke and study PD-related symptoms but greatly reduces the time window available for experimental recordings. Limiting the preparation period by limiting the number of sensors may help considerably in this regard. In addition, an excessive number of sensors may alter the natural behavior of subjects, undermining the advantages of working in ecological environments. Another crucial aspect is the cost of multiple sets of sensors. Considering that probes comprising both IMUs and EMG are generally more expensive than standalone solutions, the need for IMUs and EMG in the fine-grained evaluation of gait may be a limiting factor for many laboratories and applications in clinical routine. The use of multiple devices may also not be practical in clinical routine, as synchronization or different recording software may be needed.

Considering this, the development of novel technologies that can extract multiple types of signals from the same set of sensors is highly desirable. While the same kinematics can be produced by different muscular patterns, lower-limb kinematics can be inferred using analysis of EMG [33]. The idea of detecting gait events directly using EMG signals, circumventing additional IMUs or force plates, is gaining traction [34–38]. Ziegier and colleagues [38] reported high accuracy in classifying stance and swing phases during human gait based on EMG recordings. They first extracted a weighted signal difference that exploits the difference in EMG activity between corresponding muscles of the two legs and then trained a support vector machine to classify the gait phases. Using a deep learning approach, Morbidoni and colleagues [35] were also able to classify stance and swing phases and predict foot–floor contacts under natural walking conditions in healthy subjects. Other studies showed similar results in learned and unlearned subjects [37], and using intra-subject training only [34]. This would not only simplify future recording setups but also permit the re-analysis of EMG datasets recorded without IMUs or in cases of data loss due to technical problems with the IMU to be performed. This second scenario is particularly problematic when recordings cannot be repeated due to the patient's clinical condition. Additionally, the extraction and prediction of gait events using lower-limb EMG activity is of fundamental importance for the development of an EMG-driven prosthesis, where predicting the subsequent gait phase using muscular signals increases prosthesis efficiency and responsiveness [33].

Previous approaches aimed to predict discrete gait events (i.e., heel contact and toe-off), and little attention has been paid to reconstructing the time course of the relevant kinematic variables. Brantley and colleagues were able to predict knee and ankle kinematics, but with varying accuracy across trials and the subjects included [33]. In addition, most previous studies focused on treadmill walking, which may not capture the variability of ground walking [36–38]. Lastly, we are not aware of any approach that has been tested on unmedicated PD patients during long periods of continuous walking.

In the present study, we explore the possibility of identifying fundamental gait events from surface EMG in parkinsonian patients using a machine learning approach. Compared with previous studies, we did not frame the problem as one of detection (i.e., to identify the timings of a fixed set of events) or classification (i.e., to segment the data into contiguous gait phases). Instead, we used an innovative regression approach to approximate continuous angular velocity profiles as measured by IMUs. We consider this approach strictly more powerful and flexible than previous approaches, as access to the predicted IMU time series allows us not only to extract predetermined types of gait events but also biomechanical quantities such as joint angular velocity and further parameters on which our model has not been trained. Our study is further set apart from published work in that we focused on a clinical cohort rather than healthy participants. To our knowledge, our study is the first to demonstrate the feasibility of accurate gait parameter estimation using EMG in such a population. Remarkably, our approach accounts for the substantial across-patient variability observed in gait patterns of clinical populations, allowing it to be applied without any patient-specific calibration.

2. Materials and Methods

2.1. Participants

We recruited six patients with idiopathic PD according to the UK Brain Bank criteria who did not suffer from any other disease, including cognitive decline (i.e., Mini-Mental State Examination score of >27), vestibular disorders, and orthopedic impairments, that could interfere with walking. An additional inclusion criterion for this preliminary study was the ability of the patient to walk continuously and without assistance for at least three minutes. Disease severity was evaluated using MDS-Unified Parkinson's Disease Rating Scale motor part (UPDRS-III), and the stage of the disease was evaluated using the Hoehn and Yahr (H&Y) scale. Using items 3.15–3.17 of UPDRS-III (hands and feet), a sum rest tremor sub-score was created for the right and left sides separately. Similarly, a sum bradykinesia-rigidity score (items 3.3–3.8) was obtained for each side.

Demographic and clinical features are listed in Table 1. The study was approved by the Ethics Committee of University of Würzburg and conformed to the declaration of Helsinki. All patients gave their written informed consent to participate.

2.2. Experimental Setup and Procedure

Patients were investigated in a practical medication-off state, i.e., on the morning after overnight withdrawal (>12 h) of all dopaminergic drugs (meds-off). Kinematic data were recorded using two IMUs (Opal, APDM), at a sampling rate of 128 Hz, placed bilaterally on the outer anklebones. Each sensor was placed with its vertical axis aligned with the tibial anatomic axis. Surface leg muscle activity as measured by 10 EMG probes (FREEEMG 1000, BTS) was recorded bilaterally on tibialis anterior (Ta), soleus (S), gastrocnemius medialis (Gm), gastrocnemius lateralis (Gl), and vastus lateralis (Vl) at a sampling rate of 1000 Hz.

Two transistor–transistor logic signals (TTL) were provided at the beginning and end of each trial to both EMG and IMU devices to make data synchronization possible. Patients started walking barefoot after a verbal signal at their self-selected speed along a large ellipsoidal path of about 60 m in length (Figure 1). We recorded between three and six trials (243 ± 71 s in duration) of unperturbed, steady-state, overground walking according to the clinical condition of each subject. Overall, 26 walking trials with a total duration of 105 min were obtained.

Table 1. Demographic and clinical features. Meds-off: practical medication-off state, i.e., overnight withdrawal (>12 h) of all dopaminergic drugs. Meds-on: medication-on state 30–60 min after receiving 1 to 1.5 times the levodopa-equivalent of the morning dose. UPDRS-III is presented as total score/tremor sub-score left/tremor sub-score right/bradykinesia-rigidity sub-score left/bradykinesia-rigidity sub-score right. Abbreviations: Hoehn and Yahr stage (H&Y); Levodopa equivalent daily dose (LEDD); Unified Parkinson's Disease Rating Scale motor part (UPDRS-III).

	Gender	Age, Years	Age at Onset, Years	LEDD, mg	UPDRS-III Meds-off	UPDRS-III Meds-on	H&Y
WP1	M	46	36	1167	50/2/4/14/11	15/1/0/3/4	3
WP2	M	57	50	900	28/3/7/4/9	5/0/0/0/4	2
WP3	F	59	52	362	18/2/0/2/8	11/1/0/1/7	1
WP4	F	55	49	640	9/0/0/6/2	5/0/0/4/1	1
WP5	M	61	51	610	12/0/0/2/8	5/0/0/0/4	2
WP6	M	65	58	610	30/0/1/5/13	21/0/0/2/8	2

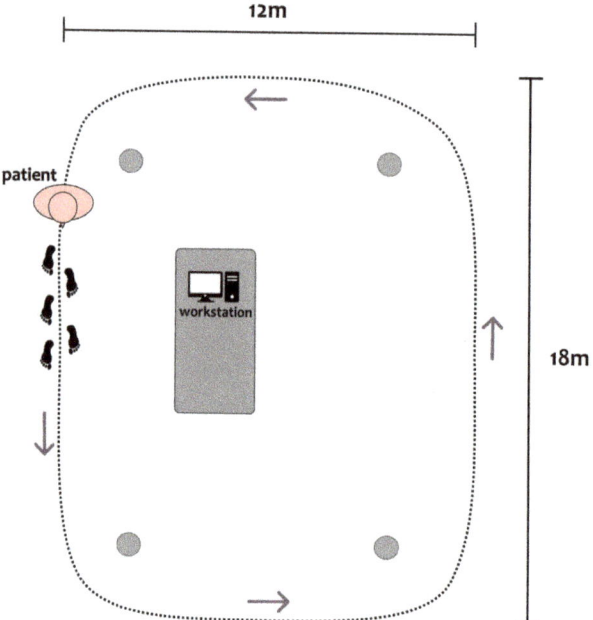

Figure 1. Top-view scheme of the experimental setup, with a patient depicted at the starting position of the circuit. Patients were asked to continuously walk along an elliptical circuit of approximately 60 m around the workstation. The inner boundary of the circuit was marked with four objects at its corners (gray dots). A clinician was close to the patient during all recordings.

2.3. Selection of EMG Channels

We focused on the muscles of the lower leg, which are highly involved during the gait cycle. Ta and S are distal monoarticular muscles with distinct and synergistic contributions to human gait [39]. According to [40], they are the most active muscles during gait and display the lowest inter-subject variability. We, therefore, hypothesized that models based on bilateral pairs of these muscles may be particularly suitable and potentially sufficient for predicting gait-related angular velocity profiles. The gastrocnemius muscle (biarticular) was added for a comprehensive evaluation of the triceps surae. Note that since medial and lateral gastrocnemii fulfill somewhat independent roles [41,42], both were added. Given the knee flexor activity of the gastrocnemius muscle, we then positioned the last available probe on the Vl, a major (monoarticular) knee extensor muscle.

Models based on different muscle combinations were compared to the model including all five pairs of muscles. We were interested in identifying minimal subsets of EMG probes that would make accurate IMU reconstruction possible. Thus, we further exhaustively tested all possible $2^5 - 1 = 31$ sets containing between one and five pairs of distinct muscles. Note that all considered models included either none or both the left and right EMG signals for each studied muscle. Thus, all models comprised an even number of muscles between two and ten.

2.4. Data Preprocessing

Figure 2 depicts a summary of data preprocessing (green box). EMG data were bandpass-filtered, rectified, and down-sampled to 200 Hz. IMU traces were up-sampled to 200 Hz using nearest-neighbor interpolation. IMU and EMG data were aligned to the rising edge of the first TTL signal for synchronization. A number of preprocessing steps were devised to facilitate the prediction of angular velocity traces from EMG data. To smooth out local extrema occurring due to noise, IMU data were processed with a moving-median filter with a 100 ms window length, followed by a moving-mean filter with a 40 ms window length. To achieve a similar degree of smoothness, EMG data were processed with a moving-median filter with a 200 ms window length, followed by a moving-mean filter with a 40 ms window length. All moving filters were centered. As a simple high-pass filter, the minimum in a moving window of 10 s in length was subtracted from the EMG data. To standardize scales across patients, EMG activation time courses were further normalized by subtracting the 1st percentile and dividing by the 95th percentile. Percentiles were estimated separately for each recording. Each recording was cropped to the exact on- and offsets of the walking period.

2.5. Extraction of Biomechanical Parameters

Swing peak velocity (SWP), heel contact (HC), and toe-off (TO) events were extracted from the angular velocity profiles measured with respect to the medio-lateral axis by the IMUs (see [43,44] for an extensive description of gait event detection using IMU data). This was performed separately for the left and right IMU sensors as follows: First, SWP events were identified as local maxima with at least 150°/s peak height and 0.7 s inter-peak distance. Two consecutive SWP events defined one gait cycle. Next, local minima within each cycle were used to define the corresponding HC and TO events. The HC event was defined as the earliest local minimum occurring in the sub-interval between 10% and 45% of the cycle. If no local minimum could be found, the global minimum within that sub-interval was used. Similarly, the TO events were defined as the latest local minimum occurring in the sub-interval between 55% and 90% of the cycle. Again, if no local minimum could be found, the global minimum within that sub-interval was used. At random, events extracted by the described algorithm were checked by an expert (C.P.) and were in agreement with manual determination based on the same IMU data. The procedure was used to define "ground-truth" gait events from recorded IMU data, as well as approximate event timings derived from reconstructed angular velocity time series based on EMG activity (see below; Figure 2, yellow and blue boxes).

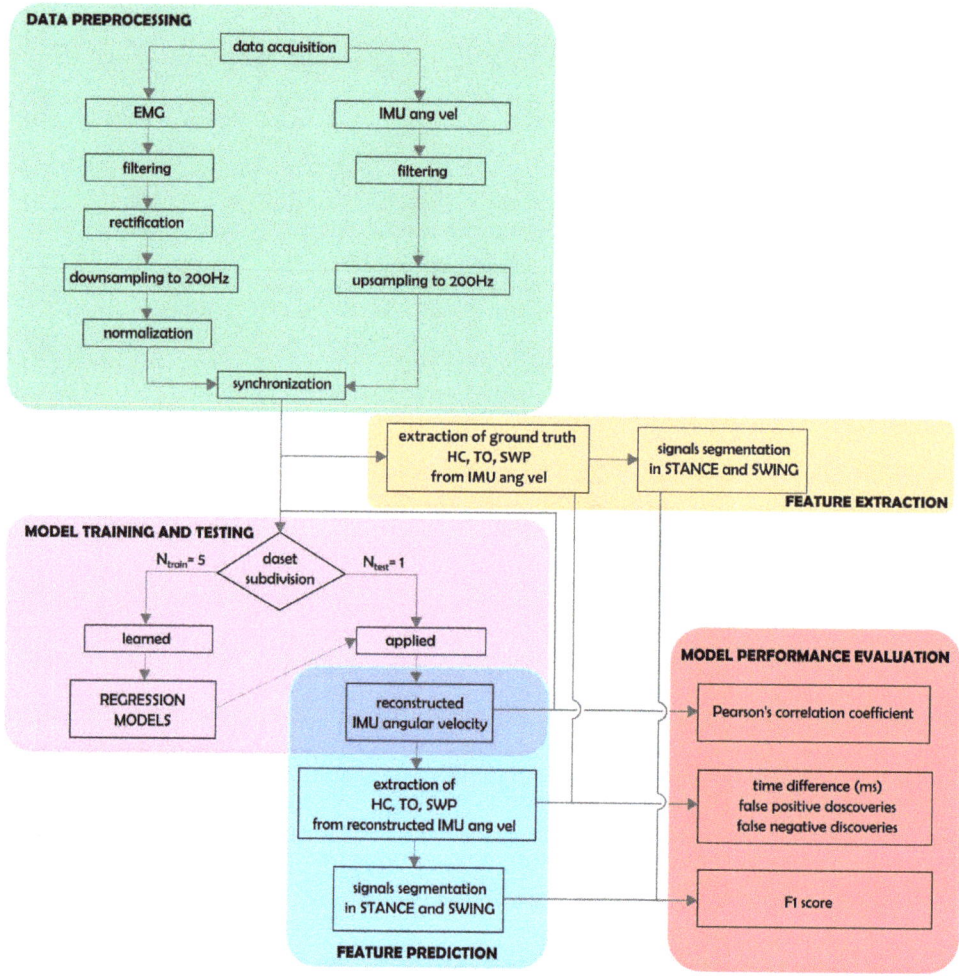

Figure 2. Schematic representation of data analysis. Thirty-one regression models corresponding to all possible muscle combinations were built and evaluated. Each model was trained on all patient data except for one, left out for the testing phase (N_{train} = 5, N_{test} = 1; pink box).

2.6. Prediction of Angular Velocity Profiles Using EMG

We used multiple linear regression to approximate the angular velocity with respect to the medio-lateral axis of the left and right ankle using the combined activation traces of multiple muscles within a window around the prediction point. The regression coefficients were fitted to minimize the mean-squared error between measured and approximated IMU traces on *training* data, consisting of pairs of IMU and EMG activity traces. To enable the prediction model to utilize the temporal dynamics of the EMG channels around the prediction time point, the temporal embedding of the EMG time series was performed. To this end, each selected EMG channel was complemented by temporally shifted versions $\tilde{x}_m(t) = [x_m(t+\tau_1), \ldots, x_m(t+\tau_K)]^T$, $m = 1, \ldots, M$, where $x_m(t+\tau)$ is the activity of the m-th EMG sensor at time $t + \tau$. Here, we used $K = 21$ equally spaced shifts, ranging from $\tau_1 = -500$ ms to $\tau_{21} = +500$ ms in steps of 50 ms. Thus, the prediction of the IMU signals at time t was based on EMG information within a window around t of one second in length. The relation between the embedded signal of all M EMG sensors,

$\tilde{x}(t) = [\tilde{x}_1(t), \ldots, \tilde{x}_M(t), 1]^T$ (including an offset term), and angular velocity $y(t)$ (either at the left or right ankle) was assumed to be linear according to the model $y(t) = \beta^T \tilde{x}(t)$. The $(K \cdot M + 1)$-dimensional coefficient vector $\beta^{OLS} = \left(\tilde{X} \tilde{X}^T \right)^{-1} \tilde{X} y^T$ was estimated using ordinary least-squares (OLS) regression, where $\tilde{X} = [\tilde{x}(1), \ldots, \tilde{x}(T)]$, $y = [y(1), \ldots, y(T)]$, and T denotes the number of available paired measurements of EMG and IMU activity in the training set. Using the fitted model, EMG-based IMU predictions were obtained as $\hat{y}(t) = \beta^{OLS^T} \tilde{x}(t)$.

2.7. Performance Analysis

Models were evaluated exclusively on hold-out data using leave-one-patient-out cross-validation (Figure 2, pink and red boxes). Models were fitted on the concatenated trials of all but one patient (training data) and were evaluated on all trials of the held-out (test) patient, where each patient served as the hold-out patient once. This evaluation scheme provided unbiased assessment of prediction performance. Model predictions $\hat{y}(t) = \beta^T \tilde{x}^*(t)$ were obtained by multiplying coefficient vector β estimated using the training data to embedded EMG data $\tilde{x}^*(t)$ from each trial of the test patient.

Predicted and ground-truth data were compared on a per-trial and leg basis using the Pearson correlation coefficient (r). Gait events (SWP, HC, and TO) were extracted from the predicted IMU time series as described in Section 2.5. Separately for each leg, ground-truth and predicted HC and TO events were used to divide each trial into alternating segments representing the swing and stance phases of the gait cycle. The resulting binary time series were compared using the F1-score (see also [34]). In addition, the absolute displacement between matching true and predicted events was measured. Matching events were defined as those being <600 ms apart from each other. Predicted events lacking a matching ground-truth counterpart were counted as false detections. The false discovery rate (FDR) was defined per event type as the number of false detections divided by the number of total event detections. Conversely, true events lacking matching prediction were counted as false negatives (misses). The false-negative rate (FNR) for each event type was defined as the number of missed events divided by the total number of true events.

3. Results

Ninety-three minutes of gait activity and 5253 full gait cycles were analyzed across the six patients. The median gait cycle duration ranged from 1045 to 1140 ms, corresponding to cadences between 51 and 59 cycles per minute (see Table 2). The gait cycle duration variability was measured as the median absolute deviation from the median duration and ranged from 10 to 30 ms.

Figure 3 illustrates the average activation patterns of individual muscles (measured by means of EMG) relative to the angular velocity profiles (measured by the IMUs). The upper panels show the average IMU and EMG activity across the gait cycles of all patients as a function of time within a cycle. All ten muscles exhibited stable activation patterns relative to the individual gait events of both legs. Importantly, due to the stable timing of the gait cycle in patients with mild PD, the left leg muscles showed precise activation in well-defined time windows regarding HC and TO events of the left and right leg, and vice versa. The Vl displayed particularly consistent timings (as indicated by dark red colors) both for the left and right legs. The lower panels depict cross-correlations (computed on the concatenated data of all trials) of temporally shifted EMG activity traces relative to the IMU signal. The same 21 lags were analyzed, ranging from −500 ms to +500 ms relative to the IMU signal reported above for the machine learning models. Thus, the depicted correlograms represent the independent linear predictive quality of each of the $10 \times 21 = 210$ EMG features considered in our models, thereby indicating the influence of each muscle and delay combination for prediction (see also [45]). The activity profiles of all ten individual muscles showed substantial positive and negative correlations with the IMU signal within a window of 1 sec. The highest absolute correlations were observed for the Vl. Specifically, left Vl activity lagged behind the left IMU trace by 150 ms (r = 0.78) and anticipated the right IMU trace by 350 ms (r = 0.76); in contrast, right Vl activity lagged behind the right IMU trace by 150 ms (r = 0.66) and anticipated the left IMU trace by 350 ms (r = 0.67). All reported cross-correlations were statistically significant ($p < 0.05$ after Bonferroni correction).

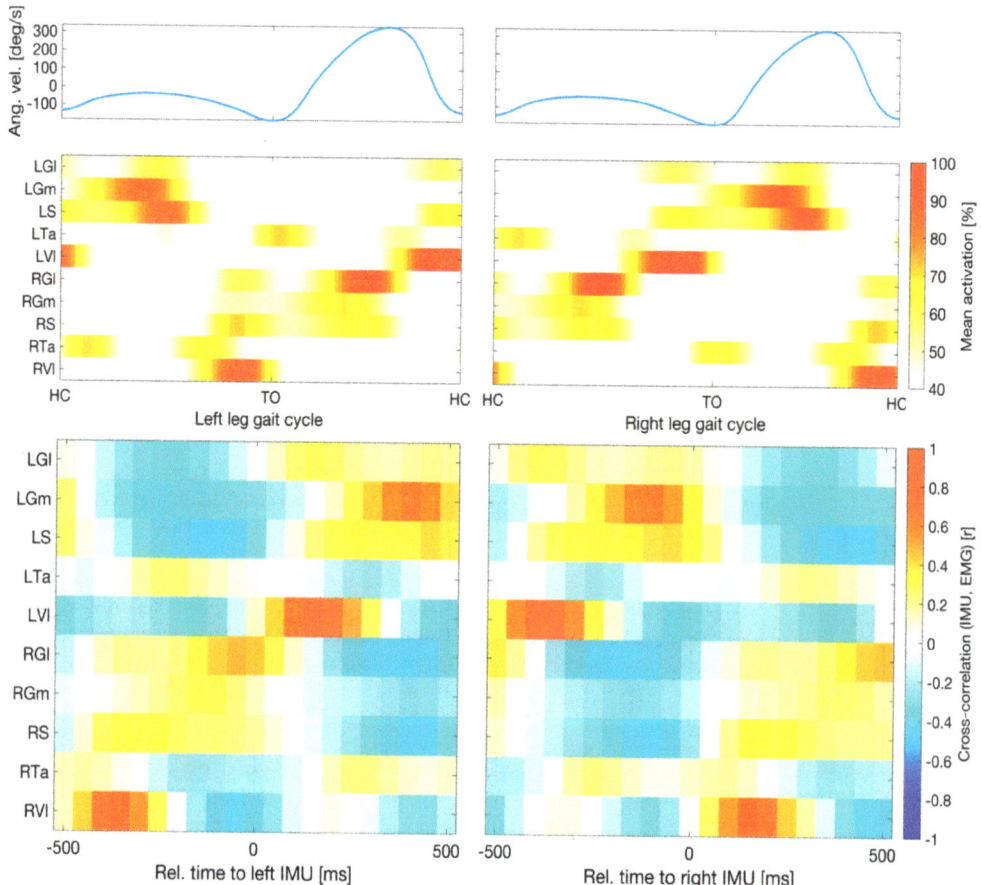

Figure 3. Relative timings of muscular and kinematic signals. Upper panels show average angular velocity measured by inertial measurement units (IMUs) and electromyographic (EMG) activity across all gait cycles of all patients as a function of time within a cycle. Percentages are relative to the 95th percentile of the raw data. Averages were cropped below 40%. All ten muscles exhibited stable activation patterns relative to the individual gait events of both legs. Lower panels depict cross-correlations (computed on the concatenated data of all trials) of temporally shifted EMG activity relative to the IMU signal. All ten muscles showed substantial absolute correlations with the IMU signal within a window of 1 sec. The highest correlations (Pearson correlation, r > 0.66) were observed for Vl activity with delays of 150 ms relative to the same leg or −350 ms relative to the opposing leg. Abbreviations: left and right gastrocnemius medialis (LGm and RGm) and lateralis (LGl and RGl); left and right soleus (LS and RS); left and right tibialis anterior (LTa and RTa); left and right vastus lateralis (LVl and RVl); TO, toe-off.

Table 2. Gait cycle statistics of individual patients.

	Median Gait Cycle Duration, ms	Cadence, Cycles/min	Gait Cycle Duration Variability, ms
WP1	1140	51	30
WP2	1050	57	15
WP3	1045	57	25
WP4	1080	54	30
WP5	1010	59	10
WP6	1095	55	25

Figure 4 shows an example segment of the preprocessed EMG and IMU data of one patient, the EMG-based predictions of the IMU time courses based on all ten available EMG probes, and the gait parameters extracted from true and predicted IMU time series. The EMG time courses of three selected individual muscles (bilateral Ta, S, and Vl) showed the clear periodic pattern of the gait cycle (bottom row). Out-of-sample predictions based on temporal embeddings of the activity of ten muscles showed a high correlation with the true IMU data (top row). Furthermore, gait events extracted from the predicted time series closely matched those extracted from the original IMU traces (top row). True and predicted gait phases based on the extracted events were consequently also closely aligned (center row). Results of similar quality were obtained when predictions were based on the left and right Vl only (see quantitative evaluation below).

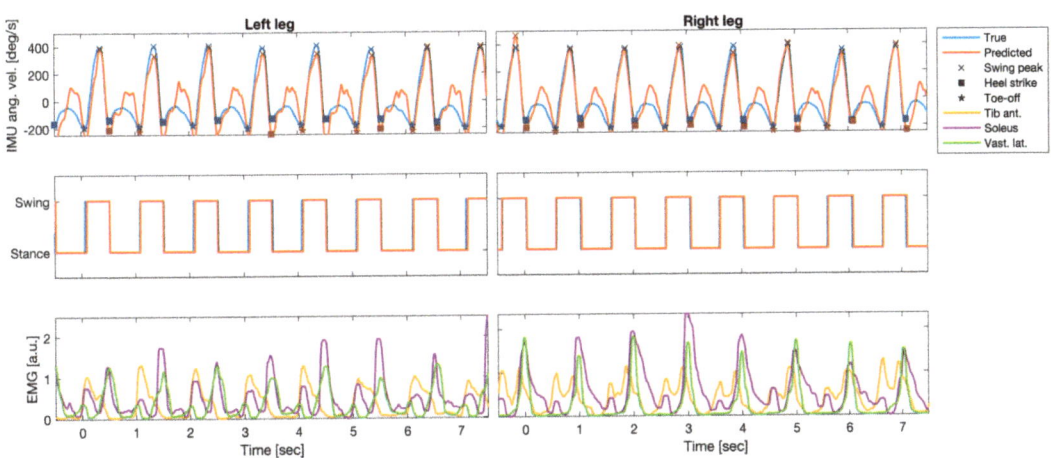

Figure 4. Example segment of preprocessed electromyography (EMG) and inertial measurement units (IMUs); angular velocity at the left and right anklebones (recordings of one patient (P5)), as well as the EMG-based predictions of the IMU time courses and the gait parameters extracted from true and predicted IMU time series. Top row: true IMU data and predictions derived from temporally embedded EMG activity of ten muscles. Predictions were derived from an ordinary least-squares regression model of fitted data of that had been fitted to data of the other five patients. Gait-related events (swing peak velocity (SWP), heel contact (HC), and toe-off (TO)) extracted from the predicted time series closely matched those extracted from the original IMU traces. Center row: True and predicted gait phases based on the extracted events were closely aligned. Bottom row: EMG time courses of three selected individual muscles (bilateral soleus, tibialis anterior, and vastus lateralis).

Figure 5 quantitatively summarizes the performance of EMG-based reconstructions of IMU time courses and gait events. The median (IQR across all 26 trials) Pearson correlation between measured and reconstructed IMU time courses, based on all ten muscles, was r = 0.80 (0.74 to 0.87) for the left ankle and r = 0.85 (0.78 to 0.90) for the right ankle. Using the left and right Vl, the performance was on par, with r = 0.86 (0.78 to 0.88) for the left IMU probe and r = 0.83 (0.80 to 0.88) for the right IMU probe. Using the left and right Ta and S muscles did not lead to competitive performance, with r = 0.47 (0.35 to 0.66) for the left IMU and r = 0.55 (0.46 to 0.66) for the right IMU. Importantly, the combination of left and right Vl was found to be on par with the full model for all the performance metrics, whereas the combination of S and Ta was competitive in none. For this reason, we restricted our reporting to the model comprising left and right Vl. With few exceptions, gait events could be reconstructed with median absolute temporal displacements of <50 ms using IMU predictions derived from this model. The median (IQR) displacement for SWP was 40 (20 to 60) ms for the left leg and 38 (25 to 60) ms for right leg. For HC events, median temporal displacements were 35 (25 to 55) ms for the left leg and 45 (30 to 60) ms for the right leg. For TO events, median displacements were 43 (30 to 100) ms for the left leg and 43 (20 to 95) ms for the right leg. Segmentations of the recordings into dichotomous gait phases based on detected HC and TO events were similar for measured and reconstructed IMU data. Median (IQR) F1-scores were 0.89 (0.87 to 0.93) for the left leg and 0.89 (0.86 to 0.93) for the right leg.

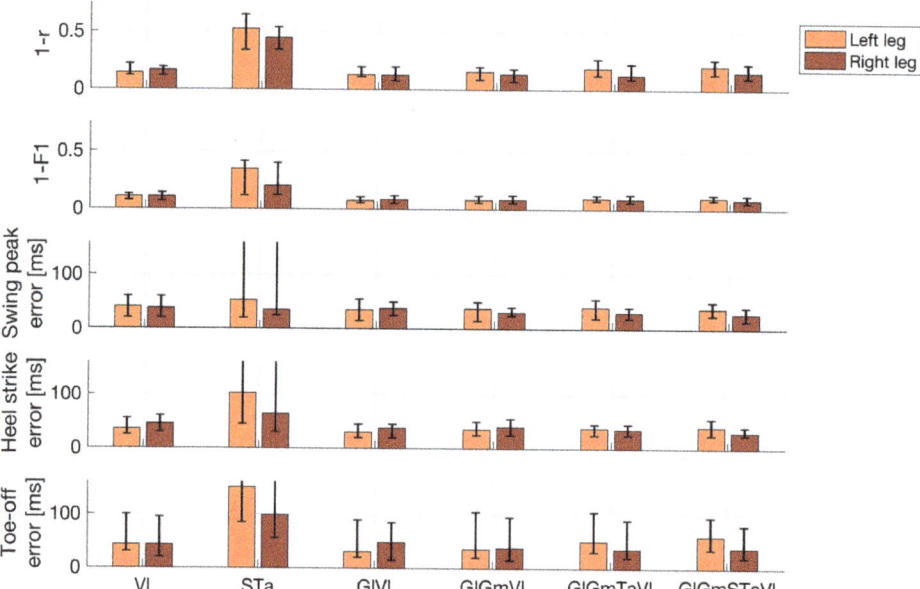

Figure 5. Performance of electromyography (EMG)-based reconstructions of inertial measurement unit (IMU) time courses and gait events. Lower numbers represent better performance. Top row: Pearson correlation (r) between measured and reconstructed angular velocity profiles of the left and right ankles. Second row: Accuracy of the reconstructed dichotomous (swing vs. stance) gait phases compared with the IMU-based ground truth, as measured by the F1-score. Bottom three rows: Absolute displacement of three types of events (swing peak velocity, heel contact, and toe-off) determined using reconstructed rather than measured IMU data. Results are shown separately for the left and right leg and for the best-performing prediction models utilizing between one and five pairs of EMG channels. In addition, results of the combination of the left and right soleus and tibialis anterior are also shown. Bar plots depict median performance across 26 walking trials of six patients in total, while overlaid whiskers depict first and third quartiles. Abbreviations: gastrocnemius medialis (Gm); lateralis (Gl); soleus (S); tibialis anterior (Ta); vastus lateralis (Vl).

Event detection errors were rare and did not occur in most trials. Across all trials, events were missed in 1.4% (n = 71; left leg) and 1.3% (n = 68; right leg) of cases. Numbers were nearly identical for all three event types, as HC and TO events were always determined relative to the two enclosing SWP events (see Section 2.5). False event discoveries were rare (<0.1% of the total events detected for both legs and all three event types). In absolute terms, between 2 and 4 out of over 5000 detected events were false discoveries.

4. Discussion

We have demonstrated the feasibility of accurately determining gait events such as HC and TO, defining the swing and stance phases of the gait cycle, in PD patients using a single pair of EMG probes placed bilaterally on the Vl muscle. Our proposed method may have substantial practical benefits in experimental setups in which EMG derivations are indispensable and where additional equipment for kinematic analysis (e.g., foot switches, IMUs, or a motion-capturing system) is either unavailable or would introduce undesired complexity, especially in severely ill patients. Furthermore, robust acquisition of EMG signals is necessary in experimental and commercial applications to achieve control of myoelectric interfaces for neuroprosthetics [29], including future adaptive DBS devices [30].

Rather than framing the prediction problem as one of binary classification [34], our approach consisted of two steps: First, the angular velocity at the left and right anklebones was predicted using the activity of between two and ten EMG probes. This mapping was learned a priori from training data for which both EMG and IMU recordings were available. Using carefully designed data features (temporally embedded, smoothed muscle activation time courses), a simple linear regression approach was found to be suitable to achieve sufficient reconstruction performance. Second, predefined rules were used to extract prominent events and the main phases of the gait cycle. These rules accommodate domain knowledge about the timing of events relative to each other, which constitutes a substantial advantage over algorithms that are completely naïve to the underlying data, framing gait cycle prediction as an abstract classification problem. Importantly, our approach does not require any calibration involving real IMU data, as models fitted a priori on a training cohort (e.g., the data reported here) can be readily applied to new patients. Due to the simplicity of our model, its application amounts to a simple linear filtering of the appropriately recorded and preprocessed EMG data and does not require any advanced machine learning software. In addition, our approach of approximating IMU time courses instead of individual events or categorial segmentation labels offers numerous additional advantages. These include the direct interpretation of the predicted time courses in terms of gait mechanics. Potential failure modes of the model (e.g., due to misplaced or noisy EMG probes) can easily be detected through visual inspection of the predicted time courses. Since SWP could be accurately detected even using reconstructed angular velocities and HC and TO were defined relative to SWP, our system achieved low numbers of event-detection errors and high overall accuracy regarding the determination of gait phases. It is also likely that our approach could be generalized to the extraction of other biomechanically relevant parameters of the upper and lower extremities.

Contrary to our prediction, the EMG profiles of the S and Ta muscles were insufficient to reliably identify major gait cycle events in parkinsonian patients. We based this hypothesis on the distinctive and synergistic activity of these two monoarticular (i.e., ankle) muscles during human locomotion. Indeed, normal EMG activity of the plantar flexors has been reported to mainly occur during the stance phase. In this phase, the triceps surae restrains the tibial rotation controlling for disequilibrium torque, which is responsible for propelling the body [46,47]. The ankle dorsi-flexors are instead mainly active during the swing phase, controlling for sufficient foot clearance, with an additional contribution in the loading response phase for the lowering of the foot to the ground after HC [48], thus assisting the forward momentum of the tibia during the heel rocker action at the ankle [49]. These muscles, however, may show large stride-to-stride variability in EMG profiles [48], especially in patients with PD [50,51]. In particular, a great intra- and inter-subject variability of Ta activity during gait has been described in parkinsonian patients in the meds-off state [50].

The prediction model did not improve when replacing the S muscle with the Gm or Gl or by adding this muscle to the S-Ta pair (data not shown). This was unexpected because while the S muscle may provide less forward propulsion with physiological aging, the gastrocnemius muscle has been shown to maintain its contribution to initiating swinging limb movement [52,53], thus possibly allowing kinematic events to be more accurately detected. Rodriguez and colleagues demonstrated a simplification of modular control of locomotion in PD with individual muscle contribution of the gastrocnemius, but not the S, among ankle plantar flexors and the semimembranosus and biceps femoris for knee flexor musculature [54].

In our study, EMG recordings of the Vl provided the most accurate prediction of IMU times series and gait events. The action pattern of this muscle during the gait cycle paralleled the activation of the Ta but was more selectively confined to the HC. This muscle controls the knee flexion that occurs after HC and ensures knee extension during terminal swing to prepare for ground contact [49,55].

In principle, there are an infinite number of different combinations of muscle activation that can be applied to maintain a particular posture or produce a given movement [56]. However, despite the apparent redundancy, four or five component activity patterns may be distributed to all the muscles that are specifically activated during locomotion; thus, the activation of each muscle involves a dynamic weighting of these basic patterns [57,58]. Interestingly, Ta, S, and Vl contributed differently to these factors [57,58]. Our results suggest that characteristic activity patterns of one pair—left and right Vl—are sufficient for the proper detection of gait events in patients with PD (H&Y: I–III).

Limitations

Our study is somewhat limited by the fact that IMU data are not considered the "gold standard" for defining ground-truth gait parameters. Force plates would have allowed the precise detection of HC and TO events, and possibly of the individual muscle contribution to ground reaction forces, to be performed [59,60]. However, it would have been impracticable to record the high number of steps and total gait time acquired in our study using force plates. IMU systems are sufficiently accurate in the assessment of fundamental gait spatiotemporal parameters [23,61] and have previously been used as ground truth for gait event detection [62]. Furthermore, they allow the SWP event to be detected, which cannot be captured by ground devices, foot switches, or insole pressure sensors.

The proposed approach was not tested on healthy control data. However, we expect our model to effectively predict gait events in healthy controls, as patient data are more heterogeneous and generally more challenging in terms of gait alterations, and inter-subject and inter-trial variability, as well as artifact contamination.

We were also only able to recruit a few patients for this study. However, it should be considered that walking for over three minutes in the meds-off state is very challenging for subjects with PD and greatly limited patient recruitment. Another limitation was the relatively homogeneous walking speed across all patients. We preferred not to alter the patients' natural speed, because we wanted to test our model in an ecological setup. In addition, the meds-off state limited the recording window and the possibility of exploring more than one gait condition. It is thus presently unclear how well our prediction model would perform for different speeds when applied out of the box. However, it is straightforward to adapt the model to different speeds by either temporally adjusting the embedding delays ($\tau_1, \ldots, \tau_K$) of test participants to their individual walking speed or retraining the model on data with matching speed.

5. Conclusions

We have demonstrated the accurate and robust detection of gait events in six parkinsonian patients using just two EMG probes placed on the left and right vastus lateralis. Unlike solutions presented in previous work, our approach proceeds in two steps: First, IMU time courses are predicted using EMG activity within a surrounding temporal window using multiple linear regressions. Second, gait parameters such as heel strike and toe-off events are extracted from the predicted time series. This approach led to accurate results and has the advantage over previous ones that discrete gait events and continuous time series of relevant kinematic quantities can be predicted. It is further expected that it could be generalized to the extraction of further gait parameters not considered here without any model retraining. Our model and an example dataset, as well as Matlab code for data preprocessing, model training, model evaluation, and plotting, have been made publicly available under https://github.com/braindatalab/EMGgaitprediction (accessed on 4 February 2023). Our approach may have practical benefits for gait studies in which the application of multiple sensing devices is considered impractical, troublesome, or too expensive. Notably, our model was validated using a leave-one-patient-out strategy. We observed very good performance in held-out patients, demonstrating that the model is able to accommodate the across-patient variability of the studied clinical population. Future work could adapt our approach to varying walking speeds and may further extend it to the prediction of other kinematic data obtained using EMG.

Author Contributions: Conceptualization, S.H. and I.U.I.; methodology, S.H., C.P. and I.U.I.; software, S.H.; formal analysis, S.H. and F.P.; investigation, C.P. and I.U.I.; resources, S.H., C.P. and I.U.I.; data curation, C.P.; writing—original draft preparation, S.H. and I.U.I.; writing—review and editing, S.H., C.P., F.P. and I.U.I.; visualization, S.H. and C.P.; supervision, C.P.; project administration, I.U.I.; funding acquisition, S.H., C.P. and I.U.I. All authors have read and agreed to the published version of the manuscript.

Funding: This study was sponsored by Deutsche Forschungsgemeinschaft (DFG; German Research Foundation) Project-ID 424778381-TRR 295 and Fondazione Grigioni per il Morbo di Parkinson. S.H. received funding from the European Research Council (ERC) under the European Union's Horizon 2020 research and innovation program (grant agreement No. 758985). C.P. was supported by a grant from German Excellence Initiative to the Graduate School of Life Sciences, University of Würzburg. I.U.I. received funding from New York University School of Medicine and The Marlene and Paolo Fresco Institute for Parkinson's and Movement Disorders, which was made possible with support from Marlene and Paolo Fresco.

Institutional Review Board Statement: The study was conducted in accordance with the Declaration of Helsinki and approved by the Ethics Committee of University of Würzburg (Nos. 103/20 and 36/17).

Informed Consent Statement: Informed consent was obtained from all subjects involved in the study.

Data Availability Statement: The data presented in this study are available upon request from the corresponding author. The data are not publicly available for privacy reasons.

Acknowledgments: We would like to thank all patients and caregivers for their participation. The draft manuscript was edited for English language by Deborah Nock (Medical WriteAway, Norwich, UK).

Conflicts of Interest: The authors declare no conflict of interest. The funders had no role in the design of the study; in the collection, analyses, or interpretation of data; in the writing of the manuscript; or in the decision to publish the results.

References

1. Wood, B.H.; Bilclough, J.A.; Bowron, A.; Walker, R.W. Incidence and Prediction of Falls in Parkinson's Disease: A Prospective Multidisciplinary Study. *J. Neurol. Neurosurg. Psychiatry* **2002**, *72*, 721–725. [CrossRef] [PubMed]
2. Giladi, N.; Balash, J.; Hausdorff, J.M. *Gait Disturbances in Parkinson's Disease BT—Mapping the Progress of Alzheimer's and Parkinson's Disease*; Mizuno, Y., Fisher, A., Hanin, I., Eds.; Springer US: Boston, MA, USA, 2002; pp. 329–335. ISBN 978-0-306-47593-1.

3. Pötter-Nerger, M.; Volkmann, J. Deep Brain Stimulation for Gait and Postural Symptoms in Parkinson's Disease. *Mov. Disord.* **2013**, *28*, 1609–1615. [CrossRef]
4. Karachi, C.; Cormier-Dequaire, F.; Grabli, D.; Lau, B.; Belaid, H.; Navarro, S.; Vidailhet, M.; Bardinet, E.; Fernandez-Vidal, S.; Welter, M.-L. Clinical and Anatomical Predictors for Freezing of Gait and Falls after Subthalamic Deep Brain Stimulation in Parkinson's Disease Patients. *Park. Relat. Disord.* **2019**, *62*, 91–97. [CrossRef]
5. Curtze, C.; Nutt, J.G.; Carlson-Kuhta, P.; Mancini, M.; Horak, F.B. Levodopa Is a Double-Edged Sword for Balance and Gait in People With Parkinson's Disease. *Mov. Disord.* **2015**, *30*, 1361–1370. [CrossRef]
6. Creaby, M.W.; Cole, M.H. Gait Characteristics and Falls in Parkinson's Disease: A Systematic Review and Meta-Analysis. *Park. Relat. Disord.* **2018**, *57*, 1–8. [CrossRef]
7. Palmisano, C.; Brandt, G.; Pozzi, N.G.; Alice, L.; Maltese, V.; Andrea, C.; Jens, V.; Pezzoli, G.; Frigo, C.A.; Isaias, I.U. Sit-to-Walk Performance in Parkinson's Disease: A Comparison between Faller and Non-Faller Patients. *Clin. Biomech.* **2019**, *63*, 140–146. [CrossRef] [PubMed]
8. Dipaola, M.; Pavan, E.E.; Cattaneo, A.; Frazzitta, G.; Pezzoli, G.; Cavallari, P.; Frigo, C.A.; Isaias, I.U. Mechanical Energy Recovery during Walking in Patients with Parkinson Disease. *PLoS ONE* **2016**, *11*, e0156420. [CrossRef] [PubMed]
9. Isaias, I.U.; Volkmann, J.; Marzegan, A.; Marotta, G.; Cavallari, P.; Pezzoli, G. The Influence of Dopaminergic Striatal Innervation on Upper Limb Locomotor Synergies. *PLoS ONE* **2012**, *7*, e51464. [CrossRef]
10. Mirelman, A.; Bonato, P.; Camicioli, R.; Ellis, T.D.; Giladi, N.; Hamilton, J.L.; Hass, C.J.; Hausdorff, J.M.; Pelosin, E.; Almeida, Q.J. Gait Impairments in Parkinson's Disease. *Lancet Neurol.* **2019**, *18*, 697–708. [CrossRef]
11. Nordin, A.D.; Hairston, W.D.; Ferris, D.P. Dual-Electrode Motion Artifact Cancellation for Mobile Electroencephalography. *J. Neural Eng.* **2018**, *15*, 056024. [CrossRef]
12. Jacobsen, N.S.J.; Blum, S.; Witt, K.; Debener, S. A Walk in the Park? Characterizing Gait-Related Artifacts in Mobile EEG Recordings. *Eur. J. Neurosci.* **2020**, *54*, 8421–8440. [CrossRef] [PubMed]
13. Arlotti, M.; Palmisano, C.; Minafra, B.; Todisco, M.; Pacchetti, C.; Canessa, A.; Pozzi, N.G.; Cilia, R.; Prenassi, M.; Marceglia, S.; et al. Monitoring Subthalamic Oscillations for 24 Hours in a Freely Moving Parkinson's Disease Patient. *Mov. Disord.* **2019**, *34*, 757–759. [CrossRef] [PubMed]
14. Canessa, A.; Pozzi, N.G.; Arnulfo, G.; Brumberg, J.; Reich, M.M.; Pezzoli, G.; Ghilardi, M.F.; Matthies, C.; Steigerwald, F.; Volkmann, J.; et al. Striatal Dopaminergic Innervation Regulates Subthalamic Beta-Oscillations and Cortical-Subcortical Coupling during Movements: Preliminary Evidence in Subjects with Parkinson's Disease. *Front. Hum. Neurosci.* **2016**, *10*, 611. [CrossRef] [PubMed]
15. Thenaisie, Y.; Palmisano, C.; Canessa, A.; Keulen, B.J.; Capetian, P.; Jiménez, M.C.; Bally, J.F.; Manferlotti, E.; Beccaria, L.; Zutt, R.; et al. Towards Adaptive Deep Brain Stimulation: Clinical and Technical Notes on a Novel Commercial Device for Chronic Brain Sensing. *J. Neural Eng.* **2021**, medRxiv:2021.03.10.21251638. [CrossRef] [PubMed]
16. Pozzi, N.G.; Canessa, A.; Palmisano, C.; Brumberg, J.; Steigerwald, F.; Reich, M.M.; Minafra, B.; Pacchetti, C.; Pezzoli, G.; Volkmann, J.; et al. Freezing of Gait in Parkinson's Disease Reflects a Sudden Derangement of Locomotor Network Dynamics. *Brain* **2019**, *142*, 2037–2050. [CrossRef]
17. Arnulfo, G.; Pozzi, N.G.; Palmisano, C.; Leporini, A.; Canessa, A.; Brumberg, J.; Pezzoli, G.; Matthies, C.; Volkmann, J.; Isaias, I.U. Phase Matters: A Role for the Subthalamic Network during Gait. *PLoS ONE* **2018**, *13*, 1–19. [CrossRef]
18. Canessa, A.; Palmisano, C.; Isaias, I.U.; Mazzoni, A. Gait-Related Frequency Modulation of Beta Oscillatory Activity in the Subthalamic Nucleus of Parkinsonian Patients. *Brain Stimulation* **2020**, *13*, 1743–1752. [CrossRef]
19. Palmisano, C.; Kullmann, P.; Hanafi, I.; Verrecchia, M.; Latoschik, M.E.; Canessa, A.; Fischbach, M.; Isaias, I.U. A Fully-Immersive Virtual Reality Setup to Study Gait Modulation. *Front. Hum. Neurosci.* **2022**, *16*, 783452. [CrossRef]
20. Dockx, K.; Bekkers, E.M.; Van den Bergh, V.; Ginis, P.; Rochester, L.; Hausdorff, J.M.; Mirelman, A.; Nieuwboer, A. Virtual Reality for Rehabilitation in Parkinson's Disease. *Cochrane Database Syst. Rev.* **2016**, *12*, CD010760. [CrossRef]
21. Sampath Dakshina Murthy, A.; Karthikeyan, T.; Vinoth Kanna, R. Gait-Based Person Fall Prediction Using Deep Learning Approach. *Soft Comput.* **2022**, *26*, 12933–12941. [CrossRef]
22. Anwary, A.R.; Yu, H.; Vassallo, M. Optimal Foot Location for Placing Wearable IMU Sensors and Automatic Feature Extraction for Gait Analysis. *IEEE Sens. J.* **2018**, *18*, 2555–2567. [CrossRef]
23. Zago, M.; Sforza, C.; Pacifici, I.; Cimolin, V.; Camerota, F.; Celletti, C.; Condoluci, C.; De Pandis, M.F.; Galli, M. Gait Evaluation Using Inertial Measurement Units in Subjects with Parkinson's Disease. *J. Electromyogr. Kinesiol.* **2018**, *42*, 44–48. [CrossRef] [PubMed]
24. Yokoyama, H.; Yoshida, T.; Zabjek, K.; Chen, R.; Masani, K. Defective Corticomuscular Connectivity during Walking in Patients with Parkinson's Disease. *J. Neurophysiol.* **2020**, *124*, 1399–1414. [CrossRef] [PubMed]
25. Wentink, E.C.; Schut, V.G.H.; Prinsen, E.C.; Rietman, J.S.; Veltink, P.H. Detection of the Onset of Gait Initiation Using Kinematic Sensors and EMG in Transfemoral Amputees. *Gait Posture* **2014**, *39*, 391–396. [CrossRef]
26. Wentink, E.C.; Beijen, S.I.; Hermens, H.J.; Rietman, J.S.; Veltink, P.H. Intention Detection of Gait Initiation Using EMG and Kinematic Data. *Gait Posture* **2013**, *37*, 223–228. [CrossRef]
27. Zhang, F.; Huang, H. Source Selection for Real-Time User Intent Recognition toward Volitional Control of Artificial Legs. *IEEE J. Biomed. Health Inform.* **2013**, *17*, 907–914. [CrossRef]

28. Huang, H.; Zhang, F.; Hargrove, L.J.; Dou, Z.; Rogers, D.R.; Englehart, K.B. Continuous Locomotion-Mode Identification for Prosthetic Legs Based on Neuromuscular-Mechanical Fusion. *IEEE Trans. Bio-Med. Eng.* **2011**, *58*, 2867–2875. [CrossRef]
29. Ison, M.; Artemiadis, P. The Role of Muscle Synergies in Myoelectric Control: Trends and Challenges for Simultaneous Multifunction Control. *J. Neural Eng.* **2014**, *11*, 051001. [CrossRef]
30. Vissani, M.; Isaias, I.U.; Mazzoni, A. Deep Brain Stimulation: A Review of the Open Neural Engineering Challenges. *J. Neural Eng.* **2020**, *17*, 051002. [CrossRef]
31. Swann, N.C.; de Hemptinne, C.; Miocinovic, S.; Qasim, S.; Ostrem, J.L.; Galifianakis, N.B.; Luciano, M.S.; Wang, S.S.; Ziman, N.; Taylor, R.; et al. Chronic Multisite Brain Recordings from a Totally Implantable Bidirectional Neural Interface: Experience in 5 Patients with Parkinson's Disease. *J. Neurosurg.* **2018**, *128*, 605–616. [CrossRef]
32. Nieuwboer, A.; Dom, R.; De Weerdt, W.; Desloovere, K.; Janssens, L.; Stijn, V. Electromyographic Profiles of Gait Prior to Onset of Freezing Episodes in Patients with Parkinson's Disease. *Brain* **2004**, *127*, 1650–1660. [CrossRef]
33. Brantley, J.A.; Luu, T.P.; Nakagome, S.; Contreras-Vidal, J.L. Prediction of Lower-Limb Joint Kinematics from Surface EMG during Overground Locomotion. In Proceedings of the 2017 IEEE International Conference on Systems, Man, and Cybernetics (SMC), Banff, AB, Canada, 5–8 October 2017; pp. 1705–1709.
34. Di Nardo, F.; Morbidoni, C.; Mascia, G.; Verdini, F.; Fioretti, S. Intra-Subject Approach for Gait-Event Prediction by Neural Network Interpretation of EMG Signals. *BioMedical Eng. Online* **2020**, *19*, 58. [CrossRef]
35. Morbidoni, C.; Cucchiarelli, A.; Fioretti, S.; Di Nardo, F. A Deep Learning Approach to EMG-Based Classification of Gait Phases during Level Ground Walking. *Electronics* **2019**, *8*, 894. [CrossRef]
36. Meng, M.; She, Q.; Gao, Y.; Luo, Z. EMG Signals Based Gait Phases Recognition Using Hidden Markov Models. In Proceedings of the 2010 IEEE International Conference on Information and Automation, ICIA 2010, Harbin, China, 20–23 June 2010; pp. 852–856. [CrossRef]
37. Nazmi, N.; Abdul Rahman, M.A.; Yamamoto, S.I.; Ahmad, S.A. Walking Gait Event Detection Based on Electromyography Signals Using Artificial Neural Network. *Biomed. Signal Process. Control* **2019**, *47*, 334–343. [CrossRef]
38. Ziegier, J.; Gattringer, H.; Mueller, A. Classification of Gait Phases Based on Bilateral EMG Data Using Support Vector Machines. In Proceedings of the IEEE RAS and EMBS International Conference on Biomedical Robotics and Biomechatronics, Enschede, The Netherlands, 26–29 August 2018; pp. 978–983. [CrossRef]
39. Crenna, P.; Frigo, C. A Motor Programme for the Initiation of Forward-Oriented Movements in Humans. *J. Physiol.* **1991**, *437*, 635–653. [CrossRef]
40. Winter, D.A.; Yack, H.J. EMG Profiles during Normal Human Walking: Stride-to-Stride and Inter-Subject Variability. *Electroencephalogr. Clin. Neurophysiol.* **1987**, *67*, 402–411. [CrossRef]
41. Ahn, A.N.; Kang, J.K.; Quitt, M.A.; Davidson, B.C.; Nguyen, C.T. Variability of Neural Activation during Walking in Humans: Short Heels and Big Calves. *Biol. Lett.* **2011**, *7*, 7539–7542. [CrossRef]
42. Hug, F.; Del Vecchio, A.; Avrillon, S.; Farina, D.; Tucker, K. Muscles from the Same Muscle Group Do Not Necessarily Share Common Drive: Evidence from the Human Triceps Surae. *J. Appl. Physiol.* **2021**, *130*, 342–354. [CrossRef]
43. Rueterbories, J.; Spaich, E.G.; Larsen, B.; Andersen, O.K. Methods for Gait Event Detection and Analysis in Ambulatory Systems. *Med. Eng. Phys.* **2010**, *32*, 545–552. [CrossRef]
44. Cereatti, A.; Trojaniello, D.; Croce, U. Della Accurately Measuring Human Movement Using Magneto-Inertial Sensors: Techniques and Challenges. In Proceedings of the 2nd IEEE International Symposium on Inertial Sensors and Systems, IEEE ISISS 2015—Proceedings, Hapuna Beach, HI, USA, 23–26 March 2015; pp. 15–18. [CrossRef]
45. Haufe, S.; Meinecke, F.; Görgen, K.; Dähne, S.; Haynes, J.D.; Blankertz, B.; Bießmann, F. On the Interpretation of Weight Vectors of Linear Models in Multivariate Neuroimaging. *NeuroImage* **2014**, *87*, 96–110. [CrossRef]
46. Honeine, J.L.; Schieppati, M.; Gagey, O.; Do, M.C. The Functional Role of the Triceps Surae Muscle during Human Locomotion. *PLoS ONE* **2013**, *8*. [CrossRef]
47. Honeine, J.-L.; Schieppati, M.; Gagey, O.; Do, M.-C. By Counteracting Gravity, Triceps Surae Sets Both Kinematics and Kinetics of Gait. *Physiol. Rep.* **2014**, *2*, e00329. [CrossRef] [PubMed]
48. Di Nardo, F.; Ghetti, G.; Fioretti, S. Assessment of the Activation Modalities of Gastrocnemius Lateralis and Tibialis Anterior during Gait: A Statistical Analysis. *J. Electromyogr. Kinesiol.* **2013**, *23*, 1428–1433. [CrossRef] [PubMed]
49. Chleboun, G.S.; Busic, A.B.; Graham, K.K.; Stuckey, H.A. Fascicle Length Change of the Human Tibialis Anterior and Vastus Lateralis during Walking. *J. Orthop. Sport. Phys. Ther.* **2007**, *37*, 372–379. [CrossRef]
50. Caliandro, P.; Ferrarin, M.; Cioni, M.; Bentivoglio, A.R.; Minciotti, I.; D'Urso, P.I.; Tonali, P.A.; Padua, L. Levodopa Effect on Electromyographic Activation Patterns of Tibialis Anterior Muscle during Walking in Parkinson's Disease. *Gait Posture* **2011**, *33*, 436–441. [CrossRef] [PubMed]
51. Islam, A.; Alcock, L.; Nazarpour, K.; Rochester, L.; Pantall, A. Effect of Parkinson's Disease and Two Therapeutic Interventions on Muscle Activity during Walking: A Systematic Review. *Npj Park. Dis.* **2020**, *6*, 22. [CrossRef]
52. Neptune, R.R.; Kautz, S.A.; Zajac, F.E. Contributions of the Individual Ankle Plantar Flexors to Support, Forward Progression and Swing Initiation during Walking. *J. Biomech.* **2001**, *34*, 1387–1398. [CrossRef]
53. Schmitz, A.; Silder, A.; Heiderscheit, B.; Mahoney, J.; Thelen, D.G. Differences in Lower-Extremity Muscular Activation during Walking between Healthy Older and Young Adults. *J. Electromyogr. Kinesiol.* **2009**, *19*, 1085–1091. [CrossRef]

54. Rodriguez, K.L.; Roemmich, R.T.; Cam, B.; Fregly, B.J.; Hass, C.J. Persons with Parkinson's Disease Exhibit Decreased Neuromuscular Complexity during Gait. *Clin. Neurophysiol.* **2013**, *124*, 1390–1397. [CrossRef] [PubMed]
55. Cioni, M.; Richards, C.L.; Malouin, F.; Bedard, P.J.; Lemieux, R. Characteristics of the Electromyographic Patterns of Lower Limb Muscles during Gait in Patients with Parkinson's Disease When OFF and ON L-Dopa Treatment. *Ital. J. Neurol. Sci.* **1997**, *18*, 195–208. [CrossRef] [PubMed]
56. Guigon, E. Models and Architectures for Motor ControlSimple or Complex? In *Motor Control*; Danion, F., Mark, L., Eds.; Oxford University Press: Oxford, UK, 2010; pp. 478–502. ISBN 978-0-19-539527-3.
57. Ivanenko, Y.P.; Poppele, R.E.; Lacquaniti, F. Five Basic Muscle Activation Patterns Account for Muscle Activity during Human Locomotion. *J. Physiol.* **2004**, *556*, 267–282. [CrossRef]
58. Roemmich, R.T.; Fregly, B.J.; Hass, C.J. Neuromuscular Complexity during Gait Is Not Responsive to Medication in Persons with Parkinson's Disease. *Ann. Biomed. Eng.* **2014**, *42*, 1901–1912. [CrossRef] [PubMed]
59. Moissenet, F.; Dumas, R. Individual Contributions of the Lower Limb Muscles to the Position of the Centre of Pressure during Gait. *Comput. Methods Biomech. Biomed. Eng.* **2017**, *20*, 137–138. [CrossRef]
60. Farinelli, V.; Hosseinzadeh, L.; Palmisano, C.; Frigo, C. An Easily Applicable Method to Analyse the Ankle-Foot Power Absorption and Production during Walking. *Gait Posture* **2019**, *71*, 56–61. [CrossRef] [PubMed]
61. Storm, F.A.; Buckley, C.J.; Mazzà, C. Gait Event Detection in Laboratory and Real Life Settings: Accuracy of Ankle and Waist Sensor Based Methods. *Gait Posture* **2016**, *50*, 42–46. [CrossRef] [PubMed]
62. Storm, F.A.; Heller, B.W.; Mazzà, C. Step Detection and Activity Recognition Accuracy of Seven Physical Activity Monitors. *PLoS ONE* **2015**, *10*, e0118723. [CrossRef]

Disclaimer/Publisher's Note: The statements, opinions and data contained in all publications are solely those of the individual author(s) and contributor(s) and not of MDPI and/or the editor(s). MDPI and/or the editor(s) disclaim responsibility for any injury to people or property resulting from any ideas, methods, instructions or products referred to in the content.

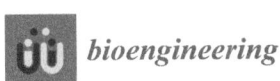

Article

Walking Speed Classification from Marker-Free Video Images in Two-Dimension Using Optimum Data and a Deep Learning Method

Tasriva Sikandar [1], Sam Matiur Rahman [2], Dilshad Islam [3], Md. Asraf Ali [4], Md. Abdullah Al Mamun [5], Mohammad Fazle Rabbi [6], Kamarul H. Ghazali [1], Omar Altwijri [7], Mohammed Almijalli [7] and Nizam U. Ahamed [8,*]

1. Faculty of Electrical and Electronics Engineering, University of Malaysia Pahang, Pekan 26600, Malaysia
2. Department of Software Engineering, Daffodil International University (DIU), Dhaka 1341, Bangladesh
3. Department of Physical and Mathematical Sciences, Chattogram Veterinary and Animal Sciences University (CVASU), Chattogram 4225, Bangladesh
4. Department of Computer Science, American International University-Bangladesh (AIUB), Dhaka 1229, Bangladesh
5. Electronics Division, Atomic Energy Centre, Dhaka 1000, Bangladesh
6. School of Health Sciences and Social Work, Griffith University, Gold Coast, QLD 4222, Australia
7. Biomedical Technology Department, College of Applied Medical Sciences, King Saud University, Riyadh 11451, Saudi Arabia
8. Department of Radiation Oncology, School of Medicine, University of Pittsburgh, Pittsburgh, PA 15232, USA
* Correspondence: nizamahamed@pitt.edu

Citation: Sikandar, T.; Rahman, S.M.; Islam, D.; Ali, M.A.; Mamun, M.A.A.; Rabbi, M.F.; Ghazali, K.H.; Altwijri, O.; Almijalli, M.; Ahamed, N.U. Walking Speed Classification from Marker-Free Video Images in Two-Dimension Using Optimum Data and a Deep Learning Method. Bioengineering 2022, 9, 715. https://doi.org/10.3390/bioengineering9110715

Academic Editors: Christina Zong-Hao Ma, Zhengrong Li, Chen He and Chunfeng Zhao

Received: 23 September 2022
Accepted: 16 November 2022
Published: 19 November 2022

Publisher's Note: MDPI stays neutral with regard to jurisdictional claims in published maps and institutional affiliations.

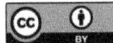

Copyright: © 2022 by the authors. Licensee MDPI, Basel, Switzerland. This article is an open access article distributed under the terms and conditions of the Creative Commons Attribution (CC BY) license (https://creativecommons.org/licenses/by/4.0/).

Abstract: Walking speed is considered a reliable assessment tool for any movement-related functional activities of an individual (i.e., patients and healthy controls) by caregivers and clinicians. Traditional video surveillance gait monitoring in clinics and aged care homes may employ modern artificial intelligence techniques to utilize walking speed as a screening indicator of various physical outcomes or accidents in individuals. Specifically, ratio-based body measurements of walking individuals are extracted from marker-free and two-dimensional video images to create a walk pattern suitable for walking speed classification using deep learning based artificial intelligence techniques. However, the development of successful and highly predictive deep learning architecture depends on the optimal use of extracted data because redundant data may overburden the deep learning architecture and hinder the classification performance. The aim of this study was to investigate the optimal combination of ratio-based body measurements needed for presenting potential information to define and predict a walk pattern in terms of speed with high classification accuracy using a deep learning-based walking speed classification model. To this end, the performance of different combinations of five ratio-based body measurements was evaluated through a correlation analysis and a deep learning-based walking speed classification test. The results show that a combination of three ratio-based body measurements can potentially define and predict a walk pattern in terms of speed with classification accuracies greater than 92% using a bidirectional long short-term memory deep learning method.

Keywords: two-dimensional (2D) image; marker-free video; walking speed; walking speed classification; bi-LSTM; deep learning; redundant feature; ratio-based body measurement; optimal feature

1. Introduction

Human gait factors of both healthy individuals and patients, such as the stride length, cadence, stance, swing periods, and hip, knee ankle and pelvic tilt joint kinematics, exhibit significant alterations in response to changes in the walking speed [1,2]. For example, healthy individuals exhibit decreases and increases in the amplitudes of cadence, step and stride lengths, stance and swing periods at slower and faster speeds, respectively [3,4].

In addition, changes in walking circumstances do not appear to alter the walking speed of healthy individuals but may have an impact on the walking speed of an individual with a physical impairment who is walking at the same speed. For instance, patients with neurological disorders such as Alzheimer's disease and neuromuscular problems, including post-stroke and cerebral palsy, exhibit a slower walking speed than healthy controls [5–7]. Additionally, in individuals older than 60 years, a slower walking speed is predictive of increased morbidity and mortality [8]. For this reason, walking speed has long been used by clinicians as a straightforward but efficient gait assessment tool for determining demographic traits (such as gender and age) and physical functions including spatiotemporal parameters as well as kinematic and kinetic patterns [5,6,9–11]. Most importantly, by combining cutting-edge artificial intelligence techniques (such as deep learning) and conventional video (i.e., two-dimensional [2D] videos or image sequences) surveillance, the walking speed can be used as an independent screening tool for several physical consequences or accidents (e.g., fall-related fear) among healthy individuals and patients with conditions such as Parkinson's disease and osteoarthritis during day-to-day gait monitoring in healthcare centres and old-age homes. Specifically, body measurement data of walking individuals (e.g., healthy or patients) extracted from 2D marker-free video image sequences can be considered sequential gait data [12,13] for the creation of walk pattern suitable for walking speed classification using artificial intelligence techniques, and the method may be applied in healthcare settings and elderly care facilities [13].

Numerous studies have researched walking gait using body measurements from 2D video or image sequence setups with a focus on speed-related factors and without the use of artificial intelligence approaches [14,15]. The extracted body measurement data from these studies include unilateral hip, knee, ankle and pelvic tilt joint kinematics [14] and body measurement data (e.g., lower-body width) of individuals [15]. However, the clothing worn (i.e., socks and undergarments) by the walking individuals has been employed as segmental markers to monitor foot and pelvic parameters in the image, which results in a significant dependence of the derived body measurement data on the clothing [14]. In addition, the body measurement data from walking individuals, such as height, width, and area, in an image exhibits inconsistent alterations based on the individual's distance from the camera in various circumstances (e.g., indoor and outdoor settings) [12,15,16]. One strategy to resolve this constraint could be scaling or resizing the video image sequences in order to equalise the walking individual's body measurements in each image, but doing so may result in visual distortion and reduced quality due to compression and stretching [16]. Another approach for overcoming this limitation could be utilizing the walking individual-to-camera distance independent body measurement data to establish steady walking speed patterns [12]. A study conducted by Zeng and Wang presented body measurement data based on a ratio (i.e., body height-width ratio data) that is steady regardless of the closeness of the individual to the camera while walking [12]. In addition, the study conducted by Zeng and Wang utilized artificial intelligence techniques for classifying walk patterns in terms of speed and established a walking pattern that could be used for classification through the use of inconsistent body measurements (e.g., body area, mid-body and lower-body width) data along with ratio-based (i.e., body height-width ratio) data [12]. Our previous published study [13] provided the first suggestion of five ratio-based body measurements, namely, (i) the ratio of the full-body height to the full-body width (HW1), (ii) the ratio of the full-body height to the mid-body width (HW2), (iii) the ratio of the full-body height to the lower-body width (HW3), (iv) the ratio of the apparent body area to the full-body area (A1), and (v) the ratio of the area between two legs to the full-body area (A2) for the definition and prediction of walk speed patterns. Our previous study [13] then proved the reliability of these five ratio-based body measurements to define and classify an individual's walking patterns in terms of speed in indoor (treadmill trial) environments using a bidirectional long short-term memory (biLSTM) deep learning-based model with a mean ± standard deviation (SD) classification accuracy of 88.05($\pm$8.85)% and a median accuracy of 89.58%. However, the development of a successful and highly predictive deep learning architecture for walking speed classification depends on the dimension of the data extracted from 2D marker-free video images [17]. Although the use of high-dimensional input features (i.e., several ratio-based body measurements) is thought to create a strong walk pattern, the use of redundant data may overburden the deep learning architecture and hinder the classification performance [18]. Therefore, the use of fewer but useful ratio-based body measurements data from 2D marker-free video images is necessary to build a successful deep learning-based model. Therefore, the current study aimed to construct walk patterns with fewer but useful ratio-based body measurements for the successful development of a deep learning architecture that would classify walking speed with the highest classification accuracy.

One of the commonly used methods for selecting the most beneficial and ideal input features (such as ratio-based body measurements) is assessing the correlations between the features and selecting those with the lowest correlation strengths because only one of two highly correlated input features is needed for a model, while the second feature does not provide any new information for target prediction [19,20]. In other words, the selection of input features with low correlations among them will provide valuable information to a model to improve its predictive ability [20]. Other commonly used methods for optimal input feature selection is fitting and assessing a deep learning-based model with several potential subsets or combinations of input features and selecting the feature subset or combination that yields the best performance [20,21]. The utilization of both methods is crucial for the development of a successful and highly predictive deep learning architecture because an analysis of the correlations among input features will yield theoretical knowledge of the quality (e.g., strong or weak) of the combination of input features, and the practical application of a deep learning-based model using different possible subsets or combinations of input features will identify the feature subset or combination that yields the best performance [19–22].

The objective of this study was to identify the optimal combination of ratio-based body measurements needed for presenting potential information that can define and predict a walk pattern in terms of speed with high classification accuracy using a deep learning-based walking speed classification model. To this end, the study analysed the correlations among five ratio-based body measurements to comprehend the relationships among ratio-based body measurements in slow, normal and fast walking speed conditions. This study also evaluated the performance (in terms of the mean ± SD classification accuracy and mean ± SD training time) of a biLSTM deep learning-based walking speed classification model using the walking speed patterns created by all possible combinations of one, two, three and four ratio-based body measurements among five ratio-based body measurements (HW1, HW2, HW3, A1, and A2). The walk pattern created by the combination of fewest ratio-based body measurements (i.e., less than five ratio-based body measurements) was defined as optimal in the study if it was able to classify the walking speed with a mean ± SD classification accuracy higher than or within 2% less [23,24] of that obtained in our previous study [13], and the ratio-based body measurements in the walk pattern showed low correlations among them. This study hypothesized that walking speed patterns identified from few ratio-based body measurements can be used to classify walking speed using deep learning-based methods with high accuracy if the correlations among the body measurements are low.

2. Methods

This study adopted lateral 2D marker-free motion image sequences from a publicly available dataset, the Osaka University-Institute of Scientific and Industrial research (OU-ISIR) dataset 'A' [25]. This is a benchmark dataset and has been used in various research areas since it was publicly published in 2012. The dataset has been used in the area human gait research focusing on speed, age, and gender [12,26], movement assessment and gait monitoring [13,27], gait-based biometric and surveillance [28,29].

2.1. Participants and Dataset

In this study, the walk speed patterns at three speeds—slow, normal, and fast—were classified using lateral 2D marker-free motion image sequences from 34 participants. The OU-ISIR dataset 'A' [25], which is available publicly, provided these image sequences (obtained using an indoor treadmill) (Figure 1). Three walking speed categories were considered: slow (2 to 3 km/h), normal (4 to 5 km/h) and fast (6 to 7 km/h) [30–32]. OU-ISIR dataset 'A' comprises of 2D image sequences recorded from 34 participants while walking at a range of speed from 2 to 7 km/h on a 550 mm wide and 2000 mm long belt area of treadmill (BIOMILL BM-2200). An increment of 1 km/h speed was maintained consistently. All participants wore standard coloured long sleeve shirt and long pants while walking. The lateral view image sequences of the participants were captured using camera (Point Grey Research Inc. Flea2 models) with 3.5 mm lens focal length, 60 fps frame rate and VGA resolution. The image sequence data were divided into the three above-mentioned categories (i.e., slow, normal, and fast). Additionally, the dataset included both male and female participants with age between 15 to 65 years who had reported no recent fall injuries, neurology or orthopaedic and gait or locomotion related issues. For each participant, 12 image sequences including two image sequences for each speed were processed, that yielded a total of 408 sequences with a minimum length of 240 frames. Three types of walk speed patterns for slow, normal and fast walking were created using quasi-periodic patterns produced from five ratio-based body measurements extracted from the minimum number of image sequences (i.e., 240 frames), which are comparable to the lengths used in previous studies [13].

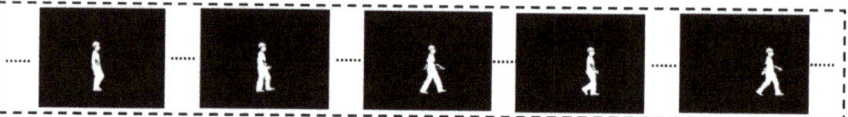

Figure 1. Example of continuous image sequences from OUISIR dataset A for one participant walking at a normal speed.

2.2. Feature Extraction

According to the procedure used in our prior study [13], which is depicted in Figure 2 and exemplified by Equations (1)–(5), data for five ratio-based body measurements (HW1, HW2, HW3, A1 and A2) were extracted from image sequences available for slow walk, normal walk, and fast walking. More specifically, among the five ratio-based body measurements defined in our previous study [13], HW1, HW2 and HW3 were calculated using the rectangular boundary box height and width. Bounding boxes were placed around the whole body, mid body and lower body locations in each image, and HW1, HW2 and HW3 were then calculated using Equations (1)–(3). The terms in the equations are presented in Figure 2a–c. A1 and A2 were measured by evaluating the white pixels in the image, boundary box area and area between two legs in each image and then using Equations (4) and (5). The terms in the equations are presented in Figure 2d,e.

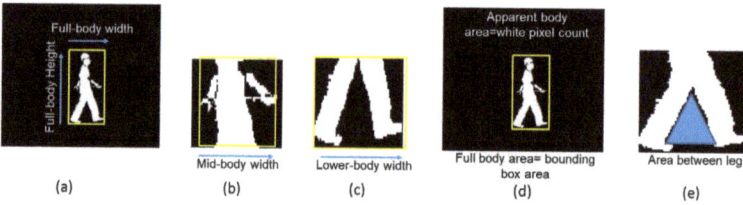

Figure 2. Detail of the terms used in Equations (1)–(5). Extraction of (**a**) full-body height (H) and full body width (W1) (**b**) mid-body width (W2) (**c**) lower-body width (W3) (**d**) full body area and apparent body area, and (**e**) area between two legs.

Ratio of the full-body height to the full-body width,

$$HW1 = \frac{Full - body\ height}{Full - body\ width} \quad (1)$$

Ratio of the full-body height to the mid-body width,

$$HW2 = \frac{Full - body\ height}{Mid - body\ width} \quad (2)$$

Ratio of the full-body height to the lower-body width,

$$HW3 = \frac{Full - body\ height}{Lower - body\ width} \quad (3)$$

Ratio of the apparent body area to the full-body area,

$$A1 = \frac{Apparent - bodyarea}{Full - bodyarea} \quad (4)$$

Ratio of the area between two legs to the full-body area,

$$A2 = \frac{Area\ between\ two\ legs}{Full - bodyarea} \quad (5)$$

After extracting data for five ratio-based body measurements from marker-free 2D image sequences, our previous research [13] discovered that each of the five ratio-based body measurements varied over time such that they created quasi-periodic patterns (Figure 3), which is an established pattern of human gait cycle motion while walking [33].

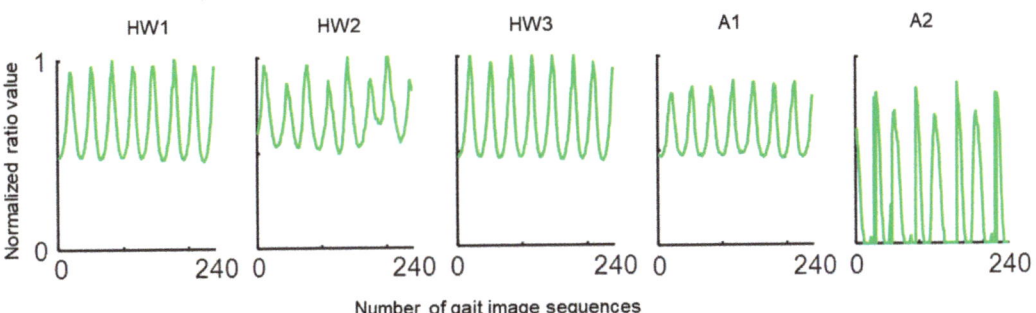

Figure 3. Quasi-periodic signals created by five ratio-based body measurements calculated from image sequences of a single individual moving normally while walking. HW1, ratio of the full-body height to the full-body width; HW2, ratio of the full-body height to the mid-body width; HW3, ratio of the full-body height to the lower-body width; A1, ratio of the apparent body area to the full-body area; and A2, ratio of the area between two legs to the full-body area.

2.3. Experiment Procedure

In the current study, for each walking speed condition, coefficient of determination (R^2) were calculated among the data of five ratio-based body measurements to determine the ratio-based body measurements with low correlation. R-Square (R^2) has been used as a state-of-the-art tool for correlation analysis [34]. The results from the correlation analysis are presented in terms of R^2 in Section 3. The quasi-periodic patterns were then used to establish three types of walk speed patterns for slow, normal and fast walking. Thirty datasets were created using three types of walk speed patterns. Among these datasets, the walk speed patterns in five, ten, ten and five datasets were established using quasi-periodic patterns from one, two, three and four of the five ratio-based body measurements, respectively. The combinations of ratio-based body measurements in the walk patterns obtained with the above-described datasets were established according to the combination rule in Equation (6), and no combinations were repeated for different orders of ratio-based body measurements. This process of creating a combination of features have been used by the current studies [35,36].

$$C_n = \frac{5!}{n!(5-n)!}, \ n = 1, 2, \ldots, 4 \quad (6)$$

In this equation, $C(n)$ is the number of combinations generated by the included ratio-based body measurements, 5 is the total number of ratio-based body measurements, n is the number of included ratio-based body measurements in the combination, and $(5 - n)$ is the number of ratio-based body measurements excluded from the combination.

Each dataset contained 136 walk speed patterns for each of the three speeds (i.e., slow, normal, and fast). Table 1 provides a description of the walk patterns in all the datasets. After datasets' construction, a biLSTM-based deep learning architecture along with k-fold (where, k = 17) cross validation [13] was performed using all ratio-based body measurements combinations (Table 1) for walking speed classification. A total of 272 cross validation experiments were performed for each deep learning-based walking speed classification task. According to the prior studies, this simple structure is adequate to produce non-overfitting and highly accurate classification problems of the same types [37,38]. Figure 4 presents workflow of the walking speed classification using different combination of ratio-based body measurements. The results from the walking speed classification are presented in terms of mean ± SD classification accuracies and mean ± SD training time in Section 3 and in Supplementary Material (Tables S1–S5).

Table 1. Description of the walk patterns in all datasets used in biLSTM-based deep learning architecture.

No. of Datasets	No. of Ratio-Based Body Measurement in Walk Speed Pattern	Combinations of Ratio-Based Body Measurement in Walk Speed Pattern	Walking Speed Pattern Dimension	No. of Walk Speed Patterns/Dataset			
				Slow Speed	Normal Speed	Fast Speed	Total
05	01	HW1	1 × 240	136	136	136	408
		HW2					
		HW3					
		A1					
		A2					
10	02	HW1, HW2	2 × 240	136	136	136	408
		HW1, HW3					
		HW2, HW3					
		HW1, A1					
		HW1, A2					
		HW2, A1					
		HW2, A2					
		HW3, A1					
		HW3, A2					
		A1, A2					

Table 1. Cont.

No. of Datasets	No. of Ratio-Based Body Measurement in Walk Speed Pattern	Combinations of Ratio-Based Body Measurement in Walk Speed Pattern	Walking Speed Pattern Dimension	No. of Walk Speed Patterns/Dataset			
				Slow Speed	Normal Speed	Fast Speed	Total
10	03	HW1, HW2, HW3	3 × 240	136	136	136	408
		HW1, HW2, A1					
		HW1, HW2, A2					
		HW1, HW3, A1					
		HW1, HW3, A2					
		HW2, HW3, A1					
		HW2, HW3, A2					
		A1, A2, HW1					
		A1, A2, HW2					
		A1, A2, HW3					
05	04	HW1, HW2, HW3, A1	4 × 240	136	136	136	408
		HW1, HW2, HW3, A2					
		HW2, HW3, A1, A2					
		HW1, HW3, A1, A2					
		HW1, HW2, A1, A2					

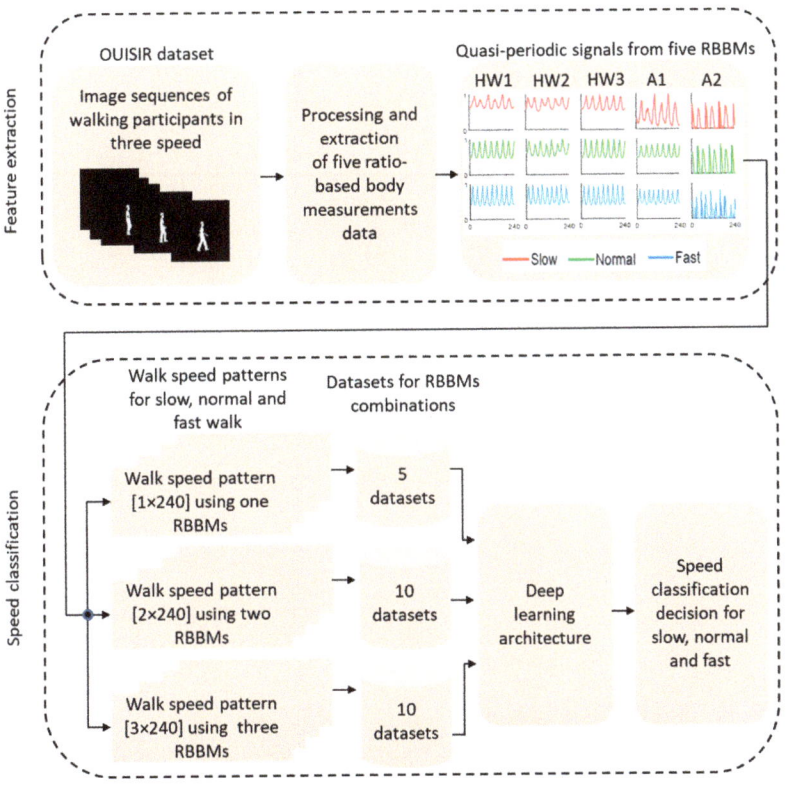

Figure 4. Workflow of the walking speed classification using different combinations of ratio-based body measurements (RBBMs).

3. Results

Figure 5 presents the results from the correlation analysis (in terms of R^2) using data of five ratio-based body measurements for slow, normal and fast walk speeds. According to the interpretations (i.e., weak correlation: 0.10–0.39 and moderate correlation: 0.40–0.69, strong correlation: 0.70–0.89, very strong correlation: 0.90–1.00) [39], the R^2 values between HW1 vs. HW2, HW2 vs. HW3, HW2 vs. A1, HW1 vs. A2, HW2 vs. A2, HW3 vs. A2 and A1 vs. A2 were generally found to be weak for slow and normal walk speeds, whereas for fast walk speeds, weak and moderate R^2 values were found between HW1 vs. A2, HW2 vs. A2, HW3 vs. A2 and A1 vs. A2 and between HW1 vs. HW2, HW2 vs. HW3, and HW2 vs. A1, respectively. In addition, moderate R^2 values were found between HW1 vs. HW3, HW1 vs. A1, and HW3 vs. A1 for slow walk speeds, but the corresponding values obtained for normal and fast walk speeds were generally strong.

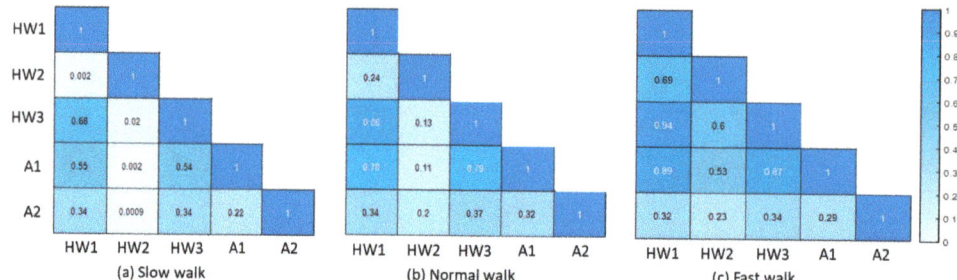

Figure 5. Coefficient of determination (R^2) among data of five ratio-based body measurements for (**a**) slow (**b**) normal and (**c**) fast walk speeds. HW1, ratio of the full-body height to the full-body width; HW2, ratio of the full-body height to the mid-body width; HW3, ratio of the full-body height to the lower-body width; A1, ratio of the apparent body area to the full-body area; and A2, ratio of the area between the legs to the full-body area. Weak correlation: 0.10–0.39, moderate correlation: 0.40–0.69, strong correlation: 0.70–0.89 and very strong correlation: 0.90–1.00.

Figure 6 presents the results from comparisons of the mean($\pm$SD) classification accuracy and mean($\pm$SD) training time for biLSTM-based walking speed classification using walk speed patterns established using one, two, three four and five ratio-based body measurements. Details of the mean($\pm$SD) classification accuracy and mean($\pm$SD) training time are provided given in the Supplementary Material (Tables S1–S5). Walking speed classification using walk speed patterns established using five ratio-based body measurements achieved a mean($\pm$SD) classification accuracy of 88.05($\pm$8.85)% (Figure 6 and Table S1 (result from our previous study [13])) and the walk speed patterns established using three ratio-based body measurements combinations such as (HW1, HW2, A2) and (HW2, HW3, A2) achieved a mean classification accuracy that was greater than that achieved with walk speed patterns established with five ratio-based body measurements (Figure 6 and Table S3). More specifically, two combinations of three ratio-based body measurements, namely, (HW1, HW2, A2) and (HW2, HW3, A2), achieved mean($\pm$SD) classification accuracies of 92.7($\pm$8.01)% and 92.79($\pm$7.8)%, respectively (Figure 6 and Table S3). In addition, the walk speed patterns established using other combinations of three ratio-based body measurements, namely, (A1, A2, HW3), (A1, A2, HW2), (HW1, HW3, A2), (HW1, HW3, A1), (HW1, HW2, A1) and (HW1, HW2, HW3), and three combinations of four ratio-based body measurements, namely, (HW1, HW2, A1, A2), (HW1, HW2, HW3, A1) and (HW1, HW2, HW3, A2), achieved mean classification accuracies that were very close (i.e., within 2% less) to the mean classification accuracy achieved with the walk speed patterns established with five ratio-based body measurements (Figure 6 and Tables S2 and S3). In contrast, the mean accuracies achieved for walking speed classification using walk speed patterns established with combinations of one and two ratio-based body measurements were less than 70% and

74%, respectively (Figure 6 and Tables S4 and S5). These results clearly show that the walk speed patterns established with combinations of three ratio-based body measurements achieved better performance in terms of the mean(±SD) classification accuracy than the walk speed patterns established with five ratio-based body measurements. Moreover, the mean training time for walking speed classification using walk speed patterns established with combinations of three ratio-based body measurements reduced to approximately 14 to 15 min (Figure 6 and Table S3) compared with the mean training time of 17.43 min for walking speed classification using walk speed patterns established with the combination of five ratio-based body measurements [Figure 6 and Table S1 (result from our previous published study [13])].

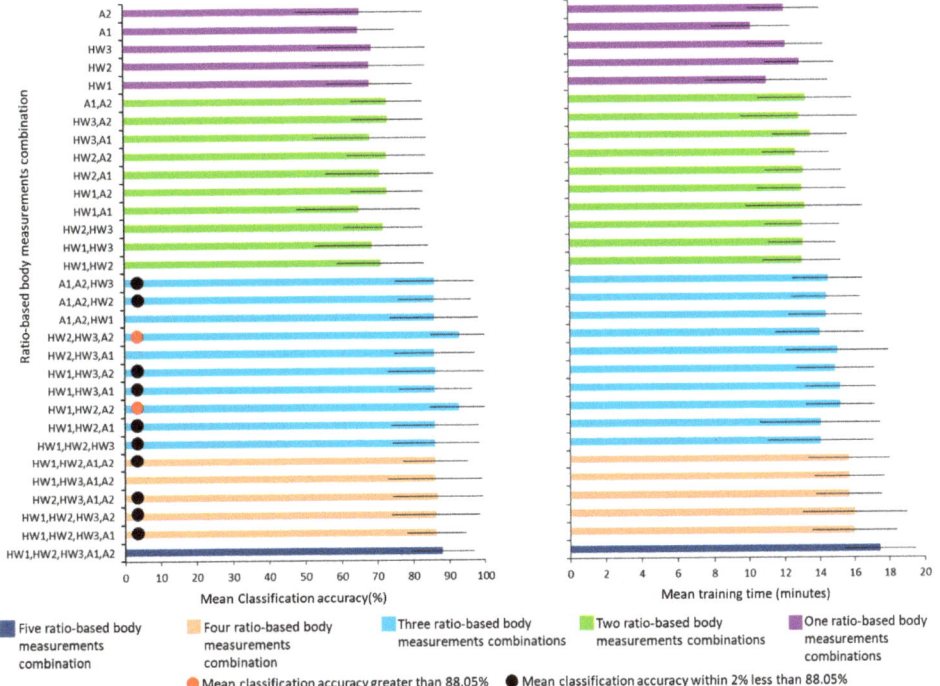

Figure 6. Mean ± SD classification accuracy and mean ± SD training time for biLSTM-based walking speed classification using walk patterns based on by one, two, three, four and five ratio-based body measurements. HW1, ratio of the full-body height to the full-body width; HW2, ratio of the full-body height to the mid-body width; HW3, ratio of the full-body height to the lower-body width; A1, ratio of the apparent body area to the full-body area; and A2, ratio of the area between the legs to the full-body area.

4. Discussion

The primary objective of this study was to determine the optimal ratio-based body measurement combination needed to present potential information that can define and predict walk patterns in terms of speed with a high classification accuracy. To accomplish the goal, this study adopted two commonly used methods of useful and optimal selection of input features (e.g., ratio-based body measurements). First, this study analysed the correlations among five ratio-based body measurements to comprehend relationships among these body measurements in slow, normal and fast walking speed conditions. Second, the performance (in terms of the mean ± SD classification accuracy and mean ± SD training time) of a biLSTM deep learning-based walking speed classification model was evaluated using walking speed patterns created using all possible combination of one, two, three and four out of five ratio-based body measurements. The combination with the fewest ratio-based body measurements (i.e., less than five ratio-based body measurements) for the establishment of walk patterns was deemed optimal if it yielded a mean ± SD classification accuracy higher than or within 2% less [23,24] of the mean ± SD classification accuracy obtained in our previous study [13], and the ratio-based body measurements used for defining the walk pattern exhibited low correlations among them.

This study utilized data for five ratio-based body measurements for the correlation analysis and biLSTM deep learning-based walking speed classification. Based on the correlation analysis and biLSTM deep learning-based walking speed classification models, this study discovered that combinations of three ratio-based body measurements with minimal correlation among them yielded the highest accuracy in terms of the mean ± SD classification accuracy for walking speed classification using the biLSTM deep learning-based model. More specifically, HW1 exhibits low correlations with HW2 and A2, and thus, the combination of these three ratio-based body measurements achieved classification accuracy of 92.7(±8.01)% (Figures 5 and 6 and Table S3). HW2 has low correlations with HW3 and A2, and the combination of these three ratio-based body measurements achieved a classification accuracy of 92.79(±7.8)% (Figures 5 and 6 and Table S3). Furthermore, the mean ± SD classification accuracies achieved with the combinations of one and two ratio-based body measurements with low correlation among them are markedly lower than the mean ± SD classification accuracy achieved in our previous study [13] (Figure 6 and Tables S4 and S5). Moreover, the other combinations of ratio-based body measurements achieved classification accuracies within 2% of the mean ± SD classification accuracy achieved in our previous study [13], and the body measurements in these combinations generally exhibited moderate to strong correlations between them (Figures 5 and 6 and Tables S1–S3). This finding implies that walking speed patterns identified from few ratio-based body measurements can produce the best performance for deep learning-based classification of walking speed if the correlation between the ratio-based body measurements is low. Additionally, full body image sequences are necessary for more accurate classification, since ratio-based body measurements (i.e., HW1, HW2 and HW3) which resulted in excellent classification accuracy required full-body height.

This study is significant in several contexts. First, video image sequences display apparent body measurements rather than real physiological dimensions of the human body [12,15,16]. It is thus crucial to examine different walking individual-to-camera distance independent body measurements (i.e., ratio-based body measurements) that can be found from video image sequences and to investigate the interactions between ratio-based body measurements in order to identify the optimal body measurements for defining and predicting a walk pattern in terms of speed [12,13]. By performing a correlation analysis and a rigorous deep learning-based assessment, the current study evaluated combinations of three out of five potential ratio-based body measurements. Combinations of these three ratio-based body measurements provided information to estimate walk patterns in terms of speed with classification accuracy greater than 92%, which is better than the results achieved in previous studies 88.57% [12], 88.05% [13]. In addition, the previous study [12] trained the model with a multiclass setting (i.e., all three types of walking speed patterns) and tested the models using a single-class setting (i.e., any one of the three walking speed patterns) while the current study used a multiclass setting as well as multiple runs for the training, validation and testing of the model, which is beneficial for achieving accurate classification accuracy and building a successful model [40,41]. It is difficult to compare our results with the previously published study [14], which used body-worn clothing for body measurement extraction, as the study only proposed extraction methods and did not experiment for classification related tasks. Additionally, the data collection procedure, experimental design, and participants' demographic characteristics of the previous study [14] are completely different from the current study. Second, earlier studies [17,18], which claim that using high-dimensional input features (such as several ratio-based body measurements) may hinder the performance of a deep learning-based architecture obtained with redundant data, support the results from the current study. In addition, previous studies [17,18], which assert that the highest performance of a deep learning-based architecture could be attained if the best data that provide information, are in agreement with the results from the current study. Furthermore, in future clinicians may utilise this method for routine gait monitoring in healthcare and old-age homes as it can be used to identify the walking speed in an indoor environment with improved classification accuracy [42]. Current patient monitoring systems include implanted devices and wearable sensors that might require invasive procedures and body attachment which are difficult and often unpleasant for patients. Therefore, remote patient monitoring using existing surveillance cameras could be a more viable option to constant observation of patient mobility. In addition, human resources and battery life of traditional sensors are critical for long term patient monitoring. As such, camera-based patient mobility monitoring might be more cost effective while alleviating the burden on resources in clinical settings [43].

Although the current study has a lot of potential for selecting the optimal ratio-based body measurements for creating walk patterns that are useful for accomplishing walking speed classification using a deep learning-based architecture with the highest classification accuracy, the study only evaluated healthy individuals. Experiments that include a gait-impaired population will be considered in the future. Additionally, this study recruited participants with a wide range of ages (15 to 65). However, the walk patterns of the participants might change according to their age [44,45]. Walk speed classification across different aged participants could be another research topic of interest in future. Additionally, this study solely used area-based and height-to-width ratio-based body measurements for the classification of walking speeds. Future studies will involve estimating additional spatiotemporal parameters, such as stride and step length, joint angles, velocity and acceleration, to gain a deeper understanding of the health of individuals and to classify typical and atypical gait patterns. Moreover, only the biLSTM approach was used in this study for the classification task. Future research will utilise more cutting-edge classification algorithms to reach the best classification accuracy.

5. Conclusions

In summary, this study found that combinations of three ratio-based body measurements extracted from lateral-view 2D images of marker-free walking individuals can potentially define and predict walk patterns in terms of speed with classification accuracies greater than 92% using a biLSTM. The excellent findings of this study support the optimal application of ratio-based body measurement data that change with variations in the walking speeds, form periodic or quasi-periodic patterns, and, more importantly, can be extracted from marker-free conventional camera images to classify walking speeds with high classification accuracy using the contemporary deep learning method. Additionally, the remarkable results obtained in this study confirm that the use of high-dimensional input features, such as multiple ratio-based body measurements, hinders the performance of deep learning-based architectures if the data are redundant. Furthermore, if the data that yield the best information are employed, the deep learning-based architecture would exhibit peak performance. This walking speed classification method using optimal data is a simple yet effective technique with a lot of potential for use in clinical settings and elderly care facilities.

Supplementary Materials: The following supporting information can be downloaded at: https://www.mdpi.com/article/10.3390/bioengineering9110715/s1, Table S1: classification accuracies for walking speed classification using walk pattern established with five RBBMs in our previous study, Table S2: classification accuracies for walking speed classification using walk pattern established with four RBBMs, Table S3: classification accuracies for walking speed classification using walk pattern established with three RBBMs, Table S4 classification accuracies for walking speed classification using walk pattern established with two RBBMs, Table S5 classification accuracies for walking speed classification using walk pattern established with one RBBMs. RBBMs refers to ratio-based body measurements.

Author Contributions: Guarantor: T.S., M.F.R., D.I. and N.U.A. are responsible for the entirety of the work and the final decision to submit the manuscript; study concept and design: all authors; data acquisition, processing, and analysis: T.S. and M.F.R.; critical review and interpretation of data: K.H.G., S.M.R., M.A.A., M.A.A.M., D.I., O.A. and M.A.; drafting of the manuscript: T.S. and M.F.R.; critical revision of the manuscript: all authors; obtaining funding: O.A. and M.A. All authors have read and agreed to the published version of the manuscript.

Funding: This research received no external funding.

Institutional Review Board Statement: Not applicable.

Informed Consent Statement: Not applicable.

Data Availability Statement: The data generated and/or analyses for the current study are available from the following publicly available databases: Osaka University-Institute of Scientific and Industrial research (OU-ISIR) Dataset 'A': (www.am.sanken.osaka-u.ac.jp/BiometricDB/GaitTM.html, access on 23 September 2022).

Acknowledgments: The authors extend their appreciation to the College of Applied Medical Sciences Research Centre and the Deanship of Scientific Research at King Saud University for funding this research.

Conflicts of Interest: The authors declare no conflict of interest.

References

1. McCrum, C.; Lucieer, F.; van de Berg, R.; Willems, P.; Pérez Fornos, A.; Guinand, N.; Karamanidis, K.; Kingma, H.; Meijer, K. The walking speed-dependency of gait variability in bilateral vestibulopathy and its association with clinical tests of vestibular function. *Sci. Rep.* **2019**, *9*, 18392. [CrossRef] [PubMed]
2. Kirtley, C.; Whittle, M.W.; Jefferson, R.J. Influence of walking speed on gait parameters. *J. Biomed. Eng.* **1985**, *7*, 282–288. [CrossRef]
3. Fukuchi, C.A.; Fukuchi, R.K.; Duarte, M. Effects of walking speed on gait biomechanics in healthy participants: A systematic review and meta-analysis. *Syst. Rev.* **2019**, *8*, 153. [CrossRef] [PubMed]
4. Mannering, N.; Young, T.; Spelman, T.; Choong, P.F. Three-dimensional knee kinematic analysis during treadmill gait: Slow imposed speed versus normal self-selected speed. *Bone Joint Res.* **2017**, *6*, 514–521. [CrossRef]
5. Carcreff, L.; Gerber, C.N.; Paraschiv-Ionescu, A.; De Coulon, G.; Aminian, K.; Newman, C.J.; Armand, S. Walking Speed of Children and Adolescents with Cerebral Palsy: Laboratory Versus Daily Life. *Front. Bioeng. Biotechnol.* **2020**, *8*, 812. [CrossRef]
6. Jarvis, H.L.; Brown, S.J.; Price, M.; Butterworth, C.; Groenevelt, R.; Jackson, K.; Walker, L.; Rees, N.; Clayton, A.; Reeves, N.D. Return to Employment After Stroke in Young Adults: How Important Is the Speed and Energy Cost of Walking? *Stroke* **2019**, *50*, 3198–3204. [CrossRef]
7. Nadkarni, N.K.; Mawji, E.; McIlroy, W.E.; Black, S.E. Spatial and temporal gait parameters in Alzheimer's disease and aging. *Gait Posture* **2009**, *30*, 452–454. [CrossRef] [PubMed]
8. Fiser, W.M.; Hays, N.P.; Rogers, S.C.; Kajkenova, O.; Williams, A.E.; Evans, C.M.; Evans, W.J. Energetics of walking in elderly people: Factors related to gait speed. *J. Gerontol. Ser. A Biomed. Sci. Med. Sci.* **2010**, *65*, 1332–1337. [CrossRef]
9. Moissenet, F.; Leboeuf, F.; Armand, S. Lower limb sagittal gait kinematics can be predicted based on walking speed, gender, age and BMI. *Sci. Rep.* **2019**, *9*, 9510. [CrossRef]
10. Xie, Y.J.; Liu, E.Y.; Anson, E.R.; Agrawal, Y. Age-related imbalance is associated with slower walking speed: Analysis from the National Health and Nutrition Examination Survey. *J. Geriatr. Phys. Ther.* **2017**, *40*, 183. [CrossRef]
11. De Cock, A.-M.; Fransen, E.; Perkisas, S.; Verhoeven, V.; Beauchet, O.; Remmen, R.; Vandewoude, M. Gait characteristics under different walking conditions: Association with the presence of cognitive impairment in community-dwelling older people. *PLoS ONE* **2017**, *12*, e0178566. [CrossRef]
12. Zeng, W.; Wang, C. Gait recognition across different walking speeds via deterministic learning. *Neurocomputing* **2015**, *152*, 139–150. [CrossRef]
13. Sikandar, T.; Rabbi, M.F.; Ghazali, K.H.; Altwijri, O.; Alqahtani, M.; Almijalli, M.; Altayyar, S.; Ahamed, N.U. Using a Deep Learning Method and Data from Two-Dimensional (2D) Marker-Less Video-Based Images for Walking Speed Classification. *Sensors* **2021**, *21*, 2836. [CrossRef] [PubMed]
14. Castelli, A.; Paolini, G.; Cereatti, A.; Della Croce, U. A 2D markerless gait analysis methodology: Validation on healthy subjects. *Comput. Math. Methods Med.* **2015**, *2015*, 186780. [CrossRef] [PubMed]
15. Verlekar, T.T.; Soares, L.D.; Correia, P.L. Automatic classification of gait impairments using a markerless 2D video-based system. *Sensors* **2018**, *18*, 2743. [CrossRef]

16. Zhang, Y.; Fang, Y.; Lin, W.; Zhang, X.; Li, L. Backward registration-based aspect ratio similarity for image retargeting quality assessment. *IEEE Trans. Image Process.* **2016**, *25*, 4286–4297. [CrossRef] [PubMed]
17. Venkatesh, B.; Anuradha, J. A review of feature selection and its methods. *Cybern. Inf. Technol.* **2019**, *19*, 3–26. [CrossRef]
18. Liew, C.S.; Abbas, A.; Jayaraman, P.P.; Wah, T.Y.; Khan, S.U. Big data reduction methods: A survey. *Data Sci. Eng.* **2016**, *1*, 265–284.
19. Ferreira, A.J.; Figueiredo, M.A.T. Efficient feature selection filters for high-dimensional data. *Pattern Recognit. Lett.* **2012**, *33*, 1794–1804. [CrossRef]
20. Kuhn, M.; Johnson, K. *Applied Predictive Modeling*; Springer: New York, NY, USA, 2013; Volume 26.
21. Murphy, K.P. *Machine Learning: A Probabilistic Perspective*; MIT press: Cambridge, MA, USA, 2012; ISBN 0262304325.
22. Sikandar, T.; Rabbi, M.F.; Ghazali, K.H.; Altwijri, O.; Almijalli, M.; Ahamed, N.U. Evaluating the difference in walk patterns among normal-weight and overweight/obese individuals in real-world surfaces using statistical analysis and deep learning methods with inertial measurement unit data. *Phys. Eng. Sci. Med.* **2022**; Online ahead of print. [CrossRef]
23. Davoudi, A.; Mardini, M.T.; Nelson, D.; Albinali, F.; Ranka, S.; Rashidi, P.; Manini, T.M. The effect of sensor placement and number on physical activity recognition and energy expenditure estimation in older adults: Validation study. *JMIR mHealth uHealth* **2021**, *9*, e23681. [CrossRef]
24. O'Day, J.; Lee, M.; Seagers, K.; Hoffman, S.; Jih-Schiff, A.; Kidziński, Ł.; Delp, S.; Bronte-Stewart, H. Assessing inertial measurement unit locations for freezing of gait detection and patient preference. *J. Neuroeng. Rehabil.* **2022**, *19*, 20. [CrossRef]
25. Makihara, Y.; Mannami, H.; Tsuji, A.; Hossain, M.A.; Sugiura, K.; Mori, A.; Yagi, Y. The OU-ISIR gait database comprising the treadmill dataset. *IPSJ Trans. Comput. Vis. Appl.* **2012**, *4*, 53–62. [CrossRef]
26. Prakash, C.; Kumar, R.; Mittal, N. Recent developments in human gait research: Parameters, approaches, applications, machine learning techniques, datasets and challenges. *Artif. Intell. Rev.* **2018**, *49*, 1–40. [CrossRef]
27. Alharthi, A.S.; Yunas, S.U.; Ozanyan, K.B. Deep learning for monitoring of human gait: A review. *IEEE Sens. J.* **2019**, *19*, 9575–9591. [CrossRef]
28. Arora, P.; Hanmandlu, M.; Srivastava, S. Gait based authentication using gait information image features. *Pattern Recognit. Lett.* **2015**, *68*, 336–342. [CrossRef]
29. Medikonda, J.; Madasu, H.; Panigrahi, B.K. Information set based gait authentication system. *Neurocomputing* **2016**, *207*, 1–14. [CrossRef]
30. Tan, D.; Huang, K.; Yu, S.; Tan, T. Efficient night gait recognition based on template matching. In Proceedings of the 18th International Conference on Pattern Recognition (ICPR'06), Hong Kong, China, 20–24 August 2006; Volume 3, pp. 1000–1003.
31. Carey, N. Establishing pedestrian walking speeds. *Portl. State Univ.* **2005**, *1*, 4.
32. Chakraborty, S.; Nandy, A.; Yamaguchi, T.; Bonnet, V.; Venture, G. Accuracy of image data stream of a markerless motion capture system in determining the local dynamic stability and joint kinematics of human gait. *J. Biomech.* **2020**, *104*, 109718. [CrossRef]
33. Khokhlova, M.; Migniot, C.; Morozov, A.; Sushkova, O.; Dipanda, A. Normal and pathological gait classification LSTM model. *Artif. Intell. Med.* **2019**, *94*, 54–66. [CrossRef]
34. Senthilnathan, S. Usefulness of Correlation Analysis. In *SSRN*; Elsevier: Amsterdam, The Netherlands, 2019.
35. Bianco, N.A.; Patten, C.; Fregly, B.J. Can measured synergy excitations accurately construct unmeasured muscle excitations? *J. Biomech. Eng.* **2018**, *140*, 011011. [CrossRef]
36. Rabbi, M.F.; Diamond, L.E.; Carty, C.P.; Lloyd, D.G.; Davico, G.; Pizzolato, C. A muscle synergy-based method to estimate muscle activation patterns of children with cerebral palsy using data collected from typically developing children. *Sci. Rep.* **2022**, *12*, 3599. [CrossRef]
37. Che, Z.; Purushotham, S.; Cho, K.; Sontag, D.; Liu, Y. Recurrent neural networks for multivariate time series with missing values. *Sci. Rep.* **2018**, *8*, 6085. [CrossRef] [PubMed]
38. Liu, T.; Bao, J.; Wang, J.; Zhang, Y. A hybrid CNN–LSTM algorithm for online defect recognition of CO2 welding. *Sensors* **2018**, *18*, 4369. [CrossRef] [PubMed]
39. Schober, P.; Boer, C.; Schwarte, L.A. Correlation coefficients: Appropriate use and interpretation. *Anesth. Analg.* **2018**, *126*, 1763–1768. [CrossRef] [PubMed]
40. Nandy, A.; Chakraborty, R.; Chakraborty, P. Cloth invariant gait recognition using pooled segmented statistical features. *Neurocomputing* **2016**, *191*, 117–140. [CrossRef]
41. Langs, G.; Menze, B.H.; Lashkari, D.; Golland, P. Detecting stable distributed patterns of brain activation using gini contrast. *Neuroimage* **2011**, *56*, 497–507. [CrossRef] [PubMed]
42. Brodie, M.A.; Coppens, M.J.; Ejupi, A.; Gschwind, Y.J.; Annegarn, J.; Schoene, D.; Wieching, R.; Lord, S.R.; Delbaere, K. Comparison between clinical gait and daily-life gait assessments of fall risk in older people. *Geriatr. Gerontol. Int.* **2017**, *17*, 2274–2282. [CrossRef] [PubMed]
43. Camera Based Patient Monitoring. Technology and Digital Health. *NIHR Oxford Biomedical Reseach Centre Newsletter.* Available online: https://oxfordbrc.nihr.ac.uk/research-themes-overview/technology-and-digital-health/camera-based-patient-monitoring/ (accessed on 1 October 2022).
44. Kung, S.M.; Fink, P.W.; Legg, S.J.; Ali, A.; Shultz, S.P. Age-dependent variability in spatiotemporal gait parameters and the walk-to-run transition. *Hum. Mov. Sci.* **2019**, *66*, 600–606. [CrossRef]
45. Chung, M.-J.; Wang, M.-J.J. The change of gait parameters during walking at different percentage of preferred walking speed for healthy adults aged 20–60 years. *Gait Posture* **2010**, *31*, 131–135. [CrossRef]

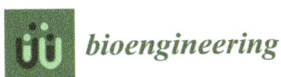

Article

Comparison of Lower Extremity Joint Moment and Power Estimated by Markerless and Marker-Based Systems during Treadmill Running

Hui Tang [1], Jiahao Pan [2], Barry Munkasy [1], Kim Duffy [3] and Li Li [1,*]

1. Georgia Southern University, Statesboro, GA 30458, USA
2. Boise State University, Boise, ID 83725, USA
3. University of Essex, Wivenhoe Park, Colchester CO4 3SQ, UK
* Correspondence: lili@georgiasouthern.edu; Tel.: +1-912-478-0200

Abstract: Background: Markerless (ML) motion capture systems have recently become available for biomechanics applications. Evidence has indicated the potential feasibility of using an ML system to analyze lower extremity kinematics. However, no research has examined ML systems' estimation of the lower extremity joint moments and powers. This study aimed to compare lower extremity joint moments and powers estimated by marker-based (MB) and ML motion capture systems. Methods: Sixteen volunteers ran on a treadmill for 120 s at 3.58 m/s. The kinematic data were simultaneously recorded by 8 infrared cameras and 8 high-resolution video cameras. The force data were recorded via an instrumented treadmill. Results: Greater peak magnitudes for hip extension and flexion moments, knee flexion moment, and ankle plantarflexion moment, along with their joint powers, were observed in the ML system compared to an MB system ($p < 0.0001$). For example, greater hip extension (MB: 1.42 ± 0.29 vs. ML: 2.27 ± 0.45) and knee flexion (MB: −0.74 vs. ML: −1.17 nm/kg) moments were observed in the late swing phase. Additionally, the ML system's estimations resulted in significantly smaller peak magnitudes for knee extension moment, along with the knee production power ($p < 0.0001$). Conclusions: These observations indicate that inconsistent estimates of joint center position and segment center of mass between the two systems may cause differences in the lower extremity joint moments and powers. However, with the progression of pose estimation in the markerless system, future applications can be promising.

Keywords: markerless motion capture system; gait analysis; joint moment; joint power

Citation: Tang, H.; Pan, J.; Munkasy, B.; Duffy, K.; Li, L. Comparison of Lower Extremity Joint Moment and Power Estimated by Markerless and Marker-Based Systems during Treadmill Running. *Bioengineering* 2022, 9, 574. https://doi.org/10.3390/bioengineering9100574

Academic Editors: Christina Zong-Hao Ma, Zhengrong Li and Chen He

Received: 9 September 2022
Accepted: 11 October 2022
Published: 19 October 2022

Publisher's Note: MDPI stays neutral with regard to jurisdictional claims in published maps and institutional affiliations.

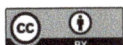

Copyright: © 2022 by the authors. Licensee MDPI, Basel, Switzerland. This article is an open access article distributed under the terms and conditions of the Creative Commons Attribution (CC BY) license (https://creativecommons.org/licenses/by/4.0/).

1. Introduction

Inverse dynamics analysis is a fundamental tool widely used for biomechanical studies to understand human movement. The inverse dynamics method combines kinematic and kinetic data with anthropometric parameters and can estimate joint moments and powers [1]. The evaluation of joint moments and powers is critical in clinical decision-making, such as gait retraining [2], treatment with insoles or orthoses [3], and even surgery [4]. Despite its widespread use, the inaccuracy of inverse dynamic analysis stemming from kinematic/kinetic/anthropometric data is well-recognized [5]. Currently, most kinematic data are provided by marker-based (MB) motion-capture systems [6]. However, inaccuracies derived from marker placements, including the center of mass locations [7,8], joint centers [9], the noise due to surface marker movement [10], and skin artifacts [11,12], can be significant barriers. In addition, using MB requires highly trained personnel to avoid human errors when placing markers on participants [13,14]. The intensive time commitment for marker placements and a controlled environment [15] also contribute to the drawbacks of MB. These all make the applications of MB systems challenging in clinical settings with clinical populations [16].

As a critical advancement in vision-based motion capture, a markerless (ML) system offers an alternative approach to measuring kinematic data. Studies have shown the applicability of the deep learning algorithm-based markerless system in gait analysis. Kanko et al. reported excellent agreement with the MB system on spatial parameters (e.g., step length, stride width, and gait speed) and slight differences in temporal parameters (swing time and double support time) [17]. In two follow-up studies, they assessed the lower extremity joint center positions and joint angles. One study emphasized the inter-session variability of joint angles. They reported that the average inter-session variability across all joint angles was 2.8° in the ML system, which is less than all previously reported values (3.0–3.6°) for the MB system [18]. Their other study presented the average systematic root-mean-square joint center differences of 2.5 cm except for the hip joint, which was 3.6 cm. The average systematic root-mean-square for all segment angle differences was 5.5°, except for the rotation angle about the longitudinal axis [19]. These strong results are approaching or superior to the accuracy of MB systems. However, we did not find any lower extremity joint moments and powers in comparison between the two types of systems in the literature. Given the fundamental quantities of interest in human motion research are the intersegmental moments acting at the joints [20], it is critical to compare joint moments estimated by the ML and MB systems.

Due to marker-based systems' weakness, markerless systems might introduce new possibilities for inverse dynamic analysis. Therefore, the purpose of the current study was to compare inverse dynamic outcomes of lower extremity joint moments and powers based on ML and MB motion capture systems.

2. Materials and Methods

2.1. Participants

Recreationally active young adults were recruited for the current study. Inclusion criteria were: (1) free of musculoskeletal injuries and operations of the lower extremity at least 6 months before the data collection and (2) experience with treadmill running. Participants were asked to be free from any intensive exercise within the 24 h before data collection. Participants signed consent forms approved by the Ethics Committee of Georgia Southern University (Approval Number: H22327) before data collection.

2.2. Experimental Setup and Procedure

Two camera systems were used in the motion capture procedure: 8 infrared cameras (Vicon Bonita, Oxford, UK) for the MB system to record marker trajectories; and 8 high-resolution video cameras (Vicon Vue, Oxford, UK) for the ML system to record movements. The resolutions of Bonita and Vue cameras are 1 megapixel (1024×1024) and 2.1 megapixels (1920×1080). Cameras were aimed at the instrumented treadmill (AMTI force-sensing tandem treadmill, Watertown, MA, USA) within a 15.5 m long by 7.6 m wide by 2.4 m tall laboratory space. Camera systems and the instrumented treadmill were synchronized using Vicon Lock+ (Vicon, Oxford, UK), where kinematics were recorded at 100 Hz, and the ground reaction forces were recorded at 1000 Hz.

Before data collection, the cameras were calibrated using an Active Wand (V1, Oxford, UK). Calibration for the Bonita cameras of the MB system and the Vue cameras of the ML system included more than 1000 frames of valid wand data and 600 frames of valid wand data, respectively. The tolerance of image error for MB and ML systems was set as 0.2 and 0.4, respectively. The three-marker option, with an origin marker and two markers for the X- and Y-axis, was used to set the MB system's global coordinate system (GCS). An MTD-3 device and CalTester software (CalTester, Motion Lab Systems Inc., Baton Rouge, LA, USA) were used to examine the spatial synchronization between the force plates and cameras, following the manufacturer's recommended protocol.

When participants arrived at the laboratory, each was introduced to the test protocol. Then, each participant changed into tight shirts and shorts provided by the lab and wore their running shoes. The investigator measured their heights and body mass. Five-minute warm-up exercise and familiarization with treadmill running followed. Following the manufacturer's suggested procedure, twenty-six 14 mm retro-reflective markers were attached to the participant's anterior superior iliac spine, posterior superior iliac spine, most lateral prominence of the greater trochanter, lateral prominence of the lateral femoral epicondyle, medial prominence of the medial femoral epicondyle, proximal tip of the head of the fibula, anterior border of the tibial tuberosity, lateral prominence of the lateral malleolus, medial prominence of the medial malleolus, dorsal margin of the first, second and fifth metatarsal head, and aspect of the Achilles tendon insertion on the calcaneus at both sides. A static trial for the MB system was recorded in advance while the participants stood on the treadmill with an anatomical posture. Each participant started walking at an initial speed of 1.12 m/s and then gradually transitioned to running at the target speed of 3.58 m/s. The participants ran on the treadmill for 120 s at 3.58 m/s, and the last 30 s of running were recorded for further analysis.

2.3. Data Analysis

2.3.1. Pre-Processing

Raw marker trajectories were interpolated using Woltring gap filling [21] by Nexus (Vicon Nexus, Oxford, UK). Raw markerless video data were pre-processed by Theia3D (Theia3Dv2022.1.0.2309, Theia Markerless, Inc., Kingston, ON, Canada), where the default IK solution was used to estimate the 3D pose [18]. The lower body kinematic chain has six degrees-of-freedom (DOF) at the pelvis, three DOF at the hip, three DOF at the knee, and six DOF at the ankle. The kinematic and ground reaction force data were filtered through Nexus using a low-pass, zero-lag, 4-order Butterworth filter with cut-off frequencies of 10 Hz and 50 Hz [22], respectively.

2.3.2. Visual3D Analyses

The pre-processed right lower extremity data were further analyzed using Visual3D (Preview v2022.06.02, C-Motion, Inc., Germantown, MD, USA).

The same Visual3D 6DOF algorithms and IK constraints for segments were adapted for both systems. IK constraints were set as six DOF at the pelvis, three at the hip, three at the knee, and six at the ankle. For the MB data, the human body was modeled by four linked segments (foot, leg, thigh, pelvis), in which a second kinematic-only foot was created as a virtual foot for kinematic estimations [23]. The segment mass estimations were based on Dempster's regression equation [24], and inertia properties were computed based on segments as geometrical shapes [25]. The hip joint center was estimated using the method proposed by Bell et al. [26]. Still, the knee and ankle joint centers were estimated using midpoints between external landmarks of the corresponding segment. The anatomical coordinate systems of segments were determined from the static calibration trial. The vertical axis was defined in the direction from distal to proximal joint center, while the anterior–posterior axis was defined as being perpendicular to the vertical axis with no mediolateral component. The third axis was the cross product of the vertical and anterior–posterior axis [27]. The model was automatically created for the ML data based on the deep learning algorithm and segment properties such as segment mass, location of the center of mass, and joint center positions were generated accordingly [19].

Resolved into the proximal coordinate system for both MB and ML data, joint angles and kinetic parameters in the sagittal plane were further calculated. The proximal segment was used as the reference when calculating joint moment and power. Internal joint moments and powers were obtained by applying Newton-Euler methods [1,28], where hip and knee extensor and ankle plantar–flexor moments were assigned to be positive. Positive power values indicated energy production through concentric muscular contractions [1].

Force-based gait events were used to identify stride cycles, in which the force threshold was set at 50 N [29]. The stride cycle was defined as two consecutive right heel contacts. The duration of each stride cycle was scaled to 101 data points.

2.3.3. Discrete Measurements

The dependent variables were extracted from the last 10 strides from both MB and ML systems. Within each stride, various positive and negative peak values (depending on joint action) in the sagittal plane were identified on moment and power profiles of the hip, knee, and ankle joints, and the relative times to the peak values were included. Presented in Figure 1, peak moments of the hip (top panel) were extension moment in the early stance phase (HM_1), flexion moment in the stance–swing transition phase (HM_2), and extension moment at the end of the swing phase (HM_3); for the knee (middle panel), the extension moment in the early stance phase (KM_1), and flexion moment at the end of the swing phase (KM_2); for the ankle (bottom panel), extension moment in the stance phase (AM_1). Presented in Figure 2, peak powers of the hip (top panel) were absorption power in the middle of the stance phase (HP_1), the production powers in the early swing phase (HP_2), and at the end of the swing phase (HP_3); for the knee (middle panel), absorption powers in the early stance phase (KP_1), in the early swing phase (KP_3), and at the end of the swing phase (KP_4), and production power in the middle of the stance phase (KP_2); for the ankle (bottom panel), absorption power in the early stance phase (AP_1), and the production power at the end of the stance phase (AP_2).

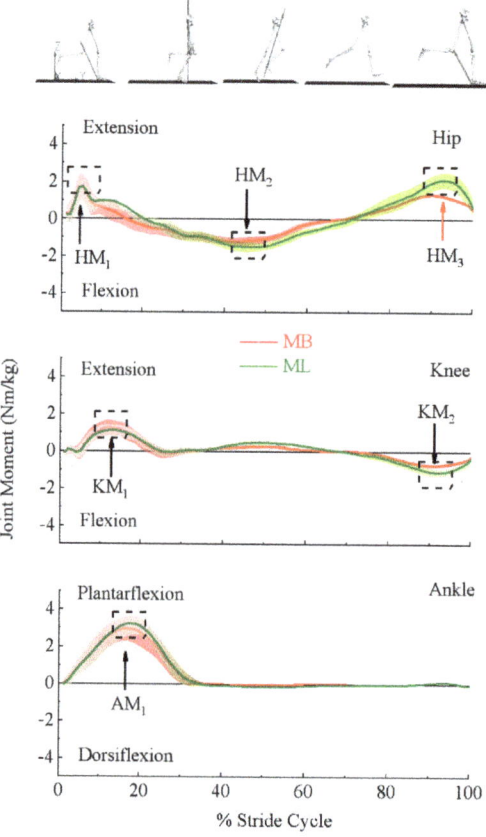

Figure 1. Labeled here are the outcome variables used to quantify the differences in the lower extremity joint moments of the hip (**top panel**), knee (**middle panel**), and ankle (**bottom panel**) (denoted under the ensemble moment curve estimated by marker-based (MB) (red) and markerless (ML) (green) motion capture systems). Joint moments were scaled to participants' body mass.

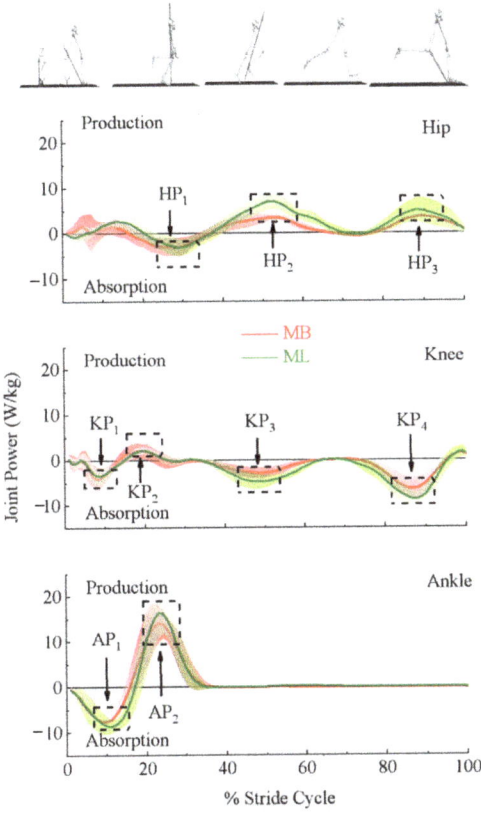

Figure 2. Labeled here are the outcome variables used to quantify the differences in the lower extremity joint powers of the hip (**top panel**), knee (**middle panel**), and ankle (**bottom panel**) (denoted under the ensemble power curve estimated by marker-based (MB) (red) and markerless (ML) (green) motion capture systems). Joint powers were scaled to participants' body mass.

2.4. Statistical Analysis

Means and standard deviations of the differences in kinematic parameters were estimated based on individual measurements between systems. All dependent variables were assessed for normality using a one-sample Kolmogorov–Smirnov test (K-S test, $\alpha = 0.05$). A two-tailed paired *t*-test was employed based on the normally distributed data to test the differences between the two systems. The effect size was assessed using Cohen's d [30]. An alpha level of 0.05 was used for statistical analysis. SPSS (22.0, IBM Inc.; Chicago, IL, USA) was used to conduct all statistical analyses. The alpha level was adjusted by 30 dependent variables using the Bonferroni correction to reduce the chances of type I error ($\alpha = 0.05/30 = 0.0017$).

3. Results

Sixteen participants (9 males and 7 females) participated. The participants' ages, body mass, and height were 23.44 ± 2.31 years, 69.72 ± 9.82 kg, and 1.73 ± 0.08 m, respectively.

3.1. Lower Extremity Joint Moments and Powers

Ensemble curves of lower extremity sagittal plane moments and powers estimated using MB and ML are presented in Figures 1 and 2, respectively. Scaled (by body mass) peak magnitudes and relative timing to the peak are presented in Tables 1 and 2, respectively.

Paired t-tests used for analysis based the results that confirmed the normality of the outcome variables. Compared to the MB system, the ML system showed significantly greater peak joint moment magnitudes at HM_2 (ML: -1.73 ± 0.27, MB: -1.38 ± 0.29), HM_3 (ML: 2.27 ± 0.45, MB: 1.42 ± 0.29), KM_2 (ML: -1.17 ± 0.24, MB: -0.74 ± 0.13), and AM_1 (ML: 3.32 ± 0.55, MB: 3.14 ± 0.51), but less peak magnitude at KM_1 (ML: 1.28 ± 0.32, MB: 1.40 ± 0.42). For the joint powers, significantly less peak magnitudes were at KP_1 (ML: -4.05 ± 1.79, MB: -5.0 ± 2.77), KP_2 (ML: 2.64 ± 1.09, MB: 3.15 ± 1.41), but were greater at HP_2 (ML: 8.07 ± 2.11, MB: 4.29 ± 1.14), HP_3 (ML: 5.68 ± 2.71, MB: 3.99 ± 2.13), KP_3 (ML: -5.42 ± 1.61, MB: -3.45 ± 1.29), KP_4 (ML: -9.65 ± 2.10, MB: -7.15 ± 1.83), AP_1 (ML: -9.44 ± 1.81, MB: -8.38 ± 2.48), as well as AP_2 (ML: 18.40 ± 4.91, MB: 16.07 ± 3.60). In addition, the relative timing to the peak was detected to be significantly different between the MB and ML systems. To be specific, the ML system took longer than the MB system to reach the HM_1 (ML: 6.74 ± 3.40, MB: 5.16 ± 1.27), HM_2 (ML: 43.59 ± 7.00, MB: 40.26 ± 6.90), HM_3 (ML: 92.73 ± 3.00, MB: 90.58 ± 3.39), KM_1 (ML: 13.53 ± 3.89, MB: 12.98 ± 2.18), KM_2 (ML: 92.19 ± 2.51, MB: 90.93 ± 2.21), HP_1 (ML: 28.30 ± 3.68, MB: 26.16 ± 4.45), and KP_1 (ML: 8.73 ± 3.01, MB: 8.19 ± 2.21). Besides, the ML system took less time than the MB system to reach the HP_3 (ML: 89.63 ± 4.15, MB: 91.23 ± 3.47). See Tables 1 and 2 for more details.

Table 1. Body mass scaled peak magnitude (Mean, SD) for joint moments and powers for the marker-based (MB) and Markerless (ML) systems.

	Parameters	MB		ML		T & p-Value	Cohen's d
		Mean	SD	Mean	SD		
Moment (Nm/kg)	Hip first peak	2.09	0.66	2.05	0.73	$t_{159} = -1.42, p < 0.2832$	0.1
	Hip second peak	*−1.38*	*0.23*	*−1.73*	*0.27*	$t_{159} = -22.99, p < 0.0001$ *	*1.8*
	Hip third peak	1.42	0.29	2.27	0.45	$t_{159} = 39.612, p < 0.0001$	3.1
	Knee first peak	**1.40**	**0.42**	**1.28**	**0.32**	$t_{159} = 5.907, p < 0.0001$ *	**0.5**
	Knee second peak	−0.74	0.13	−1.17	0.24	$t_{159} = 40.804, p < 0.0001$ *	3.2
	Ankle first peak	**3.14**	**0.51**	**3.32**	**0.55**	$t_{159} = 10.450, p < 0.0001$ *	**0.8**
Power (W/kg)	**Hip first peak**	**−5.02**	**2.60**	**−4.80**	**2.37**	$t_{159} = -1.570, p = 0.118$	**0.1**
	Hip second peak	4.29	1.14	8.07	2.11	$t_{159} = -27.082, p < 0.0001$ *	2.1
	Hip third peak	3.99	2.13	5.68	2.71	$t_{159} = -13.049, p < 0.0001$ *	1.0
	Knee first peak	**−5.00**	**2.77**	**−4.08**	**1.79**	$t_{159} = -6.138, p = 0.0229$	**0.5**
	Knee second peak	**3.15**	**1.41**	**2.64**	**1.09**	$t_{159} = 6.628, p < 0.0001$ *	**0.5**
	Knee third peak	−3.45	1.29	−5.42	1.61	$t_{159} = 21.188, p < 0.0001$ *	1.7
	Knee forth peak	−7.15	1.83	−9.65	2.10	$t_{159} = 31.515, p < 0.0001$ *	2.5
	Ankle first peak	**−8.38**	**2.48**	**−9.44**	**1.81**	$t_{159} = 7.295, p = 0.6656$	**0.6**
	Ankle second peak	16.07	3.60	18.40	4.91	$t_{159} = -10.726, p = 0.2426$	0.9

K-S tests results for peak moments and peak powers at hip, knee, and ankle joint listed here were all greater than 0.05, therefore normal distribution of the parameters listed in this table was confirmed. * Indicates significant difference; **Bold** indicates the event was observed within the stance phase; *italic with underline* indicates the event was observed during the stance–swing transition; the rest of the parameters were observed within the swing phase. For joint moment data, "+" represents the extension (ankle plantar flexion) and "−" represents the flexion (ankle dorsiflexion). For joint power data, "+" represents energy production, and "−" represents energy absorption.

Table 2. Relative Time to Peak as Percentage Stride Cycle (Mean, SD) for Joint moments and Powers for Marker-based (MB) and Markerless (ML) Systems.

	Parameters	MB Mean	MB SD	ML Mean	ML SD	T & p-Value	Cohen's d
Moment (%stride Cycle)	Hip first peak	5.16	1.27	6.74	3.40	$t_{159} = -5.946, p < 0.0001$ *	0.5
	Hip second peak	*40.26*	*6.90*	*43.59*	*7.00*	$t_{159} = -7.179, p < 0.0001$ *	*0.6*
	Hip third peak	90.58	3.39	92.73	3.00	$t_{159} = -8.637, p < 0.0001$ *	0.7
	Knee first peak	**12.98**	**2.18**	**13.53**	**3.89**	$t_{159} = -2.008, p = 0.0015$ *	0.2
	Knee second peak	90.93	2.21	92.19	2.51	$t_{159} = -10.031, p < 0.0001$ *	0.8
	Ankle first peak	**18.29**	**1.90**	**18.33**	**1.82**	$t_{159} = -0.569, p = 0.57$	0.0
Power (%Stride Cycle)	**Hip first peak**	**26.61**	**4.45**	**28.30**	**3.68**	$t_{159} = -6.983, p < 0.0001$ *	0.6
	Hip second peak	51.89	3.90	52.36	4.37	$t_{159} = -1.243, p = 0.216$	0.1
	Hip third peak	91.23	3.47	89.63	4.15	$t_{159} = 4.458, p < 0.0001$ *	0.4
	Knee first peak	**8.19**	**2.21**	**8.73**	**3.01**	$t_{159} = -2.380, p = 0.0006$ *	0.2
	Knee second peak	**19.45**	**3.09**	**21.17**	**3.51**	$t_{159} = -6.606, p < 0.0001$ *	0.5
	Knee third peak	49.31	2.77	49.06	3.30	$t_{159} = 0.860, p = 0.391$	0.1
	Knee forth peak	86.59	2.18	86.83	2.31	$t_{159} = -1.740, p = 0.084$	0.1
	Ankle first peak	**10.58**	**2.20**	**10.82**	**2.22**	$t_{159} = -1.794, p = 0.075$	0.6
	Ankle second peak	**24.10**	**2.32**	**24.21**	**2.08**	$t_{159} = -0.943, p = 0.347$	0.1

K-S tests results for relative timing to peak moments and peak powers at hip, knee, and ankle joints listed here were all greater than 0.05, therefore normal distribution of the parameters listed in this table was confirmed. * Indicates significant difference; **Bold** indicates the event was observed within the stance phase; *italic with underline* indicates the event was observed during the stance–swing transition; rest of the parameters were observed within the swing phase.

3.2. Lower Extremity Joint Center and Segment Center of Mass

Joint moments could be significantly affected by joint center position and the segment center of mass. Figures 3 and 4 demonstrate the ensemble curves of differences in joint center positions (hip, knee, ankle) and segment center of mass (thigh, leg, foot) between MB and ML.

In the mediolateral direction (Figure 3 top panel), the ankle (left) and knee (middle) joint centers were biased toward the lateral direction in the ML than the MB throughout the stride cycle. The hip joint center showed the same trend except during initial contact and the late swing phase. In the anterior–posterior direction (Figure 3 middle panel), ML showed a posterior-biased hip joint center during the stride cycle, whereas the ankle and knee joint centers varied within the stride cycle. The ML was posteriorly biased compared to the MB at initial contact for both the ankle and knee joints. For the rest of the stance phase, the ML for the ankle joint was slightly more posterior, and the knee was more anterior. While the ML for the ankle joint continued in the posterior direction in the swing phase, the ML knee continued in the anterior direction in the early swing phase but turned to the posterior direction for the rest of the swing phase. In the vertical direction (Figure 3 bottom panel), the ML of the ankle varied during the stride cycle. In the early stance and mid-swing phase, the estimated bias was toward the superior direction, while in the mid-stance and early swing, it turned to the inferior direction. The ML showed an inferior-biased knee and hip joint center in the early stance. When the ML knee joint turned to the superior direction for the rest of the stride cycle, the hip joint was superior in the mid-stance and early swing phase but moved toward the inferior direction in the rest of the swing phase. See Figure 3 for more details.

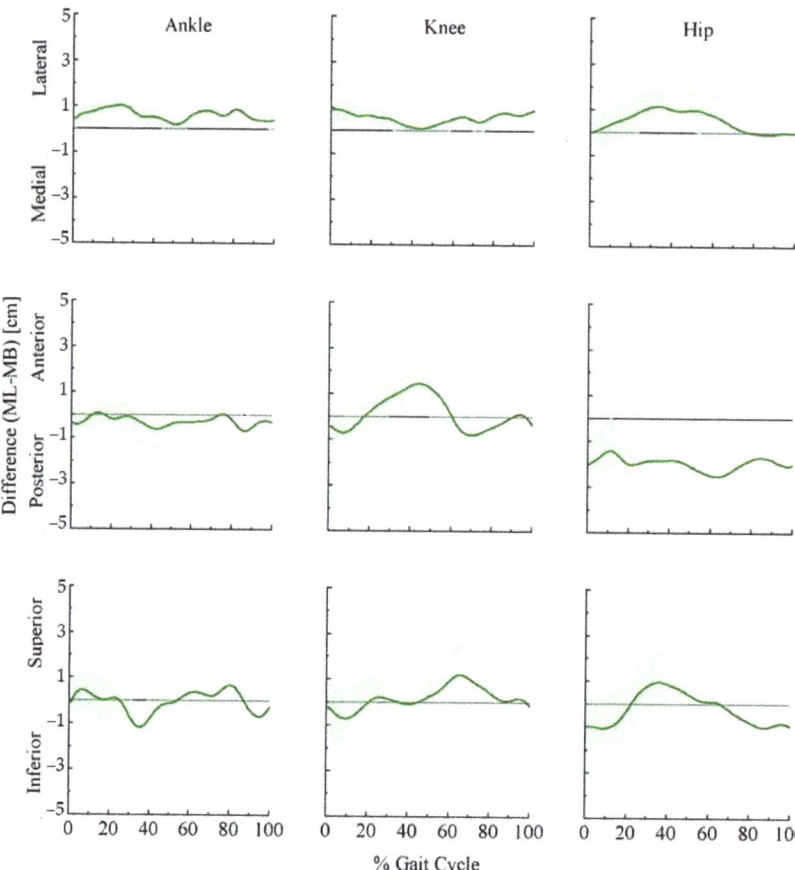

Figure 3. Ensemble curve of lower extremity joint position differences between marker-based and markerless motion capture systems across the average 10 stride cycles for 16 participants. Differences were estimated as markerless (ML) joint center position—marker-based (MB) joint center position.

In the mediolateral direction (Figure 4 top panel), the center of mass of the foot, leg, and thigh was more lateral in the ML than in the MB systems throughout the stride cycle. In the anterior–posterior direction (Figure 4 middle panel), the foot center of mass was more anterior in the ML than in the MB system during the stride cycle. For the leg center of mass, ML showed more posterior biases than the MB during the stance and swing phases except in different directions at the end of the swing phase. The thigh center of mass was mainly posterior throughout the stride cycle but briefly anterior in the swing–stance transition phase. In the vertical direction, the foot center of mass showed a higher position in the ML than in the MB system during most stance and late swing phases but was lower during the stance–swing transition and early swing phase. For the leg center of mass, the ML demonstrated lower values than the MB system during about 85% of the stride cycle but they were briefly higher during the early swing phase. The thigh center of mass from the ML showed a higher position than the MB system over the whole stride cycle.

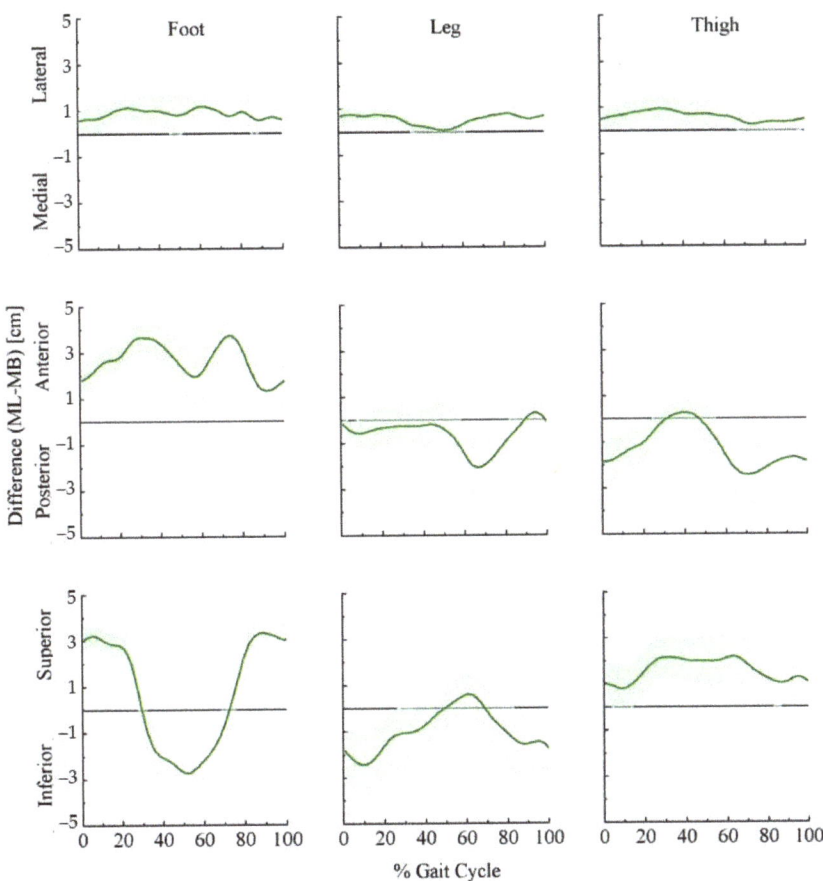

Figure 4. Ensemble curve of lower extremity segment center of mass differences between marker-based and markerless motion capture systems across the average 10 stride cycles for 16 participants. Differences were estimated as markerless (ML) center of mass position—marker-based (MB) center of mass position.

3.3. Lower Extremity Joint Angles

Ensemble curves of the difference in lower extremity joint angles (hip, knee, ankle joints) in the sagittal plane between the systems are illustrated in Figure 5.

The hip (top panel) and knee (middle panel) joint angles were biased toward the extension in the ML than MB throughout the stride cycle except briefly for the early swing phase for the hip joint, and early stance phase for the knee joint. On the other hand, ML showed a dorsiflexion-biased ankle joint angle (bottom panel) throughout the stride cycle.

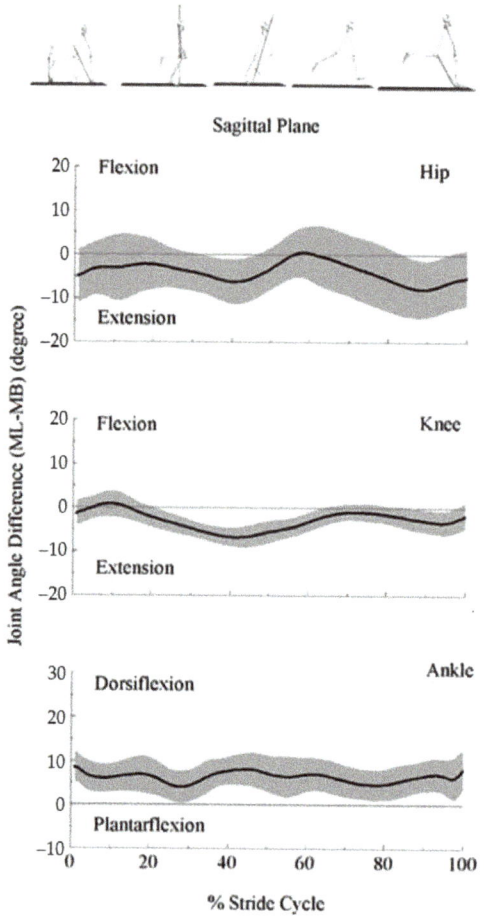

Figure 5. Ensemble curve of lower extremity joint angle differences in the sagittal plane between marker-based (MB) and markerless (ML) motion capture systems across the average 10 stride cycles for 16 participants. Differences were estimated as ML joint angles of each joint—MB joint angles of each joint.

4. Discussion

This study compared MB and ML systems with estimated lower extremity joint moments and powers during treadmill running. Significant differences were detected in the peak magnitudes for joint moments and powers and relative timings to peak estimated by the two systems. Greater peak magnitudes for hip extension and flexion moments, knee flexion moments, and ankle plantarflexion moments, along with their joint powers, were observed in the ML system. Meanwhile, significantly smaller peak magnitudes for knee extension moments coinciding with knee production power were observed.

We focused on the sagittal plane's joint angles, moments, and powers, since running is primarily a sagittal plane movement [31]. We observed greater hip and knee flexion angles and smaller ankle dorsiflexion angles in the MB system than in the ML system. The tendency was partly consistent with Kanko et al.'s study [19] (Figure 2 for lower extremity joint center, Figure 4 for segment angle and Figure 5 for joint angle), showing that the MB system's estimation resulted in greater flexion in all three joints. One possible explanation may be the model of the virtual foot. Visual3D introduces three methods to build the virtual foot, which may affect the ankle joint angles. When we chose the heel and toe targets to define the proximal and distal ends of the foot, there was no disclosure for Kanko et al.'s foot model. Different from Kanko et al.'s results, we observed larger magnitudes of systematic differences in the knee and ankle joint angles but smaller magnitudes in the hip joint. Compared to walking in Kanko et al., running in the current project is related to greater lower extremity joint motion [32]. With greater joint motion, soft tissue artifacts can also be larger, leading to an additional 3° error in the joint angles. Additionally, inconsistent marker placement can contribute to a 5° error in the joint angles [14,33].

Compared to the MB system, the ML system's estimation resulted in greater magnitudes of peak hip flexion moment in the stance–swing transition phase and extension moment in the late swing phase, knee flexion moment in the late swing phase, and ankle plantarflexion moments in the early stance phase, but smaller knee extension moments in the early stance phase. Previous studies presented similar patterns of lower extremity joint moments during running estimated by MB systems. Schache et al. (2011) and Fukuchi et al. (2017) reported lower extremity joint moments at the speed of 3.5 m/s during overground and treadmill running, respectively [34,35]. Their results showed similar peak magnitudes of hip flexion and extension moments of −1.09 and 0.91 Nm/kg (overground) and −1.15 and 1.37 Nm/kg (treadmill); knee flexion moments of −0.53 Nm/kg (overground); as well as the ankle plantarflexion moment with the values of 2.94 Nm/kg (overground) and 2.23 Nm/kg (treadmill). Besides, they reported similar knee extension moments with the values of 3.12 Nm/kg (overground) and 3.18 Nm/kg (treadmill). Consequently, joint powers also showed the same tendency. Despite the differences between overground and treadmill running, Schache et al.'s results revealed similar systematic differences to the present study. Compared to the MB system, the estimations from the ML system may result in greater hip moments and powers in the stance–swing transition and swing phase, knee moments and powers in the swing phase, as well as the ankle moments in the early stance phase, but less knee moments and power in the early stance phase.

The anthropometric model affects the results of the joint moments and powers. Once rigid body equations are set, the joint centers and moment of inertia about the center of mass eventually govern the relationships between kinetics and kinematics [20]. The systematic differences can be further explained by the variations of joint centers and segment mass centers.

It has been well-recognized that differences in hip joint center location can propagate to hip and knee kinematic and kinetic quantities, especially the hip moments concerning flexion/extension [36]. Besides, the propagation of flexion/extension moments is particularly sensitive to the anteroposterior hip joint center location. We observed that hip joint centers in the ML system were about 2 cm posterior to the MB system in the stance–swing transition and late swing phase. In addition, the sensitivity of hip moments to inertial property variations can be up to 40% [7]. Supported by our results, the thigh center of mass locations was about 2 cm superior in the ML than the MB system in the stance–swing transition phase. Similar to a previous study, greater changes occurred in the swing phase [7], and the ML system showed a biased posterior (about 2 cm) and anterior (about 1 cm) center of mass. For the knee joint, joint moments are sensitive to the differences in knee joint center locations [37]. Previous studies have reported that tibia surface movements affected the knee joint center by 1.1 cm and resulted in the most prominent joint moment in the stance phase [37]. Our results exhibited that knee joint centers differed around 1 cm in all directions and result in greater disparities in the leg center of mass in the early stance phase, which may explain the greater knee extension moment in the MB system. Moreover, our results exhibited a greater leg center of mass in the late swing phase, which may induce greater knee flexion moments. For the ankle joint, we observed less than 1 cm differences in all three directions. Previous studies indicated that average ankle joint position differences were less than 1 cm in the anteroposterior and mediolateral direction and around 2 cm in the vertical direction [19]. Plus, the foot center of mass locations varied greatly. The ML system was slightly biased in the lateral direction (<1 cm) with greater bias in the anterior and superior directions (almost 3 cm). Such a difference may be induced by the marker placements of the first and fifth metatarsal heads. While the MB system reads the markers on the side of the first and fifth metatarsal heads, the markerless system might locate the foot center of mass based on the contour of the shoe. The different joint centers could affect moment arms, and the segment center of mass could affect the estimation of the moment of inertia. Together, they could lead to greater differences in the joint moments and powers.

The methodology differences between ML and MB systems that determine the estimation of poses (body segment positions and orientations) need further attention. To ensure the consistency of the computational algorithms, Visual3D has been used for segments and inverse dynamic solutions used for both systems. However, the MB system depends heavily on physical marker placements over external/internal anatomical landmarks (hardware), and the ML system relies on deep learning-based algorithms to estimate joint center locations (software). The deep learning pose estimation algorithms learn to identify joint centers from the training data. ML in the current study includes over 500,000 manually labeled digital images of the human body and employs biomechanically applicable training data that can identify 51 salient features of the human body [17–19]. The optimization methods examine the distance between the manually labeled training data and the estimated joint centers to reduce errors. This process is repeated with the entire training data until improvements between each iteration become negligible. The pose estimation algorithm is then tested on the new image and compared to the training dataset [38]. However, any omissions or biases implicit within training datasets could propagate to situations where the training was weak [19]. Note that the inverse dynamic method is very sensitive to joint center locations, because the estimation of the net joint moments includes the cross product of forces and their moment arms, where the length of moment arms is largely affected by joint center locations [37]. A previous marker-based study has reported that 2 cm superior and 2 cm lateral placement of the hip joint center can decrease the moment of arms of the hip joint by about 28% [38]. Supported by our results, systematic differences in joint center positions have been observed, which might affect moment arms and lead to disparities in joint moments and powers. However, it remains unclear if the differences are caused by marker-based joint center errors induced by soft tissue artifacts [11] or propagations from a weak training dataset.

While the ML system may still be considered in its infancy, evidence from previous studies demonstrated its potential for clinical applications. Since pose estimation algorithms are not dependent on markers attached to the skin, soft tissue artifact errors and human errors usually induced by the MB systems can be eliminated [39]. Studies also presented that the markerless system can extract new information from old datasets [40,41]. Therefore, the ML system can be beneficial in the streamlined monitoring of changes in disease progression [41], rehabilitation [42], athletic training, and competitive sports [43]. In addition, the Theia3D markerless system has shown strong results in the inter-session joint angles variability during walking with loose clothing conditions [18], which the MB systems cannot realize. More importantly, data collection can be completed in a much shorter time than the MB systems [18]. Such benefits could facilitate data collection in a more convenient area with less effect on people's gait [44], when time is limited, and they are wearing more comfortable clothing.

However, the differences observed here could have significant implications. For example, previous studies have shown that the values of hip extension and knee flexion moments in the initial stance and late swing phase were important factors in discussing hamstrings injuries during sprinting [45,46]. The greater hip extension and knee flexion moments observed in the late swing with the ML system could impact the hamstring injury-related discussions. Similar to hamstrings, the biarticular rectus femoris plays an important role in the energy transfer between the hip and knee joints. Greater rectus femoris stress is associated with greater hip flexion and knee extension moments. We have observed, with the ML in comparison with the MB system, greater hip flexion moments in the stance to swing transition phase, greater hip power absorption in the late stance phase, and greater hip joint power production in the early swing phase, which could lead to a greater rectus femoris contraction estimation during the stance–swing transition. A previous study showed that greater rectus femoris contraction could lead to greater patellar tendon tension, a risk factor for patellofemoral pain during running [47]. Thus, joint moment/power estimated by the ML system can lead to different assessments for the risk factors of hamstring injuries, patellofemoral pain, and maybe other relevant discussions compared to the MB system. With different risk factor analyses based on the MB or ML systems, clinicians, coaches, and athletes could arrive at different decisions in their practices.

The following limitations of the current work should be noted. First, our participant pool was limited to recreationally active young adults. Different population groups may have anatomical deformities, affecting the comparison between the systems. Second, we analyzed treadmill running, where the treadmill settings may constrain the speed. Additionally, the hardware and the marker placements are unique to each lab. Despite our updated Vicon high-resolution video cameras employed for markerless data, the Vicon Bonita series infrared cameras used here do not provide us with the highest resolution available on the market. Lower camera resolution may cause trajectory errors in the identifications of landmarks [48]. Therefore, future studies should attempt to replicate the results in different populations using different speeds and hardware settings.

5. Conclusions

This study is the first to compare the inverse dynamic outcomes of lower extremity kinetics estimated by the marker-based and markerless systems. We have observed differences in joint moments and powers between the two systems, which could be partially related to the estimations of joint centers and segment center of mass (pose estimations). Although the accuracy and precision of pose estimations between the two systems require further testing, the strengths of the markerless system are apparent. The significantly less data collection and processing time contribute greatly to a more versatile application. With the progression of pose estimation software, the markerless system can be further employed in clinical biomechanics and sports medicine.

Author Contributions: Conceptualization, L.L.; methodology, L.L. and K.D.; validation, J.P. and K.D.; formal analysis, H.T., K.D. and J.P.; investigation, H.T.; data curation, J.P.; writing—original draft preparation, H.T.; writing—review and editing, L.L., K.D. and B.M.; visualization, H.T.; supervision, L.L.; project administration, L.L. All authors have read and agreed to the published version of the manuscript.

Funding: This research received no external funding.

Institutional Review Board Statement: The study was conducted in accordance with the Declaration of Helsinki, and approved by the Georgia Southern University Ethics Committee (protocol code H22732, 07/08/2022).

Informed Consent Statement: Informed consent was obtained from all subjects involved in the study. Written informed consent has been obtained from the patient(s) to publish this paper.

Data Availability Statement: Not applicable.

Conflicts of Interest: The authors declare no conflict of interest.

References

1. Winter, D.A. *Biomechanics and Motor Control of Human Movement*; John Wiley & Sons: Hoboken, NJ, USA, 2005.
2. Tate, J.J.; Milner, C. Real-Time Kinematic, Temporospatial, and Kinetic Biofeedback During Gait Retraining in Patients: A Systematic Review. *Phys. Ther.* **2010**, *90*, 1123–1134. [CrossRef] [PubMed]
3. Shaw, K.E.; Charlton, J.; Perry, C.K.L.; De Vries, C.M.; Redekopp, M.J.; White, J.A.; Hunt, M.A. The effects of shoe-worn insoles on gait biomechanics in people with knee osteoarthritis: A systematic review and meta-analysis. *Br. J. Sport. Med.* **2017**, *52*, 238–253. [CrossRef] [PubMed]
4. Hart, H.; Culvenor, A.; Collins, N.; Ackland, D.; Cowan, S.; Machotka, Z.; Crossley, K. Knee kinematics and joint moments during gait following anterior cruciate ligament reconstruction: A systematic review and meta-analysis. *Br. J. Sport. Med.* **2015**, *50*, 597–612. [CrossRef] [PubMed]

5. Riemer, R.; Hsiao-Wecksler, E.T.; Zhang, X. Uncertainties in inverse dynamics solutions: A comprehensive analysis and an application to gait. *Gait Posture* **2008**, *27*, 578–588. [CrossRef] [PubMed]
6. McLean, S.G.; Walker, K.; Ford, K.R.; Myer, G.D.; E Hewett, T.; Bogert, A.J.V.D. Evaluation of a two dimensional analysis method as a screening and evaluation tool for anterior cruciate ligament injury. *Br. J. Sport. Med.* **2005**, *39*, 355–362. [CrossRef]
7. Pearsall, D.; Costigan, P. The effect of segment parameter error on gait analysis results. *Gait Posture* **1999**, *9*, 173–183. [CrossRef]
8. Ganley, K.J.; Powers, C.M. Determination of lower extremity anthropometric parameters using dual energy X-ray absorptiometry: The influence on net joint moments during gait. *Clin. Biomech.* **2004**, *19*, 50–56. [CrossRef]
9. Schwartz, M.H.; Rozumalski, A. A new method for estimating joint parameters from motion data. *J. Biomech.* **2005**, *38*, 107–116. [CrossRef]
10. Richards, J.G. The measurement of human motion: A comparison of commercially available systems. *Hum. Mov. Sci.* **1999**, *18*, 589–602. [CrossRef]
11. Cappozzo, A.; Catani, F.; Della Croce, U.; Leardini, A. Position and orientation in space of bones during movement: Anatomical frame definition and determination. *Clin. Biomech.* **1995**, *10*, 171–178. [CrossRef]
12. Stagni, R.; Fantozzi, S.; Cappello, A.; Leardini, A. Quantification of soft tissue artefact in motion analysis by combining 3D fluoroscopy and stereophotogrammetry: A study on two subjects. *Clin. Biomech.* **2005**, *20*, 320–329. [CrossRef] [PubMed]
13. Simon, S.R. Quantification of human motion: Gait analysis—Benefits and limitations to its application to clinical problems. *J. Biomech.* **2004**, *37*, 1869–1880. [CrossRef] [PubMed]
14. Gorton, G.E., III; Hebert, D.A.; Gannotti, M.E. Assessment of the kinematic variability among 12 motion analysis laboratories. *Gait Posture* **2009**, *29*, 398–402. [CrossRef] [PubMed]
15. Buckley, C.; Alcock, L.; McArdle, R.; Rehman, R.; Del Din, S.; Mazzà, C.; Yarnall, A.; Rochester, L. The Role of Movement Analysis in Diagnosing and Monitoring Neurodegenerative Conditions: Insights from Gait and Postural Control. *Brain Sci.* **2019**, *9*, 34. [CrossRef]
16. Whittle, M.W. Clinical gait analysis: A review. *Hum. Mov. Sci.* **1996**, *15*, 369–387. [CrossRef]
17. Kanko, R.M.; Laende, E.K.; Strutzenberger, G.; Brown, M.; Selbie, W.S.; DePaul, V.; Scott, S.H.; Deluzio, K.J. Assessment of spatiotemporal gait parameters using a deep learning algorithm-based markerless motion capture system. *J. Biomech.* **2021**, *122*, 110414. [CrossRef]
18. Kanko, R.M.; Laende, E.; Selbie, W.S.; Deluzio, K.J. Inter-session repeatability of markerless motion capture gait kinematics. *J. Biomech.* **2021**, *121*, 110422. [CrossRef]
19. Kanko, R.M.; Laende, E.K.; Davis, E.M.; Selbie, W.S.; Deluzio, K.J. Concurrent assessment of gait kinematics using marker-based and markerless motion capture. *J. Biomech.* **2021**, *127*, 110665. [CrossRef]
20. Derrick, T.R.; Bogert, A.J.V.D.; Cereatti, A.; Dumas, R.; Fantozzi, S.; Leardini, A. ISB recommendations on the reporting of intersegmental forces and moments during human motion analysis. *J. Biomech.* **2019**, *99*, 109533. [CrossRef]
21. Woltring, H.J. Representation and calculation of 3-D joint movement. *Hum. Mov. Sci.* **1991**, *10*, 603–616. [CrossRef]
22. Gruber, A.H.; Zhang, S.; Pan, J.; Li, L. Leg and Joint Stiffness Adaptations to Minimalist and Maximalist Running Shoes. *J. Appl. Biomech.* **2021**, *37*, 408–414. [CrossRef] [PubMed]
23. Documentation, C.-M.W. Tutorial: Foot and Ankle Angles. 2020. Available online: https://www.c-motion.com/v3dwiki/index.php?title=Visual3D_Documentation (accessed on 12 October 2022).
24. Dempster, W.T. *Space Requirements of the Seated Operator, Geometrical, Kinematic, and Mechanical Aspects of the Body with Special Reference to the Limbs*; Michigan State University: East Lansing, MI, USA, 1955.
25. Hanavan, E.P. *A Mathematical Model of the Human Body*; AMRL Technical Report; AMRL: Tamil Nadu, India, 1964; pp. 64–102. [CrossRef]
26. Bell, A.L.; Brand, R.A.; Pedersen, D.R. Prediction of hip joint centre location from external landmarks. *Hum. Mov. Sci.* **1989**, *8*, 3–16. [CrossRef]
27. Kristianslund, E.; Krosshaug, T.; Bogert, A.J.V.D. Effect of low pass filtering on joint moments from inverse dynamics: Implications for injury prevention. *J. Biomech.* **2012**, *45*, 666–671. [CrossRef] [PubMed]
28. Robertson, D.G.E.; Caldwell, G.E.; Hamill, J.; Kamen, G.; Whittlesey, S.N. *Research Methods in Biomechanics*, 2nd ed.; Human Kinetics: Champaign, IL, USA, 2014. [CrossRef]
29. Zhang, S.; Pan, J.; Li, L. Non-linear changes of lower extremity kinetics prior to gait transition. *J. Biomech.* **2018**, *77*, 48–54. [CrossRef] [PubMed]
30. Cohen, J. *Statistical Power Analysis for the Behavioral Sciences*; Routledge: London, UK, 2013.
31. Dugan, S.A.; Bhat, K.P. Biomechanics and Analysis of Running Gait. *Phys. Med. Rehabil. Clin.* **2005**, *16*, 603–621. [CrossRef]
32. Novacheck, T.F. The biomechanics of running. *Gait Posture* **1998**, *7*, 77–95. [CrossRef]
33. Schwartz, M.H.; Trost, J.P.; Wervey, R.A. Measurement and management of errors in quantitative gait data. *Gait Posture* **2004**, *20*, 196–203. [CrossRef]
34. Fukuchi, R.K.; Fukuchi, C.A.; Duarte, M. A public dataset of running biomechanics and the effects of running speed on lower extremity kinematics and kinetics. *PeerJ* **2017**, *5*, e3298. [CrossRef]
35. Schache, A.G.; Blanch, P.D.; Dorn, T.W.; Brown, N.; Rosemond, D.; Pandy, M. Effect of Running Speed on Lower Limb Joint Kinetics. *Med. Sci. Sport. Exerc.* **2011**, *43*, 1260–1271. [CrossRef]

36. Stagni, R.; Leardini, A.; Cappozzo, A.; Benedetti, M.G.; Cappello, A. Effects of hip joint centre mislocation on gait analysis results. *J. Biomech.* **2000**, *33*, 1479–1487. [CrossRef]
37. Holden, J.P.; Stanhope, S.J. The effect of variation in knee center location estimates on net knee joint moments. *Gait Posture* **1998**, *7*, 1–6. [CrossRef]
38. Wade, L.; Needham, L.; McGuigan, P.; Bilzon, J. Applications and limitations of current markerless motion capture methods for clinical gait biomechanics. *PeerJ* **2022**, *10*, e12995. [CrossRef] [PubMed]
39. Reinschmidt, C.; Bogert, A.V.D.; Nigg, B.; Lundberg, A.; Murphy, N. Effect of skin movement on the analysis of skeletal knee joint motion during running. *J. Biomech.* **1997**, *30*, 729–732. [CrossRef]
40. Shin, J.H.; Yu, R.; Ong, J.N.; Lee, C.Y.; Jeon, S.H.; Park, H.; Kim, H.-J.; Lee, J.; Jeon, B. Quantitative Gait Analysis Using a Pose-Estimation Algorithm with a Single 2D-Video of Parkinson's Disease Patients. *J. Park. Dis.* **2021**, *11*, 1271–1283. [CrossRef] [PubMed]
41. Kidziński, Ł.; Yang, B.; Hicks, J.L.; Rajagopal, A.; Delp, S.L.; Schwartz, M.H. Deep neural networks enable quantitative movement analysis using single-camera videos. *Nat. Commun.* **2020**, *11*, 1–10. [CrossRef] [PubMed]
42. Cronin, N.J.; Rantalainen, T.; Ahtiainen, J.P.; Hynynen, E.; Waller, B. Markerless 2D kinematic analysis of underwater running: A deep learning approach. *J. Biomech.* **2019**, *87*, 75–82. [CrossRef] [PubMed]
43. Evans, M.; Colyer, S.; Cosker, D.; Salo, A. Foot Contact Timings and Step Length for Sprint Training. In Proceedings of the 2018 IEEE Winter Conference on Applications of Computer Vision (WACV), Lake Tahoe, NV, USA, 12–15 March 2018.
44. Robles-García, V.; Corral-Bergantiños, Y.; Espinosa, N.; Jácome, M.A.; García-Sancho, C.; Cudeiro, J.; Arias, P. Spatiotemporal Gait Patterns During Overt and Covert Evaluation in Patients With Parkinson's Disease and Healthy Subjects: Is There a Hawthorne Effect? *J. Appl. Biomech.* **2015**, *31*, 189–194. [CrossRef]
45. Liu, H.; Garrett, W.E.; Moorman, C.T.; Yu, B. Injury rate, mechanism, and risk factors of hamstring strain injuries in sports: A review of the literature. *J. Sport Health Sci.* **2012**, *1*, 92–101. [CrossRef]
46. Sun, Y.; Wei, S.; Zhong, Y.; Fu, W.; Li, L.; Liu, Y. How Joint Torques Affect Hamstring Injury Risk in Sprinting Swing–Stance Transition. *Med. Sci. Sport. Exerc.* **2015**, *47*, 373–380. [CrossRef]
47. Lenhart, R.L.; Thelen, D.G.; Wille, C.M.; Chumanov, E.S.; Heiderscheit, B.C. Increasing Running Step Rate Reduces Patellofemoral Joint Forces. *Med. Sci. Sport. Exerc.* **2014**, *46*, 557–564. [CrossRef]
48. Zago, M.; Luzzago, M.; Marangoni, T.; De Cecco, M.; Tarabini, M.; Galli, M. 3D Tracking of Human Motion Using Visual Skeletonization and Stereoscopic Vision. *Front. Bioeng. Biotechnol.* **2020**, *8*, 181. [CrossRef] [PubMed]

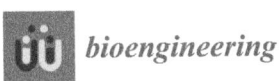

Article

Automated Student Classroom Behaviors' Perception and Identification Using Motion Sensors

Hongmin Wang [1,†], Chi Gao [2,3,†], Hong Fu [1,*], Christina Zong-Hao Ma [4,*], Quan Wang [2], Ziyu He [1] and Maojun Li [1,5]

1 Department of Mathematics and Information Technology, The Education University of Hong Kong, Hong Kong 999077, China
2 The Key Laboratory of Spectral Imaging Technology, Xi'an Institute of Optics and Precision Mechanics of the Chinese Academy of Sciences, Xi'an 710119, China
3 The University of Chinese Academy of Sciences, Beijing 100049, China
4 Department of Biomedical Engineering, The Hong Kong Polytechnic University, Hong Kong 999077, China
5 School of Information Science and Technology, Northwest University, Xi'an 710127, China
* Correspondence: hfu@eduhk.hk (H.F.); czh.ma@polyu.edu.hk (C.Z.-H.M.); Tel.: +852-2948-7535
† These authors contributed equally to this work.

Abstract: With the rapid development of artificial intelligence technology, the exploration and application in the field of intelligent education has become a research hotspot of increasing concern. In the actual classroom scenarios, students' classroom behavior is an important factor that directly affects their learning performance. Specifically, students with poor self-management abilities, particularly specific developmental disorders, may face educational and academic difficulties owing to physical or psychological factors. Therefore, the intelligent perception and identification of school-aged children's classroom behaviors are extremely valuable and significant. The traditional method for identifying students' classroom behavior relies on statistical surveys conducted by teachers, which incurs problems such as being time-consuming, labor-intensive, privacy-violating, and an inaccurate manual intervention. To address the above-mentioned issues, we constructed a motion sensor-based intelligent system to realize the perception and identification of classroom behavior in the current study. For the acquired sensor signal, we proposed a Voting-Based Dynamic Time Warping algorithm (VB-DTW) in which a voting mechanism is used to compare the similarities between adjacent clips and extract valid action segments. Subsequent experiments have verified that effective signal segments can help improve the accuracy of behavior identification. Furthermore, upon combining with the classroom motion data acquisition system, through the powerful feature extraction ability of the deep learning algorithms, the effectiveness and feasibility are verified from the perspectives of the dimensional signal characteristics and time series separately so as to realize the accurate, non-invasive and intelligent children's behavior detection. To verify the feasibility of the proposed method, a self-constructed dataset (SCB-13) was collected. Thirteen participants were invited to perform 14 common class behaviors, wearing motion sensors whose data were recorded by a program. In SCB-13, the proposed method achieved 100% identification accuracy. Based on the proposed algorithms, it is possible to provide immediate feedback on students' classroom performance and help them improve their learning performance while providing an essential reference basis and data support for constructing an intelligent digital education platform.

Keywords: intelligent system; deep learning; classroom behavior; motion identification

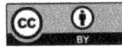

1. Introduction

1.1. Background Information on Students' Classroom Behavior

With the rapid development, penetration, and integration of artificial intelligence technologies in various areas of society, intelligent digital-based education is progressively becoming a hot issue of substantive research [1,2]. Among the many educational research carriers, the intelligent education classroom scenarios are still the commonly adopted educational method [3], which has the outstanding advantages of direct feedback and extensive interaction between teachers and students [4].

Classroom scenarios present complexity and diversity according to different participants and instructional content. Research has shown that in classroom scenarios, students' classroom behavior is one of the most important factors influencing their academic performance [5]. Compared with high-achieving students, low-achieving students typically spend a significant amount of class time engaged in non-academic work or other academic work [6]. Therefore, investigating student classroom behavior has essential research implications and applicate values for enhancing student performance and promoting instructional strategies [7].

Specifically, the study of classroom behavior through detecting and identifying students' classroom behavior patterns can provide timely and stage-specific feedback on students' classroom performance. Effective statistical analysis of students' behavior patterns will assist students in effectively understanding their learning habits, timely correcting their poor classroom behavior, improving learning strategies, adjusting learning progress, and deepening their understanding and absorption of knowledge.

Furthermore, the analysis of students' classroom behavior is especially beneficial for students with special education needs (SEN) and developmental disabilities, such as attention deficit and hyperactivity disorder (ADHD) [8], autism spectrum disorder (ASD) [9], and learning disabilities [9,10]. Conducting classroom behavior analysis is crucial to improving these students' classroom performance and enhancing their classroom concentration. The percentage of school-aged children diagnosed with developmental disorders is increasing dramatically each year due to various environmental factors such as location, level of education, and medical care. In addition, the percentage of children with developmental disorders increased to 17.8% of all children (3–17 years old, the United States). The proportion is substantial, with approximately one in six children diagnosed with a disease [11]. Specifically, ADHD has the broadest range of effects on all developmental disorders and has the most significant prevalence among children. Characteristics of children with ADHD include inattention, hyperactivity, and impulsivity. Students with developmental disorders generally suffer from academic problems due to physical or psychological issues, and their classroom performance is difficult to self-control.

The study of classroom behaviors of students with developmental disabilities can be used to detect and identify their classroom behaviors automatically to a large extent. It can help them improve their self-awareness, enhance their concentration, and effectively achieve supplementary education without external interventions [12]. Auxiliary education based on non-artificial reminders can greatly relieve their learning pressure, ease learning difficulties and anxiety, increase knowledge and improve environmental adaptability, and promote a virtuous cycle of learning [13].

Finally, due to the need to build intelligent digital education platforms for schools and parents, the study of classroom behavior can further refine students' learning performance at school [14], optimize school teaching services, improve teaching strategies, and facilitate communication and exchange among multiple parties [15]. The intelligent digital platform is designed with students as the primary body and their classroom behaviors as the principal way of measuring their classroom status in order to enhance students' learning performance and optimize the teaching services of teachers. The perception and identification of students' classroom behaviors open the door to the development of an intelligent digital education platform.

1.2. Literature Review

In this part, we review the literature from the perspectives of 'Existing methods and the limitations' and 'Advanced methods on human activity recognition' to demonstrate the previous work on the perception and identification of student classroom behaviors.

1.2.1. Existing Methods and the Limitations

The previous research on students' classroom behavior in the traditional education field is often based on statistical survey methods, requiring teachers to observe the classroom behavior of the entire class or a smaller number of people as an observer over a period within the classroom and to record their behavior [16]. In these circumstances, the teacher plays the role of the evaluator to assess the student's behavior patterns. This manual, vision-based approach is usually surpassed in identifying inappropriate classroom activities, but the teacher's one-to-many nature at the time of the count results in the poor perception of the finer classroom behaviors of most students [17]. Furthermore, this visual-based artificial approach to behavior analysis is undoubtedly time-consuming, labor-intensive, and highly subjective. It is highly likely to violate students' privacy through external interventions and create learning ancients. It cannot give objective science-based judgments, thus preventing a comprehensive classroom behavior assessment. For school-age children with developmental disabilities, classroom behavior management and interventions are the primary methods for improving their classroom performance. There are three common primary types of classroom behavior interventions: one-on-one peer help or parent coaching [18], instructional task modification [19], and self-monitoring [20]. However, while this traditional intervention method has helped children with developmental disabilities improve their classroom task completion rate and classroom behavioral performance, this behavioral intervention undoubtedly consumes many resources in terms of monitoring children's classroom behavior. It requires significant human and material resources to assist children's classroom learning process.

1.2.2. Advanced Methods on Human Activity Recognition

With the development and popularization of artificial intelligence technologies, research on scenario-based understanding and behavioral analysis has shone in practical application scenarios [21]. With the help of data-driven and algorithmic reasoning, machine learning theory provides the feasibility of achieving a one-to-one accurate understanding and assessment of students' classroom behaviors [22], especially for fine-grained behavioral analysis that is difficult to be taken into account by manual statistics. Some scholars have already implemented AI techniques with classroom scene understanding and achieved better results. For example, intelligent classroom systems that assist teachers in teaching and personalize students' learning by building front-end interactive learning environments for teachers and students and back-end intelligent learning management systems [23]. Adaptive education platforms that solve students' specific learning problems provide personalized teaching and improve students' learning experiences according to their needs and their abilities [24]. However, little research has been conducted on AI-based classroom behavioral understanding due to the immature combination of technologies and the niche nature of the educational scenario, making it almost impossible to find corresponding work for reference. Although classroom behavioral activities are too complex and refined, it still belongs to the domain of behavior recognition, so we can help build an intelligent classroom-acceptable behavior perception system by referring to the relevant theories of human activity recognition. A brief overview of the human activity recognition approach is presented in the following section.

The mainstream approaches for human activity recognition can be roughly classified into vision-based and sensor-based based on different data sources [25]. Vision-based behavioral analysis systems usually use single or multiple RGB or depth cameras to collect images or video data of participants' behavioral information, environment, and background information in a specific activity space [26]. Moreover, after feature extraction of the collected data through image processing techniques and computer vision methods, they can be used to identify participants' behavior through algorithm learning and inference. Research conducted by numerous scholars applying vision methods in the field of human activity recognition includes: identifying group behavior and classifying abnormal activities in crowded scenes for surveillance as well as public personal safety purposes [27–29], including analysis of fall detection, patient monitoring and other behavioral recognition of individuals to improve the quality of human life through vision [30,31]. However, since the vision-based data acquisition equipment for human activity behavior recognition mainly relies on cameras, it is vulnerable to environmental conditions such as light and weather, the shooting range and angle, and a large amount of acquired data storage. The reference of participants' activity is easily affected by environmental occlusion and privacy issues. Due to the influence of these factors, vision-based behavior analysis systems have not yet been widely used. In contrast, sensors have the advantages of high sensitivity, small size, accessible storage, and wide applicability to various scenarios, which can avoid various problems in using vision devices, so they are now widely embedded in mobile phones, smartwatches and bracelets, eye-tracking devices, virtual/augmented reality headsets, and various intelligent IoT devices [32]. Meanwhile, along with the widespread popularity of mobile Internet and the increasing demand for daily public use of intelligent devices, the problems of inconvenience in carrying and limited endurance of traditional sensor-based devices have been effectively solved in various application scenarios, and they have now become one of the mainstream methods for human activity recognition [25]. Scholars have applied sensing devices for intelligent activity recognition in several daily domains: Alani et al. achieved 93.67% accuracy in 2020 using a deep learning approach to recognize twenty everyday human activities in intelligent homes [33]; Kavuncuoğlu et al. used only a waist sensor to achieve accurate monitoring of fall and daily motion data, achieving 99.96% accuracy in 2520 data [34].

1.3. Contributions and Structure

The contributions of this paper include: 1. Artificial intelligent based behavior recognition is applied to the classroom environment for the first time, and an intelligent system with motion sensors to perceive and identify classroom behavior is built. 2. Based on sensor hardware devices, a classroom behavior database (SCB-13) including 14 common classroom behaviors collected from 13 participants is constructed. 3. A method of extracting valid sensor data segments based on an improved Voting-Based Dynamic Time Warping algorithm (VB-DTW) is proposed. 4. An intelligent identification method is proposed to recognize 14 common classroom behaviors based on valid behavior segments combined with a 1DCNN algorithm, and the proposed method achieved 100% recognition accuracy on a self-constructed dataset (SCB-13).

The second part of this paper describes the data hardware acquisition system and the relevant characteristics of the data; the third part gives a brief overview of the basic principles of the algorithm; the fourth part is the experimental results and comparative analysis; finally, the paper provides a conclusion.

2. Materials and Methods

2.1. Participants

In this study, we recruited 13 participants to carry out a feasibility study on the possibility of accurately identifying students' classroom behavior. The participants, aged from 20 to 26 years, were invited to participate in a classroom behavioral simulation experiment. This population consisted of 6 males and 7 females without special educational needs or developmental problems. They were culturally literate and able to comprehend, imitate, and model classroom behaviors accurately. Participants signed consent forms approved by the Ethics Committee of The Education University of Hong Kong (Approval Number: 2021-2022-0417) before data collection.

2.2. Experimental Design

For each participant, 5 sets of experimental data were gathered, and a total of 65 sets of data were collected. In each trial, participants were tasked with simulating 14 common classroom behaviors, and Table 1 shows the design of each motion. Each motion lasts for 20 s, which can be divided into the valid time duration doing the motions and the sitting still time. Except for when motion happens, the rest of the period is referred to as sitting still time.

Table 1. Motion mode design. To simulate classroom behaviors for the participants, we selected 14 typical classroom behaviors. The table lists each motion's name as well as the order in which it took place.

Serial No.	Motion Mode
1	Sitting still
2	Lying on the desktop
3	Writing notes
4	Raising a hand in the seat
5	Turning around and looking around
6	Raising a hand while standing up
7	Rocking on the seat
8	Standing up and sitting down
9	Wandering and trunk rotation
10	Playing hands
11	Turning pen in hand
12	Knocking on the desktop
13	Leaning the body and chatting
14	Shaking legs

The actual hardware system used in the acquisition system is MPU6050, the main hardware processing chip is ESP-8266, the acquisition data bit rate is 115,200 Hz, the Arduino hardware platform is used for programming control, and the sensor data is stored in a .CSV file format via the computer's USB port using Python program. Figure 1a illustrates the schematic diagram of the 3D acquisition system, and 3 cameras are respectively installed on the participant's left side, front side, and diagonal rear to record the participant's vision motion data. As depicted in Figure 1b, in order to investigate the effect of the sensor in different positions, the sensors are positioned in the middle of the spine and the right shoulder of the participant. In addition to the 14 motions, there is a 20-s system calibration time at the beginning of the experiment to reduce the initial error caused during data acquisition, and the total duration of each experiment is 5 min. The sensors generate 7 channels of data: accelerometer (x-axis, y-axis, and z-axis) data, gyroscope (x-axis, y-axis, z-axis) data, and temperature data. The participants' motion information can be measured using accelerometer data in various directions. Gyroscope data can monitor angular velocity to determine an object's position and rotational orientation. Due to their susceptibility to environmental factors, temperature data are insufficient for use in a motion recognition system.

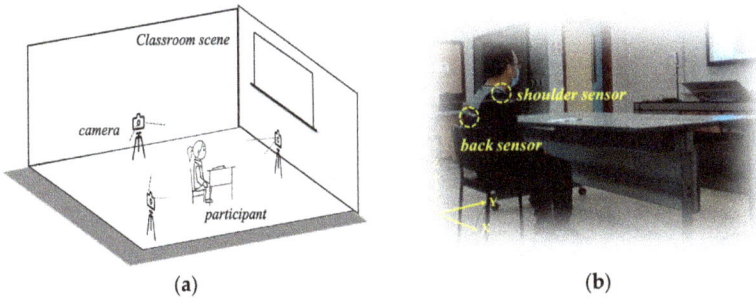

Figure 1. The acquisition system of the experiment. (**a**) The schematic diagram of the motion acquisition system in the classroom scene; (**b**) The location of the sensors. The vision information of the participants' motions is collected through cameras from three perspectives to assist in the classification. One sensor was placed in the center of the participant's spine and another one on the right shoulder to collect data on the participant's motions.

2.3. Experiment Data Introduction

SCB-13: The self-built dataset SCB-13 of this paper is made up of the above 13 participants' classroom behavior sensor data. The dataset will be used for later data analysis and model accuracy testing. Furthermore, we intend to provide a brief explanation of the experiment data of the back sensor from the perspective of an intuitive explanation.

2.3.1. Multiple Channel Data Display

After separating the gathered data by 14 given motion patterns, the 65 sets of data for the same motion are averaged to eliminate individual motion differences. Figure 2 displays the processed 6-channel data when motion 6 (raising hand while standing up) is selected as a sample motion. The data demonstrate that motion occurrence and stable state can be acquired during the valid duration of motion and sitting still time, respectively. Notably, when the students get up and raise their hands, the Z-axis data of the accelerometer change the most, which is consistent with the actual situation. It confirms the viability of using sensors for behavior identification.

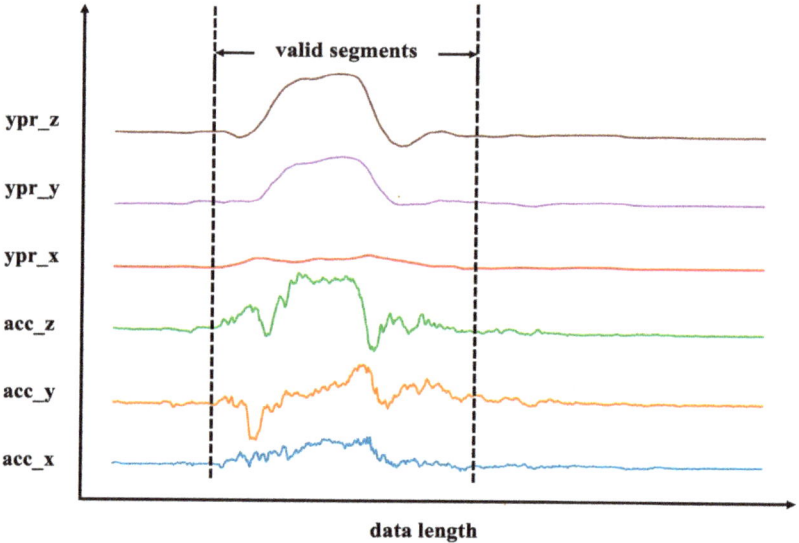

Figure 2. Take action 6 as an example to display the data of each channel of the back sensor. The lines from bottom to top represent the accelerometer x-axis(acc_x), y-axis(acc_y), z-axis(acc_z), gyroscope x-axis(ypr_x), y-axis(ypr_y), and z-axis(ypr_z). Valid segments of motions are shown within dashed lines.

2.3.2. Display of Different Motions of the Same Participant

A participant was selected randomly, and his/her 4 common classroom behaviors (motion 1 sitting still, motion 5 turning around and looking around, motion 6 raising hand while standing up, and motion 8 standing up and sitting down) were displayed in the accelerometer(acc) channel and the gyroscope(ypr) channel, as shown in Figure 3. There are observable changes in the data between different motions of the same volunteer. Nonetheless, the data patterns of motions 6 and 8 are comparable to some extent, providing the classification a challenging problem.

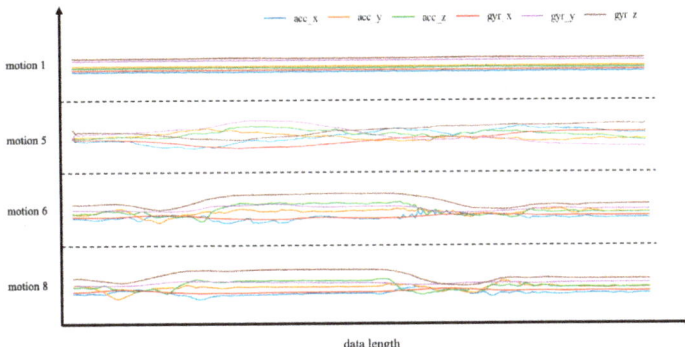

Figure 3. The randomly-selected four different actions of one of the participants and the data of the accelerometer and gyroscope data of the back sensor. The selected actions are as follows: motion 1 (sitting still), motion 5 (turning around and looking around), motion 6 (raising hand while standing up) and motion 8 (standing up and sitting down). We uniformly downsampled the data length to 200 for display clarity. Through motion sensors, we can continuously collect data about different motions, and each motion has a unique motion pattern. The relative intensity of each action is reflected in the ordinate after normalization.

2.3.3. Display of Different Participants with the Same Motion

Figure 4 shows the accelerometer data and gyroscope data of motion 6, raising hands while standing up, which were collected from 4 randomly picked individuals in order to display the differences in motion between various participants.

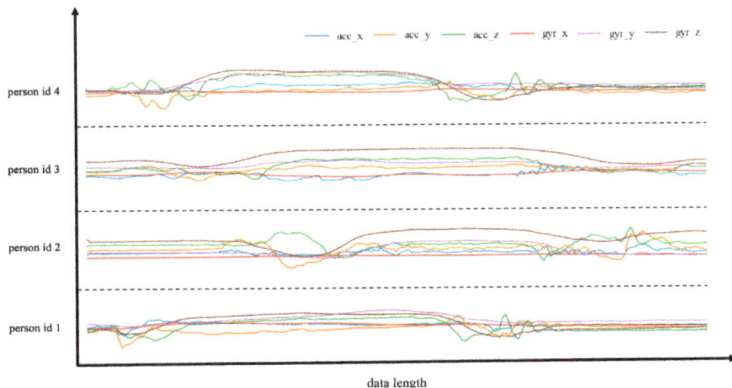

Figure 4. In the same action mode, the data of four volunteers (id1, id2, id3, id4) are randomly selected for display. We uniformly downsampled the data length to 200 for display clarity. It was challenging to classify classroom behavior since each participant carried out the same action in different ways and had unique sensor data patterns.

The preceding diagram demonstrates that various participants have distinct motion pattern characteristics, even for identical motion. It may be caused by variances in personal posture and habitual behaviors. This necessitates that the established model has robust generalization performance, capable of identifying the distinctions between the characteristics of various motion patterns while allowing for modest variations within the same motion. A comparison of the accelerometer and gyroscope data determined that the gyroscope data has more complex properties and fewer noise points, making it more ideal for the learning and reasoning of the neural network. Before generating the network's standard input, it is necessary to address the extraction and separation of valid data segments since the same motion of different participants occurs at different times and lasts varying times. Taking into account the temporal features of the data, we attempt to extract valid segments of the entire motion time in this article, which was detailed demonstrated in the identification algorithm.

2.4. Identification Algorithm

Overall, the algorithm is divided into 3 stages: the extraction of valid segments based on the Dynamic Time Warping algorithm, data augmentation, and a deep learning-based classification algorithm. The whole process of the algorithm can be shown in Figure 5. Further, about the classification algorithm, we picked the most typical Deep Neural Networks (DNNs) as the classification benchmark and investigated the classification accuracy of the RNN-based method and the CNN-based method to explore the impact of various algorithms on the precise perception and identification of classroom behaviors.

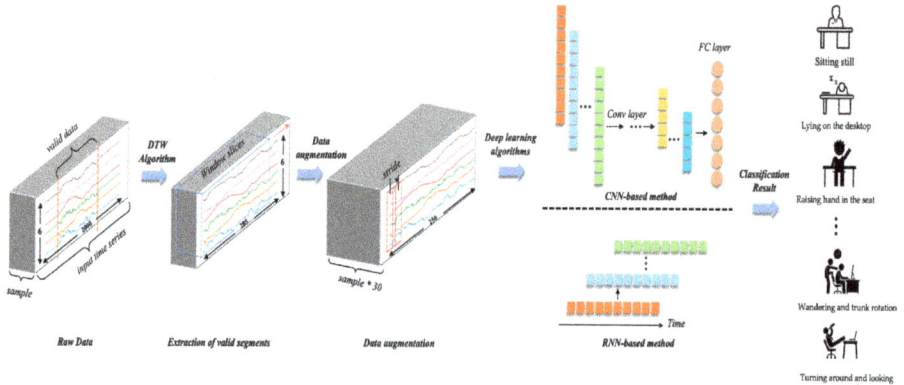

Figure 5. The framework of the whole process of the algorithm. The algorithm takes raw data as the input and outputs the most likely behavior from the 14 common classroom behaviors.

2.4.1. Voting-Based DTW (VB-DTW) Valid Segment Extraction Algorithm

Initially, we normalized the collected data to eliminate large differences in data values, which can hinder the convergence of the model. We scale the features contained in each channel by the maximum value and minimum value to the interval [0, 1] without affecting the numerical distribution:

$$X = \frac{X - Xmin}{Xmax - Xmin} \quad (1)$$

Developing a distinctive and suitable method for feature representation is necessary in order to assess if motions can be accurately distinguished from the continuous and substantial stream of sensor data. The classification accuracy is determined by the algorithm's capacity to accurately extract the features in each motion sequence, particularly for sequences having temporal properties. Even though each motion's recommended acquisition time is equal, the valid duration of each motion varies due to participant differences during the acquisition process. The ratio of the motion's valid segment to its total time segment is insufficient for some motions (such as raising a hand on a seat, standing up and raising a hand, standing up and sitting down, and knocking on a table), making it challenging to identify motion patterns and represent motion features. To accurately identify the motion mode of each motion, we must differentiate the sitting still state from the valid duration data. In this context, we proposed an improved algorithm for signal extraction based on the Dynamic Time Warping (DTW) algorithm [35], which names as Voting-Based DTW (VB-DTW) valid segment extraction algorithm.

Since the valid motion segments are surrounded by the "sitting still" data in this work, we must divide the raw motion data into tiny sequences to efficiently locate the valid segment rather than process an entire motion segment directly. To extract the valid segments, we divide the raw motion data with a length of 50, which splits the entire 2000 motion data into 40 smaller slices. Utilizing the VB-DTW algorithm, we figure out the minimum warped path of 2 adjacent slices, a total of 39 warped path values yields for each motion from a total of 40 slices. The average warped path value of the motion is utilized as the threshold, and the combined vote of 4 neighboring warped paths is used to evaluate if the slices correspond to valid motion clips. The effective segment length of the final motion is determined by connecting the extracted valid segments. In addition, to address the issue of varied lengths for each extracted valid motion segment, we uniformly downsample the extracted valid motion segments to 285 in order to make model training easier. We apply the VB-DTW algorithm on the remaining thirteen types of motions except the sitting still since the complete motion sequence of the sitting still is a valid segment of the motion. As a result, we directly downsample the sitting still data to a length of 285. The whole process of the VB-DTW-extracted valid segment algorithm can be shown in Algorithm 1.

Algorithm 1: Voting-Based DTW (VB-DTW) valid segment extraction algorithm

Input:
Segments of original data : S_i, $i = 1, 2, 3, \ldots, N$, where $N = 40$;
For each time sequence : $S_i = S_i^1, S_i^2, S_i^3, \ldots, S_i^M$, where $M = 50$.
Initialization:
$Dv = \{\ \}$, $Sv = \{\ \}$
voting set = $\{D_{j-2}, D_{j-1}, D_j, D_{j+1}, D_{j+2}\}$
1: **while** $1 \leq i \leq N - 1$ **do**
2:     $D_i \leftarrow DTW(S_i, S_{i+1})$
3: **end while**
4: $threshold \leftarrow \frac{1}{N-1} \sum_{i=1}^{N-1} D_i$
5: **while** $3 \leq j \leq N - 2$ **do**
6:     **for** D_{value} in voting set **do**
7:        $count \leftarrow 0$
8:        **if** $D_{value} > threshold$ **then**
9:           $count \leftarrow count + 1$
10:    **if** $count \geq 3$ **then**
11:       $Dv \leftarrow Dv \cup j$
12:    $j; j \leftarrow j + 1$
13: **end while**
14: **for** j in $\{1, 2, N-1, N\}$ **do**
15:    **if** $D_j > $ then
16:       $Dv \leftarrow Dv \cup j$
17: $Sv \leftarrow Sv \cup \{S_{D_v^k}, S_{D_v^k + 1}\}$ $(k = 1, 2, 3, \ldots length(Dv))$
Output:
DTW value of time series : D_j, $j = 1, 2, 3, \ldots, N - 1$;
Valid segment slices : S_v, $S_v \in S_i$.

2.4.2. Data Augmentation

Data augmentation assists in resolving the overfitting issue caused by insufficient data sets during model training. Contrary to the data augmentation methods for image data, time series data augmentation confronts several formidable obstacles, including 1. the fundamental features of time series sequences are underutilized, 2. different jobs necessitate the use of distinct data augmentation techniques, and 3. the issue of sample category imbalance.

Traditional time series data augmentation methods can be subdivided into time domain-based data enhancement to convert original data or to inject noise; frequency domain-based data enhancement converts data from the time domain to the frequency domain and then applies enhancement algorithms; and simultaneous time domain and frequency domain analysis. To prevent the issue of model overfitting caused by insufficient data, to strengthen the model's robustness, and to generate a high number of data samples, we use the window slicing-based method as the data enhancement technique. Window slicing separates the original data of length n into n − s + 1 slices with the same label as the raw segment, using S as the new slice length. During the training process, each slice is sent to the network independently as a training instance for prediction. During testing, the separated slices are also submitted to the network, and the majority vote is utilized to determine the original segment's label. In this model, we select a slice length of 256, which corresponds to approximately 90% of the original length of 285. Figure 6 depicts the data augmentation method, which divides the down-sampled valid motion sequence into 30 new slices.

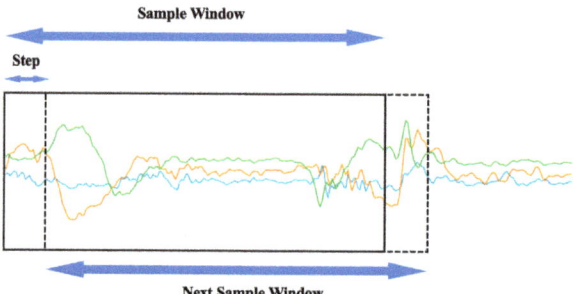

Figure 6. The detailed data augmentation procedure. The green/orange/blue lines represent the sensor data for a motion. The detailed data augmentation procedure. The green/orange/blue lines represent the sensor data for a motion. The sample window size is 256, and the stride size of the window is 1. We received 30 identical labeled data for each 285-length motion data after data augmentation.

2.4.3. Deep Learning-Based Classification Algorithm

We explored 2 categories, Recurrent Neural Networks (RNN) based methods and Convolutional Neural Network (CNN) based methods. The RNN-based method tries to represent data attributes based on temporal properties. Long Short Term Memory network (LSTM) [36] and Bidirectional Long Short Term Memory network (BiLSTM) [37] are the specific algorithms chosen for RNN-based methods. The CNN-based method can extract features by performing convolution on the data and focusing on the data's spatial characteristics. The chosen method for CNN-based methods is 1DCNN [38]. The basic deep neural network (DNN) is chosen as a simple benchmark model that aims to evaluate the performance of various algorithms from these 2 categories. The reason for comparing these four models is that this paper aimed to explore the more classical, advanced, and effective models of temporal data processing for the performance of perception and identification of students' classroom behavior tasks. The choice of these four classical models helped us to achieve the goal of presenting the best results of our model compared to the rest of the models.

(1) LSTM and BiLSTM

Recurrent neural networks (RNNs) are uniquely valuable compared to other neural networks for processing interdependent sequential data, such as text analysis, speech recognition, and machine translation. It is also widely used in the field of sensor-based motion recognition due to its property of recursion in the direction of sequence evolution, and all recurrent units are linked in a chain [39].

However, the conventional RNN has a short-term memory problem because the RNN cannot memorize and process more comprehensive sequence information, as the layers in the pre-recursive stage will stop learning due to the vanishing gradient problem or exploding gradient problem caused by backpropagation. For the problem that the later data input has more influence and the earlier data input has less influence on RNN, in 1997, Hochreiter and Schmidhuber proposed the Long Short Term Memory Network (LSTM), which successfully solved the limitation of RNN in processing long sequence data and was able to learn the long-term dependence of sequence data features. LSTM proposed the internal mechanism of 'gates' used to regulate the flow of feature information, including input gates that control the reading of data into the unit, output gates that control the output entries of the unit, and forgetting gates that reset the contents of the unit. The specific LSTM structure is shown in Figure 7, and a new vector C representing the cell state is added to the LSTM.

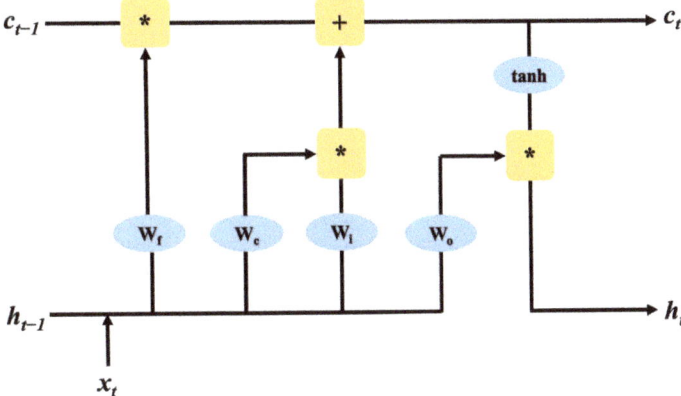

Figure 7. LSTM structure, W_f is the forgetting gate, W_i is the input gate, W_o is the output gate, x_t is the input data, h_{t-1} is the neural node of the hidden state, and W_f is used to calculate the features in c_{t-1} to obtain c_t.

Both traditional RNN and LSTM can only predict the output of the next moment based on the information of the previous moment. While in practical applications, the information of the next moment may also have a significant influence on the output state of this moment. Bi-directional LSTM (Bi-LSTM) combines 2 traditional LSTM models and uses 1 of them for forward input and the other for reverse input to fuse the information of the previous and subsequent moments for inference. Its structure is shown in Figure 8.

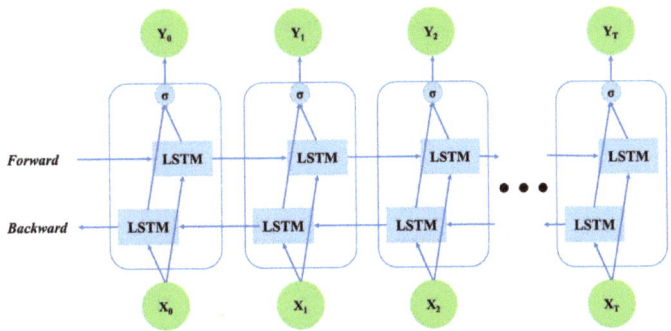

Figure 8. Bi-LSTM structure, which combines forward LSTM and backward LSTM.

(2) 1DCNN

One-dimensional convolutional neural networks (1DCNN) have strong advantages for sequence data because of the powerful ability to extract features from fixed-length segments in 1-dimensional signals. Also, the adaptive 1DCNN only performs linear 1D convolutions (scalar multiplication and addition), thus providing the possibility of real-time and low-cost intelligent control over hardware [40]. The basic structure of 1DCNN is shown in Figure 9. The kernel moves on the sequence data along the time axis to complete the feature extraction of the original data.

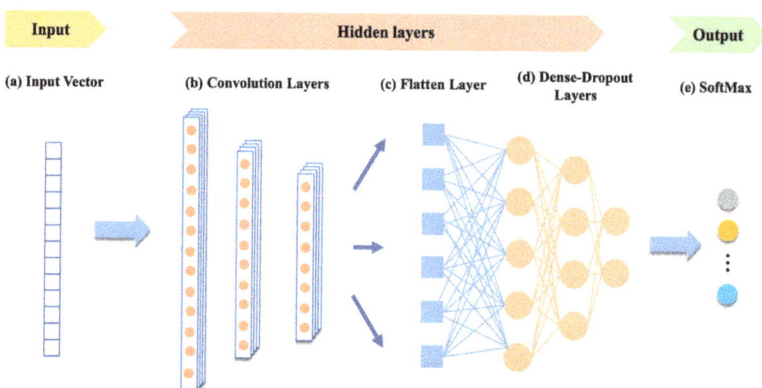

Figure 9. 1DCNN structure. The structure of 1DCNN mainly includes input, hidden layer, and output, so as to achieve the purpose of feature extraction.

In conclusion, the algorithm utilized the VB-DTW algorithm to extract valid segments, and then window slicing was used to augment the data and achieve a 30-times dataset increase. For classification, we employ 2 categories of networks. For the RNN-based method, the LSTM network and Bi-LSTM network are chosen, as well as the 1DCNN for the CNN-based method. These 2 different types of networks' abilities and contributions to percept and identify students' classroom behavior are assessed.

2.4.4. Evaluation Metrics

(1) Valid Segments Extraction

In order to demonstrate the accuracy of the valid segments obtained by the VB-DTW algorithm, we hand-crafted labeled the indices of all valid motion segments as the benchmark. We measure the similarity between the index of extracted data slices (represented as A) and the benchmark (represented as B) using the Jaccard index. The Jaccard index is used to determine the degree of similarity between limited sample data and is defined as the sample intersection size divided by the sample union size. The equation is:

$$J(A, B) = \frac{|A \cap B|}{|A \cup B|} = \frac{|A \cap B|}{|A| + |B| - |A \cap B|} \qquad (2)$$

(2) Motion Identification

In order to verify the classification performance of the model, we usually use the accuracy rate to characterize it, that is, the proportion of the number of samples with accurate classification (represented as a) to the total number of samples (represented as m) of this type. Expressed by the following formula:

$$accuracy = \frac{a}{m} \qquad (3)$$

3. Results

In summary, based on the need to understand the classroom behaviors of school children in educational scenarios, sensor-based devices provide an effective way to identify classroom behaviors intelligently. Therefore, this paper proposes the VB-DTW algorithm based on wearable sensors combined with artificial intelligence technology to achieve intelligent recognition of school children's classroom behaviors. Based on the recognition results, it is possible to provide immediate feedback on students' classroom performance and help them improve their learning performance while providing an essential reference basis and data support for constructing an intelligent digital education platform.

3.1. Identification Algorithm Valid Segmentation Results

For the 65 groups of motions with the same label, we calculate the Jaccard index of each channel of acc and ypr and then determine the average Jaccard index for each motion by averaging the six-channel values. As shown in Table 2, all the extracted valid segments' indices except lying on the desktop and writing notes are more than 88% similar to the benchmark. The Jaccard index of lying on the desktop and writing notes is worse than other motions, which may be due to the sensor data not changing significantly during motion times, as well as the warped path between the adjacent paths being near. This is a weakness in our proposed VB-DTW algorithm, which makes the algorithm inefficient for long-term recognition of a substantial portion of near-static data. We will continue to investigate the most effective approach to dealing with precise and effective segment extraction in subsequent tests.

Table 2. Jaccard index for 13 motions. All the extracted valid segments' indices except lying on the desktop and writing notes are more than 88% similar to the benchmark.

Motion Mode	Jaccard Index
Raising a hand in the seat	0.97
Turning around and looking around	0.96
Raising hand while standing up	0.96
Rocking on the seat	0.97
Stand up and sit down	0.97
Wandering and trunk rotation	0.98
Playing hands	0.87
Turning pen in hand	0.88
Knocking on the desktop	0.95
Leaning the body and chat	0.96
Shaking legs	0.94
Lying on the desktop	0.45
Writing notes	0.50

3.2. Motion Identification Results

Furthermore, the performance of the aforementioned four models in accurately classifying classroom behavior is evaluated in order to measure the influence of different classification models on the self-constructed dataset (SCB-13). A deep neural network (DNN) is chosen as a simple benchmark model for the purpose of evaluating the efficacy of various algorithms. Separately for the back sensor and shoulder sensor, the research tests the accelerometer data (acc), gyroscope data (ypr), and accelerometer and gyroscope data (acc + ypr). The research confirms the effect of classifying sensor data using LSTM and BiLSTM networks, respectively, taking into account the time-series characteristic of the data. In addition, from the perspective of one-dimensional signal feature extraction, the research uses 1DCNN to extract and classify data features in a more "intelligent" mode. The results of the experiments carried out are listed in Table 3 below.

Table 3. Main Result of four networks for the back sensor and shoulder sensor separately. Furthermore, acc represents accelerometer data, ypr represents gyroscope data, and acc + ypr represents the combination of accelerometer and gyroscope data.

Accuracy (%)	Back			Shoulder		
	acc	ypr	acc + ypr	acc	ypr	acc + ypr
DNN	81.8	91.2	93.3	89.5	86.5	91.7
LSTM	66.5	84	96.4	81.3	81.6	89.2
BiLSTM	96	98	99.8	96.4	95.9	97.2
1DCNN	99.8	99.9	100	99.6	98.3	98.8

Based on a comprehensive evaluation of the experiment outcomes, we have determined that both DNN and LSTM networks are generally useful in distinguishing classroom behaviors from the three channels' data of the accelerometer or gyroscope. However, when accelerometer and gyroscope data are incorporated into the network input, the classification effect of the DNN and LSTM network is significantly enhanced, demonstrating that more data channels are beneficial for the expression and differentiation of features.

The main experiment results show that, compared to DNN and LSTM networks, the BiLSTM network significantly improves the identification accuracy of classroom behavior. In addition, BiLSTM networks are capable of a more robust feature representation, whether for three-channel data (accelerometer, gyroscope) or six-channel data (accelerometer and gyroscope), demonstrating that the combination of forward-backward LSTM neural network for the learning of feature representation has been significantly improved.

Compared to the other three networks, the unique and potent feature extraction capabilities for sequence data demonstrated by the 1DCNN network stands out. Combining accelerometer and gyroscope data, the 1DCNN achieves classification accuracy of 100% and 98.8% for the back and shoulder sensors, respectively. In terms of model complexity and computing speed, 1DCNN is considerably superior to LSTM and BiLSTM.

In general, the data collected by the back sensor is more stable than that collected by the shoulder sensor, allowing for the differentiation of classroom activities on a wider scale. For motion classification, the gyroscope is superior to the accelerometer, despite neither being as accurate as when accelerometer and gyroscope data are used simultaneously in the classification.

4. Discussion

4.1. Ablation Study

4.1.1. Effect of VB-DTW Valid Segment Extraction

To evaluate the effectiveness of the proposed VB-DTW algorithm for valid segment extraction, we chose the data with the best classification impact (the combination of acc and ypr data) to investigate how valid segment extraction affected the action classification results. Table 4 displays the test results. According to the test results, it can be inferred that the results with VB-DTW valid segment extraction generally have higher accuracy than those without VB-DTW. The 1DCNN model outperforms the other algorithms in terms of classification accuracy for valid segment extraction.

Table 4. Test result of the effectiveness of VB-DTW valid segment extraction.

Accuracy (%)	With VB-DTW Valid Segment Extraction		Without VB-DTW Valid Segment Extraction		Improvement by VB-DTW	
	Back	Shoulder	Back	Shoulder	Back	Shoulder
DNN	93.3	91.7	89.6	82.5	3.7↑	9.2↑
LSTM	96.4	89.2	92.1	85.2	4.3↑	4.0↑
BiLSTM	99.8	97.2	93.8	90.2	5.0↑	7.0↑
1DCNN	100	98.8	98.5	95.9	1.5↑	2.9↑

4.1.2. Effect of VB-DTW Augmentation

In order to compare the accuracy of the model with and without data augmentation, we still select the data (the combination of Acc and Ypr data) with the highest level of classification accuracy. Table 5 displays the test results. The test results show that the model's classification accuracy with and without data augmentation is significantly different, and the special benefits of 1DCNN in the categorization of time series data are not reflected. These results might be brought on by the issue of data overfitting by the insufficient amount of data we gathered. As a result, for datasets with fewer data, the proposed algorithm needs to apply data augmentation on the dataset.

Table 5. Test result of the effectiveness of data augmentation.

Accuracy (%)	With VB-DTW Augmentation		Without VB-DTW Augmentation		Improvement by VB-DTW	
	Back	Shoulder	Back	Shoulder	Back	Shoulder
DNN	93.3	91.7	41.2	39.0	52.1↑	52.7↑
LSTM	96.4	89.2	49.5	51.1	46.9↑	38.1↑
BiLSTM	99.8	97.2	52.8	51.1	47.0↑	46.1↑
1DCNN	100	98.8	53.8	52.1	46.2↑	46.7↑

According to the results and discussions, the proposed VB-DTW algorithm, based on wearable sensors and artificial intelligence technology, achieves intelligent perception and identification of school-aged students' classroom behaviors. Furthermore, effective, valid segment extraction methods, as well as data augmentation in model design, are essential for the network's superior performance. Intelligent recognition of school-age children's classroom behavior can provide timely feedback, allowing the children, particularly those with special education needs, to grasp their classroom behavior in real-time and obtain assistance in the classroom without being labor-intensive.

4.2. Limitation of the Proposed Method

However, the proposed method has several limitations, particularly when students' classroom behaviors do not change significantly over time (e.g., writing notes). The proposed method cannot efficiently extract the segments of students' motions. This issue happened because the segments could not be extracted successfully due to the warped path of the DTW algorithm between adjacent paths being near since the absence of significant changes in the sensor data during motion. As a result, the proposed VB-DTW algorithm is inefficient for the long-term recognition of the majority of near-static data. In future work, we will still explore the most efficient way of dealing with precise and valid segment extraction.

5. Conclusions

The purpose of this paper is to provide auxiliary education by intelligently perceiving the behavior of students during classroom scenarios by integrating sensor equipment with AI technology. In this article, an improved algorithm which was named VB-DTW is proposed for separating valid sensor signals based on the DTW algorithm, and the effectiveness is validated using the Jaccard index. It provides the capacity to discern accurately between static and dynamic data. In addition, four classical deep learning network structures are compared for the accuracy of classroom behavior classification. It is discovered that the 1DCNN algorithm has the highest accuracy rate, particularly when accelerometer and gyroscope data are aggregated, where the recognition accuracy rate reaches 100%. We anticipate classifying more classroom activities based on hardware in real time and achieving multi-modal identification by fusing sensor data and visual data in future studies.

Author Contributions: Conceptualization, H.W., C.G., H.F., C.Z.-H.M., Q.W., Z.H. and M.L.; methodology, H.W., C.G. and H.F.; software, H.W. and C.G.; validation, H.W. and C.G.; formal analysis, H.W., C.G., H.F., C.Z.-H.M., Q.W., Z.H. and M.L.; investigation, H.W., C.G., H.F., C.Z.-H.M., Q.W., Z.H. and M.L.; resources, H.W., C.G., H.F., C.Z.-H.M., Q.W., Z.H. and M.L.; data curation, H.W. and C.G.; writing—original draft preparation, H.W., C.G., H.F., C.Z.-H.M., Q.W., Z.H. and M.L.; writing—review and editing, H.W., C.G., H.F., C.Z.-H.M., Q.W., Z.H. and M.L.; visualization, H.W. and C.G.; supervision, H.F., C.Z.-H.M. and Q.W.; project administration, H.F.; funding acquisition, H.F. All authors have read and agreed to the published version of the manuscript.

Funding: This research was supported a Dean's Reseach Fund (2021/22 DRF/SRAS-1/9th), the Education University of Hong Kong. This research was also supported by Wuxi Taihu Lake Talent Plan Supporting for Leading Talents in Medical and Health Profession, China.

Institutional Review Board Statement: The ethical review board at the Education University of Hong Kong approved this study (Protocol code: 2021-2022-0417).

Informed Consent Statement: Written informed consent was obtained from all subjects involved in the study.

Data Availability Statement: The datasets used and/or analyzed during the current study are available from the corresponding author upon reasonable request.

Acknowledgments: The authors would like to acknowledge The Education University of Hong Kong for the support in the provision of experimental sites.

Conflicts of Interest: The authors declare no conflict of interest.

References

1. Zhu, Z.-T.; Yu, M.-H.; Riezebos, P.J.S.l.e. A research framework of smart education. *Smart Learn. Environ.* **2016**, *3*, 4. [CrossRef]
2. Shoikova, E.; Nikolov, R.; Kovatcheva, E. Smart digital education enhanced by AR and IoT data. In Proceedings of the 12th International Technology, Education and Development Conference (INTED), Valencia, Spain, 5–7 March 2018; pp. 5–7.
3. Atabekov, A. Internet of things-based smart classroom environment: Student research abstract. In Proceedings of the 31st Annual ACM Symposium on Applied Computing, 2016, Pisa Italy, 4–8 April 2016, pp. 746–747.
4. Zhan, Z.; Wu, Q.; Lin, Z.; Cai, J. Smart classroom environments affect teacher-student interaction: Evidence from a behavioural sequence analysis. *Australas. J. Educ. Technol.* **2021**, *37*, 96–109. [CrossRef]
5. Alghamdi, A.; Karpinski, A.C.; Lepp, A.; Barkley, J. Online and face-to-face classroom multitasking and academic performance: Moderated mediation with self-efficacy for self-regulated learning and gender. *Comput. Hum. Behav.* **2020**, *102*, 214–222. [CrossRef]
6. Brandmiller, C.; Dumont, H.; Becker, M.J.C.E.P. Teacher perceptions of learning motivation and classroom behavior: The role of student characteristics. *Contemp. Educ. Psychol.* **2020**, *63*, 101893. [CrossRef]
7. Khan, A.; Ghosh, S.K. Student performance analysis and prediction in classroom learning: A review of educational data mining studies. *Educ. Inf. Technol.* **2020**, *26*, 205–240. [CrossRef]
8. Hopman, J.A.B.; Tick, N.T.; van der Ende, J.; Wubbels, T.; Verhulst, F.C.; Maras, A.; Breeman, L.D.; van Lier, P.A.C. Special education teachers' relationships with students and self-efficacy moderate associations between classroom-level disruptive behaviors and emotional exhaustion. *Teach. Teach. Educ.* **2018**, *75*, 21–30. [CrossRef]
9. Iadarola, S.; Shih, W.; Dean, M.; Blanch, E.; Harwood, R.; Hetherington, S.; Mandell, D.; Kasari, C.; Smith, T. Implementing a Manualized, Classroom Transition Intervention for Students with ASD in Underresourced Schools. *Behav. Modif.* **2018**, *42*, 126–147. [CrossRef] [PubMed]
10. Li, R.; Fu, H.; Zheng, Y.; Lo, W.L.; Yu, J.; Sit, H.P.; Chi, Z.R.; Song, Z.X.; Wen, D.S. Automated fine motor evaluation for developmental coordination disorder. *IEEE Trans. Neural Syst. Rehabil. Eng.* **2019**, *27*, 963–973. [CrossRef]
11. Zablotsky, B.; Black, L.I.; Maenner, M.J.; Schieve, L.A.; Danielson, M.L.; Bitsko, R.H.; Blumberg, S.J.; Kogan, M.D.; Boyle, C.A. Prevalence and Trends of Developmental Disabilities among Children in the United States: 2009–2017. *Pediatrics* **2019**, *144*, e20190811. [CrossRef]
12. Johnson, K.A.; White, M.; Wong, P.S.; Murrihy, C. Aspects of attention and inhibitory control are associated with on-task classroom behaviour and behavioural assessments, by both teachers and parents, in children with high and low symptoms of ADHD. *Child Neuropsychol.* **2020**, *26*, 219–241. [CrossRef] [PubMed]
13. Dilmurod, R.; Fazliddin, A. Prospects for the introduction of artificial intelligence technologies in higher education. *ACADEMICIA Int. Multidiscip. Res. J.* **2021**, *11*, 929–934. [CrossRef]
14. Jo, J.; Park, K.; Lee, D.; Lim, H. An Integrated Teaching and Learning Assistance System Meeting Requirements for Smart Education. *Wirel. Pers. Commun.* **2014**, *79*, 2453–2467. [CrossRef]
15. Singh, H.; Miah, S.J. Smart education literature: A theoretical analysis. *Educ. Inf. Technol.* **2020**, *25*, 3299–3328. [CrossRef]

16. Lekwa, A.J.; Reddy, L.A.; Shernoff, E.S. Measuring teacher practices and student academic engagement: A convergent validity study. *Sch. Psychol. Q.* **2019**, *34*, 109–118. [CrossRef] [PubMed]
17. Porter, L. *Student Behaviour: Theory and Practice for Teachers*; Routledge: London, UK, 2020.
18. McMichan, L.; Gibson, A.M.; Rowe, D.A. Classroom-based physical activity and sedentary behavior interventions in adolescents: A systematic review and meta-analysis. *J. Phys. Act. Health* **2018**, *15*, 383–393. [CrossRef]
19. Cox, S.K.; Root, J.R. Modified Schema-Based Instruction to Develop Flexible Mathematics Problem-Solving Strategies for Students with Autism Spectrum Disorder. *Remedial Spec. Educ.* **2018**, *41*, 139–151. [CrossRef]
20. Bertel, L.B.; Nørlem, H.L.; Azari, M. Supporting Self-Efficacy in Children with ADHD through AI-supported Self-monitoring: Initial Findings from a Case Study on Tiimood. In Proceedings of the Adjunct 15th International Conference on Persuasive Technology, Aalborg, Denmark, 20–23 April 2020.
21. Kok, V.J.; Lim, M.K.; Chan, C.S. Crowd behavior analysis: A review where physics meets biology. *Neurocomputing* **2016**, *177*, 342–362. [CrossRef]
22. Zheng, R.; Jiang, F.; Shen, R. Intelligent student behavior analysis system for real classrooms. In Proceedings of the ICASSP 2020 IEEE International Conference on Acoustics, Speech and Signal Processing (ICASSP), Barcelona, Spain, 4–8 May 2020; pp. 9244–9248.
23. Saini, M.K.; Goel, N. How Smart Are Smart Classrooms? A Review of Smart Classroom Technologies. *ACM Comput. Surv.* **2020**, *52*, 1–28. [CrossRef]
24. Kabudi, T.; Pappas, I.; Olsen, D.H.J.C.; Intelligence, E.A. AI-enabled adaptive learning systems: A systematic mapping of the literature. *Comput. Educ. Artif. Intell.* **2021**, *2*, 100017. [CrossRef]
25. Chen, K.; Zhang, D.; Yao, L.; Guo, B.; Yu, Z.; Liu, Y. Deep Learning for Sensor-based Human Activity Recognition. *ACM Comput. Surv.* **2022**, *54*, 1–40. [CrossRef]
26. Beddiar, D.R.; Nini, B.; Sabokrou, M.; Hadid, A. Vision-based human activity recognition: A survey. *Multimed. Tools Appl.* **2020**, *79*, 30509–30555. [CrossRef]
27. Bour, P.; Cribelier, E.; Argyriou, V. Crowd behavior analysis from fixed and moving cameras. In *Multimodal Behavior Analysis in the Wild*; Elsevier: Amsterdam, The Netherlands, 2019; pp. 289–322.
28. Grant, J.M.; Flynn, P.J. Crowd Scene Understanding from Video. *ACM Trans. Multimed. Comput. Commun. Appl.* **2017**, *13*, 1–23. [CrossRef]
29. Sreenu, G.; Durai, S.J.J.o.B.D. Intelligent video surveillance: A review through deep learning techniques for crowd analysis. *Big Data* **2019**, *6*, 48. [CrossRef]
30. Nguyen, T.-H.-C.; Nebel, J.-C.; Florez-Revuelta, F.J.S. Recognition of activities of daily living with egocentric vision: A review. *Sensors* **2016**, *16*, 72. [CrossRef]
31. Prati, A.; Shan, C.; Wang, K.I.K. Sensors, vision and networks: From video surveillance to activity recognition and health monitoring. *J. Ambient. Intell. Smart Environ.* **2019**, *11*, 5–22.
32. Michail, K.; Deliparaschos, K.M.; Tzafestas, S.G.; Zolotas, A.C. AI-based actuator/sensor fault detection with low computational cost for industrial applications. *IEEE Trans. Control. Syst. Technol.* **2015**, *24*, 293–301. [CrossRef]
33. Alani, A.A.; Cosma, G.; Taherkhani, A. Classifying imbalanced multi-modal sensor data for human activity recognition in a smart home using deep learning. In Proceedings of the 2020 International Joint Conference on Neural Networks (IJCNN), online, 19–24 July 2020; pp. 1–8.
34. Kavuncuoğlu, E.; Uzunhisarcıklı, E.; Barshan, B.; Özdemir, A.T.J.D.S.P. Investigating the Performance of Wearable Motion Sensors on recognizing falls and daily activities via machine learning. *Digit. Signal Process.* **2022**, *126*, 103365; [CrossRef]
35. Li, H.; Liu, J.; Yang, Z.; Liu, R.W.; Wu, K.; Wan, Y. Adaptively constrained dynamic time warping for time series classification and clustering. *Inf. Sci.* **2020**, *534*, 97–116. [CrossRef]
36. Hochreiter, S.; Schmidhuber, J. Long short-term memory. *Neural Comput.* **1997**, *9*, 1735–1780. [CrossRef]
37. Zhou, P.; Shi, W.; Tian, J.; Qi, Z.; Li, B.; Hao, H.; Xu, B. Attention-based bidirectional long short-term memory networks for relation classification. In Proceedings of the Proceedings of the 54th annual meeting of the association for computational linguistics (volume 2: Short papers), Berlin, Germany, 7–12 August 2016; pp. 207–212.
38. Cho, H.; Yoon, S.M.J.S. Divide and conquer-based 1D CNN human activity recognition using test data sharpening. *Sensors* **2018**, *18*, 1055. [CrossRef] [PubMed]
39. Goodfellow, I.; Bengio, Y.; Courville, A. *Deep Learning*; MIT Press: Cambridge, MA, USA, 2016.
40. Kiranyaz, S.; Ince, T.; Abdeljaber, O.; Avci, O.; Gabbouj, M. 1-D convolutional neural networks for signal processing applications. In Proceedings of the ICASSP 2019 IEEE International Conference on Acoustics, Speech and Signal Processing (ICASSP), Brighton, Great Britain, 12–17 May 2019; pp. 8360–8364.

Disclaimer/Publisher's Note: The statements, opinions and data contained in all publications are solely those of the individual author(s) and contributor(s) and not of MDPI and/or the editor(s). MDPI and/or the editor(s) disclaim responsibility for any injury to people or property resulting from any ideas, methods, instructions or products referred to in the content.

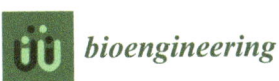

Article

Hand Exoskeleton Design and Human–Machine Interaction Strategies for Rehabilitation

Kang Xia [1,2,*], Xianglei Chen [1,*], Xuedong Chang [1], Chongshuai Liu [1], Liwei Guo [3], Xiaobin Xu [1], Fangrui Lv [1], Yimin Wang [3], Han Sun [3] and Jianfang Zhou [1]

1 College of Mechanical & Electrical Engineering, HoHai University, Nanjing 210098, China
2 School of Mechanical, Medical and Process Engineering, Queensland University of Technology (QUT), Brisbane, QLD 4001, Australia
3 Articular Orthopaedics, The Third Affiliated Hospital of Soochow University, Changzhou 213003, China
* Correspondence: xiak@hhu.edu.cn (K.X.); changei@hhu.edu.cn (X.C.)

Abstract: Stroke and related complications such as hemiplegia and disability create huge burdens for human society in the 21st century, which leads to a great need for rehabilitation and daily life assistance. To address this issue, continuous efforts are devoted in human–machine interaction (HMI) technology, which aims to capture and recognize users' intentions and fulfil their needs via physical response. Based on the physiological structure of the human hand, a dimension-adjustable linkage-driven hand exoskeleton with 10 active degrees of freedom (DoFs) and 3 passive DoFs is proposed in this study, which grants high-level synergy with the human hand. Considering the weight of the adopted linkage design, the hand exoskeleton can be mounted on the existing up-limb exoskeleton system, which greatly diminishes the burden for users. Three rehabilitation/daily life assistance modes are developed (namely, robot-in-charge, therapist-in-charge, and patient-in-charge modes) to meet specific personal needs. To realize HMI, a thin-film force sensor matrix and Inertial Measurement Units (IMUs) are installed in both the hand exoskeleton and the corresponding controller. Outstanding sensor–machine synergy is confirmed by trigger rate evaluation, Kernel Density Estimation (KDE), and a confusion matrix. To recognize user intention, a genetic algorithm (GA) is applied to search for the optimal hyperparameters of a 1D Convolutional Neural Network (CNN), and the average intention-recognition accuracy for the eight actions/gestures examined reaches 97.1% (based on K-fold cross-validation). The hand exoskeleton system provides the possibility for people with limited exercise ability to conduct self-rehabilitation and complex daily activities.

Keywords: hand exoskeleton design; motion simulation; rehabilitation; intention recognition; machine learning; deep learning

1. Introduction

In the 21st century, the aged population has increased dramatically. Among elders, a considerable number of people suffer from stroke and related complications such as hemiplegia, disability, etc., which lead to problems in daily caring [1]. To restore self-care capabilities, stroke patients usually require a long rehabilitation period after surgery [2,3]. Patients' needs at different rehabilitation stages vary, thus rehabilitation therapy should also be changed accordingly. To address this issue, human–machine interaction (HMI) technology is developed for rehabilitation exoskeletons [4–6]. In brief, all HMI technologies serve three purposes, which are intention capture, intention recognition, and physical response [7].

Capturing exoskeleton user intention traditionally relies on feedback from sensors, such as force transducers [8–10], cameras [11], strain gauges [12], and lasers [13], each of which possesses inadequate sensor–machine synergy in dealing with complex gesture/action and leads to low intention-recognition accuracy. Recently, electromyography

(EMG) and electroencephalogram (EEG) have been extensively studied for HMI due to their high intention-detection accuracy potential, which benefits from multiple signal channels [14–16]. However, EMG and EEG usually require huge data manipulation efforts, which lead to a significant delay in real-time control [17]. To balance sensor–machine synergy and real-time control performance, sensor matrices have been developed in many studies. Upon distributing a flexible skin tactile sensor array on the 'Baxter' robotic forearm, the real-time human touching detection accuracy reached 96% [18]. Moreover, by utilizing a piezoelectric force sensor matrix, the gesture recognition accuracy of a 'smart glove' could reach ~98%. In addition to the tactile sensor matrix, Inertial Measurement Units (IMU) are also renowned in wearable devices due to their compact size, high resolution, fast response, low cost, and compatibility with different systems [19]. The synergy of multiple IMUs led to successful applications in gesture recognition [20], dance mimics [21], gait analysis [22], tumble detection [23], daily life activity classifications [24], etc.

Intention recognition is another aspect of HMI, which refers to the prediction of human activities based on sensor output data [25]. In practice, the intention-recognition accuracy is affected by factors such as the resolution of the sensor, the install location of the sensor, the complexity of the gesture/action, and the types of sensors synergized for prediction [19]. In addition to sensor selection and setup, a data processing and intention prediction model is also crucial for intention-recognition accuracy. In recent years, the research on intention prediction has mainly focused on the following approaches: Statistics [26,27], machine learning [10,28], and deep learning [29–32]. Representative statistic approaches such as the least-squares method and the Kalman filtering algorithm possess advantages such as low computational complexity and good real-time control performance. However, to achieve high prediction accuracy, a linear correlation is required between data captured by the sensor and the demanded action trajectory [33]. In other words, the statistical approach is only applicable to simple motion prediction. To address this issue, machine learning and deep learning methods have been extensively studied. Representative machine learning approaches such as the Maximum Entropy Markov Model (MEMM) and the Support Vector Machine (SVM) usually require heavy data pre-processing such as Wavelet Transform (WT) or Principal Component Analysis (PCA) to optimize eigenvalues of the data sets [10,28]. Although the popular SVM model can make reasonable predictions on data sets with non-linear correlations, compared to deep learning methods such as the Convolutional Neural Network (CNN), more computational time is usually required for large sample sizes [34], and the prediction accuracy of SVM is more sample-size-dependent, due to its inferior feature-extracting capability [34].

To assist users in rehabilitation and daily life activities, a reliable mechanical structure design of hand exoskeletons is indispensable. Based on the force transmission mechanism, the hand exoskeleton can be classified as pneumatic [35], cable/tendon-driven [36,37], smart-material-based artificial muscle-driven [38–40], and linkage-driven [41,42] technology. 'Stiff hand' is usually observed in stroke patients, and significant torque force is required to perform successful rehabilitation. Artificial muscles based on smart materials such as dielectric elastomers [39] and electroactive polymers [40] are not applicable as they are usually insufficient in the generation of power, force, and deformation. Due to the compressible and temperature-sensitive nature of gas, the bending angle and bending speed of each finger joint cannot be precisely controlled by a pneumatic 'muscle' [43]. The cable-driven design reduces the weight of the exoskeleton. In practice, the cables and artificial tendons usually experience elastic deformation in operation, which may require constant calibration to avoid misalignment with the rotation center of finger joints [44,45]. Most existing cable-driven designs only drive the fingers through the stretch or bend phase, and the complete bend–stretch process cannot be repeated without the intervention of additional complex mechanisms [46]. Overall, soft design, which involves pneumatic 'muscle', artificial tendon, or smart material, provides a comfortable wear experience; however, most exoskeletons with a low-rigidity design are heavily underactuated and one active Degree of Freedom (DoF) is usually considered for each digit, which limits its applications [47].

Compared with soft exoskeletons, this design involves linkages that are bulky and rigid, which potentially provides an uncomfortable wear experience and a heavy burden for the user [48–50]. Furthermore, misalignment of the finger joint (axis) and exoskeleton joint (axis) is commonly found in current designs, which potentially leads to discomfort and skin abrasion [36,51,52]. However, the linkage-driven mechanism is still widely adopted in hand exoskeletons due to the large force transmission efficiency, precise joint trajectory control potential, and reliability of the mechanism [53].

To facilitate post-stroke rehabilitation and provide assistance for complex daily life activities, a complete smart hand exoskeleton rehabilitation system, which covers accurate digit joints' motion control, adjustable dimensions, a reliable intention-detection approach, and high intention-recognition accuracy, is proposed in this study. Based on the physiological structure of a human hand, a compact linkage-driven design with 10 active DoFs and 3 passive DoFs is proposed, which enables accurate control of a wide range of postures. Adopting the dimension-adjustable design, the device can be equipped by the majority of the population in the world. Based on the preferences of the user, the hand exoskeleton can be mounted on the existing up-limb exoskeleton system via a link module, which greatly diminishes the weight burden for the user. Three rehabilitation/daily life assistance modes are developed for various personal needs, namely, robot-in-charge, therapist-in-charge, and patient-in-charge modes. Considering HMI, a thin-film force sensor matrix and IMUs are installed in the exoskeleton, and the corresponding controller aims to capture/detect user intentions by tracing the force on the exoskeleton and the rotation angle of finger joints. The reliability of the sensor composition synergized with this device is assessed by the trigger rate, Kernel Density Estimation (KDE), and a confusion matrix. To recognize user intention, a genetic algorithm (GA) is applied to search for the optimal hyperparameters of CNN aiming for high intention-recognition accuracy.

2. Design of Hand Exoskeleton

2.1. Hand Skeleton Model Construction

The physiological structure of the hand can be revealed by analyzing the existing model of the hand skeleton in the OpenSim library. The skeleton of the hand capitates near the wrist, metacarpals, and phalanges segments. In the hand skeleton, all digits contain 1 metacarpal segment. The 4 fingers have 3 segments, namely, proximal, intermediate, and distal phalanxes. The thumb possesses 2 phalanx segments, which are proximal and distal phalanxes. The joints of the hand are named according to the bones to which they connect. Consequently, there is 1 metacarpophalangeal joint (MCP), 1 distal interphalangeal joint (DIP), and 1 proximal interphalangeal joint (PIP) for the 4 fingers, while the thumb contains only 1 MCP and 1 DIP joint (Figure 1). In addition, there is a carpometacarpal joint (CMC) for each digit near the wrist.

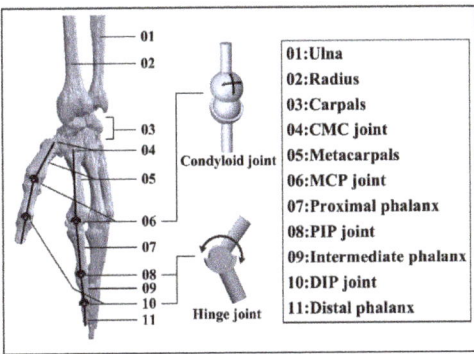

Figure 1. Constructed 3D model of hand skeleton based on anatomy.

The joint between each phalanx can be treated as a 1 DoF hinge joint, as 2 phalanges can only bend and extend along the vector direction shown in Figure 1. The MCP joint is equivalent to 2 DoFs, a ball-and-socket model that can rotate along the two directions. The CMC joints can be regarded as a 2 DoF saddle joint [54]. All digits in one hand have a total of 29 DoFs, where the thumb contains 5 DoFs and each of the four fingers has 6 DoFs. If all 29 DoFs are adopted as active DoFs, the weight of the hand exoskeleton device would be a huge burden and the reliability of the device in both motion transmission and motion control would be low. To carry out a successful grasp, each digit acts independently for flexion–extension, and the trajectory of each joint is constrained in a single plane.

Notably, the four fingers and the thumb do not share the same physiological structure. The intermediate phalanx is absent for the thumb. Moreover, the DIP joint of the thumb possesses a significantly larger active rotation range (compared with the DIP joints of fingers). However, the CMC joint (especially the CMC of the thumb) plays an essential role in grasping in terms of flexibility and force transmission. The simple grasp action can be performed with all metacarpals fixed, and rotation of the CMC joint is not mandatory. Therefore, the hand exoskeleton designed in this paper only considers the DoFs required by flexion–extension, which mainly involves PIP and MCP joints for the four fingers, while DIP and MCP joints are considered for the thumb.

2.2. Finger Kinematics

In order to conduct a finger kinematics analysis, the measurement of a volunteer is necessary. Measurements are conducted on phalanges and metacarpals with the aid of a vernier caliper. These measurements are recorded in Table 1. Note that while the exoskeleton is developed based on a single subject, the fitness for a larger population is considered, which is thoroughly discussed in Section 2.3.1. An experiment on subjects with different hand sizes is presented in Section 3.2.3.

Table 1. Parameter for subjects' fingers (units: mm).

	Thumb	Index Finger	Middle Finger	Ring Finger	Little Finger
Proximal phalanx	36	46	47	46	39
Middle phalanx	—	27	28	27	24
Distal phalanx	31	24	25	24	22
metacarpal	43	63	61	55	51

Considering all the possible gestures/actions performed by the hand, the skeleton of the hand plays an essential role in posture support, and the length of each digit stays approximately the same during the rotation process. Taking the index finger as an example, we treat the metacarpal bone as a fixed base frame and the metacarpal bone, proximal, middle, and distal phalanxes form an open-chain four-linkage mechanism. For a grasping action, the 3 DoFs in the four-linkage mechanism are all rotational, and the rotation angle ranges are 0–90°, 0–110°, and 0–70° for MCP, PIP, and DIP, respectively. Based on a modified hand skeleton model (Figure 2), D-H parameters (Table 2) of the equivalent four-linkage mechanism are established to study the kinematics of the hand, where O_0 is the coordinate system fixed at one end of the metacarpal close to carpals (CMC joint) and the O_1, O_2, O_3, and O_4 coordinate system is located at the geometric center of the MCP, PIP, DIP, and fingertip, respectively.

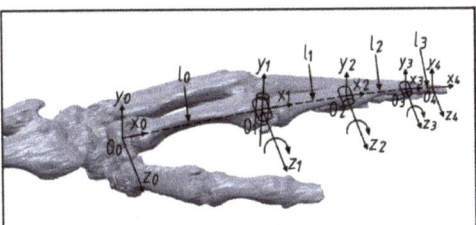

Figure 2. Coordination system of the 3D hand model.

Table 2. D-H parameters for the hand skeleton in Figure 2 (units: mm).

	l_i	α_i	d_i	θ_i
$i=0$	80	0	0	$-\theta_{CMC}$
$i=1$	46	0	0	$-\theta_{MCP}$
$i=2$	27	0	0	$-\theta_{PIP}$
$i=3$	24	0	0	$-\theta_{PID}$

In this research, the hand exoskeleton is designed to carry out rehabilitation training and aid patients in daily life activities such as object grasping. To implement the grasp action, muscles and tendons drive the MCP joint first, followed by PIP and DIP joints. In this study, workspace refers to the collection of spatial positions that a joint can reach under constraints.

Based on the Monte Carlo method [55], workspace studies on the fingertip and (the geometric center of) the DIP joint are carried out first to build and validate the initial design of the hand exoskeleton. Random valid rotation angles of each joint are substituted into a kinematics matrix based on the D-H setup to obtain the workspace cloud map of the index fingertip and DIP joint (Figure 3). As can be seen, the workspace of the DIP joint lays inside the workspace of the fingertip; however, the relatively smaller DIP joint workspace is enough for grasping large objects such as a bottle.

2.3. Design of the Exoskeleton Structure

2.3.1. Structure Analysis

In order to perform rehabilitation exercises or grasp activities, the flexion–extension motion for each digit is essential. Among all the force transmission mechanisms for rehabilitation exoskeletons, the four-linkage mechanism is simple and accurate for motion control, and thus is adopted in this study. Figure 4a presents the schematic diagram of the exoskeleton mechanism for the index finger. Rotation mechanisms for the MCP and PIP joints in the hand exoskeleton are the same. Taking the MCP joint as an example first, the metacarpal bone serves as a fixed-base frame and the proximal phalanx functions as a phantom element; together, they form a closed-chain mechanism with linear actuator 1 and exoskeleton linkages. Linear actuator 1 is an active member and dominates the flexion–extension behavior of MCP. Four constant parameters, m, n, α, and β labeled in Figure 4b,c, are adopted to describe the relationship between the actuator and angle ϕ. The relation between the length of the linear actuator 1 (l) and ϕ can be expressed as:

$$cos\phi = \frac{m^2 + n^2 - l^2}{2mn} \quad (1)$$

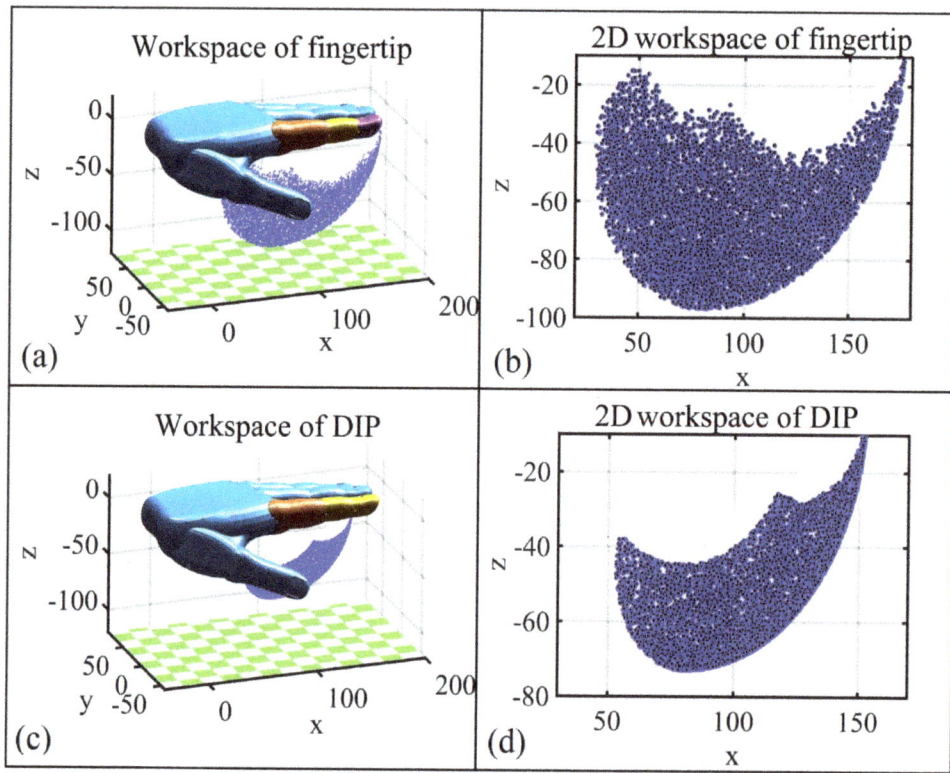

Figure 3. The workspace of the tip and DIP joint of the index finger. (**a**) The workspace of the index fingertip; (**b**) 2D view of the workspace of the index fingertip; (**c**) The workspace of the DIP joint; (**d**) 2D view of the workspace of the DIP joint.

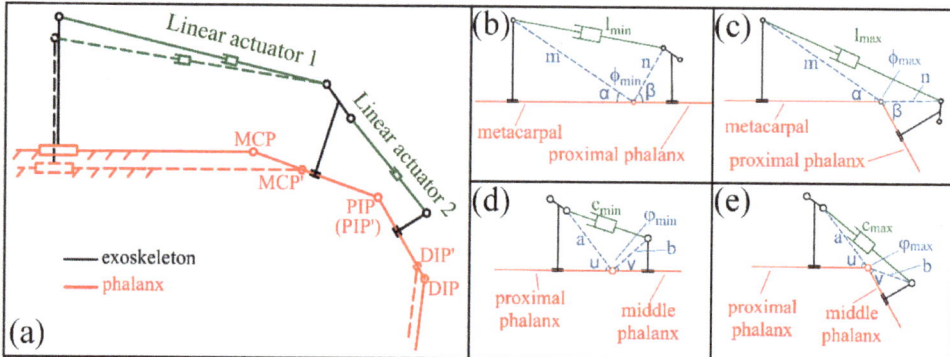

Figure 4. Sketch of exoskeleton structure for index finger. (**a**) Four-linkage mechanism of exoskeleton; (**b**) minimum angle of MCP joint; (**c**) maximum angle of the MCP joint; (**d**) minimum angle of PIP joint; (**e**) maximum angle of the PIP joint.

The rotation angle of the MCP joint can be presented as $\psi = \alpha + \beta + \phi - \pi$. Similarly, a, b, u, and v are adopted for PIP joint-related rotation and the rotation angle of the PIP joint $\omega = \alpha + \beta + \phi - \pi$. Grasping activities in daily life does not require the full rotational range of joints. To hold a cup with a diameter of ~10 cm, the angular rotation in MCP and

DIP is ~10° and ~45°, respectively, for the thumb, while the MCP and PIP joints rotate ~30° and ~60°, respectively, for the rest of the 4 fingers. In this consideration, the maximum rotation angle for MCP and PIP joints is designed to be 60°, which guarantees the safety of users and fulfills the needs for activities such as grasping and rehabilitation. With the above-mentioned understanding, Figure 4b,c illustrate the minimum and maximum lengths of the linear motor 1; meanwhile, Figure 4d,e show the minimum and maximum PIP joint rotation angles, respectively.

The overall design of the hand exoskeleton is presented in Figure 5a. Based on the preferences of the patient and suggestions of the doctor, the hand exoskeleton can either function independently or perform rehabilitation with support from the existing upper-limb exoskeleton system presented in Figure 6. The hand exoskeleton can be attached to the arm exoskeleton via a link module, which greatly diminishes the weight of the hand exoskeleton that a user needs to bear. Most components of the hand exoskeleton are realized via 3D printing utilizing polylactic acid (PLA), which is a low-density material. The strength of essential parts is verified via the FEA method (Supplementary Material, Figure S1). The structure strength meets the requirements of tasks such as rehabilitation and low-weight object holding.

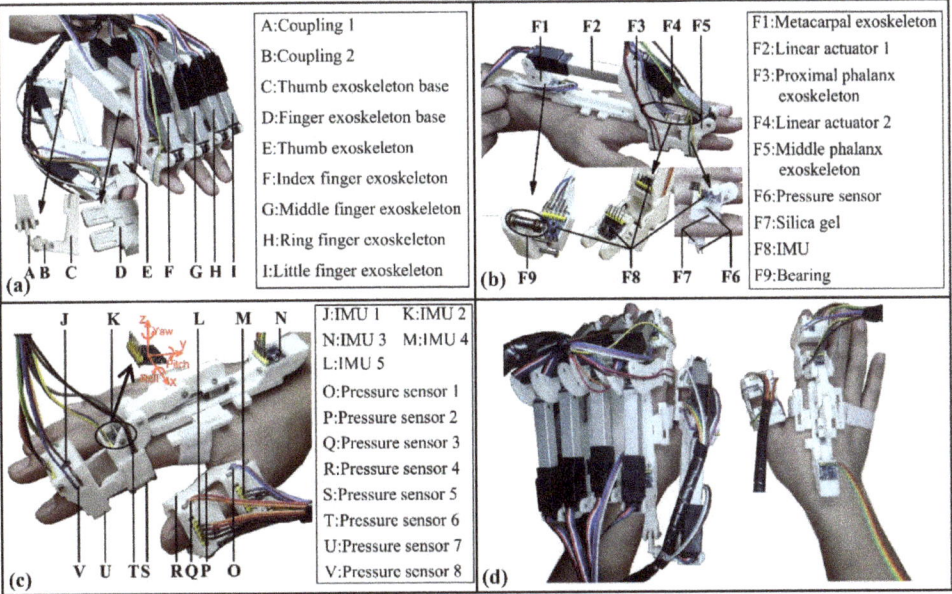

Figure 5. Hand exoskeleton rehabilitation system. (**a**) Overview of the hand exoskeleton; (**b**) components in the index finger exoskeleton; (**c**) detailed illustration of the wearable controller; (**d**) the synergy of hand exoskeleton and the wearable controller.

The hand exoskeleton contains 10 active DoFs and 3 passive DoFs in total. The motion of each digit can be controlled separately. Taking the index finger exoskeleton as an example (Figure 5b), there are 2 linear actuators selected for joint rotation, which are FIRGELLI L12-50-100-12-I (linear actuator 1) and L12-30-100-12-I (linear actuator 2). All 3 passive DoFs are shown in the insert of Figure 5a, aiming to adjust the relative position between the finger exoskeleton base and the thumb exoskeleton base. The rotation of passive joints can be constrained by tightening the bolts when comfortable angles are found for rehabilitation and grasping. More information regarding passive joints is presented in Supplementary Materials, Figure S2.

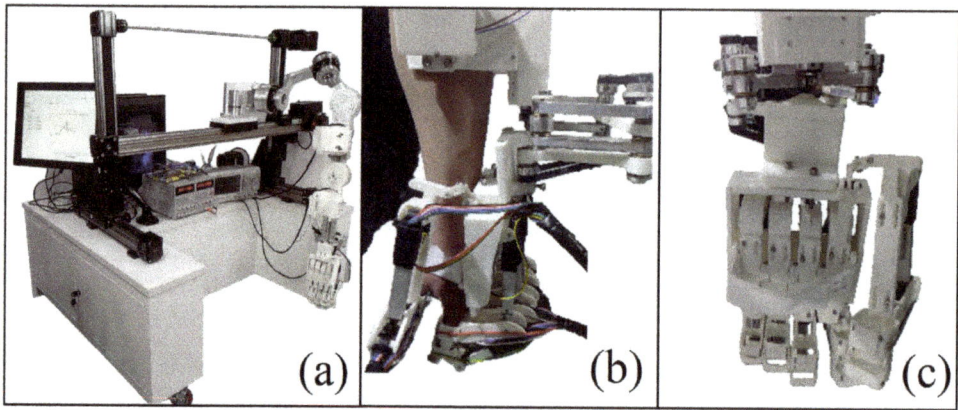

Figure 6. The combination of the hand exoskeleton and the existing upper-arm rehabilitation system. (**a**) Picture of the whole system; (**b**) side view of the hand exoskeleton mounted on upper-arm rehabilitation system; (**c**) bottom view of the hand exoskeleton mounted on upper-arm rehabilitation system.

Consider the interaction and force transmission between the hand and wearable exoskeletons, fingers and exoskeleton are tightened by the presence of elastic silica gel (inset of Figure 5b). The exoskeleton rotation axes and finger rotation axes are lined up to minimize the possible relative sliding between exoskeleton linkage and human phalanges. Regarding the friction between linkages and actuators, miniaturized bearings are adopted. For each digit, 4 thin-film pressure sensors are sandwiched between the silica gel (both dorsal and palmar sides) and digit holder. In addition, 3 IMUs are installed in the exoskeleton in the labelled position of Figure 5b. Adopting the design of the hand exoskeleton, a wearable controller without an actuator is assembled with a pressure sensor and IMUs installed in the positions labelled in Figure 5c. This wearable controller is designed for HMI, which is thoroughly discussed in Section 3.

Although the hand exoskeleton is developed based on one subject, the fitness of people with different phalanx/digit lengths is considered in this design. Representative anthropometric data are considered first; however, a complete and convincing segment data sheet is rare in the literature. Thus, the phalanx lengths of 20 subjects were measured. The height of subjects ranged from 152 to 191 cm. Based on the measurements, a length-adjustment mechanism was designed. To ensure a comfortable rehabilitation experience for different people, the rotation axes of the PIP joints (DIP joint for the thumb) of the hand exoskeleton and the human hand need to be aligned first and then the length of the metacarpal exoskeleton is adjusted via the sliding chute of the metacarpal exoskeleton (Supplementary Materials, Figures S3–S5) to align the rotation axis of the MCP joints (Figure 4a). The metacarpal exoskeleton, linear actuator 1, and proximal phalanx exoskeleton together form an open-chain mechanism. The metacarpal exoskeleton needs to be fixed to the human hand (via either a bandage or glove) to ensure the accurate control of joints.

Based on the Monte Carlo method, Figure 7 represents the DIP joint workspace (A) of the index finger, which is driven by the exoskeleton. Considering the entire workspace B of the DIP joint (Figure 3d), the two workspaces present the following relationship $A \subset B$, which guarantees the safety of the exoskeleton user in all circumstances.

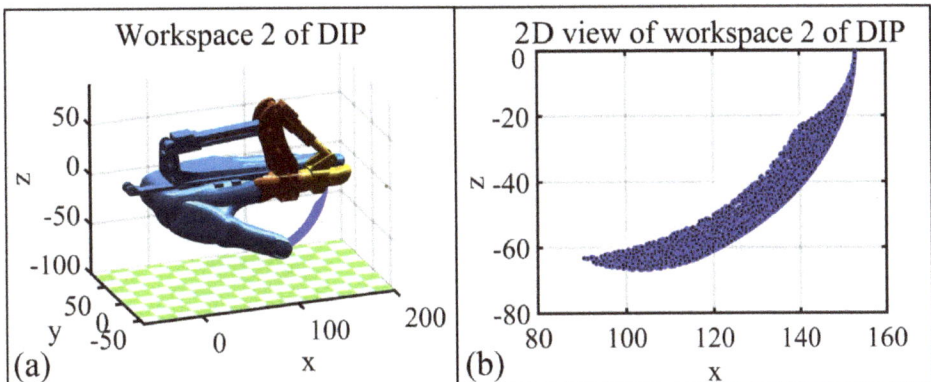

Figure 7. Workspace of exoskeleton worn by index finger. (a) The DIP joint workspace of the index finger driven by index finger exoskeleton; (b) 2D view of the DIP joint workspace for the corresponding index finger exoskeleton.

2.3.2. Kinematic Analysis

To execute rehabilitation training or grasp tasks precisely, joint space trajectory planning is needed to describe each joint angle variation with respect to time. Moreover, angular velocity and angular acceleration of both MCP and PIP joints during the rotation process need to be constrained to avoid the possibility of finger injury. To guarantee a gentle acceleration for each finger joint, a quintic polynomial is adopted for the trajectory planning of each joint. The quintic polynomial contains 6 coefficients (C_0, C_1, C_2, C_3, C_4, C_5), which constrain the angle, angular velocity, and angular acceleration. The corresponding angle, angular velocity, and angular acceleration of both joints meet the following requirements:

$$\begin{cases} \psi(t) = C_0 + C_1 t + C_2 t^2 + C_3 t^3 + C_4 t^4 + C_5 t^5 \\ \psi'(t) = C_1 + 2C_2 t + 3C_3 t^2 + 4C_4 t^3 + 5C_5 t^4 \\ \psi''(t) = 2C_2 + 6C_3 t + 12C_4 t^2 + 20C_5 t^3 \end{cases} \quad (2)$$

We assume 10 s is required for MCP and PIP joints to rotate 60°, taking t_0 and t_e as the start and end time for both joints, and the 6 parameters in Equation (3) are presented as follows:

$$\begin{cases} C_0 = 0 \\ C_1 = \psi'(t_0) \\ C_2 = \frac{\psi''(t_0)}{2} \\ C_3 = \frac{\psi''(t_e)}{20} - \frac{3\psi''(t_0)}{20} - \frac{3\psi'(t_0)}{50} - \frac{\psi'(t_e)}{25} + \frac{\pi}{300} \\ C_4 = \frac{3\psi''(t_0)}{200} - \frac{\psi''(t_e)}{100} + \frac{\psi'(t_0)}{125} + \frac{7\psi'(t_e)}{1000} - \frac{\pi}{2000} \\ C_5 = \frac{\psi''(t_e)}{2000} - \frac{\psi''(t_0)}{2000} - \frac{3\psi'(t_0)}{10000} - \frac{3\psi'(t_e)}{10000} + \frac{\pi}{50000} \end{cases} \quad (3)$$

To guarantee gentle and stable rehabilitation training with the exoskeleton, the speed and acceleration of the MCP and DIP joints are set to 0 for the start and end points. Based on the setup above, angle, angular velocity, and angular acceleration changes with respect to time are calculated for MCP and PIP joints, which are presented in Figure 8. Figure 9a presents the trajectory of the corresponding (index finger exoskeleton) DIP joint, and as can be seen, the trajectory exists completely inside the workspace of the index finger exoskeleton DIP joint (Figure 9b).

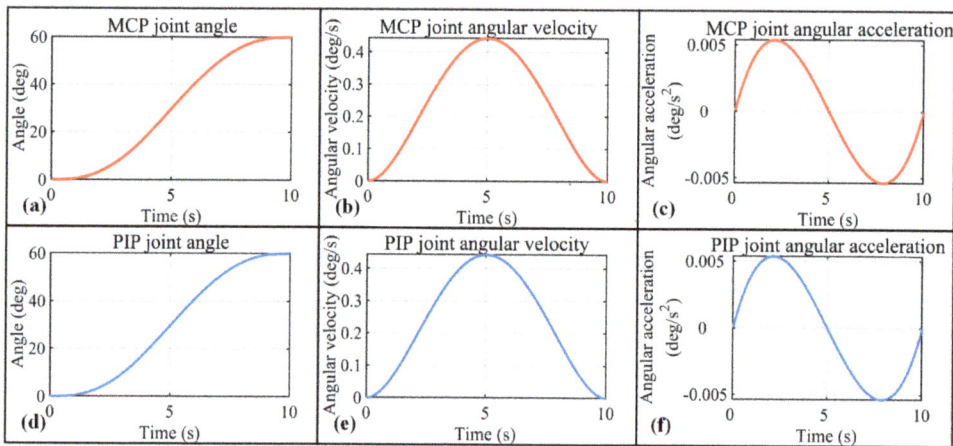

Figure 8. Trajectory planning for index finger exoskeleton MCP joint and PIP joint. (**a**–**c**) MCP joint angle, angular velocity, and angular acceleration variation with respect to time; (**d**–**f**) PIP joint angle, angular velocity, and angular acceleration variation with respect to time.

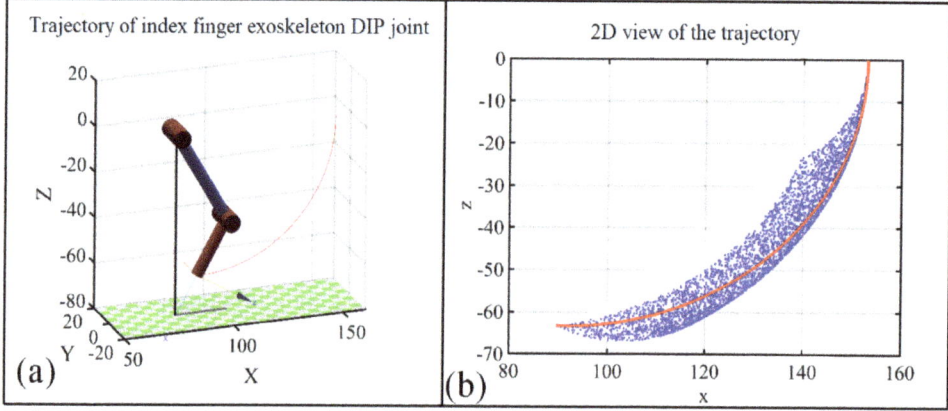

Figure 9. Trajectory of index finger exoskeleton DIP joint to accomplish a grasp action; (**a**) 3D view of the trajectory; (**b**) trajectory of index finger exoskeleton DIP joint compared with the workspace of the DIP joint.

To ensure the fingers under the control of the exoskeleton move according to the previously determined trajectory, it is necessary to control the linear actuator precisely. Based on Figure 4 and Equation (1), the length of linear actuators 1 and 2 (Figure 5b) can be expressed as:

$$\begin{cases} l(t) = \sqrt{m^2 + n^2 - 2mn\,cos[\pi - \alpha - \beta + \psi(t)]} \\ c(t) = \sqrt{a^2 + b^2 - 2ab\,cos[\pi - u - v + \psi(t)]} \end{cases} \quad (4)$$

For the grasp action defined in this section, the displacement, velocity, and acceleration for linear actuators 1 and 2 are presented in Figure 10.

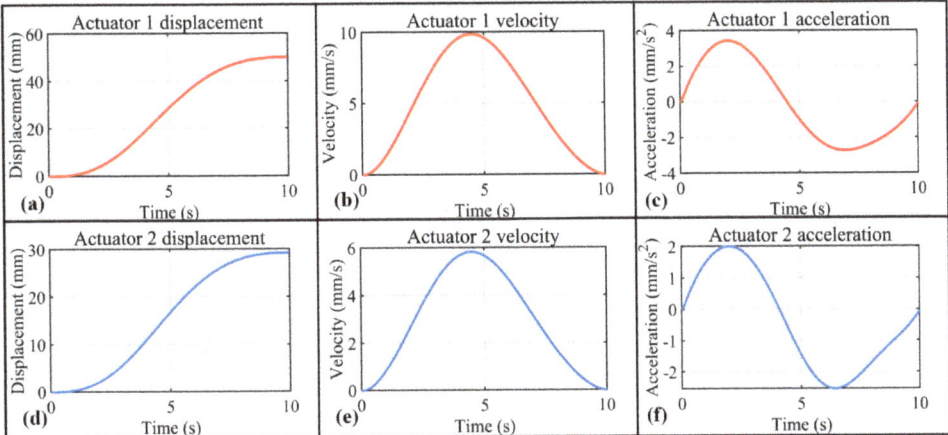

Figure 10. Displacement, velocity, and acceleration diagrams of the two actuators in order to rotate 60° in 10 s for MCP and PIP joints. (**a**) Displacement–time diagram of actuator 1; (**b**) velocity–time diagram of actuator 1; (**c**) acceleration–time diagram of actuator 1; (**d**) displacement–time diagram of actuator 2; (**e**) velocity–time diagram of actuator 2; (**f**) acceleration–time diagram of actuators 2.

3. Hand Exoskeleton HMI Strategies

3.1. Hand Exoskeleton System Overview

The overall control system is composed of four major parts, including the hand exoskeleton, host computer, slave computer (STM32-F329 microcontroller, manufactured by Zhengdianyuanzi Ltd., Guangzhou, China), and a wearable controller (Figure 11a). The host computer processes data collected by the slave computer and sends commands via the interface program developed in the QT environment. As shown in Figure 11b, the interface program possesses two basic functions including mode selection and data visualization. The slave computer integrates one analog-to-digital converter (ADC) and one serial port transmission module and controls the linear actuator via pulse width modulation (PWM).

Considering the high real-time and high-resolution requirements for rehabilitation, thin pressure sensors (RP-C18.3-ST, manufactured by Aodong Ltd., Dunhua, China) and IMUs (IMU901, manufactured by Zhengdianyuanzi Ltd.) are selected for human–machine interaction, and the distribution of these sensors is illustrated in Figure 5. The thin-film pressure sensors selected are piezoelectric and their pressure reading can be calibrated via the resistance–voltage conversion relation:

$$U_0 = \left(1 + R_{AO-RES} \times \frac{1}{R_x}\right) \times 0.1 \tag{5}$$

where R_{AO-RES} represents the adjustable resistance and R_x is the resistance that changes in real time with respect to pressure changes. The real-time pressure data collected by the sensor can be converted into an analog voltage (0~3.3 V) through the ADC module in the slave computer. The adopted IMU integrates a gyroscope, accelerometer, magnetometer, and barometer. The IMU outputs the variation of pitch, roll, and yaw angles via the Universal Synchronous Asynchronous Receiver Transmitter module (USART). In order to minimize the interference of 'abnormal data' (induced by shaking of the hand, random motion of the arm, etc.) while ensuring the reliability of data, an amplitude-limiting filtering algorithm (integrated into STM32) is utilized to constrain the steep variation in the data.

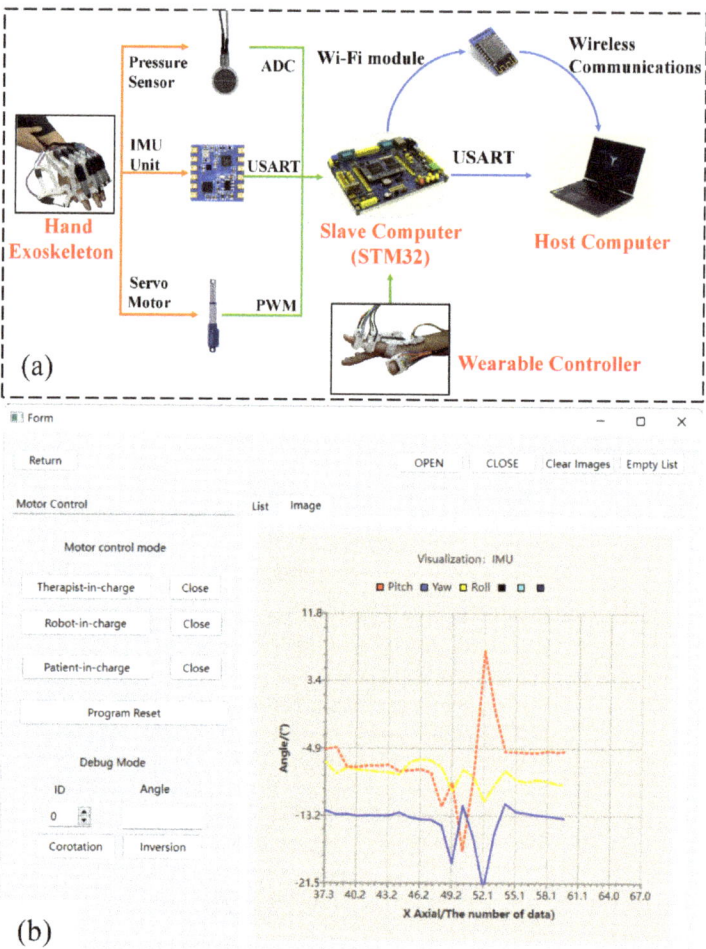

Figure 11. Control of the hand exoskeleton rehabilitation. (**a**) System overview of the hand exoskeleton; (**b**) interface program to control the hand exoskeleton.

3.2. Control Modes for Rehabilitation and Daily Life Activity Assistance

Stroke patients usually need a long rehabilitation period after surgery in order to recover from stroke-related complications such as hemiplegia. Patients' demands at different rehabilitation stages vary even for the same patient [14], thus, rehabilitation therapy should also be changed accordingly. Regarding this issue, human–machine interaction (HMI) technology is adopted to adjust rehabilitation therapy and control the motion of the hand exoskeleton based on personal needs. Three modes are designed for rehabilitation and daily life assistance, namely, robot-in-charge, therapist-in-charge, and patient-in-charge modes.

The robot-in-charge training strategy aims to help patients without the ability to move or exercise. In this mode, the hand exoskeleton guides the patient's hand along a preplanned path (proposed by doctors). The therapist-in-charge training strategy is suitable for patients in all recovery stages and requires a therapist to put on the wearable controller (Figure 5c). The angular rotation of the therapist's hand is mapped onto the patient's hand via tracking pitch, roll, and yaw angles obtained by IMUs. The patient-in-charge training strategy targets patients who are capable of low-intensity exercises. In this mode, two functions can be achieved, which are rehabilitation and daily activity assistance. A wearable controller is required to be worn by one hand, while the hand exoskeleton is equipped with the other hand (Figure 5d). Utilizing deep learning and machine learning methods, data (collected by the wearable controller) can be correlated to different pre-planned exoskeleton postures/actions. More information regarding the three modes is presented in the following sections.

3.2.1. Robot-in-Charge Rehabilitation Mode

Figure 12 illustrates the control flow diagram for the three rehabilitation modes, where the robot-in-charge mode is presented by green blocks. Based on the rehabilitation therapy suggested by the doctor, the trajectory of each exoskeleton joint can be planned with the aid of Equation (2), and the corresponding elongation in the linear attractors is calculated via Equation (4). In the rehabilitation process, the real-time data collected by the thin-film pressure sensors installed in the hand exoskeleton (Figure 5b) can be monitored by doctors and the data can be used as a recovery evaluation index.

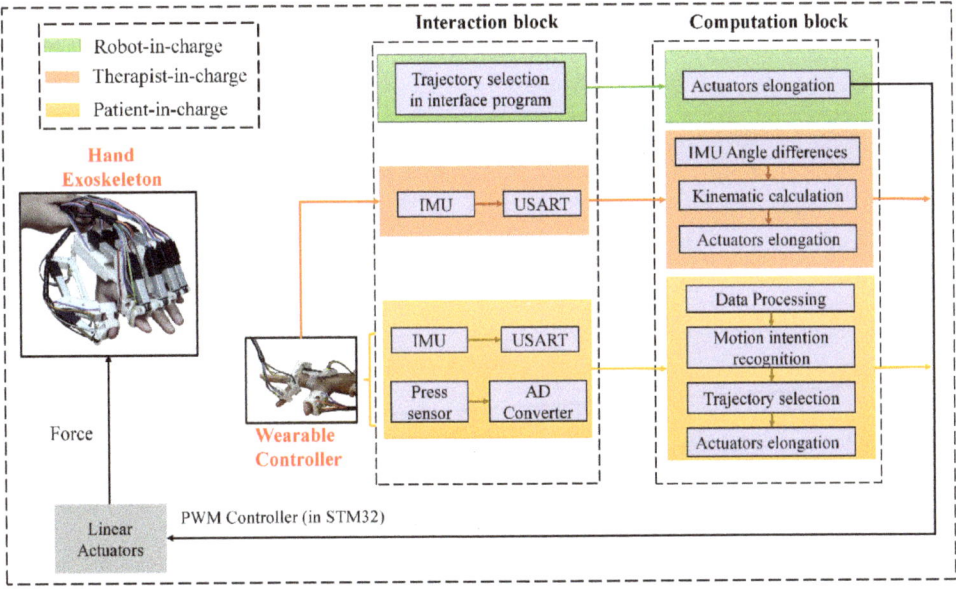

Figure 12. Hand rehabilitation exoskeleton control flow diagram for the three rehabilitation modes.

3.2.2. Therapist-in-Charge Rehabilitation Mode

The therapist-in-charge training mode is presented by the orange blocks in Figure 12. In this mode, a wearable controller is required to be equipped by the therapist. In Figure 5c, there are three IMUs (IMUs 1–3) that record the rotation of the index finder, while two IMUs (IMU 4–5) are installed to detect the motion of the thumb. The three angle readings (pitch, roll, and yaw, specified in Figure 5c) from IMU 3 mainly serve the purpose of a motion benchmark, and the rest of the angles function for hand exoskeleton motion tracking.

In the rehabilitation process, rotation in the index finger PIP or MCP joint leads to the angle variation in IMUs 1 or 2, respectively, while motion in the thumb MCP or DIP can be detected by IMUs 4 or 5, respectively. IMUs in one digit are all aligned in the same plane. For any adjacent two IMUs, differences in pitch and yaw angles are expected to be 0.

Taking the index finger PIP joint as an example, using the reading of IMU 2 as a benchmark, the PIP rotation angle can be expressed as follows:

$$\begin{bmatrix} Roll \\ Pitch \\ Yaw \end{bmatrix}_{MCP} = \begin{bmatrix} Roll \\ Pitch \\ Yaw \end{bmatrix}_{Imu1} - \begin{bmatrix} Roll \\ Pitch \\ Yaw \end{bmatrix}_{Imu2} \qquad (6)$$

With the aid of the slave computer, the real-time PIP joint angle variation of the therapist's index finger is obtained. IMUs installed in positions of the hand exoskeleton are similar to the positions in the wearable controller (Figure 5b), and the angle variation in each joint of the hand exoskeleton can also be calculated with the aid of Equation (5). Utilizing Equation (4), the demanded elongation of the linear actuator installed in the exoskeleton is calculated. Figure 13 indicates the decent real-time performance of the therapist-in-charge training mode.

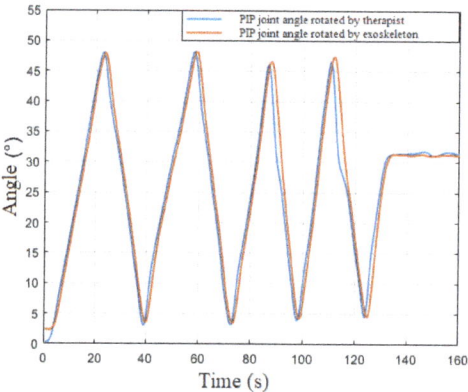

Figure 13. Real-time PIP joint angles variation for index finger of therapist and index finger exoskeleton. Blue line refers to the PIP joint rotation performed by therapist equipped with wearable controller, while the red line presents the PIP joint angle change in index finger exoskeleton.

3.2.3. Patient-in-Charge Rehabilitation Mode

The patient-in-charge training strategy designed in this research targets patients with limited exercise ability who are only able rotate digit joints at a small angle (e.g., 5°). For these patients who require self-rehabilitation and complex daily activities, intention recognition is of vital importance. 'Stiff hand' is usually observed in stroke patients, and the stiffness is unpredictable considering the vast population of stroke patients, thus recognizing one hand's posture/action to guide the other hand's motion is the best strategy. In this study, both the exoskeleton and its corresponding controller are adopted.

Compared with statistical intention-recognition methods, the deep learning approach of a CNN (Figure 14a) is adopted for its renowned training efficiency and prediction accuracy [19]. Results of the CNN model are validated and compared with the widely adopted machine learning method SVM. Gestures of the hand recognized by the wearable controller can be correlated with planned trajectories of the hand exoskeleton, and these trajectories can be planned and adjusted based on the needs of patients, utilizing Equations (2)–(4).

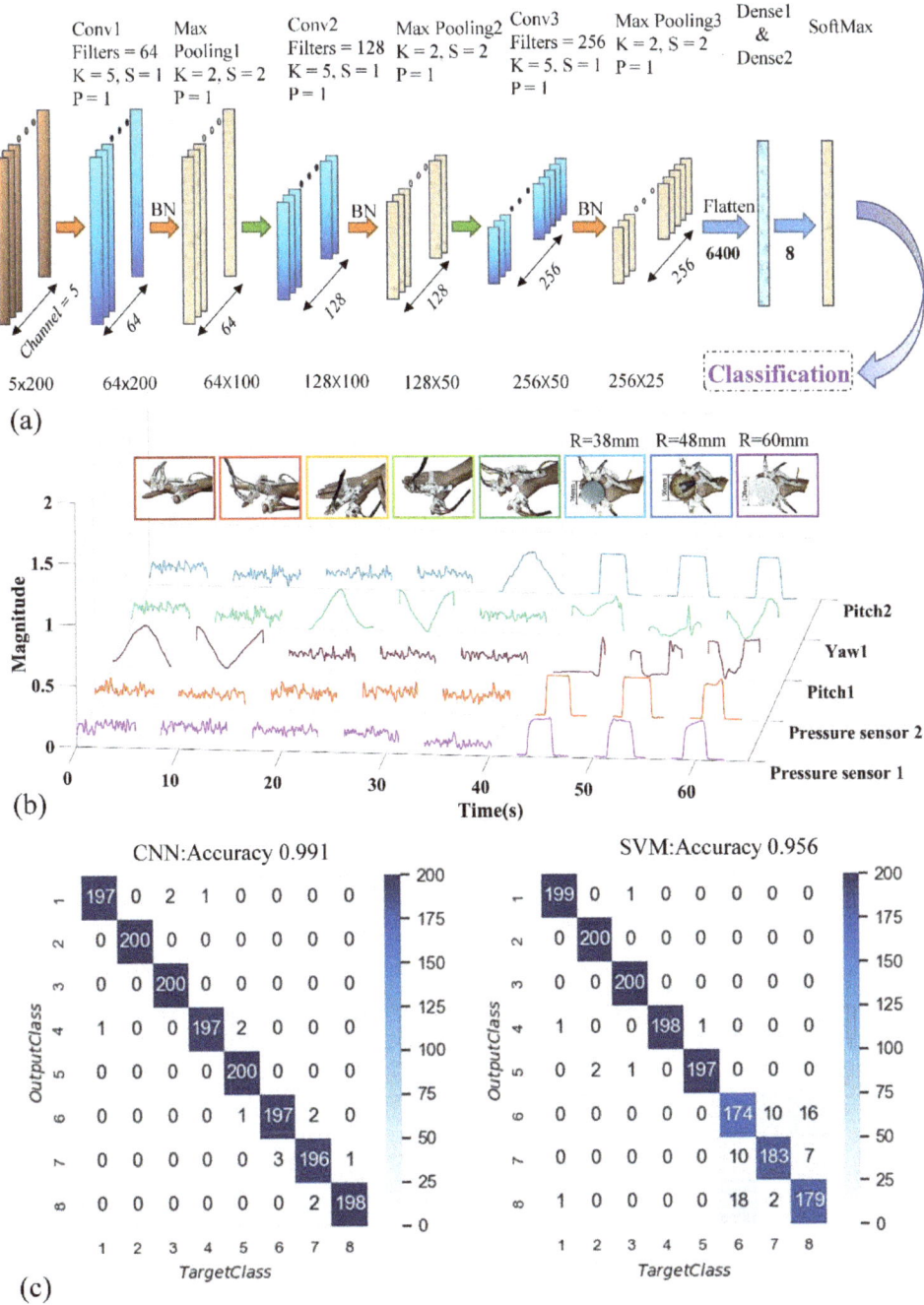

Figure 14. Deep Learning and machine-learning-based intention recognition. (**a**) 1D CNN structure diagram; (**b**) sensor output data pattern of the six actions/gestures; (**c**) confusion matrix diagrams of CNN (**left** panel) and SVM (**right** panel) models.

Data Acquisition and Processing

In this research, the wearable controller is worn by the right hand of volunteers to record data from both the IMUs and thin-film pressure sensors labelled in Figure 5c. Eight unique gestures/actions are selected for the identification experiment (inset of Figure 14b). Five healthy volunteers are involved in the data acquisition (the hand size of each volunteer is presented in Supplementary Materials Figure S5), and each gesture/action is repeated 250 times by each individual volunteer. A total of 10,000 sets of data are collected. Among all the data sets, a random 84% are utilized for training and the remaining 16% are used for testing. To mimic a real application scenario and improve intention-recognition accuracy, diversity of data sets for each gesture/action is necessary. In other words, even for the same gesture/action, the rotation angle (0 to ~60°) for each joint and the force (0 to ~3 N) exerted on the pressure sensor varies significantly for each individual repeat. In addition, during the data-acquisition process, random movement of the arm is inevitable. As such, IMU also records information related to arm rotation, shaking hand, etc. Prior to data acquisition, IMUs and pressure sensors are calibrated. The data acquisition frequency is fixed at a low value of 40 Hz, and each individual gesture/action is performed at a slow pace, which guarantees the diversity of data sets. For the actual rehabilitation process, the data collection frequency can be adjusted based on the preferences of the user.

In the data acquisition phase, the first two gestures are performed by rotating the z1 axis (Figure 2) in counterclockwise and clockwise directions, respectively. The third and fourth gestures/actions are achieved by rotating the y1 axis (Figure 2) in clockwise and counterclockwise directions, respectively. The fifth gesture refers to the bending of both MCP and PIP joints in the index finger. The last three gestures/actions are holding cylinders with a small radius (38 mm, 48 mm, and 60 mm, respectively), aiming to test the effectiveness of the whole HMI strategy. Each collected data set contains five columns, with 200 data points fitted in each column. The first two columns record measurements from pressure sensors 5 and 7 labelled in Figure 5c. The third column refers to the pitch angle change in IMU 2, which describes the up- and down-motion of the index finger dominated by the MCP joint. The roll angle variation of IMU 2 is recorded in column 4, aiming to distinguish between left and right MCP rotation. For the fifth column, the pitch angle difference between IMU 1 and IMU 2 is taken for the description of PIP joint rotation.

Data processing techniques such as normalization and feature extraction are essential for deep learning and machine learning models. Considering the range of measurements from distinct sensor types and the distribution patterns of each data set [56], extra efforts may be required for the CNN model to balance the multiple distribution centers if normalization is not applied. As a result, it slows down the training efficiency, also making the model more difficult to converge. Normalization is achieved in two steps. Firstly, all numbers in each column are scaled to fit in the range of [0, 1], utilizing $\frac{(x-x_{Min})}{x_{Max}-x_{Min}}$. Then, the data set mean value is adjusted to 0 based on $\frac{(x-\mu)}{\sigma}$. In addition, effective feature extraction reduces the correlation of irrelevant dimensions in the data sets, thereby speeding up the training process [57]. Regarding the feature extraction process, it can be achieved in the convolutional layer of the CNN model. For the SVM model, Principal Component Analysis (PCA) is required to reduce the dimensions of the original data set.

Intention-Recognition Model and Results

The structure of the one-dimensional CNN deep neural network model adopted in this research is shown in Figure 14a, which is mainly composed of convolutional, batch normalization, pooling, SoftMax, and fully connected layers. The convolutional layer is designated to extract the features of the specified data segment. The batch normalization layer ensures a decent backpropagation gradient, which alleviates the problem of vanishing gradients [58]. The pooling layer is presented for the reduction of input matrix dimensions. The SoftMax layer stabilizes the values in the backpropagation process and leads to easier convergence for the classification task. The fully connected layer links all the previous features to obtain the classification result. The key parameters, Filters (F), Kernel size (K),

Strides (S), and Padding (P), are presented in Supplementary Materials Table S1. In addition to the parameters mentioned above, the training result of the CNN model is also sensitive to the variation of hyperparameters. In the consideration of intention-recognition accuracy, GA is adopted to find the optimal hyperparameters. GA is a set of mathematical models abstracted from the process of reproduction in nature. It realizes the heuristic search of complex space by simplifying the genetic process. The flow chart of GA (more specifically, the differential evolution algorithm) is shown in Figure S6 (Supplementary Materials). The average recognition accuracy of 10-times K-fold cross-validation is taken as the fitness function of individuals in the population, and the three hyperparameters (Learning Rate, Batch Size, and Epoch) are taken as the decision variables in Table S2 (Supplementary Materials). After 10 generations of population iterations, the optimal parameters of the model were obtained and are shown in Figure S7 and Table S3 (Supplementary Materials).

SVM is a widely adopted machine learning method for classification and intention recognition. The performance of the SVM model is highly related o three hyperparameters, which are kernel function, penalty parameter C, and Gamma. In this study, the linear data dimension reduction algorithm PCA retains 98% of the key information in the original data sets, which minimizes the information loss while compressing data set dimensions significantly and accelerating training/testing. PCA processing reduces each sample data set's dimensions from 1×1000 to 1×27. The genetic algorithm is also utilized to optimize the hyperparameters of the SVM model. The average recognition accuracy of 10-times K-fold cross-validation is also taken as the fitness function of population individuals. The three hyperparameter parameters mentioned above (kernel function, parameter C, and gamma) are used as decision variables in Table S4 (Supplementary Materials). After 10 generations of population iteration, the optimal parameters of the model are obtained and shown in Figure S8 and Table S5 (Supplementary Materials).

Upon adopting the optimal hyperparameters, a confusion matrix is obtained via testing data set prediction. The confusion matrix in Figure 14c indicates that both methods reach at least 95.6% overall recognition accuracy. Featuring the confusion matrix of the CNN model, each individual posture reaches at least ~98.5% prediction accuracy, and only 15 misclassifications are observed among the total 1600 testing data sets. The SVM model presents high classification accuracy for the first five postures/actions, while significant misclassifications occur when dealing with the last three cylinder-holding tasks.

4. Discussion

4.1. Mechanical Design of the Exoskeleton

To realize accurate digit joints' motion control mechanically, joints' rotation axes of both the hand exoskeleton and the human hand need to be aligned in motion. To validate the concept, the trajectory of joints' rotation axes for both the hand exoskeleton and the human hand are simulated and compared. In a scenario in which all finger joints rotate 60°, the human hand DIP and PIP joints' trajectories obtained from Opensim fit well with the trajectories of the hand exoskeleton (Figure 15), suggesting a comfortable wear experience and potential for accurate digit joint motion control.

4.2. Intention Detection

The reliability of the sensor–device synergy is assessed by the trigger rate, Kernel Density Estimation (KDE), and the confusion matrix. The trigger rate is defined by assessing the data in each data set. For a data set correlated with action 6 (grasp a cylinder with a radius of 38 mm), all five columns of data need to be considered. If all pressure sensor readings exceed 0.2 N and all angle variations exceed 2°, a successful trigger is concluded. Assessing all 10,000 data sets, a 100% trigger rate is observed for each gesture/action (Figure 16a). Moreover, good training and estimation are more likely to be achieved based on similar testing and training data set patterns. Therefore, the KDE method is applied to illustrate the probability density distribution of a random training and testing data set. As can be seen, the two distribution patterns agree well with each other (Figure 16b).

The difference in distribution patterns is mainly due to the desired diversity of data sets (i.e., random motion of the arm, shaking of hands, different forces applied to the pressure sensor, different finger-bending angles, and digit length of volunteers). In addition, the high prediction accuracy for both CNN and SVM also suggests a reliable sensor–machine synergy and a good data acquisition process.

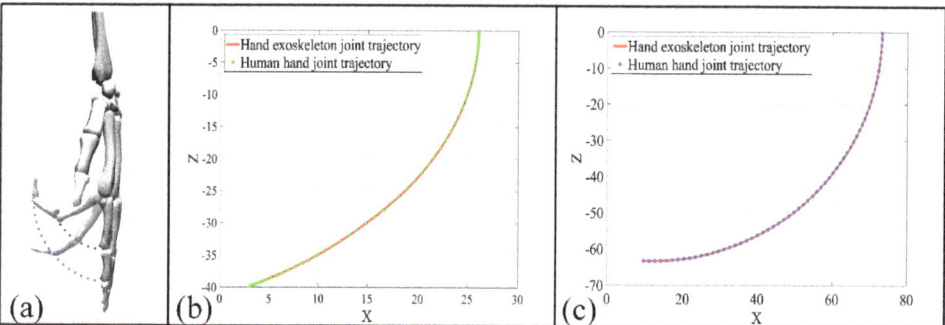

Figure 15. Exoskeleton trajectory validation for DIP and PIP joints. (**a**) Opensim simulation setup; (**b**) trajectory of DIP joints; (**c**) trajectory of PIP joints.

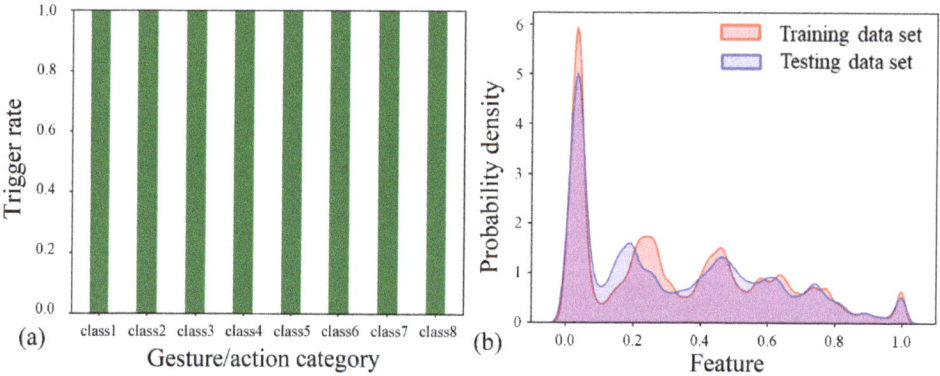

Figure 16. Reliability of the sensor-device synergy. (**a**) Trigger rate of all sensors necessary for gestures/actions; (**b**) probability density distribution for random training and testing data sets using KDE.

In the data-acquisition phase, each repeat is performed slowly, and 200 data points are collected, utilizing a low data collection frequency of 40 Hz. The data collection frequency of the system can be adjusted to a much higher level, which improves the overall system response time significantly. The low data collection frequency adopted in this study aims to guarantee data set diversity for training purposes. After thousands of repeats, the joint rotation in fingers cannot be controlled precisely with a high data collection frequency (due to the fatigue of the human hand), which may jeopardize the diversity of the data set. In a real rehabilitation scenario, the user may perform actions at a different pace; however, more training data sets with high diversity may help with intention-recognition accuracy.

4.3. Intention Recognition

Based on the results of the confusion matrix, CNN possesses 3.5% better overall prediction accuracy compared with SVM. CNN also outperforms SVM significantly in gestures/actions 6, 7, and 8, suggesting better performance in dealing with gestures/actions with high similarities. Dividing all data sets into one training set and one testing set using the leave-one-out method may have led to biased prediction results. To validate the results, k-fold cross-validation is adopted. Selecting 10 distinct random training data sets, the network is retrained 10 times and the corresponding results are recorded in Table 3. The average accuracy of CNN presents even higher superiority over SVM with a much smaller variance presented. Three possible reasons are proposed for this phenomenon. First, CNN possesses advantages in dealing with nonlinear problems [59]. In this study, volunteers with distinct digit lengths, initial hand positions, and joint motion trajectories may lead to significant non-linear correlations between data sets and the target posture, which decreases the prediction accuracy of SVM. Secondly, the convolutional layer in the CNN model extracts more deep-level features [10], while the SVM model only extracts specific features in the data pre-processing stage (using PCA). Ideally, the first five actions/gestures all experience substantial data variation in a single column with non-periodic fluctuations observed in other columns, which are mainly due to the instability of the human hand joint, random motion of the arm, and environmental noise. As these 'unwanted' amplitude fluctuations exceed a certain threshold, the rate of misclassifications rises for SVM as it is unable to effectively extract the data set feature in such a scenario. Lastly, compared with the SVM model there are more adjustable parameters in the CNN model (Supplementary Materials, Tables S1 and S2), which helps it to better adapt to the eight actions/gestures in this study. Observing each individual result, the worst prediction accuracy from SVM is only 41.1% compared with CNN's 92.2%. The low accuracy may either be a result of overfitting or the presence of substantial outliers. However, low accuracy is only observed in a single run, and outliers due to the shaking of hands and random movement of the arm are likely to be the dominant issue. Although the outliers due to arm rotation, hand shaking, etc., may violate the performance of the hand exoskeleton system, the average intention-recognition accuracy (97.1%) based on K-fold cross-validation suggests a reasonable model setup and training process. The CNN model, with its decent balance between high intention-recognition accuracy and a lightweight network structure (the prediction time consumption for both CNN and SVM models is shown in Supplementary Material Table S6), is recommended for real-time intention recognition.

Table 3. K-fold cross-validation of CNN model and SVM model.

		1	2	3	4	5	6	7	8	9	10
CNN	Run number	1	2	3	4	5	6	7	8	9	10
	Accuracy	1.0	0.991	1.0	0.922	0.951	0.958	1.0	0.951	0.973	0.964
	Average	97.1									
	Variance	0.0276									
SVM	Run number	1	2	3	4	5	6	7	8	9	10
	Accuracy	0.931	0.956	0.981	0.961	0.882	0.411	0.979	0.949	0.921	0.871
	Average	0.884									
	Variance	0.162									

In this study, a complete hand exoskeleton rehabilitation system is proposed for post-stroke rehabilitation and assistance in complex daily life activities. Three rehabilitation/daily life assistance modes are developed for various personal needs, namely, robot-in-charge, therapist-in-charge, and patient-in-charge modes. With the aid of a sensor matrix, the patient-in-charge mode allows the detection of a small rotation angle in digits and achieves high intention-recognition accuracy when dealing with similar gestures/actions. Thus, stroke patients with limited exercise ability (e.g., 5° in each joint) can conduct self-rehabilitation and complex daily activities with the proposed device. Regarding the 'stiff hand' phenomenon observed in stroke patients, the synergy of the actuator (with push force up to 43 N) and linkage can provide enough torque and an accurate trajectory for digit joints.

Note that all experiments are conducted on healthy volunteers. In future studies, the effectiveness of the hand exoskeleton system on stroke patients will be evaluated. Constrained by the size of the current electric actuator, the motion of the DIP joint is not considered. To achieve higher flexibility in the hand exoskeleton, a smaller force transmission mechanism such as voltage-sensitive composite material will be considered for the active control of finger DIP joints. The thumb CMC joint plays an essential role in grasping in terms of flexibility and force transmission. Though the current design allows the grasping of large objects (Figure S10), a mechanism with higher active DoFs for the thumb CMC joint will be designed to better service the assistive purposes. To achieve higher intention-recognition accuracy, three aspects can be considered in further study. Firstly, researchers should increase the user motion information by using more sensors in the system. Secondly, the CNN model architecture can be improved so that the model possesses stronger feature extraction capability. Thirdly, increased diversity and the number of training data sets may further improve the intention-recognition accuracy.

Supplementary Materials: The following supporting information can be downloaded at: https://www.mdpi.com/article/10.3390/bioengineering9110682/s1, Figure S1. Stress evaluation for thumb exoskeleton and index finger exoskeleton. Index finger exoskeleton base serves as fix frame with force (5 N each) applied in the direction labelled in red. The strength of the whole structure is also tested in real action. (a) For exoskeleton made by Aluminum 6061, the maximum stress is ~33.9 MPA compared with the material's yielding stress; (b) for exoskeleton made by PLA material, the maximum stress is ~31.5 MPA compared with the material's yielding stress. Figure S2. Schematic view of the three passive DoFs. Figure S3. Components in the index finger exoskeleton. There are two highlighted areas in the finger exoskeleton, which illustrate the sensor locations and the sliding chute for length adjustment. Figure S4. Hand exoskeleton worn by fingers of different phalanx lengths. (a,b) Length of proximal and intermediate phalanxes are 40 mm and 25 mm, respectively; (c,d) length of proximal and intermediate phalanxes are 46 mm and 27 mm, respectively; (e–f) length of proximal and intermediate phalanxes are 50 mm and 30 mm, respectively. Table S1. The parameters for constructing a Convolution Neural Network (CNN). Figure S5. Index finger length of the five volunteers. (a) Proximal phalanx length, middle phalanx length, and height of the volunteer are ~48 mm, ~30 mm, and ~183 cm, respectively; (b) proximal phalanx length, middle phalanx length, and height of the volunteer are ~46 mm, ~27 mm, and ~168 cm, respectively; (c) proximal phalanx length, middle phalanx length, and height of the volunteer are ~44 mm, ~24 mm, and ~170 cm, respectively; (d) proximal phalanx length, middle phalanx length, and height of the volunteer are ~43 mm, ~23 mm, and ~175 cm, respectively; (e) proximal phalanx length, middle phalanx length, and height of the volunteer are ~40 mm, ~21 mm, and ~156 cm, respectively. Figure S6. Flow chart of differential evolution algorithm. Table S2. Genetic Algorithm setup for CNN model optimization. Figure S7. Results of genetic algorithm to optimize hyperparameters of CNN model. Table S3. The optimal value of hyperparameters in the CNN model. Table S4. Genetic Algorithm setup for SVM model optimization. Figure S8. Results of Genetic Algorithm to optimize hyperparameters of SVM model. Table S5. The optimal value of hyperparameters in the SVM model. Figure S9. A demonstration of grasping objects with the passive joint setup illustrated in Figure S2. (a) A small toolbox with dimeter of ~3.5 cm; (b) water bottle with dimeter of ~6 cm; (c) Orange with dimeter of ~6 cm; A 1:35 M1A1 tank model. Figure S10. Curve of learning rate with epoch. Table S6. Prediction time using CNN model and SVM models. Figure S11. Comparison of identifiable signals with different levels of noise.

Author Contributions: Conceptualization, K.X., X.X. and X.C. (Xianglei Chenand); methodology, K.X.; software, K.X., X.C. (Xianglei Chenand), X.C. (Xuedong Chang) and C.L.; validation, K.X., X.C. (Xianglei Chenand) and X.C. (Xuedong Chang); formal analysis, K.X.; data curation, K.X., X.C. (Xianglei Chenand) and X.C. (Xuedong Chang); writing—original draft preparation, K.X., X.C. (Xianglei Chenand) and X.C. (Xuedong Chang); writing—review and editing, K.X., L.G., F.L., X.X., H.S., Y.W. and J.Z.; visualization, K.X., X.C. (Xianglei Chenand) and X.C. (Xuedong Chang); supervision, K.X. All authors have read and agreed to the published version of the manuscript.

Funding: This research is funded by the National Natural Science Foundation of China (Grant number: 12102127), Natural Science Foundation of Jiangsu Province (Grant number: BK20190164), Fundamental Research Funds for the Central Universities (Grant number: B210202125), China

Postdoctoral Science Foundation (Grant number: 2021M690872), and Changzhou Health Commission Technology Projects (Grant number: ZD202103).

Institutional Review Board Statement: Not applicable.

Informed Consent Statement: Informed consent is obtained from all subjects involved in the study.

Data Availability Statement: The data presented in this study are available in this article.

Conflicts of Interest: The authors declare no conflict of interest.

References

1. Basteris, A.; Nijenhuis, S.; Stienen, A.; Buurke, J.; Prange, G.; Amirabdollahian, F. Training modalities in robot-mediated upper limb rehabilitation in stroke: A framework for classification based on a systematic review. *J. Neuroeng. Rehabil.* **2014**, *11*, 111. [CrossRef] [PubMed]
2. Gao, X.; Liu, Z.; Li, Y.; Gu, X. A dynamic observation on the effects of rehabilitation therapy on poststroke hemiplegic patients. *Chin. J. Rehabil. Med.* **2005**, *20*, 44–46.
3. Wing, K.; Lynskey, J.; Bosch, P. Whole-Body intensive rehabilitation is feasible and effective in chronic stroke survivors: A retrospective data analysis. *Top Stroke Rehabil.* **2008**, *15*, 247–255. [CrossRef] [PubMed]
4. Santavas, N.; Kansizoglou, I.; Bampis, L.; Karakasis, E.; Gasteratos, A. Attention! A Lightweight 2D Hand Pose Estimation Approach. *IEEE Sens. J.* **2021**, *21*, 11488–11496. [CrossRef]
5. Nasri, N.; Orts-Escolano, S.; Cazorla, M. An sEMG-Controlled 3D Game for Rehabilitation Therapies: Real-Time Time Hand Gesture Recognition Using Deep Learning Techniques. *Sensors* **2020**, *20*, 12. [CrossRef] [PubMed]
6. Gordleeva, S.Y.; Lobov, S.A.; Grigorev, N.A.; Savosenkov, A.O.; Shamshin, M.O.; Lukoyanov, M.V.; Khoruzhko, M.A.; Kazantsev, V.B. Real-Time EEG-EMG Human-Machine Interface-Based Control System for a Lower-Limb Exoskeleton. *IEEE Access* **2020**, *8*, 84070–84081. [CrossRef]
7. Mortl, A.; Lawitzky, M.; Kucukyilmaz, A.; Sezgin, M.; Basdogan, C.; Hirche, S. The role of roles: Physical cooperation between humans and robots. *Int. J. Rob. Res.* **2012**, *31*, 1656–1674. [CrossRef]
8. Huang, J.; Huo, W.G.; Xu, W.X.; Mohammed, S.; Amirat, Y. Control of Upper-Limb Power-Assist Exoskeleton Using a Human-Robot Interface Based on Motion Intention Recognition. *IEEE Trans. Autom. Sci. Eng.* **2015**, *12*, 1257–1270. [CrossRef]
9. Hassan, M.; Kadone, H.; Suzuki, K.; Sankai, Y. Wearable Gait Measurement System with an Instrumented Cane for Exoskeleton Control. *Sensors* **2014**, *14*, 1705–1722. [CrossRef]
10. Zhu, M.; Sun, Z.; Zhang, Z.; Shi, Q.; Lee, C. Haptic-Feedback smart glove as a creative human-machine interface (HMI) for virtual/augmented reality applications. *Sci. Adv.* **2020**, *6*, eaaz8693. [CrossRef]
11. Abughalieh, K.M.; Alawneh, S.G. Predicting Pedestrian Intention to Cross the Road. *IEEE Access* **2020**, *8*, 72558–72569. [CrossRef]
12. Ramli, N.A.; Nordin, A.N.; Azlan, N.Z. Development of low cost screen-printed piezoresistive strain sensor for facial expressions recognition systems. *Microelectron. Eng.* **2020**, *234*, 111440. [CrossRef]
13. Zhang, H.J.; Liu, Y.J.; Wang, C.; Fu, R.; Sun, Q.Y.; Li, Z. Research on a Pedestrian Crossing Intention Recognition Model Based on Natural Observation Data. *Sensors* **2020**, *20*, 1776. [CrossRef] [PubMed]
14. Zhang, X.; Zhou, P. High-Density Myoelectric Pattern Recognition toward Improved Stroke Rehabilitation. *IEEE. Trans. Biomed. Eng.* **2012**, *59*, 1649–1657. [CrossRef] [PubMed]
15. Xiao, F.Y.; Chen, Y.Y.; Zhu, Y.H. GADF/GASF-HOG: Feature extraction methods for hand movement classification from surface electromyography. *J. Neural Eng.* **2020**, *17*, 046016. [CrossRef] [PubMed]
16. Tang, Z.C.; Zhang, L.T.; Chen, X.; Ying, J.C.; Wang, X.Y.; Wang, H. Wearable Supernumerary Robotic Limb System Using a Hybrid Control Approach Based on Motor Imagery and Object Detection. *IEEE Trans. Neural Syst. Rehabil. Eng.* **2022**, *30*, 1298–1309. [CrossRef]
17. Jaramillo-Yanez, A.; Benalcazar, M.E.; Mena-Maldonado, E. Real-Time Hand Gesture Recognition Using Surface Electromyography and Machine Learning: A Systematic Literature Review. *Sensors* **2020**, *20*, 2467. [CrossRef]
18. Albini, A.; Denei, S.; Cannata, G. Human hand recognition from robotic skin measurements in human-robot physical interactions. In Proceedings of the 2017 IEEE/RSJ International Conference on Intelligent Robots and Systems (IROS), Vancouver, BC, Canada, 24–28 September 2017; pp. 4348–4353.
19. Qiu, S.; Zhao, H.K.; Jiang, N.; Wang, Z.L.; Liu, L.; An, Y.; Zhao, H.K.; Miao, X.; Liu, R.C. Multi-Sensor information fusion based on machine learning for real applications in human activity recognition: State-of-the-art and research challenges. *Inf. Fusion* **2022**, *80*, 241–265. [CrossRef]
20. Lu, Z.; Chen, X.; Li, Q.; Zhang, X.; Zhou, P. A Hand Gesture Recognition Framework and Wearable Gesture-Based Interaction Prototype for Mobile Devices. *IEEE Trans Hum. Mach. Syst* **2017**, *44*, 293–299. [CrossRef]
21. Samprita, S.; Koshy, A.S.; Megharjun, V.N.; Talasila, V. LSTM-Based Analysis of A Hip-Hop Movement. In Proceedings of the 6th International Conference on Control, Automation and Robotics (ICCAR), Electr Network, 20–23 April 2020; pp. 519–524.
22. Mayagoitia, R.E.; Lotters, J.C.; Veltink, P.H.; Hermens, H. Standing balance evaluation using a triaxial accelerometer. *Gait. Posture* **2002**, *16*, 55–59. [CrossRef]

23. Bourke, A.K.; O'Brien, J.V.; Lyons, G.M. Evaluation of a threshold-based tri-axial accelerometer fall detection algorithm. *Gait. Posture* **2007**, *26*, 194–199. [CrossRef] [PubMed]
24. Atallah, L.; Yang, G.Z. The use of pervasive sensing for behaviour profiling—A survey. *Pervasive Mob. Comput.* **2009**, *5*, 447–464. [CrossRef]
25. Salman, A.D.; Khalaf, O.I.; Abdulsaheb, G.M. An adaptive intelligent alarm system for wireless sensor network. *Indones. J. Electr. Eng. Comput. Sci.* **2019**, *15*, 142–147. [CrossRef]
26. Tryon, J.; Trejos, A.L. Classification of Task Weight During Dynamic Motion Using EEG-EMG Fusion. *IEEE Sens. J.* **2021**, *21*, 5012–5021. [CrossRef]
27. Tunca, C.; Pehlivan, N.; Ak, N.; Arnrich, B.; Salur, G.; Ersoy, C. Inertial Sensor-Based Robust Gait Analysis in Non-Hospital Settings for Neurological Disorders. *Sensors* **2017**, *17*, 825. [CrossRef] [PubMed]
28. Tahir, S.; Jalal, A.; Kim, K. Wearable Inertial Sensors for Daily Activity Analysis Based on Adam Optimization and the Maximum Entropy Markov Model. *Entropy* **2020**, *22*, 579. [CrossRef]
29. Liu, L. Objects detection toward complicated high remote basketball sports by leveraging deep CNN architecture. *Future Gener. Comput. Syst.* **2021**, *119*, 31–36. [CrossRef]
30. Zhou, X.K.; Liang, W.; Wang, K.I.K.; Wang, H.; Yang, L.T.; Jin, Q. Deep-Learning-Enhanced Human Activity Recognition for Internet of Healthcare Things. *IEEE Internet Things J.* **2020**, *7*, 6429–6438. [CrossRef]
31. Nath, R.K.; Thapliyal, H.; Caban-Holt, A. Machine Learning Based Stress Monitoring in Older Adults Using Wearable Sensors and Cortisol as Stress Biomarker. *J. Signal Process. Syst.* **2022**, *94*, 513–525. [CrossRef]
32. Yang, J.T.; Yin, Y.H. Novel Soft Smart Shoes for Motion Intent Learning of Lower Limbs Using LSTM with a Convolutional Autoencoder. *IEEE Sens. J.* **2021**, *21*, 1906–1917. [CrossRef]
33. Chen, G.; Liu, Z.G.; Yu, G.; Liang, J.H. A New View of Multisensor Data Fusion: Research on Generalized Fusion. *Math. Probl. Eng.* **2021**, *2021*, 5471242. [CrossRef]
34. Shao, Y.; Liu, L.; Huang, L.; Deng, N. Key issues of support vector machines and future prospects. *Acta Math. Sin. Chin. Ser.* **2020**, *50*, 1233–1248.
35. Polygerinos, P.; Wang, Z.; Overvelde, J.; Galloway, K.; Wood, R.; Bertoldi, K.; Walsh, C.J. Modeling of soft fiber-reinforced bending actuators. *IEEE Trans. Robot.* **2015**, *31*, 778–789. [CrossRef]
36. Marconi, D.; Baldoni, A.; McKinney, Z.; Cempini, M.; Crea, S.; Vitiello, N. A novel hand exoskeleton with series elastic actuation for modulated torque transfer. *Mechatronics* **2019**, *61*, 69–82. [CrossRef]
37. Cempini, M.; Cortese, M.; Vitiello, N. A powered finger–thumb wearable hand exoskeleton with self-aligning joint axes. *IEEE ASME Trans. Mechatron.* **2014**, *20*, 705–716. [CrossRef]
38. Chen, Y.; Yang, Y.; Li, M.; Chen, E.; Mu, W.; Fisher, R.; Yin, R. Wearable Actuators: An Overview. *Textiles* **2021**, *1*, 283–321. [CrossRef]
39. Freni, P.; Botta, E.M.; Randazzo, L.; Ariano, P. *Innovative Hand Exoskeleton Design for Extravehicular Activities in Space*; Pernici, B., Della, S., Colosimo, T.B.M., Faravelli, T., Paolucci, R., Piardi, S., Eds.; Springer Briefs in Applied Sciences and Technology: New York, NY, USA, 2014; Volume 1, pp. 64–76.
40. Aliseichik, A.P.; Gribkov, D.A.; Efimov, A.R.; Orlov, I.A.; Pavlovsky, V.E.; Podoprosvetov, A.V.; Khaidukova, I.V. Artificial Muscles (Review Article). *J. Comput. Syst. Sci. Int.* **2022**, *61*, 270–293. [CrossRef]
41. Jo, I.; Park, Y.; Lee, J.; Bae, J. A portable and spring-guided hand exoskeleton for exercising flexion/extension of the fingers. *Mech. Mach. Theory* **2019**, *135*, 176–191. [CrossRef]
42. Taheri, H.; Rowe, J.; Gardner, D.; Chan, V.; Gray, K.; Bower, C.; Reinkensmeyer, D.; Wolbrecht, E. Design and preliminary evaluation of the FINGER rehabilitation robot: Controlling challenge and quantifying finger individuation during musical computer game play. *J. Neuroeng. Rehabil.* **2014**, *11*, 10. [CrossRef]
43. Ramos, O.; Múnera, M.; Moazen, M.; Wurdemann, H.; Cifuentes, C. Assessment of Soft Actuators for Hand Exoskeletons: Pleated Textile Actuators and Fiber-Reinforced Silicone Actuators. *Front. Bioeng. Biotechnol.* **2022**, *10*, 1149. [CrossRef]
44. Vertongen, J.; Kamper, D. Design of a 3D printed hybrid mechanical structure for a hand exoskeleton. *Curr. Dir. Biomed. Eng.* **2020**, *6*, 1–5. [CrossRef]
45. Grandi, A.; Karthikeyan, A.; Junior, E.; Covarrubias, M. Low-Cost 3D Printed Exoskeleton for Post-Stroke Hand Rehabilitation. *Comput. Aided. Des. Appl.* **2022**, *6*, 1207–1215. [CrossRef]
46. Conti, R.; Meli, E.; Ridolfi, A.; Bianchi, M.; Governi, L.; Volpe, Y.; Allotta, B. Kinematic synthesis and testing of a new portable hand exoskeleton. *Meccanica* **2017**, *52*, 2873–2897. [CrossRef]
47. Lee, J.; Kwon, K.; Yeo, W.-H. Recent advances in wearable exoskeletons for human strength augmentation. *Flex. Print. Electron.* **2022**, *7*, 023002. [CrossRef]
48. Wilhelm, N.; Haddadin, S.; Lang, J.; Micheler, C.; Hinterwimmer, F.; Reiners, A.; Burgkart, R.; Glowalla, C. Development of an Exoskeleton Platform of the Finger for Objective Patient Monitoring in Rehabilitation. *Sensors* **2022**, *22*, 4804. [CrossRef]
49. Secciani, N.; Brogi, C.; Pagliai, M.; Buonamici, F.; Gerli, F.; Vannetti, F.; Bianchini, M.; Volpe, Y.; Ridolfi, A. Wearable Robots: An Original Mechatronic Design of a Hand Exoskeleton for Assistive and Rehabilitative Purposes. *Front. Neurorobot.* **2021**, *15*, 750385. [CrossRef]
50. De la Cruz-Sánchez, B.; Arias-Montiel, M.; Lugo-González, E. Development of hand exoskeleton prototype for assisted rehabilitation. *Mech. Mach. Sci.* **2018**, *66*, 378–385.

51. Orlando, M.; Behera, L.; Dutta, A.; Saxena, A. Optimal design and redundancy resolution of a novel robotic two-fingered exoskeleton. *IEEE Trans. Nucl. Sci.* **2020**, *2*, 59–75.
52. Li, G.; Cheng, L.; Sun, N. Design, manipulability analysis and optimization of an index finger exoskeleton for stroke rehabilitation. *Mech. Mach. Theory* **2022**, *167*, 104526. [CrossRef]
53. Li, Y.; Gao, X.; Liao, B.; Peng, Y.; Chen, Y. Research Progress of Exoskeleton for Hand Rehabilitation Following Stroke. In Proceedings of the Journal of Physics: Conference Series, Atlanta, GA, USA, 15–17 January 2021; p. 012076.
54. Suarez-Escobar, M.; Rendon-Velez, E. An overview of robotic/mechanical devices for post-stroke thumb rehabilitation. *Disabil. Rehabil. Assist. Technol.* **2018**, *13*, 683–703. [CrossRef]
55. Peidró, A.; Reinoso, Ó.; Gil, A.; Marín, J.; Payá, L. An improved Monte Carlo method based on Gaussian growth to calculate the workspace of robots. *Eng. Appl. Artif. Intel.* **2017**, *64*, 197–207. [CrossRef]
56. Felix, E.A.; Lee, S.P. Systematic literature review of preprocessing techniques for imbalanced data. *IET Softw.* **2019**, *13*, 479–496. [CrossRef]
57. Mitsuhashi, T. Impact of feature extraction to accuracy of machine learning based hot spot detection. In Proceedings of the SPIE Photomask Technology Conference, Monterey, CA, USA, 11–14 September 2017; p. 104510C.
58. Ioffe, S.; Szegedy, C. Batch Normalization: Accelerating Deep Network Training by Reducing Internal Covariate Shift. In Proceedings of the 32nd International Conference on Machine Learning, Lille, France, 7–9 July 2015; pp. 448–456.
59. Park, K.; Changyi, P. Comparison of nonlinear classification methods for image data. *J. Korean Data Inf. Sci. Society* **2021**, *32*, 767–780. [CrossRef]

MDPI
St. Alban-Anlage 66
4052 Basel
Switzerland
www.mdpi.com

Bioengineering Editorial Office
E-mail: bioengineering@mdpi.com
www.mdpi.com/journal/bioengineering

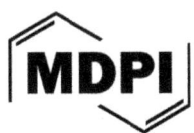

Disclaimer/Publisher's Note: The statements, opinions and data contained in all publications are solely those of the individual author(s) and contributor(s) and not of MDPI and/or the editor(s). MDPI and/or the editor(s) disclaim responsibility for any injury to people or property resulting from any ideas, methods, instructions or products referred to in the content.

www.ingramcontent.com/pod-product-compliance
Lightning Source LLC
LaVergne TN
LVHW070244100526
838202LV00015B/2178